The Evidence for
Neurosurgery

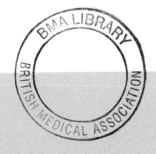

Edited by Zoher Ghogawala
Ajit A. Krishnaney
Michael P. Steinmetz
H. Hunt Batjer
Edward C. Benzel

Publisher

tfm Publishing Limited
Castle Hill Barns
Harley
Shrewsbury
SY5 6LX
UK

Tel: +44 (0)1952 510061
Fax: +44 (0)1952 510192
E-mail: info@tfmpublishing.com
Web site: www.tfmpublishing.com

Design and layout: Nikki Bramhill BSc (Hons) Dip Law
First Edition   © October 2012

Cover image of cerebrovascular bypass – courtesy of Dr. Carlos David (Lahey Clinic Medical Center)

ISBN 978 1 903378 79 3

Printed by Gutenberg Press Ltd., Gudja Road, Tarxien, PLA 19, Malta.

Tel: +356 21897037; Fax: +356 21800069.

Contents

Section 7 Neurotrauma

Contributors

Kalil G Abdullah BS Medical Student, Cleveland Clinic Lerner College of Medicine, Cleveland, Ohio, USA

Isaac Josh Abecassis BSc Medical Student, Department of Neurological Surgery, Northwestern University Feinberg School of Medicine and McGaw Medical Center, Chicago, Illinois, USA

Samuel Adediran BS Medical Student, Wright State University Medical School, Dayton, Ohio, USA

Manish K Aghi MD PhD Assistant Professor, Department of Neurological Surgery, University of California, San Francisco, California, USA

Lilyana Angelov MD Head Section of Spine Tumors and Staff Neurosurgeon, Center for Spine Health; Brain Tumor and NeuroOncology Center, Cleveland Clinic, Cleveland, Ohio, USA

Salah G Aoun MD Postdoctoral Research Fellow, Department of Neurological Surgery, Northwestern University Feinberg School of Medicine and McGaw Medical Center, Chicago, Illinois, USA

Fred G Barker II MD Associate Professor of Neurosurgery, Harvard Medical School, Massachusetts General Hospital, Boston, Massachusetts, USA

H Hunt Batjer MD FACS FAANS Michael J Marchese Professor and Chair, Department of Neurological Surgery, Northwestern University Feinberg School of Medicine and McGaw Medical Center, Chicago, Illinois, USA

Jason Beiko MD PhD Assistant Professor, Section of Neurosurgery, University of Manitoba, Winnipeg, Canada

Bernard R Bendok MD FACS FAANS FAHA Associate Professor, Departments of Neurological Surgery and Radiology, Northwestern University Feinberg School of Medicine and McGaw Medical Center, Chicago, Illinois, USA

Edward C Benzel MD Chairman, Department of Neurosurgery; Staff, Center for Spine Health, Cleveland Clinic, Cleveland, Ohio, USA; Professor of Surgery, Cleveland Clinic Lerner College of Medicine at Case Western Reserve University (CCLCM of CWRU), Cleveland, Ohio, USA

Jeffrey P Blount MD Associate Professor, Section of Pediatric Neurosurgery, Children's of Alabama, University of Alabama at Birmingham, Birmingham, Alabama, USA

David W Cadotte MSc MD Neurosurgery Resident, Division of Neurosurgery, University of Toronto, Toronto, Ontario, Canada

Daniel P Cahill MD PhD Assistant Professor; Attending Neurosurgeon, Department of Neurosurgery, Massachusetts General Hospital, Harvard Medical School, Boston, Massachusetts, USA

Bob S Carter MD PhD Professor and Chief of Neurosurgery, University of California, San Diego, California, USA

Randall M Chesnut MD FCCM FACS Integra Endowed Professor of Neurotrauma; Chief of Neurotrauma and Neurosurgical Spine Surgery, Department of Neurological Surgery; Professor, Department of Orthopaedic Surgery; Adjunct Professor, School of Global Health, Harborview Medical Center, University of Washington, Seattle, Washington, USA

E Sander Connolly MD Bennett M Stein Professor of Neurological Surgery; Vice Chairman of Neurosurgery; Director, Cerebrovascular Research Laboratory, Department of Neurological Surgery, The Neurologic Institute of New York, Columbia University, New York, USA

Celina M Crisman MD Resident, Department of Neurological Surgery, University of Medicine and Dentistry of New Jersey, Newark, New Jersey, USA

Colin P Derdeyn MD Professor of Radiology, Neurology and Neurological Surgery; Director, Stroke and Cerebrovascular Center, Washington University, St Louis, Missouri, USA

Andrea F Douglas MD Director of Spine Education and Research, Wallace Clinical Trials Center, Greenwich Hospital, Greenwich, Connecticut, USA; Clinical Assistant Professor of Neurosurgery, NYU Langone Medical Center, New York, USA

James M Drake MBBCh MSc FRCSC Professor and Neurosurgeon-in-Chief, Division of Neurosurgery, Hospital for Sick Children, University of Toronto, Toronto, Ontario, Canada

Andrew F Ducruet MD Chief Resident, Department of Neurological Surgery, The Neurologic Institute of New York, Columbia University, New York, USA

Emad N Eskandar MD Associate Professor, Director of Stereotactic and Functional Neurosurgery, Department of Neurosurgery, Massachusetts General Hospital, Harvard Medical School, Boston, Massachusetts, USA

Hamad Farhat MD Clinical Assistant Professor, Department of Neurological Surgery, NorthShore University HealthSystem, Evanston, Illinois, USA

Michael G Fehlings MD PhD FRCSC FACS Professor of Neurosurgery, Division of Neurosurgery, University of Toronto, Toronto, Ontario, Canada

Andria L Ford MD Assistant Professor of Neurology, Department of Neurology, Washington University, St Louis, Missouri, USA

Julio C Furlan MD MBA MSc PhD Neurology Resident, Division of Neurosurgery, University of Toronto, Toronto, Ontario, Canada

George M Ghobrial MD Neurological Surgery Resident, Department of Neurological Surgery, Thomas Jefferson University Hospital, Philadelphia, Pennsylvania, USA

Zoher Ghogawala MD FACS Director, Wallace Clinical Trials Center, Greenwich, Connecticut, USA; Charles A Fager Chairman of Neurosurgery, Lahey Clinic Medical Center, Burlington, Massachusetts, USA; Associate Professor of Neurosurgery, Tufts University School of Medicine, Boston, Massachusetts, USA

Michael W Groff MD Director of Spinal Neurosurgery; Co-Director Spine Center, Department of Neurosurgery, Brigham and Women's Hospital, Harvard Medical School, Boston, Massachusetts, USA

Ryder Gwinn MD Director of Epilepsy and Functional Neurosurgery, Swedish Medical Center, Swedish Neuroscience Institute, Seattle, Washington, USA

Todd C Hankinson MD MBA Assistant Professor of Neurosurgery, Children's Hospital Colorado, University of Colorado Denver, Aurora, Colorado, USA

Raqeeb Haque MD Chief Resident, Department of Neurological Surgery, The Neurologic Institute of New York, Columbia University, New York, USA

Ran Harel MD Faculty, Spine Surgery and Spine Radiosurgery, The Department of Neurosurgery and Spine Surgery, The Talpiot Medical Leadership Program, Sheba Medical Center, Israel

James Harrop MD FACS Associate Professor, Departments of Neurological and Orthopedic Surgery; Chief, Spine and Peripheral Nerve Surgery, Department of Neurological Surgery, Thomas Jefferson University Hospital, Philadelphia, Pennsylvania, USA

Brian L Hoh MD Associate Professor, University of Florida, Department of Neurological Surgery, Gainesville, Florida, USA

Brian Y Hwang MD Resident, Department of Neurological Surgery, The Johns Hopkins University, Baltimore, Maryland, USA

Steven N Kalkanis MD Co-Director, Hermelin Brain Tumor Center; Vice-Chair for Operations, Department of Neurosurgery, Henry Ford Health System, Detroit, Michigan, USA

Matthew Kimball MD Resident Physician, University of Florida, Department of Neurological Surgery, Gainesville, Florida, USA

Paul Klimo Jr MD MPH Neurosurgeon, Semmes-Murphey Neurologic & Spine Clinic, Memphis, Tennessee, USA; St Jude Children's Research Hospital, Memphis, Tennessee, USA

Ajit A Krishnaney MD Staff Neurosurgeon, Center for Spine Health, Cerebrovascular Center, Department of Neurosurgery, Cleveland Clinic, Cleveland, Ohio, USA

Abhaya V Kulkarni MD PhD FRCSC Associate Professor and Neurosurgeon, Division of Neurosurgery, Hospital for Sick Children, University of Toronto, Toronto, Ontario, Canada

Fred C Lam MD PhD FRCSC Fellow in Training, Department of Neurosurgery, Brigham and Women's Hospital, Harvard Medical School, Boston, Massachusetts, USA

Jin-Moo Lee MD PhD Associate Professor of Neurology, Radiology, and Biomedical Engineering; Director, Cerebrovascular Disease Section, Washington University, St Louis, Missouri, USA

Michael J Link MD Professor of Neurosurgery, Mayo Clinic College of Medicine, Rochester, Minnesota, USA

Geoffrey T Manley MD PhD Professor of Neurosurgery and Vice-Chairman, Department of Neurosurgery and the Brain and Spinal Injury Center (BASIC), University of California, San Francisco, California, USA

Matthew K Mian BSE Medical Student, Department of Neurosurgery, Massachusetts General Hospital, Harvard Medical School, Boston, Massachusetts, USA

Brian D Milligan MD Neurosurgical Resident, Mayo Clinic College of Medicine, Rochester, Minnesota, USA

Jacques J Morcos MD FRCS(Eng) FRCS(Ed) Professor of Clinical Neurosurgery and Otolaryngology, Department of Neurological Surgery, University of Miami, Miami, Florida, USA

Thomas E Mroz MD Director, Spine Surgery Fellowship, Cleveland Clinic, Cleveland, Ohio, USA

Praveen V Mummaneni MD Associate Professor and Vice Chairman, Department of Neurological Surgery, University of California, San Francisco, California, USA

Atsuhiro Nakagawa MD PhD Assistant Professor of Neurosurgery, Department of Neurosurgery and the Brain and Spinal Injury Center (BASIC), University of California, San Francisco, California, USA; Department of Neurosurgery, Tohoku University Hospital, Sendai, Japan

Michael C Oh MD PhD Resident Physician, Department of Neurological Surgery, University of California, San Francisco, California, USA

Alexander M Papanastassiou MD Assistant Professor of Neurosurgery, University of Texas Health Science Center, San Antonio, Texas, USA

Sanjay Patra MD Chief Resident, Neurosurgery, Department of Neurosurgery, Henry Ford Health System, Detroit, Michigan, USA

Bruce E Pollock MD Professor of Neurosurgery and Radiation Oncology, Mayo Clinic College of Medicine, Rochester, Minnesota, USA

Corey Raffel MD Neurosurgeon, Nationwide Children's Hospital, Columbus, Ohio, USA

Rudy J Rahme MD Postdoctoral Research Fellow, Department of Neurological Surgery, Northwestern University Feinberg School of Medicine and McGaw Medical Center, Chicago, Illinois, USA

Daniel K Resnick MD MS Professor and Vice Chairman, Department of Neurosurgery, University of Wisconsin, Madison, Wisconsin, USA

Rajiv Saigal MD PhD Neurotrauma Research Fellow, Department of Neurosurgery and the Brain and Spinal Injury Center (BASIC), University of California, San Francisco, California, USA

Nader Sanai MD Director, Neurosurgical Oncology, Division of Neurosurgical Oncology; Director, Barrow Brain Tumor Research Center, Barrow Neurological Institute, Phoenix, Arizona, USA

Richard Schlenk MD Neurosurgery Program Director, Cleveland Clinic Foundation, Cleveland, Ohio, USA

Stephen F Shafizadeh MD PhD Resident Physician, PGY-6 and Enfolded Cerebrovascular and Skull Base Fellow, Department of Neurological Surgery, Northwestern University Feinberg School of Medicine and McGaw Medical Center, Chicago, Illinois, USA

Sameer A Sheth MD PhD Chief Resident in Neurosurgery, Department of Neurosurgery, Massachusetts General Hospital, Harvard Medical School, Boston, Massachusetts, USA

Harminder Singh MD Clinical Assistant Professor of Neurological Surgery, Stanford Neurological Surgery, Stanford, California, USA

Edward R Smith MD Director, Pediatric Cerebrovascular Surgery, Department of Neurosurgery, Children's Hospital Boston, Massachusetts, USA; Associate Professor of Surgery, Harvard Medical School, Boston, Massachusetts, USA

Robert A Solomon MD Byron Stookey Professor of Neurosurgery; Chairman and Director of Service, Department of Neurological Surgery, The Neurologic Institute of New York, Columbia University, New York, USA

Dennis D Spencer MD Harvey and Kate Cushing Professor of Neurosurgery; Chairman, Department of Neurosurgery, Yale University, New Haven, Connecticut, USA

Michael P Steinmetz MD Chairman of Neurosciences, MetroHealth Medical Center, Cleveland, Ohio, USA; Associate Professor of Neurosurgery, Case Western Reserve University School of Medicine, Cleveland, Ohio, USA

Vartan S Tashjian MD Neurosurgeon, Department of Neurosurgery, Kaiser Permanente Medical Center – Fontana, Los Angeles, California, USA

Juan Torres-Reveron MD PhD Resident in Neurosurgery, Department of Neurosurgery, Yale University, New Haven, Connecticut, USA

R Shane Tubbs PhD PA-C Researcher, Children's of Alabama, Birmingham, Alabama, USA

Cheerag D Upadhyaya MD Fellow, Spine Surgery, Department of Neurological Surgery, University of California, San Francisco, California, USA

Shobhan Vachhrajani MD Neurosurgery Resident, Division of Neurosurgery, Hospital for Sick Children, University of Toronto, Toronto, Ontario, Canada

Alex Valadka MD Chief Executive Officer, Seton Brain and Spine Institute, Austin, Texas, USA

Gregory J Velat MD Clinical Lecturer, University of Florida, Department of Neurological Surgery, Gainesville, Florida, USA

Kenneth P Vives MD Associate Professor; Chief of Stereotactic and Functional Neurosurgery, Department of Neurosurgery, Yale University, New Haven, Connecticut, USA

Michael Y Wang MD FACS Professor of Neurological Surgery, Department of Neurological Surgery, University of Miami Miller School of Medicine, Miami, Florida, USA

John C Wellons III MD Associate Professor, Division of Neurosurgery; Division of Pediatric Neurosurgery, Children's of Alabama, University of Alabama Birmingham, Birmingham, Alabama, USA

Nicholas Wetjen MD Assistant Professor, Neurosurgeon, Mayo Clinic, Rochester, Minnesota, USA

Robert G Whitmore MD Chief Resident of Neurosurgery, Department of Neurosurgery, Hospital of the University of Pennsylvania, Philadelphia, Pennsylvania, USA; Wallace Clinical Trials Center, Greenwich, Connecticut, USA

Jau-Ching Wu MD Attending Surgeon, Department of Neurosurgery, Neurological Institute, Taipei Veterans General Hospital, Taiwan; School of Medicine, National Yang-Ming University, Taiwan

Jonathan Yun MD Resident, Department of Neurological Surgery, The Neurologic Institute of New York, Columbia University, New York, USA

Gregory J Zipfel MD Associate Professor of Neurological Surgery and Neurology; Co-Director, Stroke and Cerebrovascular Center, Washington University, St Louis, Missouri, USA

Abbreviations

5-ALA	5-aminolevulinic acid
AANS	American Association of Neurological Surgeons
ACAS	Asymptomatic Carotid Atherosclerosis Study
ACDF	anterior cervical discectomy and fusion
ACST	Asymptomatic Carotid Surgery Trial
ACT-1	Carotid Stenting versus Surgery of Severe Carotid Artery Disease and Stroke Prevention in Asymptomatic Patients (study)
ACTH	adrenocorticotrophic hormone
ADL	activities of daily living
AGF	autogenous growth factor
AHA	American Heart Association
AHRQ	Agency for Healthcare Research and Quality
AIBG	autologous iliac crest bone graft
AIS	antibiotic-impregnated shunt catheter
ALIC	anterior limbs of the internal capsules
ALIF	anterior lumbar interbody fusion
ANT	anterior nuclei of the thalamus
AOD	atlanto-occipital dislocation
ARIC	Atherosclerosis Risk in Communities (study)
ARUBA	A Randomized Trial of Unruptured Brain Arteriovenous Malformations
aSAH	aneurysmal subarachnoid hemorrhage
ASIA	American Spinal Injury Association
ATACH	Antihypertensive Treatment of Acute Cerebral Hemorrhage (study)
ATL	anterior temporal lobectomy
AVEEG	audio-video electroencephalography
AVM	arteriovenous malformation
BCNU	1,3-bis(2-chloroethyl)-1-nitrosourea
BDI	Beck Depression Inventory
BFMDRS	Burke-Fahn-Marsden Dystonia Rating Scale
BMP	bone morphogenetic protein
BP	blood pressure
CAPRIE	The Clopidogrel Versus Aspirin in Patients at Risk of Ischaemic Events (study)
CaRESS	Carotid Revascularization Using Endarterectomy or Stenting Systems (study)
CAS	carotid artery stenting
CAVATAS	Carotid and Vertebral Artery Transluminal Angioplasty Study
CBLP	chronic back and leg pain
CBTRUS	Central Brain Tumor Registry of the United States
CC	case-control study
CCB	calcium-channel blocker
CCNU	chloroethyl nitrosourea
CDC	Centers for Disease Control and Prevention
CEA	carotid endarterectomy
CHA	coralline hydroxyapatite
CHS	Cardiovascular Health Study
CI	confidence interval
CLBP	chronic low back pain

CM1	Chiari malformation type I
CM2	Chiari malformation type II
CMM	conventional medical management
CNS	Congress of Neurological Surgeons
COSS	Carotid Occlusion Surgery Study
CPC	choroid plexus cauterization
CPP	cerebral perfusion pressure
CPS	complex partial seizures
CREST	Carotid Revascularization Endarterectomy versus Stenting Trial
CRPS-I	complex regional pain syndrome type I
CS	case series
CSF	cerebrospinal fluid
CSM	cervical spondylotic myelopathy
CT	computerized tomography
CTA	computerized tomography angiography
DBM	demineralized bone matrix
DBS	deep brain stimulation
DC	decompressive craniectomy
DCI	delayed cerebral infarction
DDD	degenerative disc disease
DECRA	Decompressive Craniectomy (study)
DI	diffuse injury
DIND	delayed ischemic neurologic deficit
DPQ	Dallas Pain Questionnaire
DRG	Diagnosis-Related Group
DRI	Disability Rating Index
DSA	digital subtraction angiography
DVT	deep vein thrombosis
DWI	diffusion-weighted imaging
EAA	endocrine active adenoma
EC-IC	extracranial-intracranial
ECoG	electrocorticography
ECOG	Eastern Cooperative Oncology Group
ECST	European Carotid Surgery Trial
ED-5D	EuroQol-Five Dimensions (questionnaire)
EEG	electroencephalography
EMG	electromyography
EORTC	European Organisation for Research and Treatment of Cancer
EPD	embolic protection device
ESIT	Endoscopic Shunt Insertion Trial
ET	essential tremor
ETV	endoscopic third ventriculostomy
EVA-3S	Endarterectomy versus Angioplasty in Patients with Severe Symptomatic Carotid Stenosis (study)
EVD	external ventricular drain
FBSS	failed back surgery syndrome
FDA	US Food and Drug Administration
FdUrd	5-fluoro-2'-deoxyuridine
FLAIR	fluid attenuation inversion recovery
FOS	functional outcome scores
GBM	glioblastoma multiforme
GCS	Glasgow Coma Scale
GDC	Guglielmi detachable coil

GH	growth hormone
GOS	Glasgow Outcome Scale
GPi	globus pallidus interna
GTR	gross total resection
HA	hydroxyapatite
HAM-D	Hamilton Depressive Scale
HDE	humanitarian device exemption
HR	hazard ratio
HRQoL	health-related quality of life
HSQ	Health Status Questionnaire
IA	intra-arterial
IAP	intracarotid amytal procedure
ICD-9-CM	International Classification of Diseases, 9th Revision, Clinical Modification
ICH	intracerebral hematoma
ICP	intracranial pressure
ICSS	International Carotid Stenting Study
ICU	intensive care unit
IGF	insulin-like growth factor
INR	International Normalized Ratio
IQ	intelligence quotient
IRB	institutional review board
ISAT	International Subarachnoid Aneurysm Trial
ISS	Injury Severity Score
ISUIA	International Study of Unruptured Intracranial Aneurysms
ITG	inferior temporal gyrus
IUC	intrauterine closure
IV	intravenous
IVH	intraventricular hemorrhage
KPS	Karnofsky Performance Score
LBPR	Low Back Pain Rating Scale
LDL	low-density lipoprotein
LOS	length of stay
MA	meta-analysis
MASH	Magnesium in Aneurysmal Subarachnoid Hemorrhage (study)
MCA	middle cerebral artery
MCS	motor cortex stimulation
MDD	major depressive disorder
MEG	magnetoencephalography
MESCC	metastatic epidural spinal cord compression
MGd	motexafin gadolinium
MI	myocardial infarction
mJOA	modified Japanese Orthopedic Association (score)
MMC	myelomeningocele
MOMs	Management of Myelomeningocele Study
MPFS	malignant progression-free survival
MRA	magnetic resonance angiography
MRI	magnetic resonance imaging
mRS	modified Rankin Scale
MTG	middle temporal gyrus
MTLE	mesial temporal lobe epilepsy
MTLS	medial temporal lobe sclerosis
MTS	mesial temporal sclerosis
NASCET	North American Symptomatic Carotid Endarterectomy Trial

NCCTG	The North Central Cancer Treatment Group
NDI	Neck Disability Index
NFPA	non-functioning pituitary adenoma
NIH	National Institutes of Health
NIHSS	National Institutes of Health Stroke Scale
NOMASS	Northern Manhattan Stroke Study
NPRI	nicardipine prolonged-release implants
NSAID	non-steroidal anti-inflammatory drug
NSCLC	non-small-cell lung cancer
NSVD	normal spontaneous vaginal delivery
OCD	obsessive-compulsive disorder
ODI	Oswestry Disability Index
OEF	oxygen extraction fraction
OR	odds ratio
OS	overall survival
PAG	periaqueductal gray matter
PCS	physical component summary
PD	Parkinson's disease
PDQ	Parkinson's Disease Questionnaire
PEEK	polyether-etherketone
PET	positron emission tomography
PFS	progression-free survival
PICA	posterior inferior communicating artery
PIGD	postural instability and gait disturbance
PLF	posterolateral fusion
PLIF	posterior lumbar interbody fusion
PLL	posterior longitudinal ligament
PMMA	polymethylmethacrylate
PNC	postnatal closure
PPN	pedunculopontine nucleus
PROCESS	Prospective Randomized Controlled Multicenter Trial of the Effectiveness of Spinal Cord Stimulation
PVG	periventricular gray matter
QALY	quality-adjusted life-year
QoL	quality of life
RCT	randomized controlled trial
rFVIIa	recombinant activated factor VII
ROC	receiver operating characteristic
RR	relative risk
RSD	reflex sympathetic dystrophy
RTOG	Radiation Therapy Oncology Group
SA	selective amygdalohippocampectomy
SAH	subarachnoid hemorrhage
SAMMPRIS	Stenting vs. Aggressive Medical Management for Preventing Recurrent Stroke in Intracranial Stenosis (study)
SAPPHIRE	Stenting and Angioplasty with Protection in Patients at High Risk for Endarterectomy (study)
SBA	Spina Bifida Association
SBP	systolic blood pressure
SCI	spinal cord injury
SCLC	small-cell lung cancer
SCS	spinal cord stimulation
SEEG	stereoelectroencephalography
SF	Short Form (questionnaire)

sICD	symptomatic intracranial arterial disease
SISCOM	subtraction ictal SPECT data correlated with MRI
SIVMS	Scottish Intracranial Vascular Malformation Study
SOMI	sterno-occipital-mandibular immobilizer
SONIA	Stroke Outcomes and Neuroimaging of Intracranial Atherosclerosis (study)
SPACE	Stent-Supported Percutaneous Angioplasty of the Carotid Artery versus Endarterectomy (study)
SPECT	single photon emission computed tomography
SPORT	Spine Patient Outcomes Research Trial
SRS	stereotactic radiosurgery
SSYLVIA	Stenting of Symptomatic Atherosclerotic Lesions in the Vertebral or Intracranial Arteries (study)
STA	superficial temporal artery
sTBI	severe traumatic brain injury
STG	superior temporal gyrus
STICH	Surgical Trial in Intracerebral Hemorrhage
STN	subthalamic nucleus
STR	subtotal resection
STSG	Spine Trauma Study Group
TASS	Ticlopidine Aspirin Stroke Study
TBA	transluminal balloon angioplasty
TBI	traumatic brain injury
TCD	transcranial Doppler
TCP	tricalcium phosphate
TIA	transient ischemic attack
TLE	temporal lobe epilepsy
TLIF	transforaminal lumbar interbody fusion
TLSO	thoraco-lumbo-sacral orthosis
TMZ	temozolomide
TNP	trigeminal neuropathic pain
tPA	tissue plasminogen activator
TSC	tethered spinal cord
TS-SAH	transsylvian selective amygdalohippocampectomy
TWSTRS	Toronto Western Spasmodic Torticollis Scale
UIA	unruptured intracranial aneurysm
UPDRS	Unified Parkinson's Disease Rating Scale
VAS	Visual Analogue Scale
VC/VS	ventral capsule/ventral striatum
VIM	ventral intermediate thalamic nucleus
VNS	vagus nerve stimulation
VP	ventriculoperitoneal
VPL	ventral posterolateral nucleus
VS	vestibular schwannoma
WAD	whiplash-associated disorders
WASID	Warfarin-Aspirin in Symptomatic Intracranial Arterial Disease (study)
WBRT	whole-brain radiation therapy
WFAQ	Waddell's Fear Avoidance Questionnaire
WFNS	World Federation of Neurosurgical Societies
WHO	World Health Organization
Y-BOCS	Yale-Brown Obsessive-Compulsive Scale

Foreword

Neurosurgery represents one of the most specialized arenas in modern medicine. Today, more than ever, patients with neurological disorders seek opinions from a variety of specialists and are often treated by teams of physicians. While consensus is often reached within institutions, regional variation is found between institutions. The lack of high quality clinical evidence contributes to this problem.

This textbook aims to examine some of the most controversial areas of neurological surgery by applying the current evidence to illuminate our understanding of the pathophysiology of each disease and the outcomes from surgical and non-surgical treatments. Today's neurosurgeon must be able to apply current evidence in the clinic to determine, for example:

- which degenerative lumbar spine should be fused, decompressed, or both, and which spine deformity should be corrected and to what extent?
- which aneurysm should be treated with endovascular and/or open vascular techniques?
- whether an acoustic neuroma should be treated, followed, removed, or irradiated?

The Evidence for Neurosurgery is a textbook that challenges current dogmas in many instances, provides an organized framework for understanding where current evidence can be applied clinically, and illustrates where gaps in the evidence exist and how these deficiencies may be filled in the future.

In the first chapter, "Clinical evidence", the reader should gain an understanding of the levels of clinical evidence and will learn what types of study designs are appropriate and in which situations. The textbook is divided into six further sections: Spinal neurosurgery, Functional neurosurgery, Tumors, Pediatric neurosurgery, Vascular neurosurgery and Neurotrauma. Statements in each chapter that are supported by evidence will be followed by the level of evidence and grade of recommendation (e.g. Level IIb evidence and Grade B recommendation would be depicted as [IIb/B]). In addition, the key points of each chapter are summarized in a table with the level of evidence and grade of recommendation. Each section's editors have provided a brief synopsis of the specific challenges within each field followed by chapters that provide the current evidence in areas where clinical uncertainty lies.

Zoher Ghogawala, MD
Ajit A. Krishnaney, MD
Michael P. Steinmetz, MD
H. Hunt Batjer, MD
Edward C. Benzel, MD

The Editors

Zoher Ghogawala, MD is the Charles A. Fager Chairman of Neurosurgery at Lahey Clinic in Burlington, Massachusetts and is Associate Professor of Neurosurgery at Tufts University School of Medicine in Boston. He also serves as the Director of the Wallace Clinical Trials Center, which focuses upon comparative effectiveness research at Greenwich Hospital in Greenwich, Connecticut. Dr. Ghogawala trained in neurosurgery at the Massachusetts General Hospital in Boston, Massachusetts. Dr. Ghogawala currently serves on the Executive Committee for the Congress of Neurological Surgeons as well as the AANS/CNS Joint Section on Disorders of the Spine and Peripheral Nerves. He also serves on the Board of Directors for the North American Spine Society as well as the Neuropoint Alliance (AANS). He leads multiple non-industry funded, peer-reviewed clinical trials that aim to understand the comparative effectiveness of neurosurgical procedures.

Ajit A Krishnaney, MD is a staff neurosurgeon at the Cleveland Clinic and holds appointments in the Department of Neurological Surgery, the Center for Spine Health and the Cerebrovascular Center. He obtained his medical degree from the University of Wisconsin. He trained in neurosurgery at the Cleveland Clinic. Following residency he completed a fellowship in complex spine surgery also at the Cleveland Clinic. His clinical interests include complex spine surgery, tumors of the spine and spinal cord, and disorders of the craniocervical junction.

Michael P Steinmetz, MD is Chairman of the Department of Neuroscience at MetroHealth Medical Center and Associate Professor of Surgery at Case Western Reserve University School of Medicine in Cleveland Ohio. He trained in neurosurgery at the Cleveland Clinic followed by a fellowship in complex spine surgery at the University of Wisconsin. Following fellowship he served on the faculty of the Department of Neurosurgery and Center for Spine Health at the Cleveland Clinic for seven years prior to his appointment as Chairman of Neurosciences at MetroHealth. His clinical interests and expertise are in complex spine surgery, spine trauma and spinal cord injury.

Hunt Batjer, MD is the Michael J. Marchese Professor and Chair of the Department of Neurological Surgery at Northwestern University Feinberg School of Medicine and Northwestern Memorial Hospital in Chicago. Dr. Batjer trained at the University of Texas Southwestern Medical Center under Drs. Clark and Duke Samson and later served a fellowship at the University of London Queens Square and the University of Western Ontario under Dr. Charles Drake. He is a Past President of the Congress of Neurosurgical Surgeons and the Society of University Neurosurgeons. He is past Chairman of the AANS/CNS Section on Cerebrovascular Disease. He has served as Director and later Chair of the American Board of Neurosurgical Surgery and is currently Chair of the ACGME Neurosurgical Residency Review Committee. He is also Chairman of the Board of the Interurban and President Elect of the Neurosurgical Society of America. He is also serving as a Director at large on the Board of Directors in the AANS and Co-Chairs the NFL Committee on Head, Neck, and Spine Injuries. In 2011 he served as the Honored Guest of the Congress of Neurological Surgeons.

Edward C Benzel MD is Chairman of the Department of Neurosurgery at Cleveland Clinic, and Professor of Surgery at Cleveland Clinic Lerner College of Medicine of Case Western Reserve University (CCLCM of CWRU).

Previously, he was Chief of the Divisions of Neurosurgery at Louisiana State University ('82-'89), University of New Mexico ('89-'99) and at Lovelace Medical Center, Albuquerque, New Mexico ('93-'99). Dr. Benzel specializes in spinal biomechanics and spine surgery. He has contributed significantly to the body of literature in that field, written and edited over 20 books, and published well over 200 peer-reviewed manuscripts. In addition, he currently sits on the Editorial Review Boards of multiple journals. His career has also focused on physician education, having previously directed neurosurgery residency training programs in New Mexico and in Cleveland.

Acknowledgement

This work represents the collective effort of the leaders in the field of neurosurgery. We are especially grateful to each of the authors who systematically reviewed the literature and produced chapters that highlight the evidence to support best practice in each topic within our field.

Our Section Editors: Fred G Barker, II, MD (Tumors), Edward R Smith, MD (Pediatric neurosurgery), Alex Valadka, MD (Trauma), Bernard R Bendok, MD (Cerebrovascular), Michael P Steinmetz, MD (Spine), and Kenneth P Vives, MD (Functional) all worked to provide overall guidance to the authors in each subsection of neurosurgery and have each written separate introductions to clarify for the reader where the major challenges lie within their respective areas of expertise.

We'd also like to thank Jill N. Curran for her invaluable help throughout the editing process.

Chapter 1

Clinical evidence

Zoher Ghogawala MD FACS, Director 1; Chairman,
Department of Neurosurgery 2; Associate Professor of Neurosurgery 3
Bob S Carter MD PhD, Professor and Chief of Neurosurgery 4
Fred G Barker II MD, Associate Professor of Neurosurgery 5

1 WALLACE CLINICAL TRIALS CENTER, GREENWICH, CONNECTICUT, USA
2 LAHEY CLINIC MEDICAL CENTER, BURLINGTON, MASSACHUSETTS, USA
3 TUFTS UNIVERSITY SCHOOL OF MEDICINE, BOSTON, MASSACHUSETTS, USA
4 UNIVERSITY OF CALIFORNIA, SAN DIEGO, CALIFORNIA, USA
5 HARVARD MEDICAL SCHOOL, MASSACHUSETTS GENERAL HOSPITAL, BOSTON,
MASSACHUSETTS, USA

Introduction

The practice of neurosurgery has traditionally been taught by experienced surgeons who share their wisdom through an apprenticeship over a period of a several-year residency. While this strategy has worked well to teach surgical techniques, there has been a relative lack of instruction regarding the implementation of clinical evidence. What is clinical evidence? It is the evidentiary support that follows from the application of the scientific method to study a clinical question. Clinical evidence goes beyond one surgeon's accumulated experience and derives power from the scientific application of rigorous methods to determine the effectiveness of a treatment that applies to all surgeons and their patients.

There are several reasons why evidence-based decision-making is not inculcated into neurosurgical training; the most prominent of which is the lack of class I evidence or well-designed randomized controlled trials (RCTs) to guide our specialty [1, 2].

Second is a general lack of understanding regarding how to interpret clinical evidence of lower levels than an RCT. Making matters more complex, of the few RCTs that do reach completion, many do not provide a definitive answer to the research question or, even if they do, may fail to convince practitioners to alter their established patterns. Today, there is a growing need to supplement our education with a systematic understanding of the principles of evidence-based practice. In this chapter, we outline the key elements of clinical evidence. These elements are used throughout this textbook to aid our understanding of specific studies that might ultimately guide neurosurgical practice.

Outcomes

Well-designed clinical studies require the application of valid outcome measures. Many types of outcome instruments are available. The validation of these tools is the focus of much clinical research. The utility of outcome instruments is that they provide comprehensive data regarding the success of any clinical intervention that goes well beyond a surgeon's clinical assessment of 'good,' 'fair,' or 'poor' results. Payers, hospitals, physicians, and patients all have different perspectives when considering outcomes. In this book, we focus on the perspectives of the patient and clinician. We present five areas of outcome analyses: clinical outcomes, surrogate outcomes (e.g., imaging outcomes), functional outcomes, quality of life outcomes, and cost-effectiveness outcomes. Cost outcomes are becoming particularly important when evaluating surgical options. Clinicians will need to become more familiar with this terminology going forward.

Clinical outcomes

Clinical outcomes measure objective clinical events associated with a given disease entity. Discrete clinical events (e.g., death, stroke, specific neurological outcomes) are, by definition, clinically relevant and can be very useful in measuring the clinical efficacy of neurosurgical interventions when the natural history of a disease is associated with major morbidity or mortality. Mortality (survival) as a clinical outcome is generally used in malignant diseases where life expectancy is limited. For example, Kaplan-Meier survival curve [3] analysis has been used in malignant brain tumor trials where death is expected within months to years of the initial diagnosis [4]. For carotid occlusive disease, on the other hand, where disease-specific mortality is rare in the short term, the efficacy of carotid endarterectomy has been demonstrated largely by comparing stroke rates for different treatment strategies. NASCET (North American Symptomatic Endarterectomy Trial), for example, demonstrated that for symptomatic patients with ipsilateral carotid stenosis of 70% or greater, carotid surgery reduced the risk of ipsilateral stroke from 26% (best medical management) to 9% (carotid endarterectomy plus best medical management) at 2 years [5]. This randomized trial (comprising 2,226 patients) convincingly demonstrated the value of surgery over best medical management and has become the basis for the standard of care.

Surrogate outcomes

Surrogate outcomes are proxies for true clinical outcomes. The most commonly used surrogates in neurosurgery are radiographic outcomes (e.g., achievement of lumbar fusion as a correlate for relief of back pain, percent coil obliteration as a surrogate for preventing aneurysmal re-hemorrhage). Surrogates can also be non-radiographic, such as recording intracranial pressure monitoring data in studies of head trauma.

Imaging outcomes are often used as surrogate measures for clinical outcomes to obtain an early prediction of the eventual clinical outcome. In some situations, radiographic data might permit early intervention to modify the clinical course before symptoms are manifest. MRI evidence of tumor recurrence, for example, is an outcome measure used in many studies of malignant brain tumors where treatment effects might be modest but significant [6]. Radiographic studies for fusion, stability, or deformity assessment are often used as surrogate measures for eventual clinical outcome in spinal studies [7]. Rigorous studies using imaging outcomes often employ independent blinded reviews, with well-defined characteristics for each outcome measure.

Because imaging outcomes are often available earlier than clinical outcomes (e.g., MRI evidence of tumor recurrence usually precedes death), they avoid the confounding effect of effective salvage therapies (other than the therapy being tested in the trial). A major drawback of many imaging outcomes, however, is their failure to correlate with outcomes that are clinically significant. For example, many studies have found that radiographic spinal fusion has little or no correlation with any meaningful clinical outcome, such as pain relief [8, 9].

Functional outcomes

Functional outcomes are focused evaluations of a patient's state of function that do not attempt to summarize a patient's entire state of health. Examples of functional scores include pain perception scales (e.g., Visual Analogue Scale [10]), disability scales (e.g., Oswestry Disability Index) [11], 'return to work' status, and the Karnofsky Performance Scale [12]. Disease-specific functional outcome scales aim to quantify the degree of disease-specific impairment at baseline or to measure the change in impairment status after an intervention. When discussing changes in disease-specific outcomes scales, it is critical to address the degree of change that is clinically meaningful – that is, the minimum clinically important difference. For example, many degenerative spine trials consider a difference of 10 points on the Oswestry Disability Index to be clinically significant [13, 14].

General health-related quality of life outcomes

General health-related quality of life (HRQoL) measures are commonly used in neurosurgical studies to measure patients' overall view of their entire state of health. (The difference between 'quality of life' and HRQoL is that 'quality of life' embraces many factors outside the medical realm, such as satisfaction with work and personal relationships.) The Short Form (SF)-36, -12, and -8 instruments are all questionnaires completed by patients that are used to score HRQoL. In the SF-36, a commonly reported HRQoL instrument used in many studies, raw scores for eight categories (physical functioning, role [physical], bodily pain, general health, vitality, social functioning, role [emotional], and mental health) are linearly transformed using scoring algorithms to yield scores from 0 to 100. A physical component summary (PCS) or mental component summary is then generated using population-adjusted norms to generate normalized scores with a mean±standard deviation of 50±10. Many different medical disciplines have used the SF-36 PCS to assess the impact of an intervention on HRQoL. For example, a successful hip replacement is associated with a 9.6 point improvement in the SF-36 PCS score [15]. The minimal clinically important difference for the SF-36 PCS score has been reported by some to be at least 5 points [13, 16].

Cost-effectiveness outcomes

Cost-effectiveness analysis requires the measurement of clinical effectiveness with a preference-based HRQoL outcome score (that has been scaled to equal 0 for death and 1 for perfect health) for the purpose of calculating quality-adjusted life-years (QALYs) as a measure of the difference between two treatments. One common example of a preference-based HRQoL instrument is the EuroQol-Five Dimensions (EQ-5D) questionnaire [17].

Cost data from an intervention can be combined with QALY outcome data to generate cost-effectiveness data. In essence, the life expectancy after one treatment is multiplied by the expected HRQoL after that treatment; the same is done for the other treatment, and the difference is the QALY difference between the treatments. The cost difference between the treatments is then divided by the QALY difference to yield the cost per QALY gained. The cost of hemodialysis (arbitrarily, $50,000 per QALY gained) is often used in the USA as a benchmark for determining whether a new intervention is cost-effective [18, 19]. The specific cost-effectiveness threshold typically varies from society to society; for example, the National Institute for Health and Clinical Excellence, which advises the National Health Service in the UK, recommends a cost-effectiveness threshold of £20,000-30,000 per QALY gained for approving new therapies – often controversially [20].

The specific method used to calculate costs can greatly affect the cost-effectiveness ratio. In SPORT (Spine Patient Outcomes Research Trial), the cost-effectiveness of surgery relative to non-operative treatment for lumbar disc disease was $69,403 per QALY using overall adult surgery costs (all payers), and $34,355 per QALY using Medicare population-specific surgery costs [21]. It is common to estimate hospital costs by reporting hospital charges, which are readily available. Real hospital costs can be estimated using coding systems such as the Healthcare Common Procedure Coding System. In addition, Medicare reimbursement rates for specific hospital billing codes (International Classification of Diseases, 9th Revision [ICD-9] and Diagnosis-Related Group [DRG]) are readily available and are also used to estimate the costs of health care [22].

Randomized controlled trials

It is generally agreed that RCTs are the gold standard for determining whether an intervention is superior, equivalent, or inferior to an alternative. This is because all non-randomized experiments fail to balance important baseline prognostic variables, and thus introduce bias into the results of the trial. It is estimated, however, that fewer than 1% of published papers in leading neurosurgical journals are RCTs [23]. Why are so few trials performed? And why do so many fail to reach a conclusion that convincingly alters clinical practice?

Equipoise

Although there are many barriers to performing high-quality RCTs in surgery, one of the most common – and difficult to overcome – is lack of equipoise. This term, popularized by Freedman in a classic 1987 paper, means "genuine uncertainty within the expert medical community" on the optimal approach for a certain medical condition [24]. RCTs are ethical and feasible only when there is clinical equipoise between the treatment arms of a trial.

Lack of clinical equipoise affected the National Institutes of Health-sponsored SPORT study, which contained an RCT that compared surgery versus conservative management for symptomatic lumbar disc herniation [25]. The high cross-over rate (30% of patients crossed from the non-operative cohort to the operative cohort within 3 months) suggested that clinicians, patients, or both felt that surgery provided a higher chance of clinical benefit after 6 weeks of failed conservative management. Conversely, almost as many patients randomized to receive surgery did not undergo an operation, indicating that patients had strong opinions favoring the role of conservative treatment when symptoms were mild or improving. In retrospect, the lack of clinical equipoise limited the ability of this study to detect better outcomes from surgery [26].

One reason for this is that the intent-to-treat principle is generally used to analyze data from an RCT. That is, the outcomes are analyzed not by what treatment the patients actually received, but rather by which treatment group they were assigned to by randomization. This approach preserves the integrity of the randomized trial. For example, in the asymptomatic carotid endarterectomy trials, patients randomized to receive surgery were analyzed as such even if they had an angiographic complication following randomization or if they did not undergo surgery at all [27]. High cross-over rates in a trial should prompt questions about the reason the trial's design led to the problem, as an intent-to-treat analysis will have markedly reduced power to detect a difference between two treatments in this situation [26].

Heterogeneity

Another major barrier to performing RCTs in neurosurgery is the heterogeneity of the disease entity. The heterogeneity of the suitability of specific intracranial aneurysms for either microsurgical clipping or endovascular coiling, for example, may limit the ability to perform well-designed clinical trials comparing the two treatments. In this circumstance, trialists will need to choose entry criteria for a comparative trial with care to avoid comparing 'apples with oranges' and generating a result that has little relevance to actual practice.

Learning curve

A further challenge in studying novel neurosurgical procedures is the learning curve characteristic, both of individual practitioners and new technologies in a broader sense. The rapid changes in endovascular techniques typify the conundrum. Current techniques for coiling or stenting are changing at such a rapid pace that a trial designed today to test these newer technologies might be obsolete – and therefore irrelevant – before the trial is completed. Trials that use complication outcomes to compare newer technologies with more established approaches are particularly difficult to interpret if practitioners or centers are in the early phases of their experience with the newer technology.

In the case of the EVA-3S (Endarterectomy versus Angioplasty in Patients with Severe Symptomatic Carotid Stenosis) trial, the relative lack of experience of many participating centers (experience with only

Chapter 1

five carotid stenting procedures was required for a center to participate) might have contributed to the relatively higher complication rate that resulted in premature termination of the trial; the trial reported a stroke or mortality rate of 9.6% after stenting versus 3.9% after carotid endarterectomy [28, 29]. An RCT that directly compares a novel technology against an established technology will only guide practice if:

- There is sufficient experience with the novel technology to generate results that fairly estimate the real complication rate.
- The technology examined is comparable with what will be available after the trial is completed and its results analyzed and reported.

Understanding strengths and limitations

For the reasons outlined above, it is likely that RCTs will continue to be unable to address many of the most common neurosurgical clinical dilemmas without considerable improvements in the design and execution of trials. New approaches using modern statistical methods have improved our ability to extract meaningful conclusions from retrospective data, as well as from prospective registries. In the future, it will be critical for all neurosurgeons to understand the strengths and limitations of these types of studies, especially as policy-makers and payers use these data to develop positions on the financing of health care.

Administrative databases

Large administrative databases containing vast amounts of patient data have increased the opportunity to generate meaningful evidence using retrospective data. However, these databases sometimes introduce new problems in study design, such as the lack of specificity of decades-old coding systems for coding new treatments and disease entities, undercoding of important prognostic factors, difficulty disentangling presenting signs and symptoms of disease from treatment complications, and so on [30]. Two of the major administrative databases used for clinical research are the State Inpatient Databases (SIDs) and the Nationwide Inpatient Sample (NIS).

State Inpatient Databases

SIDs are part of the Healthcare Cost and Utilization Project sponsored by the Agency for Healthcare Research and Quality. They contain demographic data, admission and discharge dates, procedure and diagnosis codes using the ICD-9-Clinical Modification (ICD-9-CM), DRGs, hospital codes, charge data, lengths of stay, dispositions, and inpatient deaths. Five SIDs hold consistent patient identifiers across several years, permitting longitudinal follow-up of individual patients. For example, Martin *et al* have used the Washington State SID to study lumbar spine reoperation rates over time [31].

Nationwide Inpatient Sample

The Nationwide Inpatient Sample (NIS) is also part of the Healthcare Cost and Utilization Project. It represents a weighted sample from the SIDs that is readily generalizable to the entire US non-federal hospital universe. It includes data from approximately 1,000 hospitals and represents a 20% stratified probability sample of US inpatient discharges. While this database is much larger than the SIDs, it does not contain patient identifiers and analysis of individual patient data is therefore possible for one admission only. The database has been used to study inpatient complication rates and mortality in a variety of neurosurgical conditions, including cervical spondylotic myelopathy, using algorithms based on specific ICD-9-CM codes [30]. In addition, several authors have used the NIS to demonstrate the effect of hospital and surgeon volume on the morbidity and mortality of treating many neurosurgical conditions, including intracranial aneurysms, craniotomies for meningioma, and pediatric CSF shunts [32-35].

Non-randomized clinical studies

Prospective and retrospective non-randomized studies represent a major portion of the available evidence in neurological surgery. While these types of studies represent lower levels of clinical evidence (see Table 1 for how clinical evidence is used in this textbook), they nonetheless represent the bulk of neurosurgery evidence to date. Well-designed non-

Table 1. Medical levels of clinical evidence used in this textbook.

Level of evidence	Description
Ia	Systematic review of randomized controlled trials
Ib	Well-executed randomized controlled trial
IIa	Well-designed controlled study without randomization
IIb	Well-designed quasi-experimental study
III	Retrospective case-control study, comparative study, or case series
IV	Expert opinion from respected authorities or from expert committee reports

randomized prospective studies that define relevant effects of treatments on health outcomes can provide high-quality medical evidence [36-38]. There are four major types of non-randomized clinical studies: prospective cohort studies, case-control studies, nested case-control studies, and case series.

Prospective cohort studies (level II evidence)

A cohort study defines two or more groups of similar patients that are treated differently and then assessed for a specific outcome. In neurosurgery, most cohort studies are interventional in nature. That is, the efficacy of a specific intervention is tested by measuring its effect in one group of patients and comparing the results to those obtained in a similar group of patients treated in a different manner. Unlike in RCTs, assignment of patients is subject to a selection bias that can affect the results of the study. For example, the optimal management for patients with small unilateral vestibular schwannoma remains unknown partially because no large RCT has been performed to date. In an effort to generate prospective outcome data on this topic, Pollock *et al* conducted a prospective cohort study comparing 36 patients who underwent microsurgical resection with 46 patients who underwent stereotactic radiosurgery [39]. The

groups were compared using HRQoL, functional, and radiographic tumor control outcome measures. While the groups were similar with regard to preoperative tumor size, the surgical group was significantly younger. This raised questions about the generalizability of the results.

In some situations, it is advantageous to compare the outcomes from one cohort with those from a cohort treated previously. The classic paper from Fessler *et al* comparing corpectomy outcomes with those following cervical laminectomy is an example [40].

Case-control studies (level III evidence)

Case-control studies are used to identify factors that might lead to a particular outcome by retrospectively comparing 'cases' with a particular outcome to 'controls' without that outcome. The case-control method is particularly useful when the outcome is infrequent, because prospective studies would likely require large numbers of patients to have enough power to detect any differences between cohorts. Haines used the case-control approach to study craniotomy infections [41].

Nested case-control studies (level III evidence)

One variation of the case-control study is the nested case-control study. Here, patients with the condition of interest are identified from a defined cohort and, for each patient, a number of matched controls is selected from the same cohort. This strategy has the advantage of potentially limiting the costs that might be associated with conducting a large prospective trial. It also limits the confounding biases typically associated with traditional case-control studies, where the 'case' and 'control' populations can differ substantially in ways that might not be apparent to the investigators evaluating the results [42].

Case series (level III evidence)

A case series is the study of one group of patients without a comparison group. These studies tend to be descriptive and are best used to provide outcome data for new techniques or for the treatment of rare disorders.

Randomized versus non-randomized data

Non-randomized data have been reported to demonstrate significant differences between treatments 56% of the time, while RCTs show 'significant' differences only 30% of the time – suggesting that non-randomized prospective data might overestimate the treatment effect because of selection bias or other study biases, or because of publication bias (the tendency of authors and editors to favor publication of studies with 'positive' results) [43]. Systematic efforts to compare RCTs and non-randomized studies on a number of medical and surgical topics have reached different conclusions [37]. What is clear is that to match results from RCTs, non-randomized trials must be well designed with clear inclusion and exclusion criteria, and efforts must be taken to balance known prognostic factors and the utilization of objective outcome assessments [37, 38]. Although it will never be possible to complete RCTs to answer every current neurosurgical question, the RCT has the advantage of being the only known way to balance both known and unknown prognostic factors associated with the observed outcomes in a trial.

Meta-analyses

Sometimes, several clinical trials are performed in an attempt to answer the same or substantially similar clinical questions. When the individual trials are underpowered to produce a definitive answer, they can generate conflicting results or uncertainty as to the treatment effect. A meta-analysis is a mathematical combination of multiple clinical trial results to generate a conclusion based upon a larger sample of patients. A meta-analysis begins with a systematic review of the available literature. An exhaustive effort must be made to obtain results from unpublished trials. Reviews limited to published papers are skewed toward positive results, an effect called publication bias. Meta-analyses may be limited to RCTs only, but non-randomized trials are also sometimes included.

These types of analyses can easily magnify the biases of individual non-randomized trials. Meta-analysts must pay particular attention to the quality of the included studies to understand the value of its conclusions. Meta-analyses have been useful in many areas of neurosurgery. For example, the efficacy of prophylactic antibiotics has been demonstrated for both cranial and shunt surgery using meta-analyses [44-46].

Cochrane reviews

The Cochrane Collaboration (www.cochrane.org) is an organization that aims to provide systematic reviews on every medical and surgical treatment. Systematic reviews without worrisome variations or heterogeneity in the results of major studies are considered to provide class I evidence according to most classification schemas, including the well-known Oxford Classification of Medical Evidence [47]. Completed and proposed reviews are available online. Cochrane review groups that cover neurosurgical topics include the Cochrane Back, Epilepsy, Trauma, and Stroke Groups [48].

Table 2. Levels of guideline recommendation recognized by the US Preventive Services Task Force.

Level of guideline recommendation	Description
A	Clinicians should provide the service to eligible patients. There is good scientific evidence (level I) that the service improves health outcomes and the benefits substantially outweigh harms
B	Clinicians should provide the service to eligible patients. There is at least fair evidence (level II or III) that the service improves important health outcomes and that benefits outweigh harms
C	No recommendation for or against the routine utilization of the service is made. There is at least fair evidence that the service can improve health outcomes, but the balance of benefits and harms is too close to justify a general recommendation
D	Clinicians should not routinely provide the service to asymptomatic patients. There is at least fair evidence that the service is ineffective or that harms outweigh benefits
I	Evidence that the service is effective is lacking, of poor quality, or conflicting, and the balance of benefits and harms cannot be determined

Table 3. Recommendations based on clinical evidence used in this textbook.

Grade of recommendation	Description
A	At least one randomized controlled trial as part of a body of literature of overall good quality and consistency addressing the specific recommendation (evidence levels Ia and Ib)
B	Well-conducted clinical studies but no randomized clinical trials on the topic of recommendation (evidence levels IIa, IIb, III)
C	Expert committee reports or opinions and/or clinical experience of respected authorities. This grading indicates that directly applicable clinical studies of good quality are absent (evidence level IV)

Guidelines

The term 'evidence-based' first appeared in the medical literature in 1990 [49]; the phrase 'evidence-based medicine' appeared in a classic paper published in JAMA in 1992 [50]. The history becomes important because the initial papers describing the necessity for medical evidence essentially outlined a need for evidence-based guidelines. Guidelines based on published clinical evidence, as opposed to recommendations made by the consensus of an ad hoc group of experts in a particular medical specialty, have now been widely accepted as best practice. The US Preventive Services Task Force recognizes five levels of guideline recommendation (Table 2) [51].

The objective of this textbook is not to create guidelines for neurosurgical practice. Guidelines relevant to neurosurgery are currently formulated by multidisciplinary groups and are reviewed for approval by the American Association of Neurological Surgeons – Congress of Neurological Surgeons Joint Guidelines Committee. Rather, the objective of this book is to outline the available evidence on the treatment options for major clinical problems facing neurosurgeons and their patients. Grades of recommendation (A, B, or C; Table 3) are listed at the end of each chapter, based on the current level of medical evidence. Sackett, referring to the term 'evidence-based medicine,' offers a useful

perspective: "The practice of evidence-based medicine means integrating individual clinical expertise with the best available external clinical evidence from systematic research" [52].

Conclusions

RCTs, systematic reviews, and meta-analyses are all rigorous research tools that can help guide the best practice of medicine. These tools can be combined by expert groups within organized neurosurgery to create guidelines. Guidelines are useful in as much as there is good evidence to support them, but they do not themselves represent independent evidence and need updating as more data are generated. The goal of this textbook is to give neurosurgery students the tools necessary to judge the available literature for themselves, and to guide their own individual practice for individual patients.

References

1. Coffey RJ, Lozano AM. Neurostimulation for chronic noncancer pain: an evaluation of the clinical evidence and recommendations for future trial designs. *J Neurosurg* 2006; 105(2): 175-89.

2. Canadian Task Force on the Periodic Health Examination. The periodic health examination: 2. 1987 update. *CMAJ* 1988; 138(7): 618-26.

3. Kaplan E, Meier P. Nonparametric estimation from incomplete observations. *J Am Stat Assoc* 1958; 53: 457-81.

4. Hart MG, Grant R, Garside R, Rogers G, Somerville M, Stein K. Chemotherapeutic wafers for high grade glioma. *Cochrane Database Syst Rev* 2008; 3: CD007294.

5. North American Symptomatic Carotid Endarterectomy Trial Collaborators. Beneficial effect of carotid endarterectomy in symptomatic patients with high-grade carotid stenosis. *N Engl J Med* 1991; 325(7): 445-53.

6. Giese A, Kucinski T, Knopp U, *et al*. Pattern of recurrence following local chemotherapy with biodegradable carmustine (BCNU) implants in patients with glioblastoma. *J Neurooncol* 2004; 66(3): 351-60.

7. Shen FH, Samartzis D, Khanna N, Goldberg EJ, An HS. Comparison of clinical and radiographic outcome in instrumented anterior cervical discectomy and fusion with or without direct uncovertebral joint decompression. *Spine J* 2004; 4(6): 629-35.

8. Fischgrund JS, Mackay M, Herkowitz HN, Brower R, Montgomery DM, Kurz LT. 1997 Volvo Award winner in clinical studies. Degenerative lumbar spondylolisthesis with spinal stenosis: a prospective, randomized study comparing decompressive laminectomy and arthrodesis with and without spinal instrumentation. *Spine* 1997; 22(24): 2807-12.

9. Savolainen S, Rinne J, Hernesniemi J. A prospective randomized study of anterior single-level cervical disc operations with long-term follow-up: surgical fusion is unnecessary. *Neurosurgery* 1998; 43(1): 51-5.

10. Wewers ME, Lowe NK. A critical review of visual analogue scales in the measurement of clinical phenomena. *Res Nurs Health* 1990; 13 (4): 227-36.

11. Fairbank JC, Couper J, Davies JB, O'Brien JP. The Oswestry low back pain disability questionnaire. *Physiotherapy* 1980; 66(8): 271-3.

12. Karnofsky DA, Burchenal JH, Armistead GC Jr., *et al*. Triethylene melamine in the treatment of neoplastic disease; a compound with nitrogen-mustardlike activity suitable for oral and intravenous use. *AMA Arch Intern Med* 1951; 87(4): 477-516.

13. Birkmeyer NJ, Weinstein JN, Tosteson AN, *et al*. Design of the Spine Patient Outcomes Research Trial (SPORT). *Spine* 2002; 27(12): 1361-72.

14. Ostelo RW, Deyo RA, Stratford P, *et al*. Interpreting change scores for pain and functional status in low back pain: towards international consensus regarding minimal important change. *Spine* 2008; 33 (1): 90-4.

15. Katz JN, Larson MG, Phillips CB, Fossel AH, Liang MH. Comparative measurement sensitivity of short and longer health status instruments. *Med Care* 1992; 30(10): 917-25.

16. Copay AG, Glassman SD, Subach BR, Berven S, Schuler TC, Carreon LY. Minimum clinically important difference in lumbar spine surgery patients: a choice of methods using the Oswestry Disability Index, Medical Outcomes Study

questionnaire Short Form 36, and pain scales. *Spine J* 2008; 8(6): 968-74.

17. Suhonen R, Virtanen H, Heikkinen K, *et al.* Health-related quality of life of day-case surgery patients: a pre/posttest survey using the EuroQoL-5D. *Qual Life Res* 2008; 17(1): 169-77.

18. McFarlane PA. Interpreting cost-effectiveness in dialysis: can the most expensive be more expensive? *Kidney Int* 2006; 69(12): 2120-1.

19. McFarlane PA, Bayoumi AM, Pierratos A, Redelmeier DA. The impact of home nocturnal hemodialysis on end-stage renal disease therapies: a decision analysis. *Kidney Int* 2006; 69(5): 798-805.

20. McCabe C, Claxton K, Culyer AJ. The NICE cost-effectiveness threshold: what it is and what that means. *Pharmacoeconomics* 2008; 26(9): 733-44.

21. Tosteson AN, Skinner JS, Tosteson TD, *et al.* The cost effectiveness of surgical versus nonoperative treatment for lumbar disc herniation over two years: evidence from the Spine Patient Outcomes Research Trial (SPORT). *Spine* 2008; 33(19): 2108-15.

22. Rutigliano MJ. Cost effectiveness analysis: a review. *Neurosurgery* 1995; 37(3): 436-43.

23. Gnanalingham KK, Tysome J, Martinez-Canca J, Barazi SA. Quality of clinical studies in neurosurgical journals: signs of improvement over three decades. *J Neurosurg* 2005; 103(3): 439-43.

24. Freedman B. Equipoise and the ethics of clinical research. *N Engl J Med* 1987; 317(3): 141-5.

25. Weinstein JN, Tosteson TD, Lurie JD, *et al.* Surgical vs. nonoperative treatment for lumbar disk herniation: the Spine Patient Outcomes Research Trial (SPORT): a randomized trial. *JAMA* 2006; 296(20): 2441-50.

26. Ghogawala Z, Barker FG 2nd, Carter BS. Clinical equipoise and the surgical randomized controlled trial. *Neurosurgery* 2008; 62(6): N9-10.

27. Endarterectomy for asymptomatic carotid artery stenosis. Executive Committee for the Asymptomatic Carotid Atherosclerosis Study. *JAMA* 1995; 273(18): 1421-8.

28. Mas JL, Chatellier G, Beyssen B, *et al.* Endarterectomy versus stenting in patients with symptomatic severe carotid stenosis. *N Engl J Med* 2006; 355(16): 1660-71.

29. Forsting M. Shortcomings and promises of recent carotid-stenting trials. *Lancet Neurol* 2007; 6(2): 101-2.

30. Wang MC, Chan L, Maiman DJ, Kreuter W, Deyo RA. Complications and mortality associated with cervical spine surgery for degenerative disease in the United States. *Spine* 2007; 32(3): 342-7.

31. Martin BI, Mirza SK, Comstock BA, Gray DT, Kreuter W, Deyo RA. Are lumbar spine reoperation rates falling with greater use of fusion surgery and new surgical technology? *Spine* 2007; 32(19): 2119-26.

32. Barker FG, 2nd, Amin-Hanjani S, Butler WE, Ogilvy CS, Carter BS. In-hospital mortality and morbidity after surgical treatment of unruptured intracranial aneurysms in the United States, 1996-2000: the effect of hospital and surgeon volume. *Neurosurgery* 2003; 52(5): 995-1007.

33. Barker FG, 2nd, Klibanski A, Swearingen B. Transsphenoidal surgery for pituitary tumors in the United States, 1996-2000: mortality, morbidity, and the effects of hospital and surgeon volume. *J Clin Endocrinol Metab* 2003; 88(10): 4709-19.

34. Curry WT, McDermott MW, Carter BS, Barker FG, 2nd. Craniotomy for meningioma in the United States between 1988 and 2000: decreasing rate of mortality and the effect of provider caseload. *J Neurosurg* 2005; 102(6): 977-86.

35. Hoh BL, Rabinov JD, Pryor JC, Carter BS, Barker FG, 2nd. In-hospital morbidity and mortality after endovascular treatment of unruptured intracranial aneurysms in the United States, 1996-2000: effect of hospital and physician volume. *AJNR Am J Neuroradiol* 2003; 24(7): 1409-20.

36. Horwitz RI, Viscoli CM, Clemens JD, Sadock RT. Developing improved observational methods for evaluating therapeutic effectiveness. *Am J Med* 1990; 89(5): 630-8.

37. McKee M, Britton A, Black N, McPherson K, Sanderson C, Bain C. Methods in health services research. Interpreting the evidence: choosing between randomised and non-randomised studies. *BMJ* 1999; 319(7205): 312-5.

38. Concato J, Shah N, Horwitz RI. Randomized, controlled trials, observational studies, and the hierarchy of research designs. *N Engl J Med* 2000; 342(25): 1887-92.

39. Pollock BE, Driscoll CL, Foote RL, *et al.* Patient outcomes after vestibular schwannoma management: a prospective comparison of microsurgical resection and stereotactic radiosurgery. *Neurosurgery* 2006; 59(1): 77-85.

40. Fessler RG, Steck JC, Giovanini MA. Anterior cervical corpectomy for cervical spondylotic myelopathy. *Neurosurgery* 1998; 43(2): 257-65.

41. Haines SJ. Topical antibiotic prophylaxis in neurosurgery. *Neurosurgery* 1982; 11(2): 250-3.

42. Ernster VL. Nested case-control studies. *Prev Med* 1994; 23(5): 587-90.

43. Chalmers TC, Celano P, Sacks HS, Smith H Jr. Bias in treatment assignment in controlled clinical trials. *N Engl J Med* 1983; 309(22): 1358-61.

44. Haines SJ, Walters BC. Antibiotic prophylaxis for cerebrospinal fluid shunts: a meta-analysis. *Neurosurgery* 1994; 34(1): 87-92.

45. Barker FG 2nd. Efficacy of prophylactic antibiotics for craniotomy: a meta-analysis. *Neurosurgery* 1994; 35(3): 484-90.

46. Barker FG 2nd. Efficacy of prophylactic antibiotic therapy in spinal surgery: a meta-analysis. *Neurosurgery* 2002; 51(2): 391-400.

47. Oxford Centre for Evidence-based Medicine Levels of Evidence and Grades of Recommendation. 2001. Available from: www.cebm.net/index.aspx?o=1047. Accessed November 29, 2011.

48. Barker FG 2nd, Carter BS. Synthesizing medical evidence: systematic reviews and meta-analyses. *Neurosurg Focus* 2005; 19(4): E5.

49. Eddy DM. Practice policies: where do they come from? *JAMA* 1990; 263(9): 1265, 1269, 1272 passim.

50. Evidence-Based Medicine Working Group. Evidence-based medicine. A new approach to teaching the practice of medicine. *JAMA* 1992; 268(17): 2420-5.

51. U.S. Preventive Services Task Force Ratings: Grade Definitions. Agency for Healthcare Research and Quality, 2008. Available from: www.ahrq.gov/clinic/3rduspstf/ratings.htm. Accessed November 29, 2011.

52. Sackett D, Straus S, Richardson W, Rosenberg W. *Evidence-based Medicine: How to Practice and Teach EBM*, 2nd ed. New York: Churchill Livingstone, 2000.

Introduction

Spinal neurosurgery

Michael P Steinmetz MD

Chairman of Neurosciences 1

Associate Professor of Neurosurgery 2

1 METROHEALTH MEDICAL CENTER, CLEVELAND, OHIO, USA
2 CASE WESTERN RESERVE UNIVERSITY SCHOOL OF MEDICINE, CLEVELAND, OHIO, USA

Spine surgeons are often forced to make decisions without high-quality medical evidence. This lack of quality evidence has led to significant variations in practice patterns throughout the USA and the world. Expert opinion and external forces have had a significant influence in our field over the last 20 years.

Until recently, outcome measures largely focused on surrogate variables such as fusion rate and screw placement accuracy. Now, a much greater weight is being placed on validated outcome measures. The focus has shifted from metrics such as the status of bony union to true patient outcomes.

As health care costs grow and place a larger burden on society, expensive surgical procedures, including spinal procedures, have come under scrutiny. Spinal implants and bone graft alternatives (including bone morphogenic protein) are costly and might be associated with an increase in morbidity [1-3]. As the number of instrumented spinal fusions increases, with a concurrent increase in costs, governments and insurers are now demanding evidence regarding the utility of such surgical strategies.

New technology is continuously, and cautiously, applied to spine pathologies. A contemporary example is disc arthroplasty. Prospective randomized controlled trials have been performed to compare lumbar and cervical fusion with disc arthroplasty [4]. These trials were industry funded. Many now question some of the claims made from these data. For example, the cervical disc arthroplasty trials were designed as non-inferiority studies. When the data were published, however, secondary outcome measures were largely used to make claims of superiority. Significant bias on the part of investigators is a growing concern among today's spine surgeons.

This section reviews common conditions and situations faced by practicing spine surgeons. The chapters cover these topics by presenting the best available evidence as a foundation. All of the authors are noted experts in their field. Their goals are to explain how best to interpret the current evidence, and to discuss the limitations of randomized controlled trials as a solution to all clinical dilemmas.

References

1. Burkus JK, Transfeldt EE, Kitchel SH, Watkins RG, Balderston RA. Clinical and radiographic outcomes of anterior lumbar interbody fusion using recombinant human bone morphogenetic protein-2. *Spine* 2002; 27(21): 2396-408.

2. Dawson E, Bae HW, Burkus JK, Stambough JL, Glassman SD. Recombinant human bone morphogenetic protein-2 on an absorbable collagen sponge with an osteoconductive bulking agent in posterolateral arthrodesis with instrumentation. A prospective randomized trial. *J Bone Joint Surg Am* 2009; 91(7): 1604-13.

3. Polly DW Jr, Ackerman SJ, Shaffrey CI, *et al*. A cost analysis of bone morphogenetic protein versus autogenous iliac crest bone graft in single-level anterior lumbar fusion. *Orthopedics* 2003; 26(10): 1027-37.

4. Mummaneni PV, Burkus JK, Haid RW, Traynelis VC, Zdeblick TA. Clinical and radiographic analysis of cervical disc arthroplasty compared with allograft fusion: a randomized controlled clinical trial. *J Neurosurg Spine* 2007; 6(3): 198-209.

Chapter 2

Lumbar spondylolisthesis

Vartan S Tashjian MD

Neurosurgeon 1

Michael Y Wang MD FACS

Professor of Neurological Surgery 2

1 DEPARTMENT OF NEUROSURGERY, KAISER PERMANENTE MEDICAL CENTER – FONTANA, LOS ANGELES, CALIFORNIA, USA

2 DEPARTMENT OF NEUROLOGICAL SURGERY, UNIVERSITY OF MIAMI MILLER SCHOOL OF MEDICINE, MIAMI, FLORIDA, USA

Introduction

Lumbar spondylolisthesis, described as the forward slippage of one vertebra relative to the adjacent vertebrae, is estimated to affect approximately 5% of the general population [1-3]. This ventral translation of one vertebral body in relation to the next often results in significant central or lateral recess stenosis, which can manifest symptomatically with low back pain, radiculopathy, and neurogenic claudication (Figure 1). Spondylolisthesis was first described by an obstetric surgeon named Herbinaux in 1772 as a bony prominence ventral to the sacrum resulting in pelvic outlet narrowing and difficult delivery. Since then, much has been uncovered regarding the pathophysiology and etiology of the various forms of lumbar spondylolisthesis [1]. The current classification system of lumbar spondylolisthesis, as proposed by Wiltse in 1976, includes dysplastic, isthmic, degenerative, traumatic, and pathologic spondylolisthesis [4].

The recent emphasis on evidence-based practice in spinal surgery has resulted in a significant increase in the number of randomized clinical trials (RCTs) evaluating the viability of surgical interventions in the management of various lumbar degenerative conditions over the past 10 years. However, in comparison with other medical disciplines, the evidence base for the surgical management of lumbar spondylolisthesis remains relatively sparse, and clear-cut guidelines for optimal management are not currently available. This is probably because of a variety of reasons, including the inherent ethical and logistic challenges involved in designing and executing a proper blinded, randomized trial in surgical cohorts. Furthermore, as there are several distinct subtypes of lumbar spondylolisthesis, the heterogeneity of this patient population precludes the derivation of widely applicable therapeutic conclusions and guidelines.

The majority of the available literature is disproportionately related to degenerative lumbar spondylolisthesis, which therefore forms the basis of this chapter. Selective references on isthmic spondylolisthesis contribute to a lesser extent.

Methodology

A National Library of Medicine computerized literature search from 1966 through February 2010 was performed with the Medical Subject Heading

Chapter 2

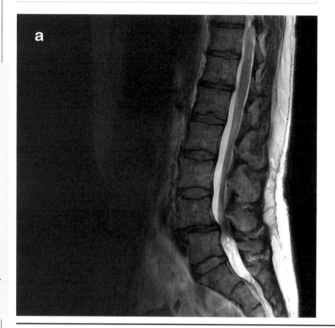
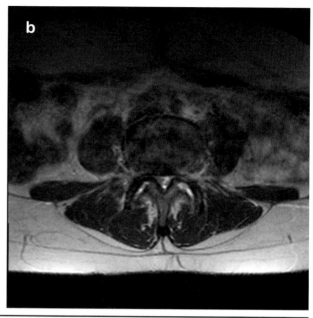

Figure 1. a) Sagittal and b) axial T2-weighted MRI demonstrating Meyerding grade I spondylolisthesis at L4-5, with resultant central/lateral recess stenosis.

'spondylolisthesis' in combination with 'surgical procedures, operative' and 'therapy,' yielding a total of 1,680 abstracts for review. The titles of the abstracts were carefully reviewed, and those indicative of management of lumbar spondylolisthesis were preferentially selected. Abstracts pertaining to conservative management versus surgical intervention were further targeted, as were articles comparing various surgical techniques in the management of spondylolisthesis. In addition, the bibliographies of selected papers were carefully reviewed to identify other related articles.

The Cochrane database was also reviewed, yielding one meta-analysis on the current management of lumbar spondylolisthesis. This extensive search resulted in a total of 67 pertinent articles, which were subsequently utilized in the writing of this chapter.

Surgical versus non-operative management of lumbar spondylolisthesis

Surgical intervention for symptomatic lumbar spondylolisthesis has long been controversial, largely because of the paucity of strong clinical evidence demonstrating a clear therapeutic benefit. Until recently, favorable outcomes following surgical intervention for spondylolisthesis were largely limited to anecdotal experience, case reports, and various low-level retrospective studies. This is despite the general consensus among orthopedic and neurospinal surgeons that symptomatic spondylolisthesis responds well to surgical management, in contrast to the surgical management of degenerative disc disease.

In an early retrospective analysis of 32 adolescent patients with Meyerding grade III-IV spondylolisthesis, Harris and Weinstein reported that 57% of patients treated with *in situ* dorsal arthrodesis were clinically asymptomatic at a mean follow-up of 24 years, as opposed to 36% of patients who were managed non-operatively [5] **(III/B)**. This was consistent with a similar study that also demonstrated better clinical results and less pain in adolescent spondylolisthesis patients treated with *in situ* fusion compared with those treated conservatively with bed rest, followed by a core-stabilizing exercise regimen [6] **(III/B)**.

Several contemporary RCTs have evaluated the efficacy of surgery in the management of lumbar spondylolisthesis (Table 1) [7-12]. The results of these trials have proven difficult to interpret for several reasons. Diagnostically speaking, the failure to distinguish patients with lumbar spondylolisthesis from those with lumbar stenosis or degenerative disc disease contributes to the issue.

stenosis and concomitant degenerative spondylolisthesis who demonstrated more favorable functional outcomes based on Oswestry Disability Index (ODI) scores, as well as more alleviation of leg and back pain at 2-year follow-up, in comparison with stenosis patients who also underwent surgery [9]. All

Table 1. Randomized controlled trials of surgery versus non-operative management of lumbar spondylolisthesis.

Reference	Intervention	n	Follow-up (years)	Primary endpoints	Randomization protocol
Möller and Hedlund, 2000 [7]	PLF:		2	DRI, VAS	Notes with interventions hand-selected
	Non-instrumented	40			
	Instrumented	37			
	1-year exercise program	34			
Ekman et al, 2005 [8]	PLF:		4	DRI, VAS	Notes with interventions hand-selected
	Non-instrumented	40			
	Instrumented	37			
	1-year exercise program	34			
Malmivaara et al, 2007 [9]	Decompression alone	40	2	ODI, VAS	Based on computer-generated random blocks of variable size
	Decompression/fusion with instrumentation	10			
	Exercise program/ NSAIDs	44			
Carreon et al, 2008 [10]	Surgical (not specified)	288	NR	ODI, SF-36	Meta-analysis of available RCTs
	Non-surgical (not specified)	130			
Weinstein et al, 2007, 2009 [11, 12]	Decompression alone	20	2, 4	ODI, SF-36	Computer-generated random treatment assignments – however, high intergroup cross-over resulted in a pseudorandomized 'as treated' analysis
	Instrumented fusion	270			
	Non-instrumented fusion	78			
	Exercise, counseling, NSAIDs	235			

DRI = Disability Rating Index; NR = not reported; NSAID = non-steroidal anti-inflammatory drug; ODI = Oswestry Disability Index; PLF = posterolateral fusion; RCT = randomized controlled trial; SF-36 = Short Form 36; VAS = Visual Analogue Scale

In a well-designed RCT comparing surgery versus non-operative treatment for degenerative lumbar stenosis, Malmivaara *et al* performed a subgroup analysis on 10 surgically treated patients with lumbar

10 patients underwent laminectomy plus dorsal pedicle screw arthrodesis, as opposed to the surgically treated stenosis patients, who underwent decompression alone. The surgical group, as a whole,

did better than the non-operative cohort in terms of functional outcome and leg and back pain scores at 2-year follow-up **(Ib/A)**; however, the subgroup analysis lacked sufficient power to explain the small outcome difference in favor of instrumented lumbar fusion in patients with concomitant degenerative spondylolisthesis [9].

This was similar to previous results reported by Möller and Hedlund, who demonstrated improved functional outcomes on the Disability Rating Index and less pain in patients with adult isthmic spondylolisthesis treated with posterolateral fusion (PLF) compared with matched cohorts enrolled in a structured exercise program [7] **(Ib/A)**. Interestingly, in a follow-up report re-evaluating outcome at 9 years post-enrollment, the degree of functional and pain improvement in the surgical cohort seemed to diminish over time. However, Disability Rating Index and pain scores were still improved over baseline as well as over the exercise group, and surgical patients still classified their global outcome as clearly better than conservatively treated patients [8] **(Ib/A)**. Carreon et al have also published an extensive systematic review of ODI and Medical Outcomes Study Short Form-36 (SF-36) outcomes in fusion (unspecified) and non-surgical treatment for symptomatic lumbar degenerative disease [10] **(Ia/A)**. As a whole, patients undergoing fusion exhibited greater improvements in ODI scores, and patients with degenerative spondylolisthesis demonstrated the greatest ODI improvements following fusion, regardless of the technique employed.

In 2009, the 4-year follow-up results of SPORT (Spine Patient Outcomes Research Trial) were made available [12]. In the pilot study published in 2007 [11], Weinstein et al sought to compare surgical versus non-surgical treatment for lumbar degenerative spondylolisthesis. The SF-36, bodily pain and physical functioning scores, and ODI were used as primary endpoints. Although the study was sufficiently powered (n=607) to detect significant statistical trends, the 1-year bidirectional cross-over rate of 40% in the randomized cohort resulted in no statistically significant effects for the primary outcomes when an intent-to-treat analysis was performed. Importantly, the as-treated analysis for both cohorts combined demonstrated a significant advantage for surgery at 3

months and 1 year postoperatively, which only diminished slightly at 2-year follow-up [11] **(IIa/B)**. This outcome advantage in surgically treated patients with degenerative spondylolisthesis was maintained at 4-year follow-up [12].

Although initially designed as an RCT, SPORT provides only level IIa/B evidence in support of surgery for the management of degenerative spondylolisthesis on the basis of the as-treated analysis. It is further limited by treatment-group heterogeneity, as there was no standardization in the conservative treatment modalities offered and surgical techniques performed. Despite these shortcomings, SPORT represents the first organized effort to specifically address the efficacy of surgery in patients with degenerative spondylolisthesis, and as such has provided valuable insight and direction for future research on the matter.

As a whole, the preponderance of the available high-level evidence suggests a clear benefit with surgery over conservative management for the management of lumbar spondylolisthesis with regard to functional outcomes and pain alleviation, especially at early postoperative time points. The degree of improvement appears to diminish over time; however, surgical patients tend to maintain improved global outcome and satisfaction scores compared with patients who are treated conservatively.

Decompression alone versus decompression plus arthrodesis

Whereas surgical decompression has historically represented an accepted, viable treatment option in the management of lumbar spondylolisthesis, the role of concomitant arthrodesis has remained unclear and controversial. In the past, various authors have reported successful results with decompressive laminectomy alone [13-19], while numerous others [20-26] have championed the utility of decompression augmented with fusion, with or without instrumentation. As only a handful of prospective trials directly comparing the two surgical interventions have been carried out, the evidence base supporting one intervention over the other is lacking.

Of the available studies, virtually all describe superior outcomes in patients undergoing decompression and fusion at the stenotic level, as opposed to decompression alone. In their landmark 1991 prospective trial, Herkowitz and Kurz were the first to demonstrate a clear benefit in patients treated with decompression plus intertransverse non-instrumented arthrodesis versus decompression alone, with regard to relief of back and leg pain [27] **(IIa/B)**. The relatively high pseudoarthrosis rate (36%) did not translate into poor clinical outcomes, similar to previously reported results [6]. Although the study design was limited by, among other things, pseudorandomization, broad pain outcome measures, and a lack of functional outcome assessment, it laid the foundation for adjunctive arthrodesis in the surgical management of lumbar spondylolisthesis.

In a relatively small (n=34), prospective, non-randomized trial, Ghogawala et al demonstrated a significant difference in the degree of ODI improvement over baseline in favor of patients treated with decompression plus posterolateral instrumented fusion as opposed to decompression alone (mean ODI difference 27.5 vs. 13.6, respectively; p=0.02) [28] **(IIa/B)**. Notably, of the 20 patients treated with laminectomy alone, 15% underwent a second operation at 1 year to fuse the level of the spondylolisthesis for delayed-onset instability. Perhaps the most compelling evidence in favor of decompression and arthrodesis for lumbar spondylolisthesis can be derived from a well-executed systematic review published by Martin et al [29]. In this study, the pooled data from two RCTs and six observational studies were examined collectively in a meta-analysis, with the data suggesting a significantly more satisfactory clinical outcome in cases where concomitant fusion was performed as opposed to decompression alone (relative risk 1.40; 95% confidence interval, 1.04-1.89; p<0.05) **(IIa/B)** [29]. In addition, there was a non-significant trend toward lower repeat operations in the fusion group compared with decompression alone.

Taken as a whole, most of the evidence in favor of decompression with fusion over decompression alone in the management of lumbar spondylolisthesis is level II. Therefore, there is moderate evidence to support adjunctive arthrodesis in the surgical management of lumbar spondylolisthesis. More high-quality RCTs should be conducted to further elucidate this advantage, and to detect any differences between the method of arthrodesis employed.

Instrumented versus non-instrumented posterolateral fusion

Pedicle screw instrumented fusion was first described by Roy-Camille in 1970. Its application to a variety of degenerative conditions of the lumbar spine increased dramatically in the early 1990s, despite a relative paucity of superior outcome and cost-effectiveness data to support its use over non-instrumented PLF. Early reports of improved outcomes with instrumentation were largely restricted to studies of questionable methodologic quality.

Chang et al retrospectively reviewed 85 cases of lumbar spondylolisthesis (57 degenerative, 28 isthmic) treated with instrumented fusion, and found that patients with degenerative spondylolisthesis had an improved clinical outcome and fusion rate with instrumentation, with 60% of patients reporting they were completely pain-free at most recent follow-up [30]. Interestingly, patients with isthmic spondylolisthesis also demonstrated an improved fusion rate; however, this did not translate into improved clinical outcomes with regard to pain relief and disability [30] **(III/B)**. Conversely, in a retrospective analysis of 57 patients with L4-5 degenerative spondylolisthesis treated with PLF with and without instrumentation, Kimura et al concluded that the addition of pedicle screw arthrodesis was of low clinical validity [31] **(III/B)**.

Several RCTs have been conducted to further elucidate the potential role of instrumentation in lumbar fusion surgery (Table 2) [32-36]. Unfortunately, the results of several of these studies are difficult to interpret with regard to applicability to lumbar spondylolisthesis, as they deal with mixed patient populations. In a meta-analysis of RCTs evaluating instrumented fusion of the degenerative lumbar spine, Mélot suggested that patients undergoing instrumented fusion demonstrated superior pain relief over non-instrumented cohorts; however, no definite

Chapter 2

Table 2. Randomized controlled trials of non-instrumented versus instrumented PLF in the surgical management of lumbar spondylolisthesis.

Reference	Intervention		n	Follow-up (years)	Primary endpoints	Randomization protocol
Fischgrund et al, 1997 [32]	Decompression + PLF			2	VAS	Withdrawal of card from envelope after decision was made to proceed with surgery
	Non-instrumented	33				
	Instrumented		35			
France et al, 1999 [33]	PLF (± decompression)			2 (mean)	VAS, DPQ	NR
	Non-instrumented	34				
	Instrumented		37			
Möller and Hedlund, 2000 [34]	PLF			2	DRI, VAS	Notes with interventions hand-selected
	Non-instrumented	40				
	Instrumented		37			
Christensen et al, 2002 [35]	PLF			5	DPQ, LBPR	20-number-per-block randomization with surgical interventions concealed in two separate envelopes
	Non-instrumented	66				
	Instrumented		64			
Anderson et al, 2008 [36]	PLF			11-13	DPQ, ODI, SF-36	20-number-per-block randomization with surgical interventions concealed in two separate envelopes
	Non-instrumented	54				
	Instrumented		53			

DPQ = Dallas Pain Questionnaire; DRI = Disability Rating Index; LBPR = Low Back Pain Rating Scale; NR = not reported; ODI = Oswestry Disability Index; PLF = posterolateral fusion; SF-36 = Short Form-36; VAS = Visual Analogue Scale

conclusion could be drawn because of the small sample size and inherent heterogeneity within the treatment group [37] **(Ia/A)**. In their RCT assessing instrumented fusion in adult isthmic spondylolisthesis with a 9-year follow-up, Ekman et al were unable to demonstrate any significant difference between instrumented and non-instrumented fusion with regard to pain relief and disability [34, 38] **(Ib/A)**, consistent with previous accounts in the literature [32]. Similarly, Christensen et al reported no significant difference in overall outcomes in patients treated with either instrumented or non-instrumented fusion, but did note that the use of pedicle screw instrumentation did increase the reoperation rate [35, 36] **(Ib/A)**. Further subgroup analysis suggested that patients with degenerative spondylolisthesis tended to improve significantly with pedicle screw instrumentation, while those with adult isthmic spondylolisthesis (grades I

and II) had superior long-term outcomes with non-instrumented fusion [35]. This is consistent with a more recent meta-analysis published in 2007, which concluded that the use of adjunctive instrumented fusion significantly increased the probability of attaining solid fusion, without any significant associated impact on clinical outcome [29] **(Ia/A)**.

While the available level I evidence suggests a higher probability of achieving solid fusion with instrumented fusion, there is no compelling evidence at the current time to suggest improved functional outcomes or pain relief with the addition of instrumentation. In limited subgroup analyses, there appears to be a trend for improved outcomes with instrumented fusion in patients with a diagnosis of degenerative lumbar spondylolisthesis.

Posterior lumbar interbody fusion versus instrumented posterolateral fusion

Although first described by Briggs and Milligan in 1944 [39], the posterior lumbar interbody fusion (PLIF) technique was later popularized by Cloward [40]. Over the ensuing 50 years, the technique further evolved to include dorsal pedicle screw fixation and, more recently, intersomatic porous spacers, as proposed by Steffe and Sitkowski [41] and Brantigan [42] (Figure 2).

In a retrospective study of 76 patients, comparing PLIF utilizing mixed autogenous or allogeneic bone chips with PLIF utilizing artificial cages packed with morselized bone chips, Yu *et al* concluded that artificial cages provide better functional outcomes (on the ODI) and radiographic improvement (with regard to maintained disc height, slip ratio, segmental lordosis, and fusion status) than PLIF with bone chips alone [43] **(III/B)**. The theoretical advantages in favor of PLIF over PLF include maintenance of disc height, anterior column support, indirect foraminal decompression, circumferential fusion, and restoration of segmental lordosis.

Similar to the widespread application of pedicle screw fixation in degenerative lumbar spine surgery, PLIF has also enjoyed a precipitous rise in popularity over the past 20 years, despite the general lack of

Chapter 2

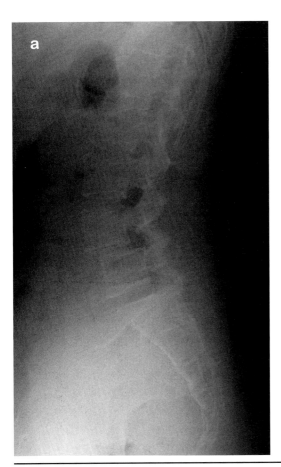
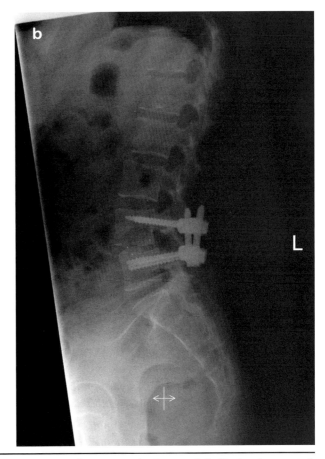

Figure 2. a) Preoperative and b) postoperative lateral X-rays of L4-5 grade I spondylolisthesis treated with transforaminal lumbar interbody fusion utilizing a single PEEK interbody graft in conjunction with percutaneous pedicle screw fixation.

high-quality outcome data supporting its use. Ha *et al* failed to demonstrate any significant difference between PLIF and PLF with regard to pain relief, ODI functional outcome, or fusion rates in 40 retrospectively studied patients [44] **(III/B)**. Dehoux *et al* reported a significant difference in functional outcome in favor of PLIF in patients with higher-grade (Meyerding III and IV) slips, which was not evident in patients with grade I and II spondylolisthesis [45] **(IIa/B)**. They also reported a higher overall fusion rate in patients undergoing PLIF, without any significant associated improvement in functional outcome. In a non-randomized, prospective study of 60 patients with adult spondylolisthesis (isthmic and degenerative), Dantas *et al* reported no statistically significant difference between PLF and PLIF on the ODI and Roland-Morris Scale [1] **(IIa/B)**, similar to results in adult patients with isthmic spondylolisthesis published elsewhere by Ekman *et al* [38] **(III/B)**. In a small RCT consisting of 20 patients, Inamdar *et al* reported improved radiographic reduction of spondylolisthesis with PLIF; however, PLF appeared to achieve better subjective clinical outcomes [46] **(Ib/A)**. In perhaps the best designed RCT on the subject, Cheng *et al* uncovered a superior fusion rate with PLIF (92.6% vs. 80.3%), without any statistical difference in clinical or functional outcomes between the two groups [47] **(Ib/A)**. Interestingly, the authors did note a higher rate of complications related to hardware biomechanics in the PLF group. A subgroup analysis of SPORT similarly demonstrated no consistent differences in clinical outcomes among patients with degenerative spondylolisthesis treated with either non-instrumented PLF, instrumented PLF, or 360° (instrumented PLF plus interbody fusion) fusion [48] **(IIb/B)**.

Currently, there is no definitive level I evidence in favor of PLIF over instrumented PLF in the surgical management of lumbar spondylolisthesis. Although there is some evidence to conclude that PLIF may indeed result in a higher fusion rate than instrumented PLF alone, the implicit clinical significance of this possibility is unclear. Additional adequately powered RCTs are needed to further elucidate the potential role of interbody fusion in the surgical treatment of lumbar spondylolisthesis.

Anterior lumbar interbody fusion versus posterior interbody fusion

The coevolution of percutaneous pedicle fixation systems and anterior lumbar interbody fusion (ALIF) techniques has led to the increasing application of anterior interbody circumferential fusion in both degenerative and isthmic spondylolisthesis. Theoretically, a ventral approach to the lumbosacral spine offers the advantages of improved slip reduction, re-establishment of near anatomic coronal balance, and unimpeded access to the intervertebral disc space, permitting the use of larger grafts and thus increasing the potential graft-to-endplate surface contact for enhanced anterior column arthrodesis.

In a retrospective analysis of 56 patients undergoing combined ALIF and instrumented PLF versus instrumented PLF alone, Suk *et al* reported almost identical fusion rates between the two groups, with less loss of postoperative slip reduction over the 2-year follow-up in the combined group [49]. Despite this radiographic advantage, no significant difference in functional or clinical outcomes was apparent [49] **(III/B)**. These findings are similar to those reported by various other retrospective analyses in the literature evaluating clinical outcomes in patients undergoing either ALIF or instrumented PLF/PLIF [50-52] **(III/B)**. Conversely, Remes *et al* reported better functional outcomes, as measured by the ODI, in patients undergoing circumferential fusion (ALIF with non-instrumented PLF) versus PLF alone [53] **(III/B)**.

In yet another retrospective study comparing ALIF with transforaminal lumbar interbody fusion (TLIF) in the surgical management of low-grade isthmic spondylolisthesis at L4-5 and L5-S1, Kim *et al* reported improved ODI scores with TLIF at the L4-5 level, and superior radiographic results with regard to restoration of disc height, whole lumbar lordosis, and the sacral slope in patients who underwent ALIF at the L5-S1 level, prompting the authors to recommend differing techniques at the respective levels [54] **(III/B)**. Yan *et al* found no significant difference in patient outcomes in a retrospective analysis of 87 patients with degenerative spondylolisthesis who underwent single-level decompression and fusion with either PLIF or TLIF [55] **(III/B)**. These results are consistent with those reported by Suh *et al* in their RCT evaluating PLIF using either one or two cages [56] **(Ib/A)**.

Currently, no level I evidence is available to support ALIF over PLIF or TLIF, or PLIF over TLIF, for the surgical management of lumbar spondylolisthesis. The limited evidence in the literature describes similar fusion rates and functional outcomes in patients undergoing circumferential fusion, regardless of the technique. There is some evidence to suggest superior radiographic outcomes with ALIF, but this does not appear to correlate with any associated clinical benefit.

Instrumented slip reduction versus *in situ* fusion

Perhaps the most controversial topic in the surgical management of lumbar spondylolisthesis is the potential role of operative slip reduction. Whereas slip reduction provides the theoretical advantages of improving biomechanical conditions to facilitate arthrodesis, providing indirect neurologic decompression, correcting lumbosacral kyphosis, and restoring sagittal lumbosacral alignment, it comes at the cost of an increased risk of neurologic deficit (typically temporary or partial L5 nerve palsies) and increased operating room time and procedural blood loss. Despite rates of associated neurologic complications ranging from 10% to 50% in the literature, the percentage of patients with lytic spondylolisthesis in whom slip reduction was performed doubled from 22% to 44% between 1996 and 2002 [2].

Early techniques for slip reduction involved non-instrumented PLF (with or without decompression), followed by staged manipulative reduction and placement in a spica cast 10-14 days postoperatively for up to 3 months [57]. Currently, the most common technique for slip reduction utilizes interbody structural grafts (placed ventrally or dorsally) in conjunction with dorsal pedicle screw reduction and fixation. The available evidence regarding the benefit of operative reduction for high-grade (Meyerding grade III/IV) spondylolisthesis is low level, as no RCTs have been conducted to directly compare functional and clinical patient outcomes between instrumented reduction and *in situ* fusion. Whereas radiographic outcome appeared superior in pediatric patients with high-grade isthmic spondylolisthesis undergoing reduction and fusion in a small retrospective analysis by Poussa *et al*, there were no significant differences compared with *in situ* fusion with regard to functional outcomes or clinical findings concerning pain relief [58] **(III/B)**. This is consistent with findings published by Transfeldt and Mehbod in their systematic review of the subject, leaving the authors unable to formulate clear guidelines because of the paucity of high-level evidence supporting the use of instrumented slip reduction in pediatric patients with high-grade spondylolisthesis [59] **(III/B)**.

The spine literature is currently devoid of sufficient level I evidence to support the use of instrumented slip reduction in the surgical management of lumbar spondylolisthesis. As the risk of neurologic compromise may indeed be higher following reduction maneuvers, RCTs comparing functional and clinical outcomes in comparison with *in situ* fusion need to be carried out. This will elucidate whether any clinical benefit justifies the inherent risks of reduction.

Motion-preservation devices for symptomatic lumbar spondylo-listhesis

In recent years, various motion-preservation devices have been advanced as viable adjuncts to decompression in the surgical management of degenerative lumbar stenosis associated with spondylolisthesis. Theoretical advantages, including a lower propensity for adjacent segment degeneration and avoidance of donor-site morbidity associated with fusion, have fostered increasing interest in this emerging technology. A useful classification scheme of dorsal dynamic stabilization devices has been published by Khoueir *et al* [60]. In comparison with symptomatic lumbar stenosis patients managed non-operatively, interspinous decompression with the X-Stop system (Medtronic Spine LLC, Memphis, TN) has been shown to provide significantly better outcomes in each domain of the Zurich Claudication

Questionnaire [61] **(Ib/A)**. Anderson *et al* similarly demonstrated statistically significant improvements in both Zurich Claudication Questionnaire and SF-36 scores in patients with degenerative lumbar spondylolisthesis implanted with the X-Stop device, with overall clinical success in 63% of implanted patients as opposed to only 13% of patients managed conservatively [62] **(Ib/A)**. Recently, the durability of these results has been called into question, as surgical reintervention rates as high as 58% have been reported in patients with degenerative lumbar spondylolisthesis implanted with X-Stop [63] **(III/B)**.

Of the available pedicle-based dynamic stabilization systems, Dynesys (Zimmer Spine, Minneapolis, MN) has been the most extensively studied in patients with symptomatic degenerative lumbar spondylolisthesis. In a prospective multicenter trial, Dynesys was found to represent a safe and effective alternative to decompression and fusion in the surgical management of degenerative spondylolisthesis [64] **(IIb/B)**. Schnake *et al* also reported clinical results with Dynesys similar to those seen in established protocols using decompression and pedicle screw fixation; however, they also observed a relatively high implant failure rate of 17% over a minimum follow-up of 2 years with the Dynesys system [65] **(III/B)**. In a follow-up publication in which patients were followed for 4 years, no further implant failure was noted; however, radiographic evidence of adjacent segment degeneration was seen in 39% of patients. Despite these findings patient satisfaction remained high, with 95% indicating they would undergo Dynesys implantation again [66] **(IIb/B)**. Conversely, in a retrospective analysis of 55 patients who underwent Dynesys implantation for symptomatic lumbar spondylolisthesis, Fakhil-Jerew *et al* reported a reoperation rate of 45% within 2 years [67] **(III/B)**.

While there is marginal level I evidence indicating that functional outcomes with dynamic stabilization may be similar to those with more traditional combined decompression and pedicle-screw arthrodesis procedures, the durability of these results is questionable. In addition, the relatively high rates of device failure and adjacent segment degeneration reported in the literature warrant further investigation. Well-designed RCTs are needed to evaluate existing dynamic stabilization devices and emerging facet replacement and resurfacing technologies. Furthermore, it should be emphasized that the available studies focused on relatively stable low-grade degenerative spondylolisthesis associated with spinal stenosis. Dynamic devices are currently contraindicated in the presence of mobile or higher-grade slips.

Conclusions

Symptomatic lumbar spondylolisthesis represents a relatively disabling condition with potentially far-reaching medico-economic implications related to associated secondary losses. Whereas conservative management may result in a modest improvement in pain symptoms over time, the natural history of the disease tends to be progressive, with complete spontaneous resolution of symptoms unlikely. Surgical intervention in the form of decompression and arthrodesis can significantly improve pain relief and functional outcomes, especially at early postoperative time points, and patients undergoing decompression and fusion tend to report satisfactory global outcomes in comparison with non-surgical cohorts. Pedicle screw fixation and interbody fusion have both been associated with higher fusion rates, but this radiographic improvement has not translated into a demonstrable clinical benefit. The role of instrumented slip reduction remains controversial, as the inherent risk of neurologic injury may not be justified by any improvements in outcomes.

Recommendations	Evidence level
◆ Surgical intervention for lumbar spondylolisthesis results in significantly improved pain relief and functional outcomes versus non-operative management.	Ia/A
◆ Decompression plus arthrodesis is superior to decompression alone in the surgical management of lumbar spondylolisthesis.	Ia/A
◆ The addition of instrumentation to PLF, in comparison with non-instrumented fusion, results in a higher rate of fusion without a significant difference in functional or clinical outcomes.	Ia/A
◆ There is no significant difference in clinical outcomes between PLF, PLF with instrumentation, and circumferential (PLF plus interbody fusion) for lumbar spondylolisthesis.	IIa/B
◆ Subgroup analysis demonstrates a trend toward improved clinical outcomes with instrumented PLF in patients with degenerative lumbar spondylolisthesis.	III/B
◆ Instrumented slip reduction does not confer any outcome benefits over *in situ* fusion, and adds an additional risk of neurologic complications.	III/B
◆ Dynamic stabilization demonstrates early outcome benefits comparable with those observed for decompression plus fusion. However, these results do not appear to be as durable as those seen with instrumented fusion.	IIb/B

Chapter 2

References

1. Dantas FL, Prandini MN, Ferreira MA. Comparison between posterior lumbar fusion with pedicle screws and posterior lumbar interbody fusion with pedicle screws in adult spondylolisthesis. *Arq Neuropsiquiatr* 2007; 65: 764-70.

2. Hakato J, Wronski J. The role of reduction in operative treatment of spondylolisthesis. *Neurologia i Neurochirurgia Polska* 2008; 42: 345-52.

3. Goyal N, Wimberley DW, Hyatt A, *et al.* Radiographic and clinical outcomes after instrumented reduction and transforaminal lumbar interbody fusion of mid and high-grade isthmic spondylolisthesis. *J Spinal Disord Tech* 2009; 22: 321-7.

4. Wiltse LL, Newman PH, Macnab I. Classification of spondylolisthesis. *Clin Orthop Relat Res* 1976; 117: 23-9.

5. Harris IE, Weinstein SL. Long-term follow-up of patients with grade-III and IV spondylolisthesis. Treatment with and without posterior fusion. *J Bone Joint Surg Am* 1987; 69: 960-9.

6. Seitsalo S. Operative and conservative treatment of moderate spondylolisthesis in young patients. *J Bone Joint Surg Am* 1990; 72: 908-13.

7. Möller H, Hedlund R. Surgery versus conservative management in adult isthmic spondylolisthesis. *Spine* 2000; 25: 1711-15.

8. Ekman P, Möller H, Hedlund R. The long-term effect of posterolateral fusion in adult isthmic spondylolisthesis: a randomized controlled study. *Spine J* 2005; 5: 36-44.

9. Malmivaara A, Slätis P, Heliövaara M, *et al.* Surgical or nonoperative treatment for lumbar spinal stenosis. *Spine* 2007; 32: 1-8.

10. Carreon LY, Glassman SD, Howard J. Fusion and nonsurgical treatment for symptomatic lumbar degenerative disease: a systematic review of Oswestry Disability Index and MOS Short Form-36 outcomes. *Spine J* 2008; 8: 747-55.

11. Weinstein JN, Lurie JD, Tosteson TD, *et al.* Surgical versus nonsurgical treatment for lumbar degenerative spondylolisthesis. *N Engl J Med* 2007; 356: 2257-70.

12. Weinstein JN, Lurie JD, Tosteson TD, *et al.* Surgical compared with nonoperative treatment for lumbar degenerative spondylolisthesis. Four-year results in the Spine Patient Outcomes Research Trial (SPORT) randomized and observational cohorts. *J Bone Joint Surg Am* 2009; 91: 1295-304.

13. Cauchoix J, Benoist M, Chassaing V. Degenerative spondylolisthesis. *Clin Orthop* 1976; 115: 122-9.

14. Dall BE, Rowe DE. Degenerative spondylolisthesis. Its surgical management. *Spine* 1985; 10: 668-72.

15. Dupuis PR, Yong-Hing K, Cassidy JD, Kirkaldy-Willis WH. Radiologic diagnosis of degenerative lumbar spinal instability. *Spine* 1985; 10: 262-76.

16. Epstein JA, Epstein BS, Lavine L. Nerve root compression associated with narrowing of the lumbar spinal canal. *J Neurol Neurosurg Psychiatry* 1962; 25: 165-76.

17. Feffer HL, Wiesel SW, Cuckler JM, Rothman RH. Degenerative spondylolisthesis. To fuse or not to fuse. *Spine* 1985; 10: 287-9.

18. Herkowitz HN, Garfin SR. Decompressive surgery for spinal stenosis. *Sem Spine Surg* 1989; 1: 163-7.

19. Spengler DM. Current concepts review. Degenerative stenosis of the lumbar spine. *J Bone Joint Surg Am* 1987; 69: 305-8.

20. Bolesta MJ, Bohlman HH. Degenerative spondylolisthesis: the role of arthrodesis. *Orthop Trans* 1989; 13: 564.

21. Brown MD, Lockwood JM. Degenerative spondylolisthesis. *Instr Course Lect* 1983; 32: 162-9.

22. Hanley EN. Decompression and distraction-derotation arthrodesis for degenerative spondylolisthesis. *Spine* 1986; 11: 269-76.

23. Kaneda K, Kazama H, Satoh S, Fujiya M. Follow-up study of medial facetectomies and posterolateral fusion with instrumentation in unstable degenerative spondylolisthesis. *Clin Orthop* 1986; 203: 159-67.

24. Lombardi JS, Wiltse LL, Reynolds J, Widell EH, Spencer C. Treatment of degenerative spondylolisthesis. *Spine* 1985; 10: 821-7.

25. Reynolds JB, Wiltse LL. Surgical treatment of degenerative spondylolisthesis. *Spine* 1979; 4: 148-9.

26. Wiltse LL. Common problems of the lumbar spine. Degenerative spondylolisthesis and spinal stenosis. *J Contin Ed Orthop* 1979; 7: 17-30.

27. Herkowitz HN, Kurz LT. Degenerative lumbar spondylolisthesis with spinal stenosis. A prospective study comparing decompression with decompression and intertransverse process arthrodesis. *J Bone Joint Surg Am* 1991; 73: 802-8.

28. Ghogawala Z, Benzel EC, Amin-Hanjani S, *et al*. Prospective outcomes evaluation after decompression with or without instrumented fusion for lumbar stenosis and degenerative grade I spondylolisthesis. *J Neurosurg Spine* 2004; 3: 267-72.

29. Martin CR, Gruszczynski AT, Braunsfurth HA, Fallatah SM, O'Neil J. The surgical management of degenerative lumbar spondylolisthesis. A systematic review. *Spine* 2007; 32: 1791-8.

30. Chang P, Seow KH, Tan SK. Comparison of the results of spinal fusion for spondylolisthesis in patients who are instrumented with patients who are not. *Singapore Med J* 1993; 34: 511-4.

31. Kimura I, Shingu H, Murata M, Hashiguchi H. Lumbar posterolateral fusion alone or with transpedicular instrumentation in L4-L5 degenerative spondylolisthesis. *J Spinal Disord* 2001; 14: 301-10.

32. Fischgrund JS, Mackay M, Herkowitz HN, Brower R, Montgomery D, Kurz LT. Degenerative lumbar spondylolisthesis with spinal stenosis: a prospective, randomized study comparing decompressive laminectomy and arthrodesis with and without spinal instrumentation. *Spine* 1997; 22: 2807-12.

33. France JC, Yaszemski MJ, Lauerman WC, *et al*. A randomized prospective study of posterolateral lumbar fusion: outcomes with and without pedicle screw instrumentation. *Spine* 1999; 24: 553-60.

34. Möller H, Hedlund R. Instrumented and noninstrumented posterolateral fusion in adult spondylolisthesis. A prospective randomized study: part 2. *Spine* 2000; 25: 1716-21.

35. Christensen FB, Hansen ES, Laursen M, Thomsen K, Bünger CE. Long-term functional outcome of pedicle screw instrumentation as a support for posterolateral spinal fusion. Randomized clinical study with a 5-year follow-up. *Spine* 2002; 27: 1269-77.

36. Anderson T, Videbaek TS, Hansen ES, Bünger C, Christensen FB. The positive effect of posterolateral lumbar spinal fusion is preserved at long-term follow-up: a RCT with 11-13-year follow-up. *Eur Spine J* 2008; 17: 272-80.

37. Mélot C. Instrumented fusion of the degenerative lumbar spine: state of the art, questions, and controversies. In: *Clinical Trends in Surgery: Methodologic and Statistical Criteria of Validity, with an Example of Meta-analysis of Randomized Trials in Spine Surgery*. Philadelphia: Lippincott-Raven, 1996: 281-9.

38. Ekman P, Möller H, Tullberg T, Neumann P, Hedlund R. Posterior lumbar interbody fusion versus posterolateral fusion in adult isthmic spondylolisthesis. *Spine* 2007; 32: 2178-83.

39. Briggs DS, Milligan PR. Chip fusion of the low back following exploration of the spinal canal. *J Bone Joint Surg Am* 1944; 26: 125-30.

40. Cloward RB. The treatment of ruptured lumbar intervertebral disc by vertebral body fusion: indications, operative technique, after care. *J Neurosurg* 1953; 10: 154-68.

41. Steffe AD, Sitkowski DJ. Posterior lumbar interbody fusions and plates. *Clin Orthop* 1988; 227: 99-102.

42. Quinn LM, Persenaire JM. Lumbar interbody fusion using the Brantigan I/F cage for posterior lumbar interbody fusion and the variable pedicle screw placement system: two-year results from a Food and Drug Administration investigational device exemption clinical trial. *Spine* (Phila Pa 1976) 2000; 25: 1437-46.

43. Yu CH, Wang CT, Chen PQ. Instrumented posterior lumbar interbody fusion in adult spondylolisthesis. *Clin Orthop Relat Res* 2008; 466: 3034-43.

44. Ha KY, Na KH, Shin JH, Kim KW. Comparison of posterolateral fusion with and without additional posterior lumbar interbody fusion for degenerative lumbar spondylolisthesis. *J Spinal Disord Tech* 2008; 21: 229-34.

45. Dehoux E, Fourati E, Madi K, Reddy B, Segal P. Posterolateral versus interbody fusion in isthmic spondylolisthesis: functional results in 52 cases with a minimum follow-up of 6 years. *Acta Orthop Belg* 2004; 70: 578-82.

46. Inamdar DN, Algappan M, Shyam L, Devadoss S, Devadoss A. Posterior lumbar interbody fusion versus intertransverse fusion in the treatment of lumbar spondylolisthesis. *J Orthop Surg* 2006; 14: 21-6.

47. Cheng L, Nie L, Zhang L. Posterior lumbar interbody fusion versus posterolateral fusion in spondylolisthesis: a prospective controlled study in the Han nationality. *Int Orthop* 2009; 33: 1043-7.

48. Abdu W, Lurie JD, Spratt KF, *et al*. Degenerative spondylolisthesis. Does fusion method influence outcome?

Four-year results of the spine patient outcomes research trial. *Spine* 2009; 34: 2351-60.

49. Suk KS, Jeon CH, Park MS, Moon SH, Kim NH, Lee HM. Comparison between posterolateral fusion with pedicle screw fixation and anterior interbody fusion with pedicle screw fixation in adult spondylolytic spondylolisthesis. *Yonsei Med J* 2001; 42: 316-23.

50. Kim JS, Kang BU, Lee SH, *et al*. Mini-transforaminal lumbar interbody fusion versus anterior lumbar interbody fusion augmented by percutaneous pedicle screw fixation. A comparison of surgical outcomes in adult low-grade isthmic spondylolisthesis. *J Spinal Disord Tech* 2009; 22: 114-21.

51. Kim NH, Lee JW. Anterior interbody fusion versus posterolateral fusion with transpedicular fixation for isthmic spondylolisthesis in adults. A comparison of clinical results. *Spine* 1999; 24: 812-7.

52. Min JH, Jang JS, Lee SH. Comparison of anterior- and posterior-approach instrumented lumbar instrumented fusion for spondylolisthesis. *J Neurosurg Spine* 2007; 7: 21-6.

53. Remes V, Lamberg T, Tervahartiala P, *et al*. Long-term outcome after posterolateral, anterior, and circumferential fusion for high-grade isthmic spondylolisthesis in children and adolescents. Magnetic resonance imaging findings after average of 17-year follow-up. *Spine* 2006; 31: 2491-9.

54. Kim JS, Lee KY, Lee SH, Lee HY. Which lumbar interbody fusion technique is better in terms of level for the treatment of unstable isthmic spondylolisthesis? *J Neurosurg Spine* 2010; 12: 171-7.

55. Yan DL, Pei FX, Li J, Soo CL. Comparative study of PLIF and TLIF treatment in adult degenerative spondylolisthesis. *Eur Spine J* 2008; 17: 1311-6.

56. Suh KT, Park WW, Kim SJ, Cho HM, Lee JS, Lee JS. Posterior lumbar interbody fusion for adult isthmic spondylolisthesis. A comparison of fusion with one or two cages. *J Bone Joint Surg Br* 2008; 90: 1352-6.

57. Burkus JK, Lonstein JE, Winter RB, Denis F. Long-term evaluation of adolescents treated operatively for spondylolisthesis. A comparison of *in situ* arthrodesis only with *in situ* arthrodesis and reduction followed by immobilization in a cast. *J Bone Joint Surg Am* 1992; 74: 693-704.

58. Poussa M, Schlenzka D, Seitsalo S, Ylikoski M, Hurri H, Osterman K. Surgical treatment of severe isthmic spondylolisthesis in adolescents. Reduction or fusion *in situ*. *Spine* 1993; 18: 894-901.

59. Transfeldt EE, Mehbod AA. Evidence-based medicine analysis of isthmic spondylolisthesis treatment including reduction versus fusion *in situ* for high-grade slips. *Spine* 2007; 32: S126-9.

60. Khoueir P, Kim KA, Wang MY. Classification of posterior dynamic stabilization devices. *Neurosurg Focus* 2007; 22: 1-8.

61. Zucherman JF, Hsu KY, Hartjen CA, *et al*. A multicenter, prospective, randomized trial evaluating the X-STOP interspinous process decompression system for the treatment of neurogenic intermittent claudication: two-year follow-up results. *Spine* 2005; 30: 1351-8.

62. Anderson PA, Tribus CB, Kitchel SH. Treatment of neurogenic claudication by interspinous decompression: application of the X-STOP device in patients with lumbar degenerative spondylolisthesis. *J Neurosurg Spine* 2006; 4: 464-71.

63. Verhoof OJ, Bron JL, Wapstra FH, van Royen BJ. High failure rate of the interspinous distraction device (X-STOP) for the treatment of lumbar spinal stenosis caused by degenerative spondylolisthesis. *Eur Spine J* 2008; 17: 188-92.

64. Stoll T, Gilles D, Schwarzenbach O. Dynamic stabilization of degenerative lumbar spondylolisthesis. *Spine J* 2004; 4: 72-3S.

65. Schnake KJ, Schaeren S, Jeanneret B, Sengupta DK. Dynamic stabilization in addition to decompression for lumbar spinal stenosis with degenerative spondylolisthesis. *Spine* 2006; 31: 442-50.

66. Schaeren S, Broger I, Jeanneret B. Dynesys stabilization in degenerative lumbar spondylolisthesis: 4 years' follow-up. *J Bone Joint Surg Br* 2009; 91: 108.

67. Fakhil-Jerew F, Haleem S, Shepperd J. Functional outcome following dynamic neurtralisation system for the treatment of spondylolisthesis without adjunct decompression. *J Bone Joint Surg Br* 2009; 91: 463.

Lumbar spondylolisthesis

Chapter 3

Cervical spondylotic myelopathy

Zoher Ghogawala MD FACS, Director 1;

Chairman, Department of Neurosurgery 2;

Associate Professor of Neurosurgery 3

1 WALLACE CLINICAL TRIALS CENTER, GREENWICH, CONNECTICUT, USA
2 LAHEY CLINIC MEDICAL CENTER, BURLINGTON, MASSACHUSETTS, USA
3 TUFTS UNIVERSITY SCHOOL OF MEDICINE, BOSTON, MASSACHUSETTS, USA

Introduction

Cervical spondylotic myelopathy (CSM) results from degenerative cervical spondylosis, one of the most common indications for cervical spine surgery in the USA. More than 112,400 cervical spine operations for degenerative spondylosis are performed annually in the USA. This represents a 100% increase in utilization over the past decade, with hospital charges now exceeding $2 billion per year [1]. Nearly a fifth of cervical spine operations in the USA are performed to treat CSM [2]. Reports suggest that surgery for CSM has a high complication rate (13-17%) [3, 4]. Some specific complications (e.g., swallowing difficulty) have a greater incidence in ventral (anterior) compared with dorsal (posterior) procedures [3].

It is widely believed that surgical decompression of the spinal cord and fusion of the spinal column permit recovery of spinal cord function and limit further dysfunction in many cases. The evidence for this is limited, but is reviewed in this chapter. Many patients with mild CSM symptoms are not treated surgically, and this approach is also supported by the evidence. Patients with CSM represent a heterogeneous population, with a range of symptom severity and a wide variety of structural spondylotic changes that result in clinical myelopathy. Many of these structural points guide clinicians to select one approach (i.e., ventral vs. dorsal) over the other. This chapter carefully reviews the evidence for the predictive ability of radiographic features with regard to outcome after different types of surgery. In addition, the evidence for differing overall morbidity with ventral versus dorsal approaches is tabulated and reviewed.

For many historical reasons, there is significant uncertainty as to the optimal surgical approach (ventral vs. dorsal) for treating CSM, especially in older patients. More comparative-effectiveness research will ultimately be needed to guide clinicians in selecting the optimal approach for specific subpopulations of patients with CSM.

Methodology

A National Library of Medicine computerized literature search was performed from 1966 to 2010 using each of the following headings: 'cervical spondylotic myelopathy,' 'cervical stenosis,' 'cervical laminectomy,' 'cervical laminoplasty,' and 'cervical corpectomy.' The titles of all articles were carefully reviewed and those indicative of the management of CSM were preferentially selected. Abstracts pertaining to the various surgical approaches in the management of CSM were further targeted and reviewed. In addition, the references from selected papers were reviewed for possible inclusion in this review.

Definition and pathophysiology

CSM is the most common cause of spinal cord dysfunction in the USA and in the world [5]. The condition presents insidiously and is defined in terms of its clinical symptoms (gait instability, bladder dysfunction, and fine finger motor difficulties) and signs (hyperreflexia, lower extremity spasticity, extensor Babinski responses, ankle clonus, weakness, and alteration of joint position sense). CSM is caused by dynamic repeated compression of the spinal cord from degenerative arthritis of the cervical spine [6]. Axonal stretch-associated injury appears to be the leading factor in explaining myelopathy in animal models [6]. Spinal cord ischemia from compression of larger vessels and impaired microcirculation is another proposed mechanism [7, 8]. The natural history of CSM is variable. Many patients with mild CSM symptoms can be carefully followed in the clinic without surgery. Surgery to decompress and fuse the spine is often advocated for severe or progressive symptoms. The results are mixed. About two-thirds of patients improve with surgery, but surgery fails to result in measurable improvement in 15-30% of cases [9]. Some series report that 10-20% of cases worsen clinically after surgery [9].

Cervical stenosis without progressive myelopathy

The normal average diameter of the cervical spinal canal is reported to be 17-18mm [10]. Not all patients with significant cervical spinal canal narrowing and compression of the spinal cord (usually to 10mm) develop myelopathy. In fact, many patients are asymptomatic and can be followed in the clinic without intervention [11]. In addition, many patients who develop mild symptoms will generally benefit from conservative treatment [12]. Some patients present with neck pain or intermittent episodes of cervical radiculopathy, resulting in arm or shoulder pain on the basis of neural foraminal narrowing from cervical spondylosis [13]. Conservative treatments for neck pain include non-steroidal anti-inflammatory drugs, muscle relaxants, and physical therapy [14]. Cervical spine epidural steroid injections are occasionally advocated for the management of cervical spondylotic radiculopathy. These are generally considered safe, although a recent review found that serious complications have been reported in many series [15]. Randomized controlled trials (RCTs) have not been performed to determine their long-term efficacy.

Table 1. Prospective controlled trials of surgery versus conservative therapy for CSM.

Reference	Study population	Patients, n	Primary outcome	Follow-up	Conclusion (level of evidence)
Kadanka et al, 2000 [16]	Mild CSM (mJOA ≥12)	48	mJOA score	2 years	Surgery was not superior to conservative therapy for mild CSM (Ib/A)
Sampath et al, 2000 [17]	CSM	43	CSRS questionnaire	11.2 months	Surgery was superior to conservative therapy for CSM (IIa/B)

CSM = cervical spondylotic myelopathy; CSRS = Cervical Spine Research Society; mJOA = modified Japanese Orthopedic Association (score)

Chapter 3

Mild cervical spondylotic myelopathy

There have been no large RCTs demonstrating that surgery is superior to non-surgical care for the treatment of CSM. A small RCT consisting of 48 patients with mild to moderate CSM, with a modified Japanese Orthopedic Association (mJOA) score (a validated disease-specific outcome measurement) of 12 or more, did not demonstrate improvements with surgery versus conservative treatment after 2 years of follow-up [16] **(Ib/A)**. In contrast, a non-randomized trial (n=43) reported a greater improvement in overall functional outcomes in CSM patients following surgery versus non-surgical treatment [17] **(IIa/B)**. It is generally agreed that patients with mild, stable symptoms may be managed without surgery, while the majority of patients with progressive myelopathy symptoms demonstrate significant improvements in validated outcome measures following surgery [18] (Table 1).

History: surgical approaches

Surgical treatment for CSM (Figure 1) was developed before studies on the pathophysiology of spinal cord dysfunction were published. Historically, CSM was treated by removing bone from the back of the cervical spine through a dorsal approach known as laminectomy (without fusion). The first cervical laminectomy for spinal cord injury was performed in 1828 [19, 20].

While laminectomy without fusion is still performed today, several factors have limited its widespread use. First, the development of instability or kyphosis in

Chapter 3

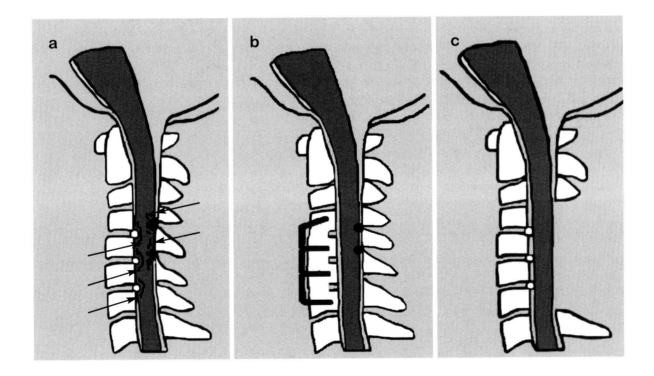

Figure 1. Schematics depicting cervical spinal compression and its surgical treatment. a) Ventral osteophytes (white) and dorsal ligamentum (black) compression of the spinal cord with sites of injury (arrows). b) Ventral surgery, showing multilevel discectomy, fusion, and plating, with removal of ventral osteophytes (white). c) Dorsal surgery, showing laminectomy with removal of dorsal ligamentum.

some cases has led many spine surgeons to add fusion to the procedure (laminectomy with fusion) or to perform a laminoplasty (which enlarges the spinal canal without fusing or removing the laminae, possibly reducing late failures). Second, the inability to remove ventral osteophytes using the dorsal laminectomy has led to the development of ventral approaches. In 1985, Fessler *et al* suggested that ventral corpectomy surgery (removal of a vertebral body from the front of the spine) might be superior to dorsal decompression [21] **(III/B)**. This study compared patient outcomes after contemporary ventral surgery with historical results obtained in dorsal surgery patients treated many years earlier. Subsequent studies, however, including a prospective non-randomized study of 316 patients from 2008, have failed to demonstrate differences in disease-specific outcomes between ventral and dorsal surgery [4] **(IIb/B)**.

Despite the mixed results from both retrospective and prospective studies examining ventral and dorsal surgery, ventral decompression might be more effective in relieving the symptoms of myelopathy in two specific clinical circumstances. According to one retrospective study, patients with preoperative kyphosis (>13°) have poorer mJOA scores after dorsal surgery (laminoplasty) [22] **(III/B)**. Another study concluded that in patients with preoperative intramedullary signal changes on MRI, ventral decompression was associated with a significantly greater improvement in motor function compared with dorsal approaches [23] **(IIb/B)**.

Enthusiasm for ventral surgery, however, has been tempered by high early postoperative complication rates. In fact, the complication rate with ventral corpectomy (29%) appears to be significantly higher than that with dorsal surgical approaches (7%) [24, 25] **(III/B)**. Early experience with multilevel corpectomy was associated with high rates of graft dislodgement and fusion failures [26, 27] **(III/B)**. This led to the development of multilevel discectomies with fusion, using plating, which has reduced the complication rate [28]. The multilevel discectomy and fusion procedure has the added advantages of improving cervical lordosis and reducing the risk of graft migration. However, pseudoarthrosis and subsidence of grafted bone remain challenges in treating patients with multilevel ventral surgery [29].

Clinical guidelines for surgical management

Professional physician organizations such as the American Association of Neurological Surgeons – Congress of Neurological Surgeons Joint Section of Disorders of the Spine and Peripheral Nerves have systematically reviewed the literature and published clinical guidelines for the surgical management of CSM [30]. These guidelines were created to assist surgeons in formulating an appropriate treatment plan, but they also identify major deficiencies in the current literature. In most situations, these clinical guidelines have been unable to issue definitive guidance because high-quality clinical research comparing treatment approaches is lacking. This is largely due to the inherent difficulties in performing clinical trials involving surgical procedures and with disorders characterized by significant heterogeneity. The recommendations of the guidelines are summarized here.

Patients with mild myelopathy symptoms may be managed with or without surgery [31] **(II/B)**. Patients with cervical stenosis without myelopathy who have either clinical or EMG findings consistent with radiculopathy should be considered for surgical decompression, because the evidence suggests that these patients might progress to symptomatic CSM [11] **(II/B)**. Surgical decompression (ventral or dorsal) is generally performed in more severe cases of myelopathy. Published series contain heterogeneous patient populations and varying approaches, and the reported outcome measures differ, making comparisons difficult [9]. Several studies have attempted to identify patient characteristics that predict improvements after surgery [32-42]. The significance of many of these variables as outcome predictors remains controversial, and their impact on the choice of surgical approach is unclear.

The higher complication rate associated with three or more levels of ventral surgery (especially corpectomy) has led some surgeons to perform ventral surgery only in those patients with two or fewer levels of disease **(III/B)**. Cervical spondylotic disease at three or more levels is usually treated with a dorsal approach [34]. In current US practice, older patients (≥75 years) are more likely to be treated using dorsal surgery according to the Nationwide Inpatient Sample [2]. This is of particular relevance because both older age (>74 years) and the dorsal surgical approach have been identified as risk factors for developing complications after cervical spine surgery [2]. Determining if the choice of approach (ventral vs. dorsal) might limit complications, especially in older patients, is an important area for future research.

Current surgical treatment

Regardless of the approach, the goal is decompression of the spinal canal to a diameter of at least 13mm with restoration of cerebrospinal fluid pulsation around the spinal cord. It is generally advisable, when positioning patients, to avoid excessive tension when taping the shoulders to prevent brachial plexus stretch injury. The use of the operative microscope is generally advocated for ventral approaches. Spinal monitoring (somatosensory evoked potential [SSEP] and/or EMG) is suggested by many surgeons, although no rigorous studies have been performed to determine the efficacy of routine spinal monitoring to prevent neurologic complications.

Ventral approaches

The presence of cervical kyphosis or kyphotic deformity has been identified as one of the major reasons for choosing a ventral surgical approach when treating CSM. There are two major approaches:

- Multilevel discectomy and fusion.
- Cervical corpectomy and fusion.

Multilevel discectomy and fusion

Ventral decompression and fusion [43] can be performed using a multilevel discectomy with fusion and plating [28, 44]. Surgeons use allograft or autograft bone spacers at each disc space and remove all compressive osteophytes using the operating microscope. Fixation is typically performed with either semi-constrained or axially dynamic (translational) titanium plates, both of which have been shown to optimize fusion and minimize complications [45-47] **(Ib/A)**. In many cases, restoration of cervical lordosis is possible using this technique (Figure 2). In some patients with marked kyphosis, it is possible to

Chapter 3

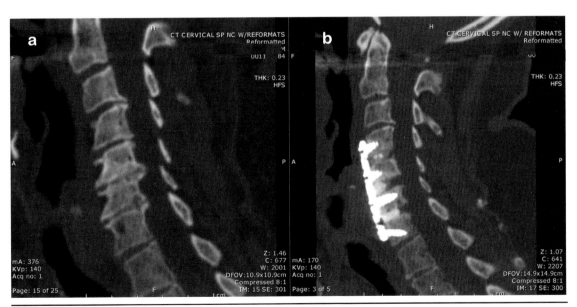

Figure 2. Multilevel discectomy and fusion for treating cervical spondylotic myelopathy. a) Sagittal cervical spine CT image, depicting loss of cervical lordosis and compressive osteophytes at two spinal levels: C5-C6 and C6-C7. b) Postoperative sagittal CT image, demonstrating satisfactory removal of compressive osteophytes and restoration of cervical lordosis.

improve the sagittal plane alignment; however, the final imaging may still reveal a straightened or kyphotic alignment in the cervical spine.

Cervical corpectomy and fusion

The degree of cervical deformity, anatomy of compression by disc or osteophyte, or presence of focal ossification of the posterior longitudinal ligament can lead many surgeons to choose to remove a portion of or the entire vertebral body to achieve the surgical goals. The technique for cervical corpectomy and fusion has been described by Cooper and others [48, 49]. Complications from multilevel corpectomy and fusion are common, and supplementation with dorsal fusion is therefore advocated by some surgeons (see the section on 'Combined ventral and dorsal approaches,' below) [49]. An additional concern with corpectomy procedures is that correction of sagittal plane malalignment is less feasible than with the multilevel discectomy and fusion approach.

Dorsal approaches

Multilevel disease (three or more levels), a developmentally narrow spinal canal (12mm anterior-posterior canal diameter at the base of C2), ossification of the posterior longitudinal ligament, and older age (>74 years) are among the many reasons to choose a dorsal approach when treating CSM.

Laminectomy

Cervical laminectomy is effective in relieving the symptoms of CSM in selected patients with preserved cervical lordosis, but is associated with progressive kyphotic deformity in 21-42% of patients [50-52]. Cervical foraminotomies are often performed for treating radiculopathy, in addition to myelopathy. In an attempt to limit the development of postoperative kyphosis, laminectomies without fusion are usually restricted to patients with preserved preoperative lordosis. Cases of congenital stenosis are the most ideal for this approach.

Laminectomy and fusion

Dorsal decompression and fusion is performed using midline cervical laminectomy with the application of lateral mass screws and rods for rigid fixation [53]. Local autograft bone or allografts are used as needed to perform a lateral mass fusion. To improve sagittal alignment, we routinely decompress the spinal cord first and then extend and dorsally translate the spine, using a Mayfield three-pin head fixation device, to correct alignment. This can only be safely performed while observing the fully decompressed spinal cord during the maneuver to assure no further neural compression will occur. This technique requires confirmation, at the conclusion of the reduction, that the spinal cord remains adequately decompressed.

Laminoplasty

Laminoplasty has been well described in the literature from Japan and carefully studied by Heller et al [54]. The open-door technique is most widely used in the USA. A laminoplasty is typically performed with a wide choice of titanium plates that are anatomically contoured for cervical laminar fixation. The surgeon can choose between ceramic or allograft laminar spacers, if it is believed they add value to the procedure. Some systems also contain 'hinge plates' to salvage displaced hinges (junction of lamina and lateral mass) in the event of excessive bone removal. Typically, 4mm or 5mm self-tapping bone screws are used to fix the plate to the lamina and to the lateral mass at each operated level.

Combined ventral and dorsal approaches

Patients with significant cervical kyphotic deformity and those in whom three or more corpectomies are being contemplated are often treated with a combined ventral and dorsal approach. The aim is to decompress the spinal cord, correct the spinal deformity, and maximize the likelihood of a successful arthrodesis [55]. These operations can be performed in a single day or staged depending on various patient factors as well as surgeon preference. Many surgeons use rigid or semi-rigid cervical collars for at least 12 weeks postoperatively in these patients.

Outcomes after surgery

Most surgical case series have shown improvements following surgery for CSM in approximately 70% of patients [18]. Although large RCTs have not been performed comparing surgical with non-surgical management for treating CSM, one prospective, non-randomized trial did demonstrate better overall functional outcomes in patients treated with surgery [17] **(IIa/B)**. Surgical management has become the accepted standard of care for progressive CSM, making any future RCTs comparing surgery to non-surgical treatment unlikely to be feasible and potentially unethical.

Several disease-specific outcome measures have been used to assess the efficacy of surgery for CSM. The mJOA scale (17-point maximum score) has been used in many studies and, in most, has improved by 2.5-4.0 points after surgery [22, 33, 36]. This disease-specific outcome measure has also been used to identify risk factors for poor outcomes after surgery for CSM. For example, Suda *et al* identified local cervical kyphosis of more than 13° as a significant predictor of poor outcomes in patients treated with one type of dorsal surgery (open-door laminoplasty) in a study using the mJOA scale [22] **(III/B)**.

CSM has a substantial negative impact on health-related quality of life. A recent Veterans Administration study found a mean physical component summary score of 27.8±8.3 (>2 standard deviations below the age-adjusted mean for normal healthy individuals) using the generic Short Form-36 (SF-36) health-related quality-of-life instrument [56]. Surgery for CSM appears to improve quality of life, measured with the SF-36, suggesting the tool might be valuable for studying the potential differential effects of surgical approaches on quality of life in CSM patients [18]. Since CSM does not have a known effect on survival, any study attempting to compare two surgical strategies for CSM should consider the effect of surgical intervention on quality of life.

In 2008, a prospective, non-randomized study of 316 patients with CSM reported that surgery resulted in significant improvements using established disease-specific (mJOA) and health-related quality of life (SF-36) outcome instruments [4] **(IIb/B)**. The high complication rate observed in this large study (17%) underscores the need to define the associations of specific procedures with types of complications and subgroups of patients [4]. In addition, this study demonstrates the well-known scenario that prospective studies will invariably report higher complication rates than retrospective reviews of surgical outcomes.

Risk of complications from surgery

In a large, retrospective, cohort review of US hospital discharges associated with cervical spine surgery using the Nationwide Inpatient Sample from 1992 to 2001, Wang *et al* reported that surgery for CSM (19% of 932,009 admissions) was associated with higher complication rates than other types of cervical spine surgery [2]. Dorsal surgery was utilized more frequently in older patients and was independently associated with higher complication rates. Age greater than 74 years was also an independent predictor of the development of complications [2] **(IIb/B)**. Similarly, another study reported a complication rate of 38% in patients older than 75 years compared with 6% in younger patients [57] **(IIb/B)**. This particular analysis, however, did not directly compare the complication rates of ventral and dorsal surgery and was not limited to patients with CSM. Boakye *et al*, on the other hand, used the Nationwide Inpatient Sample from 1993 to 2002 to compare complication rates between ventral and dorsal fusion procedures for CSM (58,115 admissions). Their retrospective analysis identified a complication rate of 12% for ventral fusion surgery versus 16% for dorsal fusion surgery [3] **(IIb/B)**.

In a retrospective review of 83 patients treated for CSM using either corpectomy and strut grafting (ventral surgery) or laminoplasty (dorsal surgery), Yonenobu *et al* found no significant differences in patient outcomes as measured by the JOA scale [24]. However, patients treated with a laminoplasty experienced fewer complications (7%) than patients in the corpectomy group (29%) **(III/B)**. Similarly, Edwards *et al* found no differences in outcomes between patients treated with corpectomy versus laminoplasty, although the laminoplasty group

Table 2. Complications of surgical management for cervical spondylotic myelopathy: ventral versus dorsal surgery.

Reference	Study population	n	Intervention	Complication rate, %	Evidence level/ recommendation
Yonenobu et al, 1992 [24]	Study design Retrospective, comparative	41 42	Corpectomy Laminoplasty	29.3 7.1	III/B
Edwards et al, 2002 [25]	Retrospective, case-control	13 13	Corpectomy Laminoplasty	69 7.7	III/B
Boakye et al, 2008 [3]	Retrospective, administrative database	46,562 8,112	Ventral fusion Dorsal fusion	11.9 16.4	IIb/B

Chapter 3

experienced fewer complications [25] **(III/B)**. These studies are summarized in Table 2.

Two types of surgical complications are generally observed after operations for treating CSM:

* Dysphagia (difficulty with swallowing), which is more common after ventral surgery.
* C5 nerve root paresis (temporary but sometimes permanent weakness of the shoulder), which is seen after both ventral and (more often) dorsal surgery.

Edwards et al reported a 31% rate of persistent dysphagia or dysphonia (hoarseness) after ventral surgery, and noted that this complication is often under-reported [58]. Published rates of C5 paresis range from 12% (ventral procedures) to 30% (dorsal procedures) [59]. This complication is often disabling for several months and might be related to traction on the C5 root caused by spinal cord shift after decompression [60]. No study to date has prospectively compared C5 paresis rates after ventral and dorsal surgery.

Administrative hospital discharge databases are unlikely to capture these complication rates accurately, and are not able to estimate their severity or impact on a patient's quality of life [2]. Prospective studies using quality-of-life instruments are more

likely to provide useful information for clinicians and patients on complication rates after ventral and dorsal surgery and on the overall impact of these complications on patients' lives. Furthermore, the varying definitions for these conditions have led to marked discrepancies in the reporting of each of these disabling postoperative situations.

Deformity and late failures

The development of progressive kyphotic deformity after cervical laminectomy has been reported by several groups [50, 51] **(III/B)**. In some cases, the deformity results in clinical deterioration and poor outcomes [61]. Reoperation is sometimes required to correct deformity. The reoperation rate after initial cervical laminectomy is not known, although studies using administrative state inpatient databases should, in the near future, provide useful information on the clinical magnitude of the problem.

A need for randomized controlled trials

While an RCT comparing the ventral and dorsal approaches has been advocated by many, the heterogeneity of the patient population and individual surgeon bias favoring either approach has discouraged the performance of an RCT to date.

Our previous work suggests that most US cervical spine experts (both orthopedic and neurologic) believe there is sufficient clinical equipoise to justify a comparative trial if the study population is carefully defined [62]. Several other important factors justify a trial at this time. First, the complication rate for CSM surgery is very high (17% in one prospective study) [4] and particularly so in patients older than 74 years [2], a growing segment of the US population [63]. Second, outcomes are unsatisfactory in 30% of cases [9]. Third, the costs of dorsal decompression and fusion appear to be significantly higher than those of ventral surgery, suggesting that even if the approaches have similar outcomes, an understanding of the differential in hospital costs will be relevant [64].

Conclusions

CSM is the most common cause of spinal cord dysfunction in the USA. Decompressive surgery can stabilize or sometimes improve its disabling symptoms. There is, however, controversy surrounding the choice of approach: ventral (anterior) or dorsal (posterior). These two main surgical approaches have been used for nearly 50 years and yet, to date, no RCT has been performed to compare their effectiveness. Furthermore, comparative-effectiveness studies evaluating the addition of arthrodesis when performing dorsal surgery have not been undertaken. Published data now demonstrate that complications from CSM surgery (and reoperations for late failures) are prevalent and differ between the ventral and dorsal approaches. Definitive studies that can help to establish scientifically based guidelines are likely to improve the results of CSM treatment.

Chapter 3

Recommendations	Evidence level
• Surgery for CSM is associated with improved outcomes compared with non-surgical conservative treatment.	II/B
• Patients with mild CSM symptoms can be managed without surgery.	II/B
• Patients older than 75 years have higher complication rates than younger patients following surgery for CSM.	IIb/B
• Preoperative kyphosis of more than 13° is associated with poorer disease-specific outcomes after laminoplasty.	III/B
• Ventral surgery is associated with improved outcomes in patients with preoperative MRI intramedullary signal changes.	IIb/B
• Three-level ventral corpectomy is associated with a higher complication rate than one- or two-level constructs.	III/B
• Multilevel ventral corpectomy is associated with a higher graft complication rate than multilevel discectomy and fusion.	III/B
• Ventral corpectomy is associated with more complications than laminoplasty.	III/B
• Ventral fusion is associated with fewer complications than dorsal fusion following surgery for CSM.	IIb/B
• Cervical laminectomy without fusion is associated with progressive kyphotic deformity.	III/B
• Dynamic plating systems are associated with lower rates of complications than rigid cervical plating systems following ventral cervical procedures.	Ib/A

References

1. Patil PG, Turner DA, Pietrobon R. National trends in surgical procedures for degenerative cervical spine disease: 1990-2000. *Neurosurgery* 2005; 57(4): 753-8.

2. Wang MC, Chan L, Maiman DJ, Kreuter W, Deyo RA. Complications and mortality associated with cervical spine surgery for degenerative disease in the United States. *Spine* 2007; 32(3): 342-7.

3. Boakye M, Patil CG, Santarelli J, Ho C, Tian W, Lad SP. Cervical spondylotic myelopathy: complications and outcomes after spinal fusion. *Neurosurgery* 2008; 62(2): 455-61.

4. Fehlings MG, Sasso RC, Kopjar B, *et al*. Anterior vs. posterior surgery of cervical spondylotic myelopathy: a large prospective multi-center clinical trial. Presented at the 24th Annual Meeting of the AANS/CNS Section on Disorders of the Spine and Peripheral Nerves. Orlando, FL, 2008.

5. Young WF. Cervical spondylotic myelopathy: a common cause of spinal cord dysfunction in older persons. *Am Fam Physician* 2000; 62(5): 1064-70, 73.

6. Henderson FC, Geddes JF, Vaccaro AR, Woodard E, Berry KJ, Benzel EC. Stretch-associated injury in cervical spondylotic myelopathy: new concept and review. *Neurosurgery* 2005; 56(5): 1101-13.

7. al-Mefty O, Harkey HL, Marawi I, *et al*. Experimental chronic compressive cervical myelopathy. *J Neurosurg* 1993; 79(4): 550-61.

8. Baron EM, Young WF. Cervical spondylotic myelopathy: a brief review of its pathophysiology, clinical course, and diagnosis. *Neurosurgery* 2007; 60 (1 Suppl. 1): S35-41.

9. Rowland LP. Surgical treatment of cervical spondylotic myelopathy: time for a controlled trial. *Neurology* 1992; 42(1): 5-13.

10. Bohlman HH, Emery SE. The pathophysiology of cervical spondylosis and myelopathy. *Spine* 1988; 13(7): 843-6.

11. Bednarik J, Kadanka Z, Dusek L, *et al*. Presymptomatic spondylotic cervical cord compression. *Spine* 2004; 29(20): 2260-9.

12. Lees F, Turner JW. Natural history and prognosis of cervical spondylosis. *BMJ* 1963; 2(5373): 1607-10.

13. Rao R. Neck pain, cervical radiculopathy, and cervical myelopathy: pathophysiology, natural history, and clinical evaluation. *J Bone Joint Surg* 2002; 84-A(10): 1872-81.

14. Mazanec D, Reddy A. Medical management of cervical spondylosis. *Neurosurgery* 2007; 60 (1 Suppl. 1): S43-50.

15. Abbasi A, Malhotra G, Malanga G, Elovic EP, Kahn S. Complications of interlaminar cervical epidural steroid injections: a review of the literature. *Spine* 2007; 32(19): 2144-51.

16. Kadanka Z, Bednarik J, Vohanka S, *et al*. Conservative treatment versus surgery in spondylotic cervical myelopathy: a prospective randomised study. *Eur Spine J* 2000; 9(6): 538-44.

17. Sampath P, Bendebba M, Davis JD, Ducker TB. Outcome of patients treated for cervical myelopathy. A prospective, multicenter study with independent clinical review. *Spine* 2000; 25(6): 670-6.

18. Latimer M, Haden N, Seeley HM, Laing RJ. Measurement of outcome in patients with cervical spondylotic myelopathy treated surgically. *Br J Neurosurg* 2002; 16(6): 545-9.

19. Wiggins GC, Shaffrey CI. Dorsal surgery for myelopathy and myeloradiculopathy. *Neurosurgery* 2007; 60 (1 Suppl. 1): S71-81.

20. Smith AG. Account of a case in which portions of three dorsal vertebrae were removed for the relief of paralysis from fracture, with partial success. *N Am Med Surg* 1829; 8: 94-7.

21. Fessler RG, Steck JC, Giovanini MA. Anterior cervical corpectomy for cervical spondylotic myelopathy. *Neurosurgery* 1998; 43(2): 257-65.

22. Suda K, Abumi K, Ito M, Shono Y, Kaneda K, Fujiya M. Local kyphosis reduces surgical outcomes of expansive open-door laminoplasty for cervical spondylotic myelopathy. *Spine* 2003; 28(12): 1258-62.

23. Suri A, Chabbra RP, Mehta VS, Gaikwad S, Pandey RM. Effect of intramedullary signal changes on the surgical outcome of patients with cervical spondylotic myelopathy. *Spine J* 2003; 3(1): 33-45.

24. Yonenobu K, Hosono N, Iwasaki M, Asano M, Ono K. Laminoplasty versus subtotal corpectomy. A comparative study of results in multisegmental cervical spondylotic myelopathy. *Spine* 1992; 17(11): 1281-4.

25. Edwards CC 2nd, Heller JG, Murakami H. Corpectomy versus laminoplasty for multilevel cervical myelopathy: an independent matched-cohort analysis. *Spine* 2002; 27(11): 1168-75.

26. Sasso RC, Ruggiero RA Jr., Reilly TM, Hall PV. Early reconstruction failures after multilevel cervical corpectomy. *Spine* 2003; 28(2): 140-2.

27. Wang JC, Hart RA, Emery SE, Bohlman HH. Graft migration or displacement after multilevel cervical corpectomy and strut grafting. *Spine* 2003; 28(10): 1016-21.

28. Stewart TJ, Schlenk RP, Benzel EC. Multiple level discectomy and fusion. *Neurosurgery* 2007; 60 (1 Suppl. 1): S143-8.

29. Zdeblick TA, Hughes SS, Riew KD, Bohlman HH. Failed anterior cervical discectomy and arthrodesis. Analysis and treatment of thirty-five patients. *J Bone Joint Surg* 1997; 79(4): 523-32.

30. Mummaneni PV, Kaiser MG, Matz PG, *et al*. Cervical surgical techniques for the treatment of cervical spondylotic myelopathy. *J Neurosurg Spine* 2009; 11(2): 130-41.

31. Matz PG, Anderson PA, Holly LT, *et al*. The natural history of cervical spondylotic myelopathy. *J Neurosurg Spine* 2009; 11(2): 104-11.

32. Bucciero A, Vizioli L, Carangelo B, Tedeschi G. MR signal enhancement in cervical spondylotic myelopathy. Correlation with surgical results in 35 cases. *J Neurosurg Sci* 1993; 37(4): 217-22.

33. Chiles BW, 3rd, Leonard MA, Choudhri HF, Cooper PR. Cervical spondylotic myelopathy: patterns of neurological deficit and recovery after anterior cervical decompression. *Neurosurgery* 1999; 44(4): 762-9.

34. Ebersold MJ, Pare MC, Quast LM. Surgical treatment for cervical spondylitic myelopathy. *J Neurosurg* 1995; 82(5): 745-51.

35. Fukushima T, Ikata T, Taoka Y, Takata S. Magnetic resonance imaging study on spinal cord plasticity in patients with cervical compression myelopathy. *Spine* 1991; 16(10 Suppl.): S534-8.

36. Kohno K, Kumon Y, Oka Y, Matsui S, Ohue S, Sakaki S. Evaluation of prognostic factors following expansive laminoplasty for cervical spinal stenotic myelopathy. *Surg Neurol* 1997; 48(3): 237-45.

37. Mehalic TF, Pezzuti RT, Applebaum BI. Magnetic resonance imaging and cervical spondylotic myelopathy. *Neurosurgery* 1990; 26(2): 217-26.

38. Morio Y, Yamamoto K, Kuranobu K, Murata M, Tuda K. Does increased signal intensity of the spinal cord on MR images due to cervical myelopathy predict prognosis? *Arch Orthop Trauma Surg* 1994; 113(5): 254-9.

39. Okada Y, Ikata T, Yamada H, Sakamoto R, Katoh S. Magnetic resonance imaging study on the results of surgery for cervical compression myelopathy. *Spine* 1993; 18(14): 2024-9.

40. Wada E, Ohmura M, Yonenobu K. Intramedullary changes of the spinal cord in cervical spondylotic myelopathy. *Spine* 1995; 20(20): 2226-32.

41. Watabe N, Tominaga T, Shimizu H, Koshu K, Yoshimoto T. Quantitative analysis of cerebrospinal fluid flow in patients with cervical spondylosis using cine phase-contrast magnetic resonance imaging. *Neurosurgery* 1999; 44(4): 779-84.

42. Yone K, Sakou T, Yanase M, Ijiri K. Preoperative and postoperative magnetic resonance image evaluations of the spinal cord in cervical myelopathy. *Spine* 1992; 17(10 Suppl.): S388-92.

43. Smith GW, Robinson RA. The treatment of certain cervical-spine disorders by anterior removal of the intervertebral disc and interbody fusion. *J Bone Joint Surg* 1958; 40-A(3): 607-24.

44. Hillard VH, Apfelbaum RI. Surgical management of cervical myelopathy: indications and techniques for multilevel cervical discectomy. *Spine J* 2006; 6(6 Suppl.): 242-51S.

45. Brodke DS, Zdeblick TA. Modified Smith-Robinson procedure for anterior cervical discectomy and fusion. *Spine* 1992; 17(10 Suppl.): S427-30.

46. Kwon BK, Vaccaro AR, Grauer JN, Beiner JM. The use of rigid internal fixation in the surgical management of cervical spondylosis. *Neurosurgery* 2007; 60 (1 Suppl. 1): S118-29.

47. Pitzen TR, Chrobok J, Stulik J, *et al.* Implant complications, fusion, loss of lordosis, and outcome after anterior cervical plating with dynamic or rigid plates: two-year results of a multi-centric, randomized, controlled study. *Spine* 2009; 34(7): 641-6.

48. Cooper PR. Anterior cervical vertebrectomy: tips and traps. *Neurosurgery* 2001; 49(5): 1129-32.

49. Douglas AF, Cooper PR. Cervical corpectomy and strut grafting. *Neurosurgery* 2007; 60(1 Suppl. 1): S137-42.

50. Lu JJ. Cervical laminectomy: technique. *Neurosurgery* 2007; 60(1 Suppl. 1): S149-53.

51. Mikawa Y, Shikata J, Yamamuro T. Spinal deformity and instability after multilevel cervical laminectomy. *Spine* 1987; 12(1): 6-11.

52. Guigui P, Benoist M, Deburge A. Spinal deformity and instability after multilevel cervical laminectomy for spondylotic myelopathy. *Spine* 1998; 23(4): 440-7.

53. Huang RC, Girardi FP, Poynton AR, Cammisa Jr FP. Treatment of multilevel cervical spondylotic myeloradiculopathy with posterior decompression and fusion with lateral mass plate fixation and local bone graft. *J Spinal Disord Tech* 2003; 16(2): 123-9.

54. Heller JG, Edwards CC 2nd, Murakami H, Rodts GE. Laminoplasty versus laminectomy and fusion for multilevel cervical myelopathy: an independent matched cohort analysis. *Spine* 2001; 26(12): 1330-6.

55. Mummaneni PV, Haid RW, Rodts GE Jr. Combined ventral and dorsal surgery for myelopathy and myeloradiculopathy. *Neurosurgery* 2007; 60 (1 Suppl. 1): S82-9.

56. King JT Jr., McGinnis KA, Roberts MS. Quality of life assessment with the Medical Outcomes Study Short Form-36 among patients with cervical spondylotic myelopathy. *Neurosurgery* 2003; 52(1): 113-20.

57. Holly LT, Moftakhar P, Khoo LT, Shamie AN, Wang JC. Surgical outcomes of elderly patients with cervical spondylotic myelopathy. *Surg Neurol* 2008; 69(3): 233-40.

58. Edwards CC 2nd, Karpitskaya Y, Cha C, *et al.* Accurate identification of adverse outcomes after cervical spine surgery. *J Bone Joint Surg* 2004; 86-A(2): 251-6.

59. Bose B, Sestokas AK, Schwartz DM. Neurophysiological detection of iatrogenic C-5 nerve deficit during anterior cervical spinal surgery. *J Neurosurg Spine* 2007; 6(5): 381-5.

60. Saunders RL. On the pathogenesis of the radiculopathy complicating multilevel corpectomy. *Neurosurgery* 1995; 37(3): 408-12.

61. Yonenobu K, Okada K, Fuji T, Fujiwara K, Yamashita K, Ono K. Causes of neurologic deterioration following surgical treatment of cervical myelopathy. *Spine* 1986; 11(8): 818-23.

62. Ghogawala Z, Coumans JV, Benzel EC, Stabile LM, Barker FG 2nd. Ventral versus dorsal decompression for cervical spondylotic myelopathy: surgeons' assessment of eligibility for randomization in a proposed randomized controlled trial: results of a survey of the Cervical Spine Research Society. *Spine* 2007; 32(4): 429-36.

63. Riggs BL, Melton LJ, 3rd. The worldwide problem of osteoporosis: insights afforded by epidemiology. *Bone* 1995; 17(5 Suppl.): 505S-11.

64. Ghogawala Z, Wasserberger E, Potter R, Barker FG. Ventral surgery versus dorsal decompression with fusion for cervical spondylotic myelopathy: a cost analysis. Presented at the 76th Annual Meeting of the American Association of Neurological Surgeons. Chicago, Illinois, 2008.

Cervical spondylotic myelopathy

Chapter 4

Lumbar fusion for low back pain without neurologic symptoms or spinal deformity

Daniel K Resnick MD MS

Professor and Vice Chairman

DEPARTMENT OF NEUROSURGERY, UNIVERSITY OF WISCONSIN, MADISON, WISCONSIN, USA

Introduction

The use of lumbar fusion as a treatment for low back pain without neurologic symptoms or spinal deformity is an area of intense scrutiny and controversy. Low back pain is extremely common, and patients with chronic low back pain (CLBP) consume an inordinate proportion of health care resources. Multiple papers in the professional and lay press have attacked the use of lumbar fusion for low back pain, citing lack of effectiveness, high complication rates, and high costs [1-3]. Recent national coverage decisions by private insurers in the USA, targeting the use of lumbar fusion for low back pain, have significantly limited the ability of surgeons to offer these procedures to their patients. Confusing the issue, a number of meta-analyses, systematic reviews, and technology assessments have been performed with often conflicting conclusions regarding the same body of evidence [4-10].

This review discusses the highest-quality evidence available relating to fusion for CLBP without neurologic symptoms or spinal deformity. The reasons for the disparate conclusions reached by various author groups based on similar data are discussed,

and the strengths and weaknesses of the available data are described.

Methodology

A computerized search of the database of the National Library of Medicine was performed using PubMed. The Cochrane Database and the National Guidelines Clearinghouse were also searched using computerized search engines. Previously published systematic reviews from the Cochrane Group, the American Association of Neurological Surgeons, and the American Pain Society were also used to identify relevant literature.

The initial PubMed search was performed in February 2010. Using the search term 'lumbar fusion AND randomized trial AND human' and restricting results to the English language yielded 286 references. The titles and, when appropriate, abstracts of these references were reviewed. This resulted in four randomized trials examining the treatment of patients with CLBP caused by degenerative disease with lumbar fusion compared with no specific treatment or alternative non-operative

Table 1. Randomized controlled trials comparing the treatment of patients with chronic low back pain caused by degenerative disease of the lumbar spine without neurologic symptoms or deformity.

Study	Study design	Patient selection	Groups compared	Results
Fritzell et al, 2001 [11]	Ib Randomized Power analysis described a priori Excellent follow-up Validated outcome instruments Statistical analysis complete Intent-to-treat analysis with relatively few cross-overs (25 total)	294 patients randomized with low back pain thought to be due to DDD at L4-5, L5-S1, or both levels Mean duration off work approximately 3 years in both groups Groups had similar characteristics	Three fusion techniques vs. 'different kinds of physical therapy'	At 2 years (98% follow-up), surgical results were superior for Million, ODI, Zung, General Function Score, return to work, and subjective rating scales The differences were statistically and clinically significant The non-operative group did not improve
Brox et al, 2003 [12]	Ib Randomized, single-blinded Short follow-up and lack of power given efficacy of both treatments	64 patients randomized with low back pain of at least 1 year duration, thought to be caused by DDD diagnosed by X-ray at L4-5, L5-S1, or both levels	Instrumented PLF was compared with a multiweek inpatient structured cognitive and physical therapy program	At 1 year, both groups improved Cognitive and physical therapy group showed more improvement in fear avoidance behavior and fingertip-floor distance Surgical patients showed more improvement in back and leg pain Patient satisfaction was similar in both groups
Brox et al, 2006 [13]	Ib Restrictive patient population, short follow-up, and lack of power given documented efficacy of both treatments	60 patients with low back pain following a previous lumbar discectomy were randomized Follow-up was 1 year	Instrumented PLF was compared with a multiweek inpatient structured cognitive and physical therapy program	At 1 year, both groups improved ODI improvements were similar between groups Patient satisfaction was similar in both groups Success rates were equivalent between groups (~50%)
Fairbank et al, 2005 [14]	IIb Patient selection criteria, degree of cross-over and LTF precludes any conclusions based on data presented Intent-to-treat analysis performed despite cross-over and LTF issues	349 patients with low back pain whose physicians felt uncertain as to whether they needed surgery were randomized without further description of diagnostic criteria	A structured cognitive and physical therapy program was compared with a variety of surgical approaches Approximately 20% of patients operated on did not undergo fusion LTF of ~25-30% of patients ~20-25% of patients crossed over or otherwise did not receive assigned therapies	No conclusions regarding the efficacy of lumbar fusion versus any alternative therapy can be drawn Patients in both groups improved from baseline

DDD = degenerative disc disease; LTF = loss to follow-up; PLF = posterolateral fusion treatments. Studies involving different patient populations (e.g., isthmic spondylolisthesis), trials comparing fusion techniques or fusion with other surgical techniques (e.g., disc arthroplasty), and previously published systematic reviews were identified and used as supporting materials.

Chronic low back pain

The results of four randomized controlled clinical trials comparing the treatment of patients with CLBP caused by degenerative disease of the lumbar spine without neurologic symptoms or deformity were available for review (Table 1) [11-14]. These studies have been previously discussed in a number of systematic reviews [4-10].

Fusion versus natural history

The first trial was published by Fritzell *et al* and involved 294 patients who were randomized to receive one of three types of lumbar fusion versus continuation of usual non-operative care [11]. Adult patients were required to have had at least 2 years of debilitating low back pain thought to be caused by degenerative changes at L4-5, L5-S1, or both levels (Figure 1).

Surgical and non-surgical groups were comparable in almost all preoperative demographics, with a median duration of preoperative symptoms of approximately 8 years in both groups. Approximately 20% of patients in both groups were still working full time, and 60% of patients in both groups were involved in litigation. The only statistically significant difference noted between groups was a higher incidence of medical comorbidities in the surgical group (p=0.02).

Outcome measures were a mix of general and disease-specific, including the Oswestry Disability Index (ODI), the Million Visual Analogue Score, the General Function Score, a depression inventory (Zung), a Visual Analogue Scale (VAS) for back and leg pain, and overall satisfaction scores. Follow-up was through 2 years and excellent follow-up rates were achieved (approximately 97%). An intent-to-treat

analysis was performed and there were very few cross-overs (25 total group changers).

Outcomes were superior in the surgically treated patients on all measures, including return to work, and the differences were statistically and clinically relevant. However, while significant improvements in pain and disability did occur in the fusion group,

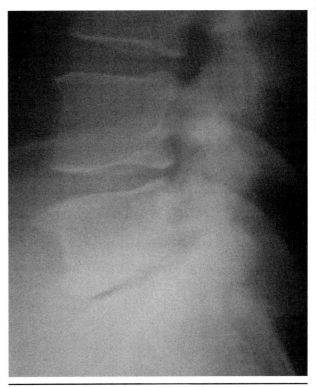

Figure 1. A typical radiograph image from a patient with degenerative disease of the lumbar spine. This patient would have been a candidate for the Fritzell *et al* or Brox *et al* studies [11, 12] if he had disabling back pain.

surgery was not universally beneficial and patients in the surgical group did report ongoing pain and disability. Only 63% reported feeling 'much better' or 'better' at 2 years following surgery. An important consideration when interpreting the results of this study is that the control group did not improve at all from baseline. This is probably explained by the fact that no new treatments were attempted with the control group – they were simply offered more of the same medications, therapies, and interventions that had failed previously [11]. It is therefore best to consider this trial as a comparison of lumbar fusion with the natural history of patients with disabling CLBP treated in the community. For this comparison, the Fritzell paper is considered to provide level I medical evidence **(Ib/A)**.

Fusion versus cognitive and physical therapy: I

In 2003, Brox *et al* published a randomized study designed to explore the differential effectiveness of lumbar fusion versus a specific structured cognitive and physical therapy regimen [12]. They randomized 64 patients to instrumented dorsolateral fusion (Figure 2) or an intensive 5-week program of cognitive and

physical therapy (averaging 25 hours/week) followed by outpatient counseling and physical therapy. Patients selected for the study were required to have had 1 year of pain, an ODI of at least 30, and degenerative changes on plain radiographs at L4-5 and at L5-S1.

Patients were followed for 1 year, and the primary outcome measure was the ODI. Secondary outcome measures were a pain VAS, pain medication use, a depression inventory, General Function Score, the Prolo scale, fingertip-to-floor distance, work status, and Waddell's Fear Avoidance Questionnaire (WFAQ; a measure of the patient's aversion to activities due to fear of exacerbating symptoms). A power analysis was performed, which assumed, based on a pilot study, that minimal improvement in the ODI would be seen in the cognitive and physical

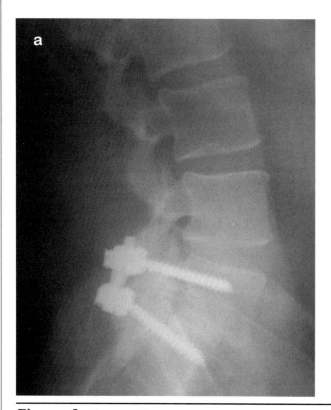
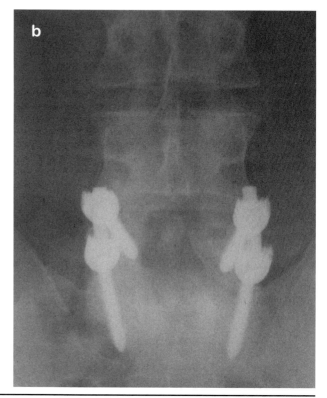

Figure 2. a) Lateral and b) anteroposterior radiographs from a patient treated with posterior lumbar interbody fusion for back pain associated with degenerative disc disease. This patient had concomitant radiculopathy because of foraminal stenosis. Note that the addition of the interbody graft was not performed in the Brox *et al* studies, but was performed in one of the surgical arms of the Fritzell *et al* study [11].

therapy group. Follow-up was excellent (97%), cross-over was minimal, and an intent-to-treat analysis was performed.

Both groups enjoyed statistically and clinically significant improvements in the ODI, with the surgical group improving from a mean of 42 pre-intervention to 26 post-intervention, and the cognitive and physical therapy group improving from a mean of 43 to 30 [12]. In addition, improvements were seen in almost all secondary measures in both groups, with significant differences in favor of the cognitive and physical therapy group in the WFAQ and fingertip-to-floor distance, and in favor of surgery for leg pain. Again, only 60-70% of patients judged their treatment to be a 'success.' This study loses power because the initial analysis assumed no improvement in the control group – an assumption that was false **(Ib/A)**.

Brox repeated this study using a more select patient group – patients with CLBP following discectomy – in 2006 [13]. The statistical methods, outcome measures, and results were essentially the same as in the 2003 study, with the exception that only about half of the patients in either group felt their treatment resulted in 'fair' or better results, illustrating the difficulties in dealing with this patient population. It is interesting that the authors used the same assumptions in the power analysis for this study, despite the fact that their cognitive and physical therapy regimen was shown to result in significant improvements in the ODI in the 2003 study **(Ib/A)**.

In the Brox studies [12, 13], lumbar fusion is not being compared with the natural history of patients with CLBP, but with an intensive 5-week, 25 hours/week program of highly structured and personalized cognitive and physical therapy. Brox demonstrates convincingly that the program used results in improvements in ODI and other outcome measures that are comparable with improvements seen in patients undergoing fusion. The added improvement in the WFAQ in the cognitive therapy groups is not at all surprising, given the fusion patients did not receive any treatment for fear-avoidance behavior. This study does not indicate that fusion is ineffective – rather, it indicates that other treatments may also be effective. It should be noted that 'effective' is a relative term, as

half of the patients treated did not feel that their treatment was successful and return to work rates were minimal in all groups.

Fusion versus cognitive and physical therapy: II

In 2005, Fairbank *et al* published the results of a highly publicized but highly flawed randomized study looking at surgical intervention for CLBP [14]. These authors randomized 349 patients with CLBP to surgical intervention versus the previously described structured cognitive and physical therapy treatments [12]. An important distinction in this study was that patients were only eligible for inclusion if the treating physician and the patient were both undecided regarding the appropriate treatment. Therefore, patients with severe degenerative changes and straightforward symptoms would have been excluded. Another difference in this study was that patients assigned to surgical intervention did not necessarily undergo fusion, with approximately 15% actually undergoing 'dynamic stabilization.' Valid outcome parameters including the ODI and VAS pain scores were used and the authors attempted to follow patients for 2 years [14]. An intent-to-treat analysis was performed.

Unfortunately, there was significant cross-over from the non-surgical to the surgical arm of the study. Nearly 30% of patients assigned to non-operative therapy had surgery, while 37 of the 176 patients (21%) assigned to surgery did not undergo a procedure, and only four of these patients received the structured therapy. An additional 19% of patients in both groups were lost to follow-up. This degree of cross-over causes homogeneity between the assigned treatment groups and completely destroys the utility of an intent-to-treat analysis, as was seen and described in the SPORT (Spine Patient Outcomes Research Trial) studies from North America [15-17]. Despite this limitation, patients assigned to the surgery group still demonstrated statistically significant improvements in the ODI compared with patients assigned to the structured therapy; however, the difference was not clinically relevant [14]. Because of the patient selection criteria, the degree of cross-over, and the fact that non-fusion

Chapter 4

Chapter 4

surgical interventions were included in the surgical arm, no conclusions regarding the relative efficacy of any treatment can be drawn from this study (IIb/B).

Interpreting the evidence

These four studies represent the best evidence available comparing lumbar fusion with either usual management (or natural history) or a structured, intensive, 5-week cognitive and physical therapy program. All of these studies have design characteristics that limit their applicability to the North American CLBP population.

First, patient selection criteria varied between the studies and were primarily based on plain films. It is possible that the patients randomized into these studies may not have met criteria for lumbar fusion in North American practice, where there is more intensive use of advanced imaging techniques for patient selection (for better or worse). Furthermore, the degree of improvement seen in the surgical patients in the European studies is much less than that described for patients treated with lumbar fusion in North American investigational device exemption studies where fusion was used as a control procedure [18, 19]. Another concern relates to the relatively short (1 year) duration of follow-up in both of the Brox studies, especially given the recalcitrance of low back pain over time. Perhaps the most important factor regarding the applicability of the Brox studies, however, is the fact that the structured program used is currently not available in the USA. It is important to remember that 'multidisciplinary' pain centers in the USA are largely procedure-based, and that treatment at such centers is not associated with the same benefits as those described for the structured regimen [20-22].

Because of the costs and controversies associated with the treatment of CLBP, there have been more structured reviews published on the topic than there have been controlled clinical trials. Resnick et al reviewed the Fritzell study and the first Brox study and recommended that fusion be considered as a treatment option for patients with CLPB based on the best evidence available at the time [5]. Gibson and Waddell reviewed a similar body of literature and determined that there was essentially no evidence to support the performance of lumbar fusion [6]. Mirza and Deyo reviewed the same four studies described herein, and determined that surgery may be more efficacious than usual care but may not be more effective than structured cognitive and physical therapy [4]. These authors specifically cited the difficulty in generalizing results from European studies to the North American population. Ibrahim et al published a meta-analysis using pooled data from the above studies and found little evidence to support lumbar fusion because of marginal improvements in the ODI and known costs and complications [8]. Chou et al found that fusion for CLBP was associated with small to moderate benefits compared with traditional non-surgical treatments, and was equivalent to structured intensive cognitive and physical therapy as described in the European studies [10].

It is apparent from the disparate results of randomized trials and the disparate conclusions of structured reviews that there is disagreement regarding the role of lumbar fusion for CLBP without radiculopathy, neurogenic claudication, or deformity. It is clear that compared with the natural history or 'usual care' of CLBP, lumbar fusion is associated with significant improvements in low back pain, leg pain, and functional disability. While clinically significant, the degree of improvement is not miraculous and a significant proportion of patients (30-50%) will continue to report significant dissatisfaction and disability related to their low back pain. A structured, intensive, 5-week, 25-hour/week course of cognitive and physical therapy followed by ongoing counseling for up to 1 year is associated with similar benefits in functional outcomes and improved fear avoidance behavior, but is associated with more back and leg pain. Again, a large proportion of patients (30-50%) treated with this intensive regimen will continue to complain of significant dissatisfaction and disability.

In conclusion, a uniformly safe and effective treatment for patients with CLBP caused by degenerative changes at L4-5 or L5-S1 does not exist. The available literature suggests that certain patients will benefit from either fusion or structured intensive cognitive and physical therapy. At the present time, either treatment is associated with better outcomes than the usual care afforded to patients in North America **(Ib/A)**. Choice of treatment should be based on consideration of the available therapies, costs and potential complications, and patient preference.

Directions for future research

Based on the experiences of the SPORT investigators [15-17], it is unrealistic to expect a successful North American randomized study investigating the efficacy of lumbar fusion for CLBP. In addition, patient selection criteria and the availability of alternative treatments vary regionally. A large-scale prospective registry project with the participation of community practitioners would provide important information regarding the comparative effectiveness of various treatment strategies for CLBP for patients with a variety of presenting complaints, anatomic features, and treatment histories.

Conclusions

Lumbar fusion should be offered to select patients with CLBP caused by degenerative changes at L4-5 or L5-S1 without neurologic symptoms or spinal deformity who have failed to improve despite a comprehensive course of non-operative management. Lumbar fusion has been shown to be associated with better outcomes than the natural history of CLBP in this patient population **(Ib/A)**.

Lumbar fusion or intensive structured cognitive and physical therapy should be offered to patients with CLBP caused by degenerative changes at L4-5 or L5-S1 without neurologic symptoms or spinal deformity who have failed to improve despite a comprehensive course of usual non-operative management. Both strategies are associated with improvements compared with the natural history of CLBP in this patient population, and similar degrees of functional improvement are associated with both treatments **(Ib/A)**.

Recommendations	Evidence level
◆ Lumbar fusion is associated with significant improvements in low back pain, leg pain, and functional disability compared with the natural history or 'usual care' of CLBP.	Ib/A
◆ A structured, intensive, 5-week, 25 hours/week course of cognitive and physical therapy followed by counseling for up to 1 year is associated with significant improvements in functional outcomes and fear avoidance behavior when compared with the natural history or 'usual care' of CLBP.	Ib/A

References

1. Deyo RA, Mirza SK, Turner JA, Martin BI. Overtreating chronic back pain: time to back off? *J Am Board Fam Med* 2009; 22(1): 62-8.

2. Deyo RA. Back surgery - who needs it? *N Engl J Med* 2007; 356(22): 2239-43.

3. Abelson R, Peterson M. An operation to ease back pain bolsters the bottom line, too. New York Times, 31 December 2003.

4. Mirza SK, Deyo RA. Systematic review of randomized trials comparing lumbar fusion surgery to nonoperative care for treatment of chronic back pain. *Spine* (Phila Pa 1976) 2007; 32(7): 816-23.

5. Resnick DK, Choudhri TF, Dailey AT, *et al.* Guidelines for the performance of fusion procedures for degenerative disease of the lumbar spine. Part 7: intractable low-back pain without stenosis or spondylolisthesis. *J Neurosurg Spine* 2005; 2(6): 670-2.

6. Gibson JN, Waddell G. Surgery for degenerative lumbar spondylosis: updated Cochrane Review. *Spine* (Phila Pa 1976) 2005; 30(20): 2312-20.

7. Carreon LY, Glassman SD, Howard J. Fusion and nonsurgical treatment for symptomatic lumbar degenerative disease: a systematic review of Oswestry Disability Index and MOS Short Form-36 outcomes. *Spine J* 2008; 8(5): 747-55.

8. Ibrahim T, Tleyjeh IM, Gabbar O. Surgical versus non-surgical treatment of chronic low back pain: a meta-analysis of randomised trials. *Int Orthop* 2008; 32(1): 107-13.

9. Allen RT, Rihn JA, Glassman SD, Currier B, Albert TJ, Phillips FM. An evidence-based approach to spine surgery. *Am J Med Qual* 2009; 24(6 Suppl.): 15-24S.

10. Chou R, Baisden J, Carragee EJ, Resnick DK, Shaffer WO, Loeser JD. Surgery for low back pain: a review of the evidence for an American Pain Society Clinical Practice Guideline. *Spine* (Phila Pa 1976) 2009; 34(10): 1094-109.

11. Fritzell P, Hagg O, Wessberg P, Nordwall A. 2001 Volvo Award Winner in Clinical Studies: lumbar fusion versus nonsurgical treatment for chronic low back pain: a multicenter randomized controlled trial from the Swedish Lumbar Spine Study Group. *Spine* (Phila Pa 1976) 2001; 26(23): 2521-32; discussion 32-4.

12. Brox JI, Sorensen R, Friis A, *et al.* Randomized clinical trial of lumbar instrumented fusion and cognitive intervention and exercises in patients with chronic low back pain and disc degeneration. *Spine* (Phila Pa 1976) 2003; 28(17): 1913-21.

13. Brox JI, Reikeras O, Nygaard O, *et al.* Lumbar instrumented fusion compared with cognitive intervention and exercises in patients with chronic back pain after previous surgery for disc herniation: a prospective randomized controlled study. *Pain* 2006; 122(1-2): 145-55.

14. Fairbank J, Frost H, Wilson-MacDonald J, Yu LM, Barker K, Collins R. Randomised controlled trial to compare surgical stabilisation of the lumbar spine with an intensive rehabilitation programme for patients with chronic low back pain: the MRC spine stabilisation trial. *BMJ* 2005; 330(7502): 1233.

15. Weinstein JN, Tosteson TD, Lurie JD, *et al.* Surgical vs. nonoperative treatment for lumbar disk herniation: the Spine Patient Outcomes Research Trial (SPORT): a randomized trial. *JAMA* 2006; 296(20): 2441-50.

16. Weinstein JN, Lurie JD, Tosteson TD, *et al.* Surgical versus nonsurgical treatment for lumbar degenerative spondylolisthesis. *N Engl J Med* 2007; 356(22): 2257-70.

17. Weinstein JN, Tosteson TD, Lurie JD, *et al.* Surgical versus nonsurgical therapy for lumbar spinal stenosis. *N Engl J Med* 2008; 358(8): 794-810.

18. Blumenthal S, McAfee PC, Guyer RD, *et al.* A prospective, randomized, multicenter Food and Drug Administration investigational device exemptions study of lumbar total disc replacement with the CHARITE artificial disc versus lumbar fusion: part I: evaluation of clinical outcomes. *Spine* (Phila Pa 1976) 2005; 30(14): 1565-75; discussion E387-91.

19. Burkus JK, Transfeldt EE, Kitchel SH, Watkins RG, Balderston RA. Clinical and radiographic outcomes of anterior lumbar interbody fusion using recombinant human bone morphogenetic protein-2. *Spine* 2002; 27: 2396-408.

20. Robinson JP, Allen T, Fulton LD, Martin DC. Perceived efficacy of pain clinics in the rehabilitation of injured workers. *Clin J Pain* 1998; 14(3): 202-8.

21. Robinson JP, Fulton-Kehoe D, Martin DC, Franklin GM. Outcomes of pain center treatment in Washington State workers' compensation. *Am J Ind Med* 2001; 39(2): 227-36.

22. Robinson JP, Fulton-Kehoe D, Franklin GM, Wu R. Multidisciplinary pain center outcomes in Washington State Workers' Compensation. *J Occup Environ Med* 2004; 46(5): 473-8.

Chapter 4

Chapter 5

Thoracolumbar spine fractures

George M Ghobrial MD, Neurological Surgery Resident 1
Harminder Singh MD, Clinical Assistant Professor of Neurological Surgery 2
James Harrop MD FACS, Associate Professor, Departments of Neurological and Orthopedic Surgery; Chief, Spine and Peripheral Nerve Surgery 1

1 DEPARTMENT OF NEUROLOGICAL SURGERY, THOMAS JEFFERSON UNIVERSITY HOSPITAL, PHILADELPHIA, PENNSYLVANIA, USA
2 STANFORD NEUROLOGICAL SURGERY, STANFORD, CALIFORNIA, USA

Introduction

Traumatic spinal column injuries affect approximately 160,000 patients a year in the USA, with 10-30% having a concurrent spinal cord injury. Overall, 15-20% of traumatic fractures occur at the thoracolumbar junction (T11-L2). The mortality rate of patients with paraplegia secondary to thoracic fractures is greater than 7%, which illustrates the devastating effects of thoracolumbar trauma [1]. This high mortality rate is related to the traumatic forces and mechanisms required to produce an injury to the thoracic and lumbar spine.

The unique regional anatomy of the thoracic spine and thoracolumbar junction consists of a transition from a fixed kyphotic spinal segment to a mobile lordotic one, which predisposes this region to injury from trauma. Primary goals in the management of patients with thoracolumbar trauma are prompt recognition and treatment of associated injuries and expeditious stabilization of the spine to protect and maximize recovery of the neural elements.

Optimal management algorithms for thoracolumbar spine fractures are controversial and a clear consensus is lacking because of the shortage of definitive studies. No large, prospective, randomized controlled trials (RCTs) exist for surgical treatment of thoracolumbar junction trauma [1]. This is partly due to difficulties with recruitment and follow-up of trauma patients, as well as the diversity of injuries and mechanisms of injury to the spine. Most treatment recommendations are based upon grade B evidence and expert panels. A definitive treatment algorithm based on clinical trials has not been universally accepted for this spinal disorder, partially due to the numerous classification systems that exist (Table 1). A consensus of international experts from the Spine Trauma Study Group (STSG) offers general advice for treating injuries based on injury morphology, neurologic status, and the presence of compromise in the dorsal ligamentous complex [1]. The STSG consists of 22 spine surgeons from level I trauma centers in the USA, Canada, Australia, Germany, Mexico, India, and the Netherlands [1].

Methodology

A National Library of Medicine computerized advanced search was undertaken in October 2011. Articles published between 1966 and October 2011 with the subjects 'thoracolumbar' and 'fracture' were

Table 1. Common thoracolumbar injury classification schemes.

Classification system	Type	Description	Points
Magerl (AO Classification System)	A	Compression of vertebral body alone	-
	B	Distraction injury of anterior and posterior element	-
	C	Axial torque/multidirectional injury of anterior and posterior elements	-
Denis (Burst Fracture System)	A	No endplates fractured	-
	B	Superior endplate fracture only	-
	C	Inferior endplate fracture only	-
	D	Superior and inferior endplates fractured	-
Thoracolumbar Injury Severity Score	1. Injury mechanism	Compression	1
		Translation	3
		Rotation	4
	2. Posterior ligamentous complex disruption	Intact	0
		Suspicion for/indeterminate	2
		Injured	4
	3. Neurologic status	Nerve root involvement	2
		Cord involvement (incomplete)	3
		Cord involvement (complete)	2
		Cauda equina involvement	2

queried, totaling 1,500. Upon careful evaluation, relevant abstracts were selected pertaining to operative management, excluding case reports. A preference was given to evaluating clinical trials and prospective studies. In addition, further relevant papers were identified from select bibliographies contained in the aforementioned search.

Conservative management

Thoracolumbar spine injuries without the potential for progressive deformity, no neurologic findings on examination, and lacking damage to the dorsal ligamentous complex can be managed non-surgically [1]. Vertebral compression fractures classified as one-column injuries in the absence of kyphotic deformity and isolated dorsal element fractures are stable by definition and can also be treated non-operatively. The three-column model of stability (Figure 1), as

described by Denis [2], defines the anterior column as the ventral half of the disc and vertebral body; the middle column as the dorsal half of the disc and vertebral body and the posterior longitudinal ligament (PLL); and the posterior column as the dorsal elements. Where excessive kyphosis is present, or greater than 20° angulation at one segment [3, 4], the propensity for increased pain and deformity is a primary concern. To an extent, minimal kyphosis is expected to develop after one-column ventral injury and the use of a brace is recommended to limit progressive deformity, although studies have questioned the benefits of a bracing program [5].

Burst fractures (AO type A) (Figure 2), which are two-column injuries by definition in the Denis classification system, are for the most part non-operative in the absence of neurologic signs and injury to the dorsal ligamentous complex [2, 4] **(III/B)**. As defined by Denis, burst fractures are vertebral body

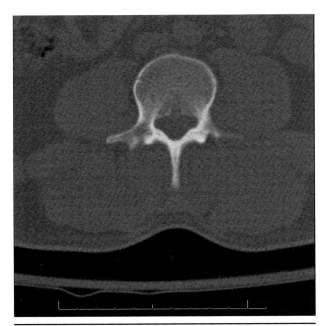

Figure 1. CT of the lumbar spine in the axial view, showing the normal anatomy in an adult. The three columns of the spine are separated into the anterior, middle, and posterior. The anterior column is defined as the anterior longitudinal ligament and the anterior half of the vertebral body. The middle column is marked by the posterior half of the vertebral body and the posterior longitudinal ligament. The posterior column consists of the facet joints and posterior elements.

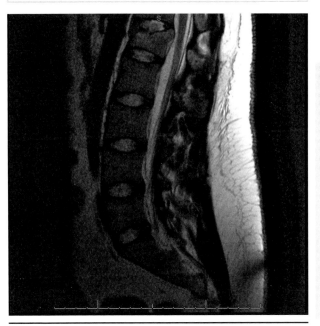

Figure 2. T2-weighted MRI of the lumbar spine in the sagittal view, demonstrating an L1 burst fracture with minimal retropulsion resulting in dural impression.

fractures involving the anterior and middle columns. The vertebral body (including the anterior longitudinal ligament) and the dorsal vertebral body cortex are involved, while the PLL is usually intact. Bed rest and early mobilization in a TLSO brace are the mainstays of treatment, while close monitoring for increased kyphosis is continued in follow-up visits [4, 5]. The most worrying risk of non-operative treatment is the potential for neurologic deterioration. Chronic or glacial instability usually presents as mechanical pain, but can also present as an acute or chronic neurologic deficit.

Various authors have proposed guidelines for intervention. Brown *et al* and Cantor *et al* advocate conservative management of burst fractures with less than 50% loss of height, less than 30° kyphosis, and less than 3cm of sagittal malalignment [6, 7] **(III/B)**.

However, these recommendations are not based on clinical or biomechanical studies.

The absence of neurologic deficit is more valuable information than the extent of canal compromise from retropulsed bone fragments, particularly when the fracture is below the conus medullaris, and many take this as an indication for non-operative management. If, however, neurologic status declines during follow-up or canal stenosis is greater than 50% then operative intervention is indicated [8, 9] **(IV/C)**. As long as the dorsal ligamentous complex is intact and the patient does not exhibit neurologic compromise, the consensus of the STSG is for non-surgical management [1].

Most level I evidence in thoracolumbar injury is seen in the management of stable burst fractures without neurologic deficit. Level I and II evidence supports the non-operative treatment of burst fractures. Because of these studies, the recommendations of the STSG favor conservative management.

Chapter 5

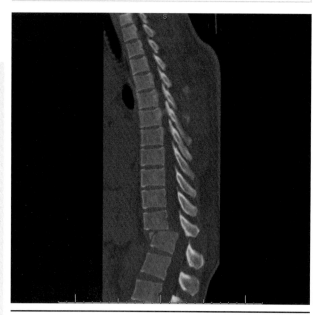

Figure 3. CT of the thoracolumbar spine in the sagittal, midline view, demonstrating a T11-12 flexion-distraction injury with resulting kyphotic deformity. Although not visualized, the facets are jumped bilaterally.

Surgical indications

Dorsal approach

Spinal flexion-distraction injuries are defined by disruption of the posterior and middle columns in tension, and these injuries typically are accompanied by neurologic deficits (AO type B) [10]. Figure 3 shows a radiographic example of a flexion-distraction injury at T11-12 in a motorist. The anterior column of the spine often remains intact. Surgical intervention for these fractures is through re-creating the dorsal tension band through spinal instrumentation. Ventral approaches are not routinely used since the anterior column is typically intact [11] **(Ib/A)**. However, this approach is based on limited literature and evidence, as no large RCTs have been conducted.

Expert opinion may guide the use of a dorsal approach for stabilization in neurologically intact patients with significant disruption of the dorsal ligamentous complex only. Dai et al randomized 73 patients to the dorsolateral approach with and without fusion for the treatment of Denis type B burst fractures (involving superior endplate fracture only) without neurologic deficits, and found no significant difference between the two groups [12]. The study reported excellent results in correcting the deformity and functional outcome scores were improved **(Ib/A)**. In a retrospective review, Tezer et al evaluated 48 patients with flexion-distraction injuries who received dorsal stabilization alone, with short-segment pedicle screw instrumentation, and reported similar excellent results with regards to functional outcome, pain, and return to work [13] **(III/B)**. Inamasu et al reported surgical results from a case series of 32 patients with unstable burst fractures, fracture-dislocation injuries, and flexion-distraction injuries [14]. All patients were treated with dorsal instrumented stabilization, with satisfactory radiographic results and some improvement in neurologic function observed in incomplete injuries **(III/B)**.

Siebenga et al randomized 34 neurologically intact patients with compression fractures to short-segment dorsal stabilization versus immobilization in an orthosis alone for injury at the thoracolumbar junction [10]. The degree of correction of the kyphotic deformity, functional outcome scores, Visual Analogue Scale pain score, and days to return to work were found to be improved in the surgical arm at follow-up **(Ib/A)**. This paper was the first to show the utility of open surgery over non-operative strategies. This differed from the earlier works of Wood et al, who found no difference in outcomes when comparing operative and non-operative treatment of neurologically intact burst fractures [5] **(Ib/A)**. Given the lack of prospective RCTs, the physician can counsel the patient for or against surgery in the case of thoracolumbar burst fractures without neurologic deficit, citing the findings of Siebenga et al for improved functional outcome scores, decreased deformity, and an earlier return to work as a case for surgery [10].

A meta-analysis of four RCTs evaluating 79 patients at an average of 4 years' follow-up found that surgery had a slight advantage over non-operative treatment in the correction of kyphotic deformities. Otherwise, surgical outcomes were equivalent to non-surgical outcomes, but at a higher cost [15]. A Cochrane review identified only one RCT (involving 53 patients) meeting the inclusion criteria, and found no significant difference between the surgical and non-surgical

Table 2. Thoracolumbar surgical trials.

Study	Design	Comparison	Fracture type	n	Surgery	Conclusion	Evidence level/ recommendation
Yi et al, 2006 [15]	Meta-analysis	Surgery vs. brace	TL burst	53	Posterior vs. orthosis	No significant difference	Ia/A
Gnanenthiran et al, 2011 [16]	Meta-analysis	Surgery vs. brace	TL burst	79	Posterior vs. orthosis	No significant difference	Ia/A
Dai et al, 2009 [12]	RCT	Fusion vs. non-fusion	Denis type B burst	73	Posterolateral approach	No significant difference ($p<0.05$)	Ib/A
Bailey et al, 2009 [22]	RCT	Orthosis vs. no orthosis	AO type 3 T11-L3	69	NA	No significant difference ($p<0.05$)	Ib/A
Dai et al, 2009 [20]	RCT	Anterior only	TL burst, LSS >6, and three column	65	Anterior (iliac crest vs. titanium mesh cage)	All fused, no significant deformity (no significant difference between groups)	Ib/A
Siebenga et al, 2006 [10]	RCT	Posterior vs. orthosis	AO type A	34	Posterior vs. orthosis	Surgery: decreased deformity, higher FOS	Ib/A
Wood et al, 2003 [5]	RCT	Surgery vs. orthosis	Stable burst, no neurologic deficit	47	Anterior or posterior vs. orthosis	No significant difference	Ib/A
Reinhold et al, 2010 [18]	RCT	Varied	Acute T1-L5	733	Anterior vs. posterior vs. anterior or posterior	Anterior/posterior: better radiographic deformity correction Posterior: better functional and subjective outcomes	IIa/B
Marco and Kushwaha, 2009 [23]	Cohort	Posterior surgery	Unstable burst	38	Kyphoplasty preceding post short-segment instrumentation	2-year improved ambulation, neurologic function	IIb/B
Defino and Canto, 2007 [24]	Cohort	Bracing	Stable burst, compression	20	NA	Endpoints achieved, deformity corrected	IIb/B
Stancic et al, 2001 [19]	Cohort	Anterior vs. posterior	Stable burst	25	Anterior decompression or fixation vs. post-fixation	No significant difference in neurologic improvement and FOS, decreased morbidity with a posterior approach	IIb/B
Sasso et al, 2006 [17]	Retrospective review	Anterior only	Unstable three-column TL	40	Anterior decompression, graft, plating	Improved FOS, arthrodesis achieved	III/B
McDonough et al, 2004 [21]	Retrospective review	Anterior only	Unstable three-column TL	35	Anterior corpectomy, instrumented fusion	Improved neurologic function	III/B
Tezer et al, 2005 [13]	Retrospective review	Posterior only	Flexion-distraction (Chance)	48	Posterior short-segment instrumentation	Arthrodesis in all cases	III/B
Inamasu et al, 2008 [14]	Retrospective review	Posterior only	17 unstable burst, 15 fracture-dislocation or flexion-distraction	32	Stability, limited recovery	Improved radiographic results, improved neurologic outcomes in ASIA B-D	III/B
McAfee et al, 1985 [25]	Case series	Anterior only	TL burst (stable or unstable)	71	Anterior decompression	Improved neurologic outcomes for incomplete injury	III/B
Vaccaro et al, 2006 [1]	Expert opinion	NA	TL spine injuries	NA	NA	Guidelines for surgical management	IV/C

ASIA = American Spinal Injury Association; FOS = functional outcome scores; NA = not applicable; RCT = randomized controlled trial; TL = thoracolumbar

Chapter 5

arms [16] **(Ia/A)**. These meta-analyses are based on a very small patient population; larger patient populations will be needed to make further conclusions.

Non-randomized studies have shown that dorsal fixation surgery results in superior functional outcome scores and improved neurologic recovery following treatment of unstable burst fractures when compared with ventral-alone approaches [17-19] **(II/B)**. Largely, dorsal fixation has been demonstrated as a tool for the treatment of acute thoracolumbar fractures in which damage to the dorsal ligamentous complex is illustrated radiographically (Table 2) [1, 5, 10, 12-25] **(III/B)**.

Ventral approach

The ventral and ventrolateral approaches are commonly utilized for stabilization and treatment of anterior and middle column thoracolumbar fractures, which cannot be completely accessed dorsally. The STSG advocates the use of the ventral approach in neurologically incomplete patients with burst fractures and intact dorsal ligaments [1]. Moreover, surgery is warranted in patients who are neurologically intact but who show evidence of loss of disruption of the PLL, inferred from more than 25° of kyphosis on radiographs or direct visualization of rupture of the PLL on fat-suppressed sagittal T2-weighted MRI [1] **(IV/C)**.

Dai *et al* reported on a prospective randomized study of 65 patients with severe thoracolumbar burst fractures and three-column injury who were treated with the ventral-only approach [20]. Dividing the subjects into iliac crest bone grafts and titanium mesh strut grafts did not alter the rate of fusion or deformity **(Ib/A)**. Sasso *et al* treated unstable three-column thoracolumbar fractures with ventral decompression, strut graft, and Z-type plating [17], while McDonough *et al* treated three-column thoracolumbar fractures with corpectomy followed by instrumentation and plating [21]. Both studies reported positive results in all endpoints **(III/B)**.

In the case of neurologically complete injuries with intact dorsal ligaments, the STSG could not reach a majority treatment algorithm consensus, arguing for either the ventral (45% of experts) or dorsal approach (55% of experts). Those favoring the ventral approach noted that removing the ventral kyphotic segments would decompress the neural elements and spinal fluid pathways, potentially limiting the occurrence of post-traumatic syringomyelia [1] **(IV/C)**.

In conclusion, most evidence for the use of ventral-approach surgery is based on the expert consensus **(IV/C)**. Ventral-alone surgery at the thoracolumbar junction for the treatment of trauma is uncommon and no level I evidence is available. Most evidence for ventral-alone surgery is level III, consisting of retrospective reviews of three-column injuries in patients with incomplete neurologic injury. The experience of many surgeons is that good outcomes can be achieved; however, rigorous studies comparing ventral-only with dorsal or combined approaches have not been completed to date (Table 2).

Combined ventral and dorsal approach

Distraction injuries, seatbelt injuries, and Chance fractures may require surgical stabilization to restore the dorsal tension band following loss of integrity of the posterior column. Typically, surgical stabilization is required for translation injuries, rotational injuries, and those that destroy spinal integrity with disruption through the disc space and ligamentous complexes. Fracture-dislocation injuries have a significant distraction component. The additional rotatory component separates this injury from seatbelt-type (flexion-dislocation) injuries, in that the disruption of all three spinal columns is commonly seen [26]. These traumatic injuries with severe rotational components carry a high risk of complete spinal cord injury (loss of motor function and sensation below the injury).

In complete spinal cord injury patients with disruption of the dorsal ligaments, the STSG advocates for dorsal stabilization only [1]. In this, the main objective of surgical intervention is to provide dorsal stabilization for early rehabilitation of the patient. Ventral decompression and stabilization is performed following dorsal surgical realignment of the fracture in the rare instances in which partial neurologic deficit exists in the presence of significant ventral neural compression [26-28] **(III/B)**.

When partial neurologic deficit is present, improving residual canal compromise is a further goal of surgery; this is often seen with burst fractures. Canal clearance can be achieved through a dorsal approach via transpedicular decompression and laminectomy, while the ventral approach is particularly useful for decompressing midline ventral lesions and correcting severe kyphotic deformities [29-31].

Dorsal decompression via multilevel laminectomy alone after thoracic and thoracolumbar injuries has been shown to be ineffective and is no longer used as an isolated treatment strategy [31-37]. Loss of the dorsal tension band and instability, along with potential progression of a kyphotic deformity, may ensue, with the added risk of dorsal migration of the spinal cord. In a prospective analysis of 733 patients with acute thoracolumbar spinal injuries, 319 of whom received combined surgery, Reinhold *et al* demonstrated good correction of deformity but with decreased functional outcome scores, higher pain scores, and increased time to ambulation compared with dorsal-alone surgery [18] **(IIb/B)**.

In summary, large cohorts of patients undergoing combined surgery are easily found in the literature [18], but no randomized trials have compared combined surgery with ventral or dorsal surgery alone.

Conclusions

The care of patients with thoracolumbar spine trauma with or without neurologic deficits has evolved dramatically over the past 30 years. The development of more effective instrumentation techniques, coupled with the establishment of spinal injury care and a greater understanding of spinal biomechanics, has definitely improved the care of these patients. Despite these advances, most patients with thoracolumbar injuries who are neurologically intact are still treated non-operatively with cast or brace immobilization and early ambulation. In complete neurologic injury, the goal of surgery is to aid in early rehabilitation of the patient through spinal stabilization. In incomplete neurologic injury, the goal of surgery is to decompress the neural elements and provide stabilization.

With a paucity of RCTs, the majority of guidelines to date on the treatment of thoracolumbar spine fractures are based on expert consensus.

Chapter 5

Recommendations	Evidence level
◆ Stable burst fractures in the absence of neurologic signs and injury to the dorsal ligamentous complex can be treated non-operatively or operatively. No significant difference has been demonstrated between the two, except with a slight surgical advantage for deformity correction.	Ia/A
◆ Patients with acute thoracolumbar fractures with damage to the dorsal ligamentous complex can be treated with dorsal fixation.	III/B
◆ Ventral- or dorsal-approach surgery for unstable burst fractures results in satisfactory functional and radiographic outcomes.	III/B
◆ Combined ventral-dorsal surgery for unstable three-column thoracolumbar injuries results in less kyphotic deformity than dorsal surgery alone.	IIb/B

References

1. Vaccaro AR, Lim MR, Hurlbert RJ, *et al*, for the Spine Trauma Study Group. Surgical decision making for unstable thoracolumbar spine injuries. *J Spinal Disord Tech* 2006; 19(1): 1-10.

2. Denis F. The three column spine and its significance in the classification of acute thoracolumbar spinal injuries. *Spine* 1983; 8(8): 817-31.

3. Verlaan JJ, Diekerhof CH, Busken E, *et al*. Surgical treatment of traumatic fractures of the thoracic and lumbar spine: a systematic review of the literature on techniques, complications, and outcome. *Spine* 2004; 29(7): 803-14.

4. White AA, Panjabi MM. *Clinical Biomechanics of the Spine*. Philadelphia: JB Lippincott, 1978.

5. Wood K, Buttermann G, Mehbo A, Garvey T, Jhanjee R, Sechriest V. Operative compared with nonoperative treatment of a thoracolumbar burst fracture without neurological deficit. *J Bone Joint Surg Am* 2003; 85-A(5): 773-81.

6. Brown CW, Gorup JM, Chow GH. Nonsurgical treatment of thoracic burst fractures in controversies in spine surgery. In: *Spine Surgery*. Zdeblick TA, Benzel EC, Anderson PA, Stillennan CB, Eds. St. Louis: Quality Medical Publishing, 1999; 86-96.

7. Cantor JB, Lebwohl NH, Garvey T, Eismont FJ. Non-operative management of stable thoracolumbar burst fractures with early ambulation and bracing. *Spine* 1993; 19: 1731-40.

8. Cotler JM, Vernace JV, Michalski JA. The use of Harrington rods in thoracolumbar fractures. *Orthop Clin North Am* 1986; 17: 87-103.

9. Tezer M, Erturer RE, Ozturk C, *et al*. Conservative treatment of fractures of the thoracic spine. *Int Orthop* 2005; 29: 78-82.

10. Siebenga J, Leferink VJ, Segers MJ, *et al*. Treatment of traumatic thoracolumbar spine fractures: a multicenter prospective randomized study of operative versus nonsurgical treatment. *Spine* 2006; 31: 2881-90.

11. Gertzbein SD, Court-Brown CM. Flexion-distraction injuries of the lumbar spine: mechanism of injury and classification. *Clin Orthop* 1988; 227: 52-60.

12. Dai LY, Jiang LS, Jiang SD. Posterior short-segment fixation with or without fusion for thoracolumbar burst fractures. A five to seven-year prospective randomized study. *J Bone Joint Surg Am* 2009; 91(5): 1033-41.

13. Tezer M, Ozturk C, Aydogan M, *et al*. Surgical outcome of thoracolumbar burst fractures with flexion-distraction injury of the posterior elements. *Int Orthop* 2005; 29(6): 347-50.

14. Inamasu J, Guiot BH, Najatsukasa M. Posterior instrumentation surgery for thoracolumbar junction injury causing neurologic deficit. *Neurol Med Chir* (Tokyo) 2008; 48(1): 15-21.

15. Yi L, Jingping B, Gele J, Baoleri X, Taixiang W. Operative versus non-operative treatment for thoracolumbar burst fractures without neurological deficit. *Cochrane Database Syst Rev* 2006; 18(4): CD005079.

16. Gnanenthiran SR, Adie S, Harris IA. Nonoperative versus operative treatment for thoracolumbar burst fractures without neurologic deficit: a meta-analysis. *Clin Orthop Relat Res* 2012; 470(2): 567-77.

17. Sasso RC, Renkens K, Hanson D, Reilly T, Mcguire RA Jr, Best NM. Unstable thoracolumbar burst fractures: anterior-only versus short-segment posterior fixation. *J Spinal Disord Tech* 2006; 19(4): 242-8.

18. Reinhold M, Knop C, Beisse R, *et al*. Operative treatment of 733 patients with acute thoracolumbar spinal injuries: comprehensive results from the second, prospective, internet-based multicenter study of the Spine Study Group of the German Association of Trauma Surgery. *Eur Spine J* 2010; 19(10): 1657-76.

19. Stancic MF, Gregorovic E, Nozica E, Penezic L. Anterior decompression and fixation versus posterior reposition and semirigid fixation in the treatment of unstable burst thoracolumbar fracture: prospective clinical trial. *Croat Med J* 2001; 42(1): 49-53.

20. Dai LY, Jiang LS, Jiang SD. Anterior-only stabilization using plating with bone structural autograft versus titanium mesh cages for two- or three-column thoracolumbar burst fractures: a prospective randomized study. *Spine* 2009; 34(14): 1429-35.

21. McDonough PW, Davis R, Tribus C, Zdeblick TA. The management of acute thoracolumbar burst fractures with anterior corpectomy and Z-plate fixation. *Spine* 2004; 29(17): 1901-8, discussion 1909.

22. Bailey CS, Dvorak MF, Thomas KC, *et al*. Comparison of thoracolumbosacral orthosis and no orthosis for the treatment of thoracolumbar burst fractures: interim analysis of a multicenter randomized clinical equivalence trial. *J Neurosurg Spine* 2009; 11(3): 295-303.

23. Marco RA, Kushwaha VP. Thoracolumbar burst fractures treated with posterior decompression and pedicle screw instrumentation supplemented with balloon-assisted vertebroplasty and calcium phosphate reconstruction. *J Bone Joint Surg Am* 2009; 91(1): 20-8.

24. Defino HL, Canto FR. Low thoracic and lumbar burst fractures: radiographic and functional outcomes. *Eur Spine J* 2007; 16(11): 1934-43.

25. McAfee PC, Bohlman HH, Yuan HA. Anterior decompression of traumatic thoracolumbar fractures with incomplete neurological deficit using a retroperitoneal approach. *J Bone Joint Surg Am* 1985; 67(1): 89-104.

26. Chapman JR, Agel J, Jurkovich GJ, *et al*. Thoracolumbar flexion-distraction injuries: associated morbidity and neurological outcomes. *Spine* 2008; 33(6): 648-57.

27. Convery FR, Minteer MA, Smith RW, Emerson SM. Fracture-dislocation of the dorsal-lumbar spine: acute operative stabilization by Harrington instrumentation. *Spine* 1978; 3: 160-6.

28. Denis F, Armstrong GW, Searls K, Matta L. Acute thoracolumbar burst fractures in the absence of neurologic deficit. *Clin Orthop Relat Res* 1984; 189: 142-9.

29. Berry JL, Moran JM, Berg WS, Steffee AD. A morphological study of human lumbar and selected thoracic vertebrae. *Spine* 1987; 12: 362-6.

30. Bohlman HH. Traumatic fractures of the upper thoracic spine with paralysis. *J Bone Joint Surg Am* 1974; 56: 1299.

31. Bohlman HH, Freehafer A, Dejak J. The results of treatment of acute injuries of the upper thoracic spine with paralysis. *J Bone Joint Surg Am* 1985; 67: 360-9.

32. Morgan TH, Wharton GW, Austin GN. The results of laminectomy in incomplete spinal cord injury. *J Bone Joint Surg Am* 1970; 52: 1115-30.

33. Rampersaud YR, Annand N, Dekutoski MB. Use of minimally invasive techniques in the management of thoracolumbar trauma. *Spine* 2006; 33(11): S96-102.

34. Cosar M, Sasani M, Oktenoglu T, *et al*. The major complications of transpedicular vertebroplasty. *J Neurosurg Spine* 2009; 11: 607-13.

35. McCullen G, Vaccaro AR, Garfin SR. Thoracic and lumbar trauma: rationale for selecting the appropriate fusion technique. *Orthop Clin North Am* 1998; 29(4): 813-28.

36. Kaneda K, Abumi K, Jujiya M. Burst fractures with neurologic deficits of the thoracolumbar-lumbar spine. Results of anterior decompression and stabilization with anterior instrumentation. *Spine* 1984; 9: 788-95.

37. Boerger TO, Limb D, Dickson RA. Does 'canal clearance' affect neurological outcome after thoracolumbar burst fractures? *J Bone Joint Surg Br* 2000; 82(5): 629-35.

Chapter 5

Thoracolumbar spine fractures

Chapter 6

Transpedicular instrumentation for lumbar fusion

Thomas E Mroz MD

Director, Spine Surgery Fellowship 1

Kalil G Abdullah BS

Medical Student 2

1 CLEVELAND CLINIC, CLEVELAND, OHIO, USA
2 CLEVELAND CLINIC LERNER COLLEGE OF MEDICINE, CLEVELAND, OHIO, USA

Introduction

There are a multitude of indications for lumbar spine fusion, including a degenerative condition (e.g., spondylolisthesis, degenerative disc disease), deformity, and following reconstruction for infection, tumor, trauma, or infection. Regardless of the indication, the primary goal of this surgery is to achieve fusion. Lumbar fusion and graft substrate technology have evolved a great deal over the past several decades. Not only have new types of fusion procedures been developed (e.g., anterior lumbar interbody fusion [ALIF], direct lateral lumbar fusion, transforaminal interbody fusion), but there has also been a flood of new types of fusion implants and graft substrates into the market.

Transpedicular instrumentation was first reported by Boucher in 1959 and was popularized in the late 1970s by Roy-Camille, who was the first to connect pedicle screws with rods and plates. Much research has been aimed intentionally or unintentionally at defining the efficacy of pedicle screws in promoting fusion. This chapter reviews the literature on transpedicular fixation in fusion surgery for degenerative conditions and collates it according to

levels of evidence and recommendations laid out in Chapter 1.

Each of the predominant lumbar fusion procedures (i.e., ALIF, posterior lumbar interbody fusion [PLIF], transforaminal lumbar interbody fusion, posterolateral fusion) is unique with regard to biology and biomechanics, and each is considered separately in this chapter. It is important to note that this chapter focuses on pedicular fixation on fusion rates and, by design, does not analyze other clinical outcomes.

Methodology

A PubMed search of English-language literature from 1970 to May 2010 was conducted. Search strings included permutations of the following terms: 'pedicle screw,' 'transpedicular,' 'transpedicular screw,' 'pedicle screw fixation,' 'transpedicular fusion,' and 'pedicle screw instrumentation.' The resulting literature was then parsed for duplicates and preclinical studies, and the resulting articles of immediate clinical relevance were qualitatively evaluated.

Table 1. Posterolateral fusion with and without pedicle screws.

Study	Pedicle screws	n	Fusion rate, %	Evidence level/recommendation
Marjedtko et al, 1994 [1]	No	84	86	IIa/B
Bridwell et al, 1993 [2]	No	10	30	IIa/B
Feffer et al, 1985 [3]	No	8	100	III/B
Herkowitz and Kurz, 1991 [4]	No	25	64	IIa/B
Lombardi et al, 1985 [5]	No	21	90	III/B
Postacchini and Cinotti, 1992 [6]	No	10	60	III/B
Zdeblick, 1993 [7]	No	10	60	Ib/A
Marjedtko et al, 1994 [1]	Yes	101	93	IIa/B
Bridwell et al, 1993 [2]	Yes	24	87	IIa/B
Zdeblick, 1993 [7]	Yes	8	88	Ib/A
Chang and McAfee, 1988 [8]	Yes	14	100	III/B
Hirabayashi et al, 1991 [9]	Yes	32	94	III/B
Simmons and Capicotto, 1998 [10]	Yes	15	100	III/B
Fischgrund et al, 1997 [11]	No	45	15	Ib/A
	Yes	83	29	
Kimura et al, 2001 [12]	No	24	82	III/B
	Yes	26	92	
Mochida et al, 1999 [14]	No	35	65	III/B
	Yes	34	91	
Kakiuchi and Ono, 1998 [15]	No	14	85	IIb/B
	Yes	19	100	
France et al, 1999 [16]	No	28	64	Ib/A
	Yes	29	76	
Fritzell et al, 2002 [17]	No	67	72	Ib/A
	Yes	62	87	

Posterolateral fusion

Some of the best data that evaluate the effectiveness of pedicle screws for posterolateral fusion have come from studies of degenerative spondylolisthesis. Marjedtko *et al* performed a meta-analysis of studies published between 1970 and 1993 that included an evaluation of lumbar fusion surgery with and without pedicle screws for degenerative spondylolisthesis [1]. The weighted fusion rate from six studies [2-7] and including 86 patients who underwent decompression and fusion without pedicle screws was 86%; the range, however, was wide at 30-100% (Table 1). In the same meta-analysis, Marjedtko *et al* reported on five studies [2, 7, 8-10] and 101 patients who underwent decompression with pedicle screw instrumentation (Table 1) [1]. The weighted fusion rate was 93%, with a range of 87-100% **(IIa/B)**.

In 1997, Fischgrund *et al* presented clinical and radiographic results from a prospective randomized controlled clinical trial on 76 patients who underwent decompression and fusion with iliac crest bone graft, and with or without pedicle screws for degenerative spondylolisthesis [11]. Two-year follow-up data were available for 88% of patients (67/76); 45% of patients (15/33) without instrumentation were deemed fused, compared with 83% of patients (29/35) with pedicle screws (p<0.0015) **(Ib/A)**.

Kimura *et al* retrospectively compared clinical and radiographic outcomes in 57 patients who underwent decompression and fusion with iliac crest bone graft with and without pedicle screws for degenerative spondylolisthesis [12]. Fusion rates were higher in patients treated with pedicle screws (93%, 26/28 patients) compared with those fused *in situ* (83%, 24/29 patients) **(III/B)**.

In 2007, Martin *et al* published a systematic review of five studies published between 1966 and 2005 that compared fusion rates between patients treated with (n=126) and without (n=112) pedicle screws after decompression for lumbar degenerative spondylolisthesis [13]. Importantly, no study reported lower fusion rates with the use of transpedicular screws. Of the five included studies, two were randomized clinical trials [2, 11] and three were comparative observational studies [12, 14, 15] (Table 1).

Use of pedicle screws was associated with a higher relative risk (RR) of achieving fusion than fusion without screws (RR 1.37; 95% confidence interval [CI], 1.07-1.75; p<0.05). A higher probability of achieving fusion with instrumentation was reported by randomized controlled trials (RR 1.96; 95% CI, 1.35-2.84; p<0.05) than by observational, comparative studies (RR 1.20; 95% CI, 1.05-1.36; p<0.05). Fusion rates of the individual studies are provided in Table 1.

In a randomized controlled trial, France *et al* compared the fusion rates in patients who underwent single- or two-level posterolateral fusion with iliac crest bone graft with pedicle screws versus without screws for the treatment of symptomatic degenerative disc disease [16]. A substantial number of patients (n=26) were lost to follow-up, and there was only a 69% radiographic follow-up rate (57 of the original 83 patients). Combining the single- and two-level fusions, patients with pedicular fixation (n=29) had fusion rates of 76% versus 64% in those who underwent uninstrumented fusion (n=28). Overall, 86% of patients who underwent single-level fusion with pedicle screws fused, compared with 71% of the patients without screws. In contrast, patients who underwent two-level fusion without pedicle screws (n=12) had a higher fusion rate than patients with screws (n=7) (58% vs. 43%). Follow-up in this study was again suboptimal, weakening its strength **(IIb/B)**.

In an often-cited randomized controlled trial, Fritzell *et al* reported fusion rates for patients who underwent one- and two-level posterolateral fusion with iliac crest autogenous bone with and without pedicle screws for the treatment of symptomatic degenerative disc disease [17]. In the single-level fusion group, 78% of patients in the uninstrumented group fused, compared with 94% in the pedicle screw group. Similarly, 65% of patients without pedicular fixation fused, compared with 78% of those treated with pedicle screws in the two-level group. Combining both single- and two-level fusions, the patients with pedicle screws had higher fusion rates compared with their uninstrumented counterparts (87% vs. 72%) **(Ib/A)**.

In summary, a multitude of studies have presented various levels and grades of evidence (Table 1) and quite thoroughly evaluated the efficacy of

Chapter 6

transpedicular fixation on fusion rates following posterolateral lumbar fusion. Almost uniformly, fusion rates are improved with pedicle screws. The use of iliac crest bone graft in the controlled trials adds weight to this notion. This is particularly important because a variety of graft substrates in the form of allograft, demineralized bone matrices, and bone morphogenetic protein-2 have all been used for posterolateral fusion. More research is necessary to completely define the posterolateral fusion rates with and without pedicle screws with these products. Furthermore, there is a paucity of literature that defines the fusion rates for posterolateral fusion with more non-rigid pedicle screw-rod systems, and meaningful conclusions about this cannot be drawn at this time.

Anterior lumbar interbody fusion

ALIF is a common procedure used to treat a variety of spinal pathologies, including degenerative disk disease, spondylolisthesis, and spinal stenosis. There are a multitude of variations of ALIF surgery with regard to the types of interbody graft (e.g., autogenous or allograft bone, metallic cage) and fixation devices (e.g., ventral plate, pedicle screws, translaminar screws) used, with implications for biological fusion. The aim of this chapter is to define the utility of pedicle screws; therefore, only the literature on stand-alone ALIF and ALIF with pedicle screws is considered.

Gill and Blumenthal have reported on 53 patients who underwent ALIF with allograft bone (n=48) or iliac crest bone (n=5) as a stand-alone device for the treatment of degenerative disc disease [18]. The fusion rate was 80%, as measured by radiographs **(III/B)**. In 1988, Blumenthal et al reported a fusion rate of only 73% in their retrospective analysis of 34 patients undergoing stand-alone ALIF with allograft (n=27) or autograft (n=7) bone [19]. In another retrospective study with 85 patients (128 levels), Loguidice et al demonstrated a union rate of 75% for ALIF procedures without pedicle screws, with no significant difference in the fusion rate between autogenous or cadaveric bone [20]. They also reported pseudoarthrosis rates of 16%, 21%, and 31% for L5-S1, L4-5, and L3-4, respectively **(III/B)**. Newman and

Grinstead retrospectively analyzed data from 36 patients who underwent stand-alone ALIF for disc degeneration using an autogenous corticocancellous double-dowel graft [21]. Fusion was assessed by flexion and extension radiographs and was reported to be 88.9% **(III/B)**.

In 1993, Kumar et al used femoral ring allograft for stand-alone ALIF and reported a 66% solid fusion rate assessed by radiographs [22] **(III/B)**. In 1997, Penta and Fraser published a retrospective analysis of 103 patients who underwent ALIF using either autologous corticocancellous bone blocks (n=65) or two corticocancellous dowel allografts (n=65) [23]. The fusion rates for the autograft and allograft groups were 73% and 83%, respectively. It should be noted, however, that 38 patients were lost to radiographic follow-up, and the reported fusion rates represented only 69% of the surgical cohort **(III/B)**. Finally, Greenough et al retrospectively reviewed 151 patients who underwent stand-alone ALIF with autogenous bone dowels and reported a fusion rate of only 76% [24] **(III/B)**. The level of evidence for stand-alone ALIF surgery is limited, and level I evidence is not available. A careful consideration of the available studies demonstrates a fusion rate for stand-alone ALIF with allograft or autograft of 60-89%. Clearly, this wide range of fusion reflects the heterogeneity of available studies with regard to the design, execution, and reporting of results (Table 2).

The low fusion rates reported for ALIF surgery without pedicle screws prompted the investigation of supplemental fixation with pedicle screws to add stability and enhance fusion. In an in vitro cadaveric model, Beaubien et al tested 12 lumbar spines with 5Nm loading in torsion, lateral bending, and flexion and extension for the intact spine, ALIF, and ALIF with pedicle screws [25]. Pedicle screws significantly reduced the range of motion and the neutral zone compared with both the intact spine and ALIF alone (p<0.05). In 2004, Lee et al retrospectively reviewed 73 patients who underwent ALIF for isthmic spondylolisthesis with metallic cages followed by same-day placement of percutaneous pedicle screws [26]. Static and dynamic radiographs were reviewed by an independent radiologist, and fusion was reported to be 97% (71/73 patients) **(III/B)**. This is substantially higher than the fusion rates reported for stand-alone

Table 2. ALIF surgery with and without pedicle screws.

Study	Pedicle screws	Interbody graft	n	Fusion rate, %	Evidence level/recommendation
Gill and Blumenthal, 1992 [18]	No	Allograft (n=48) Autograft (n=5)	53	80	III/B
Blumenthal et al, 1988 [19]	No	Allograft (n=27) Autograft (n=7)	34	73	III/B
Loguidice et al, 1988 [20]	No	Autograft Allograft	85	75	III/B
Newman and Grinstead, 1992 [21]	No	Autograft	36	89	III/B
Kumar et al, 1993 [22]	No	Allograft	32	60	III/B
Penta and Fraser, 1997 [23]	No	Allograft dowel (n=65) Autograft block (n=60)	65 60	82 72	III/B
Greenough et al, 1994 [24]	No	Autograft dowels	151	76	III/B
Lee et al, 2004 [26]	Yes	Cages, graft not specified	73	97	III/B
Pavlov et al, 2004 [27]	Yes	SynCage with autogenous bone	52	98	III/B
Anjarwalla et al, 2006 [28]	Yes	Carbon fiber cage with autogenous bone	81	88	III/B
El Masry et al, 2004 [29]	Yes	Autogenous bone graft	47	97	III/B
Lee et al, 2006 [30]	Yes	Cages with allograft or autograft	54	96	III/B

ALIF = anterior lumbar interbody fusion

ALIF [18-24]. In the same year, Pavlov et al reported fusion rates on a cohort of 52 ALIF patients treated with a metallic cage (SynCage, Mathys AG Bettlach, Switzerland) packed with iliac crest bone graft with dorsal fixation [27]. A total of 32 patients underwent single-level ALIF, and 19 patients received two-level surgery. The authors used either translaminar or transpedicular fixation (n=10 patients). Unfortunately, the fusion rate (99%) was reported for both groups together. All one-level ALIFs fused, while 97% of the two-level ALIFs fused **(III/B)**.

In an interesting study, Anjarwalla et al retrospectively reviewed 81 patients who underwent a variety of procedures (stand-alone ALIF, n=25; ALIF plus translaminar screws, n=15; ALIF plus unilateral pedicle screws, n=17; ALIF plus bilateral pedicle screws, n=24) [28]. Each ALIF was performed using a carbon fiber/PEEK cage (DePuy Spine, Raynham, MA, USA) that was packed with iliac crest autogenous bone graft. Fusion analysis was performed using thin-slice CT, and was reviewed independently. Patients who underwent stand-alone

Chapter 6

ALIF had the lowest fusion rate (32%), while bilateral pedicles resulted in the highest fusion rate (88%). Translaminar screws and unilateral pedicle screws were associated with fusion rates of 47% and 82%, respectively **(III/B)**. El Masry *et al* retrospectively reviewed 47 patients who underwent ALIF with autogenous bone graft with transpedicular fixation with supplemental dorsal fusion [29]. They reported a fusion rate of 97%, which again is higher than most reported fusion rates for stand-alone ALIF in the literature **(III/B)**. Lee *et al* retrospectively evaluated the utility of ALIF and percutaneous pedicle screw fixation for revision lumbar surgery in 54 patients [30]. Metallic cages were used in all cases with either allograft or iliac crest bone graft. A total of 52 of 54 patients (96%) were deemed to have achieved fusion **(III/B)**.

Fusion rates of 88-98% have been published for ALIF surgery supplemented with dorsal pedicle screws. These rates are higher than those reported for stand-alone ALIF (60-89%). Overall, the strength of the evidence that has evaluated either stand-alone ALIF or ALIF with pedicle screws is low **(III/B)**. Even so, the bulk of the evidence strongly supports the use of pedicle fixation in terms of higher fusion rates.

As mentioned, there are many permutations of ALIF surgery with regard to structural grafts (e.g., allograft, PEEK, carbon fiber, metallic), graft substrates (e.g., demineralized bone matrix, bone morphogenetic protein-2, various ceramic formulations, local or iliac crest bone, allograft bone chips), fixation methods (e.g., ventral plates, graft-screw hybrids, translaminar, transfacet, and pedicle screws), and the addition of posterior or posterolateral fusion. All of these variables can affect ventral fusion rates. Unfortunately, level I evidence does not exist that compares the 'purest' type ALIF surgery: ALIF with autogenous bone, with or without pedicle screws, without dorsal fusion. The studies reviewed in this chapter compared stand-alone ALIF with dorsal pedicle screws without fusion, and hence provide the best available evidence on the utility of pedicle screws to enhance fusion. The addition of pedicle screws has been shown biomechanically to be more stable *in vitro*, and this added stability promotes biological union.

Posterior lumbar interbody fusion

The technique of PLIF has evolved substantially over the past decades. The procedure usually involves the placement of two interbody cages dorsally. This requires the removal of a substantial portion of both facet joints in order to provide a corridor to deploy the cages without excessive retraction of the neural elements. The removal of the facets results in relative segmental instability despite the support of the interbody cages. Thus, stand-alone PLIF has been challenged both biomechanically and clinically. Tsantrizos *et al* performed a biomechanical study with human cadaveric spines that evaluated three different cage designs (i.e., threaded cylindrical titanium cages, allograft cages, and a fenestrated rectangular 'contact fusion' cage) as stand-alone constructs and then with pedicle screw fixation [31]. The specimens were tested in axial rotation, lateral bending, and flexion and extension. Stand-alone cages all decreased the range of motion in lateral bending and flexion, but axial rotation increased relative to the intact specimens. The use of pedicle screws was superior to all stand-alone constructs in all loading directions, and there was no difference between the various cage designs when pedicle screws were used.

Several authors have reported clinical results for PLIF with and without pedicle fixation (Table 3). Hacker retrospectively reviewed a series of 54 patients who were treated with stand-alone PLIF utilizing BAK cages, which are cylindrical threaded metallic devices [32]. The fusion analysis was performed with flexion and extension radiographs; however, only 24 of 54 patients had these studies performed. This substantially weakens this evidence for fusion rates. Nonetheless, the author reported a fusion rate of 96% **(III/B)**. In another study, Chitnavis *et al* reported on a series of 50 PLIF patients, 40 of whom were treated with stand-alone procedures [33]. The authors did not report fusion rates separately for patients with and without screws, and a fusion assessment was reported for only 39 patients. In this series (80% stand-alone), the fusion rate was 95% **(III/B)**. Zhao *et al* compared a single BAK placed unilaterally (n=13) with two BAK cages placed bilaterally (n=12) in a randomized trial [34]. The fusion rates were assessed using static and dynamic radiographs and were

Table 3. PLIF with and without pedicle screws.

Study	Pedicle screws	n	Fusion rate, %	Evidence level/recommendation
Hacker, 1997 [32]	No	54[a]	96	III/B
Chitnavis et al, 2001 [33]	No[b]	50	95	III/B
Zhao et al, 2002 [34]	No (one cage)	13	92.3	Ib/A
	No (two cages)	12	91.7	
Elias et al, 2000 [35]	No	67	82	III/B
Fuji et al, 2003 [36]	No	25	28	III/B
Steffee and Sitkowski, 1988 [37]	Yes	67	100	III/B
Yashiro et al, 1991 [38]	Yes	25 (one level)	92	III/B
		5 (two level)	100	
Brantigan et al, 2000 [39]	Yes	178	99	IIb/B
Barnes et al, 2001 [40]	Yes	22	95	III/B
Suh et al, 2008 [41c]	Yes	47 (one cage)	91	IIb/B
		44 (two cages)	93	

[a] = fusion rates only reported for 24 of the 54 patients in the study. [b] = the cohort was mixed: 40/50 patients had a stand-alone procedure; 10/50 patients had pedicle screws. [c] = this study was PLIF with posterolateral fusion. Fusion rates are reported for ventral fusion; PLIF = posterior lumbar interbody fusion

reviewed by an independent assessor. Fusion rates were reported to be 92.3% and 91.7% for the unilateral and bilateral cage groups, respectively (p>0.09) **(Ib/A)**. However, not all fusion results have been favorable. Elias et al published a retrospective analysis of 67 patients who underwent stand-alone PLIF with a titanium threaded cage [35]. They reported a pseudoarthrosis rate of 28%, as suggested by 10 patients with interval motion on flexion and extension radiographs, seven with lucency around the cage(s), and two with cage migration **(III/B)**. Similarly, Fuji et al also reported suboptimal fusion rates using threaded cylindrical cages as a stand-alone construct [36]. In this retrospective analysis of 25 consecutive patients, fusion was assessed using flexion and extension radiographs. The fusion rate was a dismal 28% (7/25 patients) **(III/B)**. Based upon the data available for

stand-alone PLIF, fusion rates range from 28% to 96%. Clearly this is a huge range, and reflects the heterogeneity of the published reports with regard to study design, execution, reporting, and the types of fusion analysis performed.

Many authors have published clinical trials for PLIF with pedicle fixation. On a historical note, Steffee and Sitkowski provided an early account of PLIF with pedicle screws for various degenerative conditions in 1988 [37]. This study included 36 patients (104 levels) and reported "no dislocations of any interbody grafts, no indication of absorption or pseudarthrosis..." Presumably this means a 100% fusion rate, but the specifics of the fusion analysis were not explained in the report **(III/B)**. Yashiro et al retrospectively reviewed 30 patients who underwent single- (n=25) and two-level (n=5) PLIF with screws [38]. The authors reported fusion rates of 92% and 100% for single- and two-level PLIF, respectively **(III/B)**. In a large prospective study, Brantigan *et al* performed PLIF with pedicle screws using the Brantigan cage (rectangular carbon fiber) packed with autogenous bone [39]. The study included 221 patients, with 2-year fusion data reported for 178 patients. Fusion was assessed at regular intervals for this investigational device exemption study, and was reported to be 98.9% (176/178 patients) at 2 years **(IIb/B)**. Barnes *et al* reported a fusion rate of 95% in their retrospective study with 22 patients who underwent PLIF with pedicle screws [40] **(III/B)**. More recently, Suh *et al* reported on PLIF using one or two non-threaded interbody cages with pedicle screws and posterolateral fusion for 91 patients with isthmic spondylolisthesis (47 patients with one cage, 44 patients with two cages) [41]. Ventral and dorsal fusion

were assessed separately in this prospective study. Fusion rates were 91% for the one cage procedure and 93% for two cages **(IIb/B)**. Among the reports of PLIF with transpedicular fixation, the fusion rate range is 91-100%, and is less variable in the literature when compared with PLIF without pedicle screws. Based upon this review of the available data for PLIF, the addition of pedicle screws results in more consistent radiographic fusion.

Conclusions

The evidence suggests that the use of pedicle screws results in increased fusion rates for posterolateral fusion, ALIF, and PLIF. Most published reports on this topic provide level III/B evidence, and there is a paucity of higher-level publications.

Recommendations	Evidence level
◆ Posterolateral lumbar fusion with pedicle screws improves fusion rates in patients compared with posterolateral fusion without pedicle screws.	Ib/A
◆ ALIF surgery supplemented with dorsal pedicle screws results in higher fusion rates compared with stand-alone ALIF.	III/B
◆ PLIF with transpedicular fixation results in more consistent radiographic fusion compared with PLIF without pedicle screws.	IIb/B

References

1. Marjedtko SM, Connolly PJ, Shott S. Degenerative lumbar spondylolisthesis. A meta-analysis of literature 1970-1993. *Spine* (Phila Pa 1976) 1994; 19(20 Suppl.): 2256-65S.

2. Bridwell KH, Sedgewick TA, O'Brien MF, Lenke LG, Baldus C. The role of fusion and instrumentation in the treatment of degenerative spondylolisthesis with spinal stenosis. *J Spinal Disord* 1993; 6(6): 462-72.

3. Feffer HL, Wiesel SW, Cuckler JM, Rothman RH. Degenerative spondylolisthesis. To fuse or not to fuse. *Spine* (Phila Pa 1976) 1985; 10(3): 287-9.

4. Herkowitz H, Kurz L. Degenerative lumbar spondylolisthesis with spinal stenosis: a prospective study comparing decompression with decompression and intertransverse process arthrodesis. *J Bone Joint Surg Am* 1991; 73(6): 802-8.

5. Lombardi JS, Wiltse LL, Reynolds J, Widell EH, Spencer C 3rd. Treatment of degenerative spondylolisthesis. *Spine* (Phila Pa 1976) 1985; 10(9): 821-7.

6. Postacchini F, Cinotti G. Bone regrowth after surgical decompression for lumbar stenosis. *J Bone Joint Surg Br* 1992; 74(6): 862-9.

7. Zdeblick T. A prospective, randomized study of lumbar fusion: prelimary results. *Spine* (Phila Pa 1976) 1993; 18(8): 983-91.

8. Chang K, McAfee P. Degenerative spondylolisthesis and degenerative scoliosis treated with a combination segmental rod-plate and transpedicular screw instrumentation system: a preliminary report. *J Spinal Disord* 1988; 1(4): 247-56.

9. Hirabayashi S, Kumano K, Kuroki T. Cotrel-Dubousset pedicle screw system for various spinal disorders. Merits and problems. *Spine* (Phila Pa 1976) 1991; 16(11): 1298-304.

10. Simmons E, Capicotto W. Posterior transpedicular Zielke instrumentation of the lumbar spine. *Clin Orthop Relat Res* 1988; 236: 180-91.

11. Fischgrund JS, Mackay M, Herkowitz HN, Brower R, Montgomery DM, Kurz LT. 1997 Volvo Award Winner in clinical studies. Degenerative lumbar spondylolisthesis with spinal stenosis: a prospective, randomized study comparing decompressive laminectomy and arthrodesis with and without spinal instrumentation. *Spine* (Phila Pa 1976) 1997; 22(24): 2807-12.

12. Kimura I, Shingu H, Murata M, Hashiguchi H. Lumbar posterolateral fusion alone or with transpedicular instrumentation in L4-L5 degenerative spondylolisthesis. *J Spinal Disord* 2001; 14(4): 301-10.

13. Martin CR, Gruszczynski AT, Braunsfurth HA, Fallatah SM, O'Neil J, Wai EK. The surgical management of degenerative lumbar spondylolisthesis: a systematic review. *Spine* (Phila Pa 1976) 2007; 32(16): 1791-8.

14. Mochida J, Suzuki K, Chiba M. How to stabilize a single level lesion of degenerative lumbar spondylolisthesis. *Clin Orthop Relat Res* 1999; 368: 126-34.

15. Kakiuchi M, Ono K. Defatted, gas-sterilised cortical bone allograft for posterior lumbar interbody vertebral fusion. *Int Orthop* 1998; 22(2): 69-76.

16. France J, Yaszemski M, Lauerman W, *et al*. A randomized prospective study of posterolateral lumbar fusion. Outcomes with and without pedicle screw instrumentation. *Spine* (Phila Pa 1976) 1999; 24(6): 553-60.

17. Fritzell P, Hagg O, Wessberg P, *et al*. Chronic low back pain and fusion: a comparison of three surgical techniques. A prospective multicenter randomized study from the Swedish lumbar spine study group. *Spine* (Phila Pa 1976) 2002; 27(11): 1131-41.

18. Gill K, Blumenthal S. Functional results after anterior lumbar fusion at L5-S1 in patients with normal and abnormal MRI scans. *Spine* (Phila Pa 1976) 1992; 17(8): 940-2.

19. Blumenthal SL, Baker J, Dossett A, Selby DK. The role of anterior lumbar fusion for internal disc disruption. *Spine* (Phila Pa 1976) 1988; 13(5): 566-9.

20. Loguidice VA, Johnson RG, Guyer RD, *et al*. Anterior lumbar interbody fusion. *Spine* (Phila Pa 1976) 1988; 13(3): 366-9.

21. Newman MH, Grinstead GL. Anterior lumbar interbody fusion for internal disc disruption. *Spine* (Phila Pa 1976) 1992; 17(7): 831-3.

22. Kumar A, Kozak JA, Doherty BJ, *et al*. Interspace distraction and graft subsidence after anterior lumbar fusion with femoral strut allograft. *Spine* (Phila Pa 1976) 1993; 18(16): 2393-400.

23. Penta M, Fraser RD. Anterior lumbar interbody fusion. A minimum 10-year follow-up. *Spine* (Phila Pa 1976) 1997; 22(20): 2429-34.

24. Greenough CG, Taylor LJ, Fraser RD. Anterior lumbar fusion: a comparison of noncompensation patients with compensation patients. *Clin Orthop Relat Res* 1994; 300: 30-7.

25. Beaubien BP, Mehbod AA, Kallemeier PM, *et al*. Posterior augmentation of an anterior lumbar interbody fusion. Minimally invasive fixation versus pedicle screws in vitro. *Spine* (Phila Pa 1976) 2004; 29(19): E406-12.

26. Lee SH, Choi WG, Lim SR, Kang HY, Shin SW. Minimally invasive anterior lumbar interbody fusion followed by percutaneous pedicle screw fixation for insthmic spondylolisthesis. *Spine J* 2004; 4(6): 644-9.

27. Pavlov PW, Meijers H, van Limbeek J, *et al*. Good outcome and restoration of lordosis after anterior lumbar interbody fusion with additional posterior fixation. *Spine* (Phila Pa 1976) 2004; 29(17): 1893-900.

28. Anjarwalla NK, Morcom RK, Fraser RD. Supplementary stabilization with anterior lumbar intervertebral fusion - a radiographic review. *Spine* (Phila Pa 1976) 2006; 31(11): 1281-7.

29. El Masry M, Badawy W, Rajendran P, Chan D. Combined anterior interbody fusion and posterior pedicle screw fixation in patients with degenerative lumbar disc disease. *Int Orthop* 2004; 28(5): 294-7.

30. Lee SH, Kang BU, Jeon SH, *et al*. Revision surgery of the lumbar spine: anterior lumbar interbody fusion followed by percutaneous pedicle screw fixation. *J Neurosurg Spine* 2006; 5(3): 228-33.

31. Tsantrizos A, Baramki HG, Zeidman S, Steffen T. Segmental stability and compressive strength of posterior lumbar interbody fusion implants. *Spine* (Phila Pa 1976) 2000; 25(15): 1899-907.

32. Hacker RJ. Comparison of interbody fusion approaches for disabling low back pain. *Spine* (Phila Pa 1976) 1997; 22(6): 660-6.

33. Chitnavis B, Barbagallo G, Selway R, Dardis R, Hussain A, Gullan R. Posterior lumbar interbody fusion for revision disc surgery: review of 50 cases in which carbon fiber cages were implanted. *J Neurosurg* 2001; 95(2 Suppl.): 190-5.

34. Zhao J, Wang X, Hou T, He S. One versus two BAK fusion cages in posterior lumbar interbody fusion to L4-L5 degenerative spondylolisthesis: a randomized, controlled prospective study in 25 patients with minimum two-year follow-up. *Spine* (Phila Pa 1976) 2002; 27(24): 2753-7.

35. Elias WJ, Simmons NE, Kaptain GJ, Chadduck JB, Whitehill R. Complications of posterior lumbar interbody fusion when using a titanium threaded cage device. *J Neurosurg* 2000; 93(1 Suppl.): 45-52.

36. Fuji T, Oda T, Kato Y, Fujita S, Tanaka M. Posterior lumbar interbody fusion using titanium cylindrical threaded cages: is optimal interbody fusion possible without other instrumentation. *J Orthop Sci* 2003; 8(2): 142-7.

37. Steffee AD, Sitkowski DJ. Posterior lumbar interbody fusion and plates. *Clin Orthop Relat Res* 1988; 227: 99-102.

38. Yashiro K, Homma T, Hokari Y, Katsumi Y, Okumura H, Hirano A. The Steffee variable screw placement system using different methods of bone grafting. *Spine* (Phila Pa 1976) 1991; 16(11): 1329-34.

39. Brantigan JW, Steffee AD, Lewis ML, Quinn LM, Persenaire JM. Lumbar interbody fusion using the Brantigan I/F cage for posterior lumbar interbody fusion and the variable pedicle screw placement system: two-year results from a Food and Drug Administration investigational device exemption clinical trial. *Spine* (Phila Pa 1976) 2000; 25(11): 1437-46.

40. Barnes B, Rodts GE, McLaughlin MR, Haid RW Jr. Threaded cortical bone dowels for lumbar interbody fusion: over 1-year mean follow-up in 28 patients. *J Neurosurg* 2001; 95(1 Suppl.): 1-4.

41. Suh KT, Park WW, Kim SJ, Cho HM, Lee JS, Lee JS. Posterior lumbar interbody fusion for adult isthmic spondylolisthesis. A comparison of fusion with one or two cages. *J Bone Joint Surg Br* 2008; 90(10): 1352-6.

Chapter 7

Graft extenders in spinal surgery

Andrea F Douglas MD

Director of Spine Education and Research 1

Clinical Assistant Professor of Neurosurgery 2

1 WALLACE CLINICAL TRIALS CENTER, GREENWICH HOSPITAL,
GREENWICH, CONNECTICUT, USA
2 NYU LANGONE MEDICAL CENTER, NEW YORK, USA

Introduction

The use of spinal fusion for the treatment of degenerative spinal pathologies has increased dramatically over the last three decades. Health care spending on spinal fusion surgeries increased five-fold from 1992 to 2003 [1]. The rate of complex fusion procedures in the Medicare population increased 15-fold from 2002 to 2007 [2], a trend that is expected to continue.

Autologous iliac crest bone graft (AIBG) has traditionally been the gold standard for achieving bony fusion of the spine. It is, however, associated with significant morbidities, including prolonged operative time, increased intraoperative blood loss, and postoperative graft site pain [3, 4]. The incidence of major and minor graft site morbidity has been reported to range from 2.1% to 20.6% [3, 4]. Furthermore, the pseudoarthrosis rate is 0-8%, 10-20%, and 30-56% for one-, two-, and three-level cervical fusions with AIBG [5-7]. The pseudoarthrosis rate for lumbar dorsolateral spinal fusions (posterolateral fusion [PLF]) with AIBG is also high, ranging from 10% to 50% [8, 9]. The use of allograft or local autogenous bone graft in spinal fusion surgeries is associated with even higher pseudoarthrosis rates [10, 11].

Pseudoarthrosis remains one of the most common reasons for revision spinal fusion surgery. Spinal surgeons have therefore been charged with finding reasonable graft alternatives for improving the rate of spinal fusion, without increasing surgical morbidity. The ideal bone graft should be biocompatible, bioresorbable, osteoconductive or osteoinductive, compression-resistant, and cost-effective.

This chapter reviews the relevant medical literature (published in English) on bone graft extenders available for use in spinal fusion, stratified by quality and class of study design. It is hoped that this will encourage evidence-based judgment in our clinical practice as spinal surgeons.

Methodology

A National Library of Medicine computerized literature search from 1966 through to February 2010 was performed with the medical subject headings

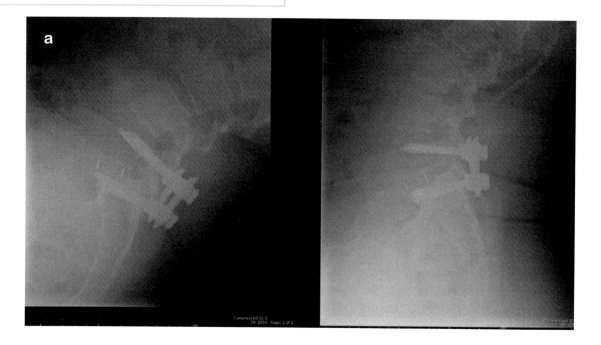

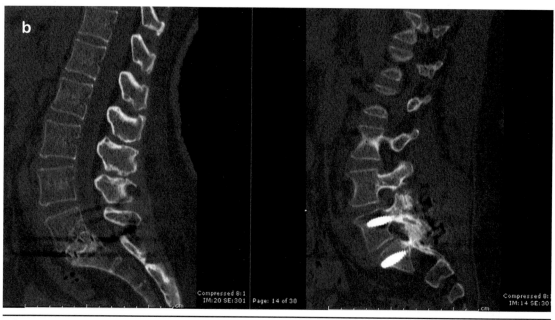

Figure 1. Dynamic X-rays and lumbar spine CT illustrating interbody and posterolateral fusion. a) Flexion and extension X-rays of the lumbar spine in a patient 6 months after pedicle instrumented fusion at L5-S1, showing no evidence of dynamic instability. b) Sagittal lumbar spine CT scan of the same patient showing completed interbody and facet arthrodesis.

'spinal fusion,' 'spinal arthrodesis,' and 'allograft.' The titles of the abstracts were carefully reviewed, and those evaluating the efficacy of spinal fusion allografts on spinal fusion and patient outcomes (clinical and functional) were preferentially selected. A variety of industry-generated 'white papers' specifically evaluating the efficacy of certain products on spinal fusion or arthrodesis were also reviewed.

Assessment of fusion

Bridwell *et al* devised a scale, the Bridwell-Lenke grading system, for determining lumbar dorsolateral spinal fusion using plain radiographs of the lumbar spine [12] (Table 1). One study presented here used surgical and histologic assessment to compare fusion rates with bone morphogenetic protein (BMP)-7 versus hydroxyapatite (HA)-tricalcium phosphate (TCP) [13]. However, spinal fusion is typically assessed with static and dynamic radiographs with or without CT scans, using the following well-established criteria [14-16]:

◆ Complete bridging bone seen between the transverse processes at the level of fusion.
◆ Less than 5° of angulation on lateral flexion-extension X-rays, measured using digital calipers.
◆ Less than 2-3mm of translation on lateral flexion-extension X-rays, measured using digital calipers.
◆ Absence of radiolucent lines around more than 50% of the graft.

Table 1. The Bridwell-Lenke grading system for lumbar dorsolateral spinal fusion.

Fusion grade	Degree of spinal fusion
I	Complete healing and complete incorporation of the allograft into the vertebral endplate
II	Incomplete or partial incorporation of the allograft
III	Failure of incorporation of the allograft with maintenance of the graft
IV	Failure of fusion with resorption of the graft

Dynamic X-rays and lumbar spine CT illustrating interbody and posterolateral fusion are shown in Figure 1.

Osteoconductive graft extenders

Osteoconductive graft extenders reproduce a porous scaffold that mimics human cancellous bone. They are often combined with bone marrow aspirate or local or allograft bone, since they are biomechanically compressible and weak. Table 2 summarizes the class I and II data on this group of graft extenders.

Tricalcium phosphate

Initial human clinical experience with TCP was gained from the adolescent idiopathic scoliosis population, with a randomized controlled trial (RCT) comparing the use of TCP in combination with local bone with that of AIBG [17] **(Ib/A)**. The statistically equal fusion rates for TCP and AIBG seen in these patients has been supported by similar findings in a retrospective review [18] **(III/B)** and a subsequent RCT by Lerner *et al* [19] **(Ib/A)**.

Dai and Jiang have reported the only RCT examining the relative efficacy of TCP and AIBG for instrumented lumbar PLF [20] **(Ib/A)**. The fusion rate was 100% in both groups, with no significant differences in functional and clinical outcomes after 36 months of follow-up. Prospective cohort and retrospective studies examining fusion rates for TCP in both non-instrumented and instrumented lumbar PLF have also reported favorable fusion rates of 85% and 89-96%, respectively [21-23].

One retrospective review evaluating the use of TCP combined with local bone in posterior lumbar interbody fusion (PLIF) also reported 100% fusion, although two patients fused in a collapsed position [24] **(III/B)**.

Hydroxyapatite-enhanced options

Human bone has 70% HA by weight. Collagen-HA matrices are designed to mimic the three-dimensional structure of native bone and, when mixed with bone marrow aspirate, are believed to provide an environment for osteoprogenitor cell attachment, proliferation, and differentiation. The HA extenders

Table 2. Osteoconductive agents as graft extenders in spinal fusion. *Continued overleaf.*

Reference	Graft extender	Study type	Study design	n	Follow-up, months	Fusion assessment	Fusion rate	Other outcomes	Fusion type	Evidence level/ recommendation
Moro-Barrero et al, 2007 [23]	β-TCP (60HA-40TCP)	Prospective, each patient was own control	I: Local on left II: TCP on right spine	1 level: 22 ≥2 levels: 13	24	X-ray and CT, spine surgeon and radiologist	I: 80% (28/35) II: 88.6% (31/35)	NA	Instrumented PLF	IIb/B
Dai and Jiang, 2008 [20]	β-TCP (BioLu)	Prospective RCT	I: AIBG + local II: TCP + local	I: 30 II: 32	36	Two independent radiologists with X-ray	I/II: 100%	mJOA, SF-36: p>0.05 for I and II	Instrumented lumbar PLF	Ib/A
Acharya et al, 2008 [29]	HA-Bg	Prospective, controlled	I: AIBG on right II: HA-Bg on left spine	24	12 (22/24 patients); early termination, HA-Bg resorption	X-ray ± CT	I: 95% (21/22) II: 5% (21/22) with 75% HA-Bg resorption	NA	Instrumented lumbar PLF	IIb/B
Chen et al, 2005 [31]	CaSO$_4$ (OsteoSet)	Prospective, internal control	I: AIBG one side II: local + CaSO$_4$ contra	74	32.5	Two independent orthopedists, dynamic X-rays	I: 87.7% (one-level 89.7%, two-level 85.7%) II: 85.1% (one-level 87.2%, two-level 82.9%)	ODI	Instrumented PLF	IIa/B
Niu et al, 2009 [30]	CaSO$_4$ (OsteoSet)	RCT, each patient served as own control	I: local + BMA vs. AIBG II: local + TCP + BMA vs. AIBG	I: 21 II: 22	I: 24.6 II: 24.1	Two blinded surgeons; X-ray ± CT	I: local 85.7%; AIBG 90.5% (p>0.05) II: TCP 45.5%; AIBG 90.9% (p<0.05)	NA	Instrumented lumbar PLF	Ib/A
Hsu et al, 2005 [34]	CHA	Prospective, case-controlled	Left: AIBG Right: I: local + AIBG II: CHA + AIBG III: local + CHA	I: 20 II: 19 III: 19	12	Dynamic X-ray, two independent orthopedists	AIBG: 89.7% I: 90% II: 78.9% III: 57.9%	NA	Instrumented lumbar PLF	IIa/B

Table 2. Osteoconductive agents as graft extenders in spinal fusion. *Continued.*

Reference	Graft extender	Study type	Study design	n	Follow-up, months	Fusion assessment	Fusion rate	Other outcomes	Fusion type	Evidence level/recommendation
Delecrin et al, 2000 [17]	TCP (Triosite)	RCT	I: AIBG II: TCP-HA + local	I: 30 II: 28	24-48	X-ray, maintenance of corrected deformity	I: 2.3° loss of correction II: 3.2° loss of correction	NA	AIS thoracic PLF	Ib/A
Lerner et al, 2009 [19]	TCP (Vitoss)	RCT	I: AIBG II: TCP-HA + local	I: 20 (8 with anterior) II: 20 (9 with anterior)	20	X-ray	I: 100% (4.2° loss of correction) II: 95% (2.6° loss of correction)	VAS back, donor site. 20% AIBG with 2/10 pain	AIS thoracic PLF	Ib/A
McConnell et al, 2003 [36]	CHA	RCT	I: AIBG II: CHA	I: 16 II: 14	24	X-ray, independent spine surgeon and radiologist	I: 89% II: 11% (non-fragmented graft healing)	ODI, SF-36; no significant difference	Plated ACDF	Ib/A

ACDF = anterior cervical discectomy and fusion; AIBG = autologous iliac crest bone graft; AIS = adolescent idiopathic scoliosis; Bg = bioglass; BMA = bone marrow aspirate; CHA = coralline hydroxyapatite; HA = hydroxyapatite; mJOA = modified Japanese Orthopedics Association Scale; NA = not applicable; ODI = Oswestry Disability Index; PLF = posterolateral fusion; RCT = randomized controlled trial; SF = Short Form; TCP = tricalcium phosphate; VAS = Visual Analogue Scale

Chapter 7

71

also resorb relatively slowly, making radiographic assessment of fusion a challenge.

The efficacy of a collagen-HA graft extender versus AIBG in patients undergoing instrumented PLF (with anterior lumbar interbody fusion [ALIF] or PLIF) was evaluated in a retrospective case-controlled series by Neen et al, who reported a fusion rate of 94% and 84% for the AIBG and HA groups, respectively [25] (III/B). These results are comparable to the 95% fusion rate reported by Carter et al, who retrospectively evaluated patients undergoing lumbar PLF and transforaminal lumbar interbody fusion (TLIF) with the same graft extender [26] (III/B). Similarly, for anterior cervical spinal fusion, Khoueir et al reported a 97% fusion rate using a fibular strut allograft packed with collagen-HA [27] (III/B) and Cosar et al reported 94% fusion with a TCP-HA graft extender [28] (III/B).

These data contradict the findings of Acharya et al who examined the use of an HA-bioglass (HA-Bg) extender versus AIBG in lumbar PLF [29] (IIb/B). Although they achieved a 95% fusion rate with AIBG, there was a 75% graft resorption rate with HA-bioglass and a 5% fusion rate overall for the extender, suggesting that HA-bioglass is an inappropriate graft extender for lumbar spinal fusion.

Calcium sulfate

Calcium sulfate pellets act as osteoconductors, and are believed to resorb at a rate similar to that of new bone growth. The use of calcium sulfate relative to AIBG in lumbar fusion was examined in a RCT performed by Niu et al with 43 patients who underwent instrumented PLF [30] (Ib/A). The AIBG fusion rate averaged 90.7%, while the calcium sulfate fusion rate was 45.5% (p<0.05). These data contradict those presented by Chen et al (IIa/B) and Chang et al (III/B), who performed instrumented PLF with the same graft extender and reported overall fusion rates of 85-92.3% for calcium sulfate and 87.7% for AIBG [31, 32].

Coral

Zdeblick et al first reported the animal experience with coralline HA (CHA) in the cervical spine with a non-rigid plate fixation [33]. CHA is a synthetic derivative of sea coral (mainly composed of calcium carbonate) that is then converted to calcium HA. It is relatively dense, with a three-dimensional structure similar to that of cortical bone, making radiographic assessment of fusion after its use challenging.

The efficacy of CHA in comparison with AIBG has been prospectively evaluated in instrumented lumbar PLF by Hsu et al who, at 1 year, reported a statistically significant AIBG fusion rate of 90% versus a CHA/local bone fusion rate of 58% [34] (IIb/B). In patients with adolescent idiopathic scoliosis, Mashoof et al retrospectively observed an expectedly superior 100% fusion rate for CHA/local bone after 27 months [35] (III/B).

McConnell et al examined the efficacy of CHA in anterior cervical fusion using an RCT, comparing its use relative to AIBG. They reported no significant difference in clinical outcome or fusion rates between the two groups [36] (Ib/A). Based on statistically significant differences in graft fragmentation (CHA 89%, AIBG 11%) and settling (CHA 50%, AIBG 11%), the authors concluded that CHA does not possess adequate structural integrity to achieve anterior cervical fusion. This directly contradicts an earlier retrospective review of 26 patients followed for an average of 30 months, which reported a 100% fusion rate for anterior cervical discectomy and fusion (ACDF) with CHA [37] (III/B).

Bioglass (silicated options)

The tissue-bonding properties of calcium-phosphate silicated materials are based on the availability of silanol radicals on the surface of the glass, which promotes the precipitation of hydroxyl-carbonate-apatite on its surface. These compounds are thought to be bioactive and are believed to promote rapid growth of new bone. Ilharreborde et al performed a retrospective review of 88 patients with adolescent idiopathic scoliosis undergoing instrumented thoracic PLF, and reported no statistically significant difference between the 88% and 81% fusion rates for the AIBG and bioglass groups, respectively [38] (III/B).

Osteoinductive graft extenders

There are more class I data for the osteoinductive category of spinal allograft extenders than for any other. Agarwal *et al* presented a comprehensive meta-analysis of 17 studies that compared the efficacy and safety of all commercially available osteoinductive bone graft substitutes for lumbar fusion [39] **(Ia/A)**. The authors examined 10 RCTs: eight compared the efficacy of the graft extenders to AIBG; nine were industry sponsored; and nine had at least one investigator with a conflict of interest related to the funding source for the study [39]. The authors concluded that BMP-2 may be an effective alternative to AIBG in lumbar fusion, as Resnick *et al* had suggested several years previously [40] **(IV/C)**.

Bone morphogenetic proteins

BMPs were first described by Urist and Strates, who discovered that demineralized, lyophilized segments of bone induced new bone formation when implanted in muscle pouches in rabbits [41]. Cahill *et al* performed a retrospective cohort study of nearly 328,500 patients from the Nationwide Inpatient Sample Database and found that the prevalence of BMP use increased from 0.69% of all fusions in 2002 to 24.89% in 2006 [42] **(III/B)**. The use of BMPs has been more frequent for lumbar spinal fusion, multilevel spinal fusion, and in non-teaching hospitals, with the highest use seen in the western US states [42]. The use of BMPs was associated with an 11-41% increase in total hospital charges, with the greatest increase seen in anterior cervical fusions [42].

Systematic reviews by Garrison *et al* and Mussano *et al* have reported on the superior efficacy of BMPs for spinal fusion [43, 44] **(Ia/A)**. Papakostidis *et al* performed a meta-analysis of all RCTs comparing BMPs with AIBG for dorsolateral lumbar fusion [45] **(Ia/A)**. They concluded that BMP-2 was more efficacious than AIBG in promoting fusion (relative risk 0.29; 95% CI, 0.18-0.47; p<0.00001), whereas BMP-7 may be equivalent to AIBG (relative risk 1.17; 95% CI, 0.54-2.54; p=0.70) [45]. BMPs also appeared more efficient in instrumented than non-instrumented dorsolateral fusions [45].

Some clinical series have suggested that the vertebral endplate remodeling observed with BMPs for lumbar interbody fusion may have a substantial effect on fusion rates. McClellan *et al* retrospectively reviewed data from 26 patients undergoing TLIF with BMP and identified osteolytic vertebral endplate defects in 69% of fused levels [46] **(III/B)**. Burkus *et al* and Pradhan *et al* have also reported a significant degree of temporary vertebral endplate remodeling in their series [47, 48]. The former reported no effect on fusion or clinical outcome, while the latter attributed a reduced fusion rate to the vertebral remodeling seen in their patients who underwent fusion using BMP-2. The class I and II data on BMP graft extenders are presented in Table 3.

BMP-2

In 2002, the US Food and Drug Administration (FDA) approved the use of BMP-2 in a tapered interbody cage for ALIF in adult patients based on the fusion rates reported by Boden *et al* of 100% for BMP-2 versus 66.7% for AIBG [49] **(Ib/A)**. Burkus *et al* substantiated this data, presenting the two largest cohorts to date (279 and 131 patients) in multicenter RCTs comparing the use of BMP-2 with AIBG for patients undergoing single-level ALIF [47, 50] **(Ib/A)**. In both studies, patients were followed for 24 months and the BMP-2 fusion rate (95-100%) remained higher than that of the control group (82-89%). Later prospective reports of pedicle screw instrumented ALIF have also shown a BMP-2 fusion rate of 100%, compared with 89% for femoral allograft [51] **(IIa/B)**.

The use of BMP-2 in the dorsolateral, posterior interbody lumbar spine and the cervical spine is 'off-label' and solely at the discretion of the spine surgeon. Boden *et al*, Dimar *et al*, and Dawson *et al* designed RCTs to examine the use of BMP-2 versus AIBG for patients undergoing instrumented and non-instrumented lumbar PLF and reported statistically significant differences in fusion rates: 88-100% for BMP-2 and 40-74% for AIBG [52-54] **(Ib/A)**. A prospective cohort study examining the use of BMP-2 versus AIBG for instrumented lumbar PLF has reported comparable fusion rates of 77% for the AIBG group, compared with 97% for the BMP-2 group (p<0.05) [55]

Table 3. Osteoinductive agents as graft extenders: BMP. *Continued overleaf.*

Reference	Graft extender	Study type	Study design	n	Follow-up, months	Fusion assessment	Fusion rate	Other outcomes	Fusion type	Evidence level/ recommendation
Boden et al, 2000 [49]	BMP-2	Single-center RCT	I: AIBG II: BMP-2 (titanium cage)	14	24	X-ray and CT, three independent radiologists	I: 66.7% (2/3) II: 100% (11/11)	ODI and SF-36	ALIF	II/B
Burkus et al, 2002 [50]	BMP-2	Multicenter RCT	I: AIBG II: BMP-2 (titanium cage)	I: 136 II: 143	24	X-ray and CT, independent radiologist	I: 88.7% II: 94.5%	VAS, ODI, SF-36 improved No difference between groups	ALIF	Ib/A
Burkus et al, 2006 [47]	BMP-2	Multicenter RCT	I: AIBG II: BMP-2 (both with bone dowel allograft)	I: 52 II: 79	12 and 24	X-ray and CT; independent radiologist; Bidwell-Lenke grades	12 months: I: 89% II: 100% 24 months: I: 81.5% II: 100% ($p<0.05$)	ODI, SF-36 improved No significant difference between groups	Stand alone ALIF	Ib/A
Slosar et al, 2007 [51]	BMP-2	Prospective controlled	I: FRA II: FRA + BMP-2	I: 30 II: 45	24	X-ray and CT, Molinari-Bridwell Scale	I: 89% II: 100%	NRS, ODI significantly improved in BMP-2 group	Instrumented ALIF	IIa/B
Boden et al, 2002 [52]	BMP-2 (with 60% HA, 40% TCP carrier)	Single-center RCT	I: AIBG + screws II: BMP + screws III: BMP	I: 5 II: 11 III: 9	17 (12-27)	Two blinded radiologists; X-ray ± CT as necessary	I: 40% (2/5) II/III: 100%	ODI: I: -17.3 at 6 months II: -17.0 at 3 months III: -17.6 at 6 weeks and -28.7 at 17 months (all significant)	Instrumented /non-instrumented lumbar PLF	Ib/A
Dimar et al, 2006 [53]	BMP-2	RCT	I: AIBG II: BMP-2	I: 53 II: 45	24	CT, independent neuroradiologist	I: 73% (39/53) II: 88% (40/45)	VAS, ODI, SF-36 all improved No significant difference	Instrumented lumbar PLF	Ib/A

Table 3. Osteoinductive agents as graft extenders: **BMP.** *Continued overleaf.*

Reference	Graft extender	Study type	Study design	n	Follow-up, months	Fusion assessment	Fusion rate	Other outcomes	Fusion type	Evidence level/ recommendation
Singh *et al*, 2006 [55]	BMP-2	Prospective cohort	I: AIBG II: BMP-2 (+ lamina bone)	I: 11 II: 41	24	CT, three independent radiologists	I: 77% II: 97%	NA	Instrumented lumbar PLF	IIa/B
Dawson *et al*, 2009 [54]	BMP-2	Multicenter RCT	I: AIBG II: BMP-2 + ceramic	I: 21 II: 25	24	X-ray	I: 70% (14/20) II: 95% (18/19)	ODI, SF-36, VAS No significant difference	Instrumented lumbar PLF	Ib/A
Haid *et al*, 2004 [66]	BMP-2	Multicenter RCT	I: AIBG II: BMP-2 (two cages)	I: 33 II: 34	24	X-ray	I: 77.8% II: 92.3%	VAS, ODI, SF-36 VAS back significantly improved for BMP group	PLIF	Ib/A
Mummaneni *et al*, 2004 [67]	BMP-2	Prospective, controlled	I: AIBG + cage II: BMP-2 + cage	I: 19 II: 21	9	Dynamic X-ray	I: 94.7% (18/19) II: 95.2% (20/21)	VAS: 58% of AIBG patients with 5/10 pain at 6 months (from donor site)	Instrumented TLIF	IIb/B
Anand *et al*, 2006 [68]	BMP-2	Prospective cohort	I: FRA + AIBG II: BMP + FRA + local + Grafton	76 single-level, 24 two-level I: 15 II: 85	30	X-ray and CT where necessary, Lenke or Brantigan and Steffee criteria	I: 93% (1/15) II: 100% (85/85)	VAS 9→3 (p<0.05) ODI 35→12 (p<0.05) SF-36 improved, not statistically significant	Instrumented C-TLIF	IIb/B
Baskin *et al*, 2003 [75]	BMP-2	Multicenter RCT	I: AIBG II: BMP-2 (both in fibular allograft)	I: 15 II: 18	12 and 24	X-ray and CT, two blinded radiologists	I: 100% II: 100% at 12 and 24 months	SF-36 and NDI BMP group had significantly improved NDI at 24 months	Instrumented ACDF	Ib/A

Table 3. Osteoinductive agents as graft extenders: BMP. *Continued.*

Reference	Graft extender	Study type	Study design	n	Follow-up, months	Fusion assessment	Fusion rate	Other outcomes	Fusion type	Evidence level/ recommendation
Butterman, 2008 [69]	BMP-2	Prospective	I: AIBG II: BMP + allograft	I: 36 II: 30	24	X-ray and CT	I: 94%, two donor site complications II: 96.7%, neck swelling and dysphagia in 50%	ODI, VAS No significant difference	Instrumented ACDF	IIb/B
Johnsson et al, 2002 [79]	BMP-7	Single-center RCT	I: AIBG II: BMP-7	I: 10 II: 10	12	X-ray	I: 80% (8/10) II: 60% (6/10)	NA	Non-instrumented lumbar PLF	Ib/A
Kanayama et al, 2006 [13]	BMP-7 vs. HA-TCP/local	Single-center RCT	I: BMP-7 II: local + HA-TCP	I: 9 II: 10	12	X-ray, CT; histology for fused patients	I: 77% (7/9) on X-ray and 86% (6/7) histology; overall 67% (6/9) II: 90% (9/10) X-ray and 100% (9/9) histology; overall 90%	ODI improved; no difference between I and II	Instrumented PLF	Ib/A
Vaccaro et al, 2008 [76]	BMP-7 (OP-1)	Multicenter RCT	I: AIBG II: BMP	I: 12 II: 24	48 (22/36 patients with radiographic follow-up; 25/36 patients with clinical follow-up)	Two blinded neuroradiologists, dynamic X-ray	I: 50% II: 68%	ODI (>20% improved): I: 57% II: 73.7%	Non-instrumented lumbar PLF	Ib/A

ACDF = anterior cervical discectomy and fusion; AIBG = autologous iliac crest bone graft; ALIF = anterior lumbar interbody fusion; BMP = bone morphogenetic protein; FRA = femoral ring allograft; NA = not applicable; NDI = Neck Disability Index; NRS = Numeric Rating Scale; ODI = Oswestry Disability Index; PLF = posterolateral fusion; PLIF = posterior lumbar interbody fusion; RCT = randomized controlled trial; SF = Short Form; TLIF = transforaminal lumbar interbody fusion; VAS = Visual Analogue Scale

(IIa/B). Similarly, for multilevel instrumented 360° thoracolumbar fusions for degenerative scoliosis, BMP-2 fusion rates are reportedly superior to AIBG, at 95% versus 72%, respectively [56, 57].

The use of BMP-2 has also been shown to improve fusion rates in smokers and the elderly undergoing instrumented lumbar PLF [58-60] **(III/B)**. Boden *et al* found a transient 4.5% rate of antibody conversion in the BMP-2-treated group, a finding that may be insignificant based on recent data showing that re-exposure to BMP in revision lumbar surgery is not associated with increased wound complications or clinically allergic reactions [52, 61] **(III/B)**.

Complications associated with the use of BMP-2 in the lumbar spine have included heterotopic epidural and foraminal bone formation (up to 20% incidence) [53, 62] and postoperative radiculitis (up to 11% incidence) [63], particularly with PLIF and TLIF procedures [64, 65]. Haid *et al* have performed the only multicenter RCT for patients undergoing instrumented PLIF, and reported 79% versus 94% fusion rates for AIBG and BMP-2, respectively [66] **(Ib/A)**. Other prospective reports have supported their finding that BMP-2 is non-inferior to AIBG for TLIF/PLIF surgery: 95-100% fusion rate versus 93-95%, respectively [67, 68] **(IIb/B)**.

The use of BMP-2 in ventral cervical surgery has been linked to an increased incidence of postoperative complications, including hematomas, swelling, and airway compromise (up to 50% of patients) [69-72]. In July 2008, the FDA issued a public health warning about life-threatening complications with the use of BMP in the cervical spine [73]. Cahill *et al* found that the use of BMP-2 in anterior cervical fusion procedures was associated with a 7.1% complication rate versus 4.7% without BMP [42]. Crawford *et al* have also reported a 14.6% incidence of wound complications with the use of BMP-2 versus 2.8% with AIBG for instrumented dorsolateral cervical fusion [74] **(III/B)**. Baskin *et al* have performed the only RCT comparing the efficacy of AIBG versus BMP-2 for patients undergoing plated ACDF with a 100% fusion rate in both groups [75] **(Ib/A)**. Another prospective report supports the finding that BMP-2 is non-inferior to AIBG for ACDF, with rates of 96.7% versus 94%, respectively [69] **(IIb/B)**.

BMP-7

In 2004, the FDA approved OP-1 Putty (BMP-7) under a Humanitarian Device Exemption for revision dorsolateral lumbar spinal fusions where autograft and bone marrow harvest are not feasible or are not expected to promote fusion due to compromising factors including osteoporosis, smoking, and diabetes. Vaccaro *et al* performed a multicenter RCT with 36 patients comparing BMP-7 and AIBG for non-instrumented lumbar PLF. At 48 months, solid fusion was reported for 68.8% and 50% of the BMP-7 and the AIBG patients, respectively [76] **(Ib/A)**. These results appear to validate the previously published short-term results, which reported fusion rates of 74% and 55% for BMP-7 at 12 and 24 months, respectively, and rates of 60% and 40% for AIBG at the same intervals [77, 78] **(Ib/A)**. Johnsson *et al*, also with an RCT for non-instrumented lumbar PLF, reported similar fusion rates of 60% and 80% for BMP-7 and AIBG, respectively [79] **(Ib/A)**. Instrumented lumbar PLF with BMP-7 compared with HA-TCP was also examined in a RCT by Kanayama *et al*. They reported similar fusion rates of 67% in the BMP-7 group versus 90% in the HA-TCP and local autograft group [13] **(Ib/A)**.

Demineralized bone matrix

Bae *et al* and Wang *et al* have reported a significant degree of osteoinductive variability among and within individual production lots of commercially available demineralized bone matrix (DBM) [80, 81]. Table 4 presents Class I or II data on the use of DBM in spinal fusion.

The use of DBM for instrumented lumbar PLF was examined and compared with AIBG in prospective trials by Cammisa *et al* [82] **(IIa/B)** and Vaccaro *et al* [83] **(IIb/B)**. They reported fusion rates of 52-70% for DBM and 54-70% for AIBG. Retrospective case-controlled and clinical series have reported higher fusion rates (60-95%) for DBM, and overall there appears to be no statistically significant difference compared with the use of AIBG in a similar surgical population [22, 84, 85] **(III/B)**.

Chapter 7

Table 4. Osteoinductive agents as graft extenders: DBM.

Reference	Graft extender	Study type	Study design	n	Follow-up, months	Fusion assessment	Fusion rate	Other outcomes	Fusion type	Evidence level/ recommendation
Cammisa et al, 2004 [82]	DBM (Grafton)	Multicenter, prospective, internal control	I: AIBG one side II: autologous + DBM (1:2 ratio) contra side	120, each patient own control	24 Only 81/120 patients with follow-up (70%)	Static and dynamic X-rays, independent, blinded radiologist	I: 54% (44/81) II: 52% (42/81) Bilateral fusion: 75%	NA	Instrumented lumbar PLF	IIa/B
Vaccaro et al, 2007 [83]	DBM (Grafton)	Prospective, controlled	I: AIBG II: DBM + AIBG III: DBM + BMA	I: 27 II: 27 III: 19	24	Dynamic X-ray	I: 67% II: 70% III: 63%	NA	Instrumented lumbar PLF	IIb/B
An et al, 1995 [86]	DBM (Grafton)	Prospective	I: AIBG II: allograft + DBM	I: 38 patients, 59 levels; II: 39 patients, 63 levels	12	X-ray, blinded radiologist	I: 78% of levels II: 66.7% of levels	NA	ACDF	IIa/B

ACDF = anterior cervical discectomy and fusion; AIBG = autologous iliac crest bone graft; BMA = bone marrow aspirate; DBM = demineralized bone matrix; NA = not applicable; PLF = posterolateral fusion

Table 5. Osteoinductive agents as graft extenders: platelet gel/AGF.

Reference	Graft extender	Study type	Study design	n	Follow-up, months	Fusion assessment	Fusion rate	Other outcomes	Fusion type	Evidence level/ recommendation
Jenis et al, 2006 [90]	Platelet gel (AGF)	Prospective, controlled	I: AIBG II: allograft + AGF	I: 22 patients, 32 levels II: 15 patients, 25 levels	24	CT at 6 months, and X-ray at 12 and 24 months	I: 85% II: 89%	ODI, VAS, SF-36 No significant difference	Instrumented 360 lumbar fusion	IIa/B
Feiz-Erfan et al, 2007 [91]	Platelet gel (Symphony)	Randomized, blinded	I: allograft II: allograft + gel	50 patients, 81 levels I: 39 levels II: 42 levels (42% one-level, 58% two-level fusion)	12-24 90% for 1 year, 84% for 2 years	X-ray, independent physicians	12 months: I: 85% (33/39) II: 79% 24 months: I: 87% II: 79%	NDI, VAS, SF-36	Instrumented ACDF	Ib/A

ACDF = anterior cervical discectomy and fusion; AIBG = autologous iliac crest bone graft; BMA = bone marrow aspirate; DBM = demineralized bone matrix; NA = not applicable; PLF = posterolateral fusion

In contrast, for ACDF surgeries, prospective series have reported statistically significant differences between the fusion rates achievable with DBM (67-97%) compared with AIBG (78%) [86-88].

Platelet gel/autogenous growth factor

The activation of platelets is thought to release growth factors contained within the cells that initiate tissue repair. It is theorized that the fibrin mesh initiated by platelet activation may provide a framework for mesenchymal cells and osteoblast adherence, thus initiating bone formation. Table 5 summarizes the class I and II data addressing the use of platelets or autogenous growth factor (AGF) in spinal fusion.

In a retrospective case-controlled study of 152 patients undergoing instrumented PLF, Carreon et al reported fusion rates of 83% with AIBG and 75% with AGF [89] **(III/B)**. Jenis et al prospectively examined the efficacy of AGFs in patients with grade 1 isthmic spondylolisthesis who underwent 360° lumbar fusions, and reported 85% and 89% fusion rates for the AIBG and AGF groups, respectively [90] **(IIa/B)**.

Most recently, Feiz-Erfan et al performed a double-blind RCT to examine the efficacy of platelet gel concentrate added to a cervical allograft in ACDF [91] **(Ib/A)**. The fusion rates at 24 months for allograft and AGF were 87% and 79%, respectively.

Conclusions

Based on class I data, BMP-2 is the only graft extender superior to AIBG for lumbar fusion. TCP and BMP-7 are non-inferior to AIBG for lumbar fusion. Calcium sulfate and CHA are inferior to AIBG for lumbar fusion and anterior cervical fusion, respectively.

Based on class II data, BMP-2, DBM, and AGF (mixed with allograft) are non-inferior to AIBG for lumbar fusion, while HA-bioglass and CHA are inappropriate for use in lumbar fusion.

The key points below summarize the various conclusions that one might draw for each of the presented graft extenders based on the class of data discussed.

Recommendations	Evidence level
◆ TCP is non-inferior to AIBG for PLF in adolescent idiopathic scoliosis and lumbar degenerative disc disease.	I/A
◆ HA-bioglass graft is inappropriate for lumbar PLF.	II/B
◆ HA-collagen is non-inferior to AIBG for lumber fusion and ACDF.	III/B
◆ TCP-HA is non-inferior to AIBG for anterior cervical fusion.	III/B
◆ AIBG is superior to calcium sulfate for lumbar PLF.	I/A
◆ AIBG is superior to CHA for ACDF and for PLF.	I/A, II/B
◆ CHA is non-inferior to AIBG for thoracolumbar PLF for adolescent idiopathic scoliosis.	III/B
◆ Bioglass is possibly non-inferior to AIBG for adolescent idiopathic scoliosis.	III/B
◆ BMP-2 is superior to AIBG for lumbar ALIF, PLF, and PLIF/TLIF.	I/A
◆ BMP-2 is non-inferior to AIBG for lumbar PLIF/TLIF and for ACDF.	II/B, I/A
◆ BMP-7 is non-inferior to AIBG.	I/A
◆ DBM is non-inferior to AIBG for ACDF and PLF.	II/B
◆ AGF is non-inferior to allograft alone.	I/A
◆ AGF mixed with allograft is non-inferior to AIBG.	II/B

References

1. Weinstein JN, Lurie JD, Olson PR, Bronner KK, Fisher ES. United States' trends and regional variations in lumbar spine surgery: 1992-2003. *Spine* 2006; 31(23): 2707-14.

2. Deyo RA, Mirza SK, Martin BI, Kreuter W, Goodman DC, Jarvik JG. Trends, major medical complications, and charges associated with surgery for lumbar spinal stenosis in older adults. *JAMA* 2010; 303(13): 1259-65.

3. Kurtz LT, Garfin SR, Booth RE. Iliac bone grafting: techniques of harvesting and complications. In: *Complications of Spinal Surgery*. Garfin SR, Ed. Baltimore: Williams & Wilkins, 1989; 323-41.

4. Younger III EW, Chapman MW. Morbidity at bone graft donor sites. *Orthop Trans* 1986; 10: 494.

5. Bishop RC, Moore KA, Hadley MN. Anterior cervical interbody fusion using autogenic and allogenic bone graft substrate: a prospective comparative analysis. *J Neurosurg* 1999; 85: 206-10.

6. Eck KR, Lenke LG, Bridwell KH, *et al*. Radiographic assessment of anterior titanium mesh cages. *J Spinal Disord* 2000; 13: 501-9.

7. Emery SE, Fisher JR, Bohlman HH. Three-level anterior cervical diskectomy and fusion: radiographic and clinical results. *Spine* 1997; 22: 2622-4.

8. Katz JN. Lumbar spinal fusion: surgical rates, costs and complications. *Spine* 1995; 20: 78-83S.

9. Videback TS, Christensen FB, Soegaard R, *et al*. Circumferential fusion improves outcome in comparison with instrumented posterolateral fusion: long-term results of randomized clinical trial. *Spine* 2006; 31: 2875-80.

10. Jorgenson SS, Lowe TG, France J, Sabin J. A prospective analysis of autograft versus allograft in posterolateral lumbar fusion in the same patient. A minimum of 1-year follow-up in 144 patients. *Spine* 1994; 19(18): 2048-53.

11. Putzier M, Strube P, Funk JF, *et al*. Allogenic versus autologous cancellous bone in lumbar segmental spondylodesis: a randomized prospective study. *Eur Spine J* 2009; 18: 687-95.

12. Bridwell KH, Lenke LG, McEnery KW, Baldus C, Blanke K. Anterior fresh frozen structural allografts in the thoracic and lumbar spine. Do they work if combined with posterior fusion and instrumentation in adult patients with kyphosis or anterior column defects? *Spine* 1995; 20(12): 1410-8.

13. Kanayama M, Hashimoto T, Shigenobu K, Yamane S, Bauer TW, Togawa D. A prospective randomized study of posterolateral lumbar fusion using osteogenic protein-1 (OP-1) versus local autograft with ceramic bone substitute: emphasis of surgical exploration and histologic assessment. *Spine* 2006; 31(10): 1067-74.

14. Brodsky AE, Kovalsky ES, Khalil MA. Correlation of radiologic assessment of lumbar fusions with surgical exploration. *Spine* 1991; 16: S261-5.

15. Chotivichit A, Fujita T, Wong TH, Kostuik JP, Sieber AN. Role of femoral ring allograft in anterior interbody fusion of the spine. *J Orthop Surg* 2001; 9(2): 1-5.

16. Burkus JK, Foley K, Haid RW, LeHuec JC. Surgical Interbody Research Group - radiographic assessment of interbody fusion devices: fusion criteria for anterior lumbar interbody surgery. *Neurosurg Focus* 2001; 10(4): E11.

17. Delecrin J, Takahashi S, Gouin F, Passuti N. A synthetic porous ceramic as a bone graft substitute in the surgical management of scoliosis: a prospective, randomized study. *Spine* 2000; 25(5): 563-9.

18. Muschik M, Ludwig R, Halbhubner S, Bursche K, Stoll T. Beta-tricalcium phosphate as a bone substitute for dorsal spinal fusion in adolescent idiopathic scoliosis: preliminary results of a prospective clinical study. *Eur Spine J* 2001; 10(Suppl. 2): S178-84.

19. Lerner T, Bullmann V, Schulte TL, Schneider M, Liljenqvist U. A level-1 pilot study to evaluate ultraporous beta-tricalcium phosphate as a graft extender in the posterior correction of adolescent idiopathic scoliosis. *Eur Spine J* 2009; 18(2): 170-9.

20. Dai LY, Jiang LS. Single-level instrumented posterolateral fusion of lumbar spine with beta-tricalcium phosphate versus autograft: a prospective, randomized study with 3-year follow-up. *Spine* 2008; 33(12): 1299-304.

21. Epstein NE. A preliminary study of the efficacy of beta tricalcium phosphate as a bone expander for instrumented posterolateral lumbar fusions. *J Spinal Disord Tech* 2006; 19(6): 424-9.

22. Epstein NE, Epstein JA. SF-36 outcomes and fusion rates after multilevel laminectomies and 1 and 2-level instrumented posterolateral fusions using lamina autograft and demineralized bone matrix. *J Spinal Disord Tech* 2007; 20(2): 139-45.

23. Moro-Barrero L, Acebal-Cortina G, Suarez-Suarez M, Perez-Redondo J, Murcia-Mazon A, Lopez-Muniz A. Radiographic analysis of fusion mass using fresh autologous bone marrow with ceramic composites as an alternative to autologous bone graft. *J Spinal Disord Tech* 2007; 20(6): 409-15.

24. Hashimoto T, Shigenobu K, Kanayama M, *et al*. Clinical results of single-level posterior lumbar interbody fusion using the Brantigan I/F carbon cage filled with a mixture of local morselized bone and bioactive ceramic granules. *Spine* 2002; 27(3): 258-62.

25. Neen D, Noyes D, Shaw M, Gwilym S, Fairlie N, Birch N. Healos and bone marrow aspirate used for lumbar spine fusion: a case controlled study comparing healos with autograft. *Spine* 2006; 31(18): E636-40.

26. Carter JD, Swearingen AB, Chaput CD, Rahm MD. Clinical and radiographic assessment of transforaminal lumbar interbody fusion using HEALOS collagen-hydroxyapatite sponge with autologous bone marrow aspirate. *Spine J* 2009; 9(6): 434-8.

27. Khoueir P, Oh BC, DiRisio DJ, Wang MY. Multilevel anterior cervical fusion using a collagen-hydroxyapatite matrix with iliac crest bone marrow aspirate: an 18-month follow-up study. *Neurosurgery* 2007; 61(5): 963-71.

28. Cosar M, Ozer AF, Iplikcioglu AC, *et al*. The results of beta-tricalcium phosphate coated hydroxyapatite (beta-TCP/HA) grafts for interbody fusion after anterior cervical discectomy. *J Spinal Disord Tech* 2008; 21(6): 436-41.

Chapter 7

29. Acharya NK, Kumar RJ, Varma HK, Menon VK. Hydroxyapatite-bioactive glass ceramic composite as stand-alone graft substitute for posterolateral fusion of lumbar spine: a prospective, matched, and controlled study. *J Spinal Disord Tech* 2008; 21(2): 106-11.

30. Niu CC, Tsai TT, Fu TS, Lai PL, Chen LH, Chen WJ. A comparison of posterolateral lumbar fusion comparing autograft, autogenous laminectomy bone with bone marrow aspirate, and calcium sulphate with bone marrow aspirate: a prospective randomized study. *Spine* 2009; 34(25): 2715-9.

31. Chen WJ, Tsai TT, Chen LH, *et al*. The fusion rate of calcium sulfate with local autograft bone compared with autologous iliac bone graft for instrumented short-segment spinal fusion. *Spine* 2005; 30(20): 2293-7.

32. Chang CH, Lin MZ, Chen YJ, Hsu HC, Chen HT. Local autogenous bone mixed with bone expander: an optimal option of bone graft in single-segment posterolateral lumbar fusion. *Surg Neurol* 2008; 70(Suppl. 1): 47-9.

33. Zdeblick TA, Cooke ME, Kunz DN, Wilson D, McCabe RP. Anterior cervical discectomy and fusion using a porous hydroxyapatite bone graft substitute. *Spine* 1994; 19(20): 2348-57.

34. Hsu CJ, Chou WY, Teng HP, Chang WN, Chou YJ. Coralline hydroxyapatite and laminectomy-derived bone as adjuvant graft material for lumbar posterolateral fusion. *J Neurosurg Spine* 2005; 3(4): 271-5.

35. Mashoof AA, Siddiqui SA, Otero M, Tucci JJ. Supplementation of autogenous bone graft with coralline hydroxyapatite in posterior spine fusion for idiopathic adolescent scoliosis. *Orthopedics* 2002; 25(10): 1073-6.

36. McConnell JR, Freeman BJ, Debnath UK, Grevitt MP, Prince HG, Webb JK. A prospective randomized comparison of coralline hydroxyapatite with autograft in cervical interbody fusion. *Spine* 2003; 28(4): 317-23.

37. Thalgott JS, Fritts K, Giuffre JM, Timlin M. Anterior interbody fusion of the cervical spine with coralline hydroxyapatite. *Spine* 1999; 24(13): 1295-9.

38. Ilharreborde B, Morel E, Fitoussi F, *et al*. Bioactive glass as a bone substitute for spinal fusion in adolescent idiopathic scoliosis: a comparative study with iliac crest autograft. *J Pediatr Orthop* 2008; 28(3): 347-51.

39. Agarwal R, Williams K, Umscheid CA, Welch WC. Osteoinductive bone graft substitutes for lumbar fusion: a systematic review. *J Neurosurg Spine* 2009; 11(6): 729-40.

40. Resnick DK, Choudhri TF, Dailey AT, *et al*; for the American Association of Neurological Surgeons/Congress of Neurological Surgeons. Guidelines for the performance of fusion procedures for degenerative disease of the lumbar spine. Part 16: bone graft extenders and substitutes. *J Neurosurg Spine* 2005; 2(6): 733-6.

41. Urist MR, Strates BS. Bone morphogenetic protein. *J Dent Res* 1971; 50(6): 1392-406.

42. Cahill KS, Chi JH, Day A, Claus EB. Prevalence, complications, and hospital charges associated with use of bone-morphogenetic proteins in spinal fusion procedures. *JAMA* 2009; 302(1): 58-66.

43. Garrison KR, Donell S, Ryder J, *et al*. Clinical effectiveness and cost-effectiveness of bone morphogenetic proteins in the non-healing of fractures and spinal fusion: a systematic review. *Health Technol Assess* 2007; 11(30): 1-150, iii-iv.

44. Mussano F, Ciccone G, Ceccarelli M, Baldi I, Bassi F. Bone morphogenetic proteins and bone defects: a systematic review. *Spine* 2007; 32(7): 824-30.

45. Papakostidis C, Kontakis G, Bhandari M, Giannoudis PV. Efficacy of autologous iliac crest bone graft and bone morphogenetic proteins for posterolateral fusion of lumbar spine: a meta-analysis of the results. *Spine* 2008; 33(19): E680-92.

46. McClellan JW, Mulconrey DS, Forbes RJ, Fullmer N. Vertebral bone resorption after transforaminal lumbar interbody fusion with bone morphogenetic protein (rhBMP-2). *J Spinal Disord Tech* 2006; 19(7): 483-6.

47. Burkus JK, Sandhu HS, Gornet, MF. Influence of rhBMP-2 on the healing patterns associated with allograft interbody constructs in comparison with autograft. *Spine* 2006; 31(7): 775-81.

48. Pradhan BB, Bae HW, Dawson EG, Patel VV, Delamarter RB. Graft resorption with the use of bone morphogenetic protein: lessons from anterior lumbar interbody fusion using femoral ring allografts and recombinant human bone morphogenetic protein-2. *Spine* 2006; 31(10): E277-84.

49. Boden SD, Zdeblick TA, Sandhu HS, Heim SE. The use of rhBMP-2 in interbody fusion cages. Definitive evidence of osteoinduction in humans: a preliminary report. *Spine* 2000; 25(3): 376-81.

50. Burkus JK, Gornet MF, Dickman CA, Zdeblick TA. Anterior lumbar interbody fusion using rhBMP-2 with tapered interbody cages. *J Spinal Disord Tech* 2002: 15(5): 337-49.

51. Slosar PJ, Josey R, Reynolds J. Accelerating lumbar fusions by combining rhBMP-2 with allograft bone: a prospective analysis of interbody fusion rates and clinical outcomes. *Spine J* 2007; 7(3): 301-7.

52. Boden SD, Kang J, Sandhu H, Heller JG. Use of recombinant human bone morphogenetic protein-2 to achieve posterolateral lumbar spine fusion in humans: a prospective, randomized clinical pilot trial: 2002 Volvo Award in clinical studies. *Spine* 2002; 27(23): 2662-73.

53. Dimar JR, Glassman SD, Burkus KJ, Carreon LY. Clinical outcomes and fusion success at 2 years of single-level instrumented posterolateral fusions with recombinant human bone morphogenetic protein-2/compression resistant matrix versus iliac crest bone graft. *Spine* 2006; 31(22): 2534-40.

54. Dawson E, Bae HW, Burkus JK, Stambough JL, Glassman SD. Recombinant human bone morphogenetic protein-2 on an absorbable collagen sponge with an osteoconductive bulking agent in posterolateral arthrodesis with instrumentation. A prospective randomized trial. *J Bone Joint Surg Am* 2009; 91(7): 1604-13.

55. Singh K, Smucker JD, Gill S, Boden SD. Use of recombinant human bone morphogenetic protein-2 as an adjunct in posterolateral lumbar spine fusion: a prospective CT-scan analysis at one and two years. *J Spinal Disord Tech* 2006; 19(6): 416-23.

56. Mulconrey DS, Bridwell KH, Flynn J, Cronen GA, Rose PS. Bone morphogenetic protein (RhBMP-2) as a substitute for iliac crest bone graft in multilevel adult spinal deformity

surgery: minimum two-year evaluation of fusion. *Spine* 2008; 33(20): 2153-9.

57. Maeda T, Buchowski JM, Kim YJ, Mishiro T, Bridwell KH. Long adult spinal deformity fusion to the sacrum using rhBMP-2 versus autogenous iliac crest bone graft. *Spine* 2009; 34(20): 2205-12.

58. Glassman SD, Dimar JR 3rd, Burkus K, *et al.* The efficacy of rhBMP-2 for posterolateral lumbar fusion in smokers. *Spine* 2007; 32(15): 1693-8.

59. Hamilton DK, Jones-Quaidoo SM, Sansur C, Shaffrey CI, Oskouian R, Jane JA Sr. Outcomes of bone morphogenetic protein-2 in mature adults: posterolateral non-instrument-assisted lumbar decompression and fusion. *Surg Neurol* 2008; 69(5): 457-61; discussion 461-2.

60. Lee KB, Taghavi CE, Hsu MS, *et al.* The efficacy of rhBMP-2 versus autograft for posterolateral lumbar spine fusion in elderly patients. *Eur Spine J* 2010; 19(6): 924-30.

61. Carreon LY, Glassman SD, Brock DC, Dimar JR, Puno RM, Campbell MJ. Adverse events in patients re-exposed to bone morphogenetic protein for spine surgery. *Spine* 2008; 33(4): 391-3.

62. Joseph V, Rampersaud YR. Heterotopic bone formation with the use of rhBMP2 in posterior minimal access interbody fusion: a CT analysis. *Spine* 2007; 32(25): 2885-90.

63. Mindea SA, Shih P, Song JK. Recombinant human bone morphogenetic protein-2-induced radiculitis in elective minimally invasive transforaminal lumbar interbody fusions: a series review. *Spine* 2009; 34(14): 1480-5.

64. Villavicencio AT, Burneikiene S, Nelson EL, Bulsara KR, Favors M, Thramann J. Safety of transforaminal lumbar interbody fusion and intervertebral recombinant human bone morphogenetic protein-2. *J Neurosurg Spine* 2005; 3(6): 436-43.

65. Wong DA, Kumar A, Jatana S, Ghiselli G, Wong K. Neurologic impairment from ectopic bone in the lumbar canal: a potential complication of off-label PLIF/TLIF use of bone morphogenetic protein-2 (BMP-2). *Spine J* 2008; 8(6): 1011-8.

66. Haid RW Jr, Branch CL Jr, Alexander JT, Burkus JK. Posterior lumbar interbody fusion using recombinant human bone morphogenetic protein type 2 with cylindrical interbody cages. *Spine J* 2004; 4(5): 527-38; discussion 538-9.

67. Mummaneni PV, Pan J, Haid RW, Rodts GE. Contribution of recombinant human bone morphogenetic protein-2 to the rapid creation of interbody fusion when used in transforaminal lumbar interbody fusion: a preliminary report. Invited submission from the Joint Section Meeting on Disorders of the Spine and Peripheral Nerves, March 2004. *J Neurosurg Spine* 2004: 1(1): 19-23.

68. Anand N, Hamilton JF, Perri B, Miraliakbar H, Goldstein T. Cantilever TLIF with structural allograft and RhBMP2 for correction and maintenance of segmental sagittal lordosis: long-term clinical, radiographic, and functional outcome. *Spine* 2006; 31(20): E748-53.

69. Buttermann GR. Prospective nonrandomized comparison of an allograft with bone morphogenic protein versus an iliac-crest autograft in anterior cervical discectomy and fusion. *Spine J* 2008; 8(3): 426-35.

70. Shields LB, Raque GH, Glassman SD, *et al.* Adverse effects associated with high-dose recombinant human bone morphogenetic protein-2 use in anterior cervical spine fusion. *Spine* 2006; 31(5): 542-7.

71. Smucker JD, Rhee JM, Singh K, Yoon ST, Heller JG. Increased swelling complications associated with off-label usage of rhBMP-2 in the anterior cervical spine. *Spine* 2006; 31(24): 2813-9.

72. Vaidya R, Carp J, Sethi A, Bartol S, Craig J, Les CM. Complications of anterior cervical discectomy and fusion using recombinant human bone morphogenetic protein-2. *Eur Spine J* 2007; 16(8): 1257-65.

73. FDA public health notification: life-threatening complications associated with recombinant bone morphogenetic protein in cervical spine fusion. Issued July 1, 2008. Available from: http://www.fda.gov/cdrh/safety/070108-rhbmp.html. Accessed March 30, 2010.

74. Crawford CH 3rd, Carreon LY, McGinnis MD, Campbell MJ, Glassman SD. Perioperative complications of recombinant human bone morphogenetic protein-2 on an absorbable collagen sponge versus iliac crest bone graft for posterior cervical arthrodesis. *Spine* 2009; 34(13): 1390-4.

75. Baskin DS, Ryan P, Sonntag V, Westmark R, Widmayer MA. A prospective, randomized, controlled cervical fusion study using recombinant human bone morphogenetic protein-2 with the CORNERSTONE-SR allograft ring and the ATLANTIS anterior cervical plate. *Spine* 2003; 28(12): 1219-25.

76. Vaccaro AR, Whang PG, Patel T, *et al.* The safety and efficacy of OP-1 (rhBMP-7) as a replacement for iliac crest autograft for posterolateral lumbar arthrodesis: minimum 4-year follow-up of a pilot study. *Spine J* 2008; 8(3): 457-65.

77. Vaccaro AR, Patel T, Fischgrund J, *et al.* A pilot study evaluating the safety and efficacy of OP-1 Putty (rhBMP-7) as a replacement for iliac crest autograft in posterolateral lumbar arthrodesis for degenerative spondylolisthesis. *Spine* 2004; 29(17): 1885-92.

78. Vaccaro AR, Patel T, Fischgrund J, *et al.* A 2-year follow-up pilot study evaluating the safety and efficacy of op-1 putty (rhbmp-7) as an adjunct to iliac crest autograft in posterolateral lumbar fusions. *Eur Spine J* 2005; 14(7): 623-9.

79. Johnsson R, Stromqvist B, Aspenberg P. Randomized radiostereometric study comparing osteogenic protein-1 (BMP-7) and autograft bone in human noninstrumented posterolateral lumbar fusion: 2002 Volvo Award in clinical studies. *Spine* 2002; 27(23): 2654-61.

80. Bae HW, Zhao L, Kanim LE, Wong P, Delamarter RB, Dawson EG. Intervariability and intravariability of bone morphogenetic proteins in commercially available demineralized bone matrix products. *Spine* 2006, 31(12): 1299-08.

81. Wang JC, Alanay A, Mark D, *et al.* A comparison of commercially available demineralized bone matrix for spinal fusion. *Eur Spine J* 2007; 16(8): 1233-40.

82. Cammisa FP Jr, Lowery G, Garfin SR, *et al.* Two-year fusion rate equivalency between Grafton DBM gel and autograft in posterolateral spine fusion: a prospective controlled trial

employing a side-by-side comparison in the same patient. *Spine* 2004; 29(6): 660-6.

83.   Vaccaro AR, Stubbs HA, Block JE. Demineralized bone matrix composite grafting for posterolateral spinal fusion. *Orthopedics* 2007; 30(7): 567-70.

84.   Sassard WR, Eidman DK, Gray PM, *et al.* Augmenting local bone with Grafton demineralized bone matrix for posterolateral lumbar spine fusion: avoiding second site autologous bone harvest. *Orthopedics* 2000; 23(10): 1059-64; discussion 1064-5.

85.   Schizas C, Triantafyllopoulos D, Kosmopoulos V, Tzinieris N, Stafylas K. Posterolateral lumbar spine fusion using a novel demineralized bone matrix: a controlled case pilot study. *Arch Orthop Trauma Surg* 2008; 128(6): 621-5.

86.   An HS, Simpson JM, Glover JM, Stephany J. Comparison between allograft plus demineralized bone matrix versus autograft in anterior cervical fusion. A prospective multicenter study. *Spine* 1995; 20(20): 2211-6.

87.   Topuz K, Colak A, Kaya S, *et al.* Two-level contiguous cervical disc disease treated with peek cages packed with demineralized bone matrix: results of 3-year follow-up. *Eur Spine J* 2009; 18(2): 238-43.

88.   Park HW, Lee JK, Moon SJ, Seo SK, Lee JH, Kim SH. The efficacy of the synthetic interbody cage and Grafton for anterior cervical fusion. *Spine* 2009; 34(17): E591-5.

89.   Carreon LY, Glassman SD, Anekstein Y, Puno RM. Platelet gel (AGF) fails to increase fusion rates in instrumented posterolateral fusions. *Spine* 2005; 30(9): E243-7.

90.   Jenis LG, Banco RJ, Kwon B. A prospective study of autologous growth factors (AGF) in lumbar interbody fusion. *Spine J* 2006; 6(1): 14-20.

91.   Feiz-Erfan I, Harrigan M, Sonntag VK, Harrington TR. Effect of autologous platelet gel on early and late graft fusion in anterior cervical spine surgery. *J Neurosurg Spine* 2007; 7(5): 496-502.

Chapter 7

Chapter 8

Orthoses

Fred C Lam MD PhD FRCSC, Fellow in Training

Michael W Groff MD, Director of Spinal Neurosurgery;
Co-Director Spine Center

DEPARTMENT OF NEUROSURGERY, BRIGHAM AND WOMEN'S HOSPITAL,
HARVARD MEDICAL SCHOOL, BOSTON, MASSACHUSETTS, USA

Introduction

The use of spinal orthotics can be dated back as early as 2750 BC in Egypt [1]. Current principles of orthoses have evolved from devices used by Hippocrates and armorers of the Middle Ages [2]. The main goal when employing orthoses is to maintain spinal alignment through the application of external forces, allowing for immobilization and stabilization. Morris and Lucas described four biomechanical effects of spinal orthoses [3]:

- Motion control.
- Spinal realignment.
- Trunk support (with lumbar orthoses).
- Weight transfer (with cervical and lumbar orthoses).

The efficacy of an orthotic depends on its design, the tightness with which it is worn, its ability to resist the patient's attempts to move against it, and the patient's body shape [2]. The spine surgeon should have a good understanding of the nature of the spinal disorder being treated in order to select the most appropriate orthotic device.

Cervical orthoses (occiput to T3) can be classified into four basic types, listed from the least to the most restrictive: the cervical collar, poster-type orthosis, cervicothoracic orthosis, and halo orthosis [4]. Cervical collars, including the soft collar, hard collar, and Philadelphia collar, are inexpensive and convenient, but are poor at restricting motion and weight transfer. Poster-type orthoses such as the Guilford and the sterno-occipital-mandibular immobilizer (SOMI) braces restrict flexion in the middle cervical spine, but are poor at limiting axial rotation, lateral bending, and flexion at C1 and C2. Cervicothoracic orthoses such as the Yale cervical orthosis control motion and can provide at least 90% restriction of flexion, extension, and rotation [5-7]. Halo orthoses are superior at controlling rotation, lateral bending, and flexion-extension motion over the upper cervical spine (limiting flexion-extension most effectively at the atlanto-occipital joint) and the second and third cervical vertebrae, compared with other orthoses [6]. In contrast, cervicothoracic orthoses are more effective at limiting movement at the middle and lower cervical levels [6]. Disadvantages of the halo include the potential to create a snaking effect in the cervical spine [8], risks of penetration of the skull by pins, delayed development of brain abscesses [9], and cranial nerve palsies [2].

Thoracolumbar orthoses (T3-L3) are used to immobilize the spine in the settings of fractures and neoplastic and/or infectious disorders that cause spinal instability, and as an adjunct following surgical correction of spinal instability or deformity. These orthoses are also used for treating children suffering from progressive scoliosis or kyphosis. Such orthoses include thoracic corsets, dorsolumbar braces, hyperextension braces, the Milwaukee brace, and Risser plaster jackets. Thoracic corsets offer some restriction of movement but are generally limited to the treatment of chronic, benign, thoracolumbar pain syndromes. Similarly, dorsolumbar braces, such as the Taylor brace, offer some resistance to flexion-extension, but are poor at resisting lateral bending or rotational motions and, as such, have limited usage. Hyperextension braces, such as the Jewitt brace, resist motion primarily in flexion, but offer little resistance to motion in all other planes. Hypothetically, by placing the spine in hyperextension, load sharing is shifted to the dorsal elements, which may decrease the stress on the vertebral bodies in the setting of fractures; however, this does not seem to prevent additional vertebral collapse in patients with severely comminuted thoracolumbar fractures or osteoporosis. The Milwaukee brace is used in the correction of progressive kyphoscoliosis and deformity.

Lumbosacral orthoses (L3-S1) are used as a supportive tool in the treatment of low back pain disorders, for immobilization and support of the spine following trauma, and as an adjunct following spinal fusion. Corsets are mainly used for supportive therapy in stable spinal orders causing low back pain. The flexion body jacket provides lumbar support by increasing abdominal pressure and immobilization. Lumbosacral spicas extend from 2cm below the shoulder blade to the midportion of the sacrum dorsally, and ventrally from the xiphisternum to the pubis. Addition of a thigh extension allows for secure fixation of the pelvis and substantially restricts movement through the L3-S1 region.

It can therefore be seen that a wide variety of orthoses are at the spine surgeon's disposal. This chapter reviews the evidence for the use of orthoses in the treatment of common spinal disorders.

Methodology

A National Library of Medicine computerized literature search was performed of publications from 1966 to 2010 using each of the following headings separately to build a wide database of articles: 'cervical orthosis,' 'thoracic orthosis,' 'thoracolumbar orthosis,' and 'lumbosacral orthosis.' These headings were then combined with the heading 'evidence-based' to select articles of that nature. The bibliographies of these articles were reviewed for other possible inclusions.

Cervical orthosis versus active mobilization for whiplash injury

Whiplash is an acceleration-deceleration mechanism of energy transfer to the neck. This causes bony or soft tissue injury, which can lead to a variety of symptoms termed whiplash-associated disorders (WAD). It has been reported that the incidence of whiplash injury in the USA ranges from 70 to 325 per 100,000 population [10, 11]. Patients with WAD develop chronic pain and psychosocial problems, leading to decreased social productivity, absenteeism from work, and increased workers' compensation [11].

Treatment for WAD involves a number of modalities, ranging from neck immobilization to cervical orthosis and multimodal rehabilitation. Several randomized controlled clinical trials advocate for active intervention versus rest and immobilization [11-13] **(Ib/A)**. A recent randomized controlled outcome study specifically addressing active mobilization compared with collar therapy for whiplash showed that early exercise therapy was superior to a cervical orthosis in reducing pain intensity and disability [13] **(Ib/A)**. Thus, while it remains undecided as to which of the several active treatment modalities are more effective in treating WAD, one randomized control study advocates against the use of a cervical orthosis in this setting.

Cervical orthosis for the treatment of upper cervical spine injuries (occiput to C2)

Injuries of the upper cervical spine can be categorized according to level, namely:

◆ Atlanto-occipital dislocation (AOD).
◆ Occipital condyle fractures.
◆ Atlantoaxial instability (or transverse atlantal ligamentous insufficiency).
◆ Atlantoaxial rotator subluxation.
◆ Atlas fractures.
◆ Odontoid fractures.
◆ Traumatic spondylolisthesis of the axis.

Review of the literature shows insufficient evidence to support treatment standards for these injuries, with a large body of level III evidence reporting success using a cervical orthosis, fusion, or both.

Atlanto-occipital dislocation

AOD is a rare injury, and there is an absence of high-level evidence outlining a standard of treatment. Although uncommon, the failure to recognize this type of injury will delay treatment and may lead to poor patient outcomes [14]. Review of the literature shows level III/B evidence consisting of single case studies or small case series. Specifically pertaining to the use of cervical orthoses in the treatment of AOD, a thorough review was performed by the spine section of the American Association of Neurological Surgeons (AANS) and Congress of Neurological Surgeons (CNS) in their 2001 recommendations (www.spinesection.org/education.php).

The AANS/CNS identified a total of 79 cases of AOD reported in the literature between 1966 and 2001. Of these, 19 patients were initially treated with external immobilization excluding traction. Eight of the 19 patients were immobilized preoperatively, and did not worsen, prior to undergoing craniocervical fusion [15-20]. Of the other 11 patients, four worsened and were subsequently fused, while the remaining seven patients were managed in cervical orthoses; two patients in a collar and one in a halo were

subsequently unstable at follow-up and were fused. Only four patients were successfully treated with a cervical orthosis alone. A total of 21 patients were initially treated with traction. Six were subsequently managed with external immobilization, with two remaining unstable and requiring fusion.

In summary, 11 of 40 patients (28%) with AOD managed with a cervical orthosis either deteriorated neurologically or failed to achieve craniocervical stability and required fusion. Thus, treatment of AOD with a cervical orthosis alone should be considered with caution **(III/B)**. Because AOD is a distraction-type injury, traction or orthoses are contraindicated. General consensus advocates early rigid immobilization in halo fixation to prevent further worsening of instability [21-24] **(IV/C)**.

Occipital condyle fractures

Bell first described the occipital condyle fracture in 1817 [25]. Improvements in imaging, including CT scanning at the skull base, have increased recognition of this fracture pattern over the last two decades [26, 27]. Apart from two prospective studies outlining clinical criteria to prompt CT imaging through the skull base [26, 27], all published literature to date are level III studies.

The 1966-2001 literature review conducted by the AANS/CNS in the formulation of their 2001 recommendations on the treatment of occipital condyle fractures (www.spinesection.org/education.php) identified reports of 91 patients with fractures. Of these, 23 initially went untreated, 44 were managed in a collar orthosis, and 13 were managed in a halo or Minerva jacket. Five patients received surgery, and six underwent unreported treatments. Of the 23 patients who initially went untreated, two developed lower cranial nerve palsies [28], one developed vertigo [29], and one developed a lateral rectus palsy [30]. All patients responded to treatment in a cervical collar. Nine other patients who were also initially untreated developed cranial nerve deficits in a delayed manner [31-39]. Because 12 of 23 patients developed delayed deficits without treatment and another developed deficits following the premature discontinuation of external immobilization, it is suggested that patients with type III fractures (using the classification system of Anderson and Montesano [40]) should be treated with a cervical orthosis, the choice of which type appears to be at the clinician's discretion **(III/B)**.

Atlantoaxial instability

Atlantoaxial instability was classified by Fielding *et al* into three types [41]:

* Type I – due to a deficient odontoid process.
* Type II – secondary to a deficient transverse atlantal ligamentous complex.
* Type III – encompasses rotatory fixation.

Instability may be isolated to the ligamentous complex alone, as is seen in infectious processes such as Grisel's syndrome [42] and congenital laxity such as in Down's syndrome [43], or may involve a combination of bony, ligamentous, and vascular injuries, as seen in trauma. Biomechanical cadaveric studies have shown that an intact transverse ligament restricts the ventral displacement of C1 on C2 to approximately 3mm, while 3-5mm implies disruption of the ligament, and displacement exceeding 5mm implies disruption of the remainder of the transverse atlantal ligamentous complex [44]. Instability should be suspected if the predental space is larger than 5mm in children younger than 8 years and larger than 3mm in children 8 years and older and in adults [45].

To date, only level III data outline the management of atlantoaxial instability. Perhaps the most extensive body of pediatric clinical cases has been compiled by review of 2,100 patients and the establishment of a treatment algorithm proposed in 1977 by Menezes [45, 46]. In Menezes' case series of 54 children with Grisel's syndrome, all were managed conservatively in a SOMI brace until clearance of the infection, without a need for surgical fusion [42] **(III/B)**. However, there have also been reports of failed conservative management in a halo vest requiring surgical decompression and fusion [47, 48] **(III/B)**. Two other case series reviewing the use of a halo orthosis in ligamentous injuries of the upper cervical spine both concluded that orthosis alone was insufficient, but

served to prevent neurological deterioration in the interim period leading up to surgical fixation [49, 50] **(III/B)**. A third case series reviewed 10 patients with ligamentous instability, half of whom required surgical stabilization. Only three of the 10 were treated with an external orthosis: two in a halo for 3 months, and one in a collar for 6 weeks [51].

Atlantoaxial rotatory fixation was categorized into four types by Fielding and Hawkins [52] and later into types A, B, and C by White and Panjabi [53]. There is insufficient evidence to support treatment standards, with case studies or series advocating maintaining spinal alignment once the subluxation is reduced in a cervical orthosis [49, 51, 52, 54-60] **(III/B)**. There is no consensus as to which type of orthosis is superior, but most studies have preferred halo immobilization, probably secondary to its ability to achieve immobilization at the C1-C2 joint.

The use of halo fixation is now deemed safe in children younger than 3 years. Multiple pins and appropriate pin pressure are used to evenly distribute loading and prevent puncture through the thin cranium [61, 62]. Alternatively, a pinless halo system, consisting of a silicone non-allergenic facemask that adheres to the skin to prevent slippage and a dorsal occipital support that holds the head against the frontal and mandibular supports, has also been used with good efficacy [63, 64].

Atlas fractures

Fractures of the C1 vertebra account for approximately 2% of all spinal injuries [65-68] and are combined with fracture of the C2 vertebra in 40% of cases [69, 70]. Several classification systems of atlas fractures exist. The earliest, proposed by Jefferson in 1920 [71], was later modified by Gehweiler *et al* [72] and further elaborated upon by Landells and Van Peteghem [68]. In the current era of MRI and CT imaging, a published series found that the 'Rule of Spence' [73], which indicates rupture of the transverse ligament if the sum of the displacement of lateral masses exceeds 6.9mm, in fact missed 61% of transverse ligamentous ruptures [74].

A 2010 review by Kakarla *et al*, based on treatment recommendations from several case series, outlined an algorithm for the treatment of atlas fractures either in isolation or combined with fracture of the axis [75] **(III/B)**. In summary, isolated atlas fractures with an intact transverse ligament on MRI and less than 7mm lateral mass displacement can be managed in a cervical collar for 3 months followed by dynamic X-rays. Those with greater than 7mm displacement should be immobilized in a halo vest for 3 months with follow-up dynamic X-rays. Isolated fractures with a disrupted ligament and a bony avulsion (Dickman type II fracture) should also be placed in a halo vest for 3 months followed by dynamic X-rays. A failed trial of rigid immobilization mandates fusion **(III/B)**.

Combined fractures of the atlas and axis

Odontoid fractures occur concurrently with C1 fractures in up to 53% of reported cases [66, 76-78], while traumatic spondylolisthesis of C2 combined with C1 fracture has been reported in up to 26% of cases [78-82]. There are currently no established standards or guidelines for the treatment of combined C1-C2 fractures; typically, treatment of the C2 fracture drives the decision-making for the combined fracture [69]. Patients should be maintained in a rigid orthosis and followed with supine and upright X-rays to ensure correct alignment [65, 66, 76, 83, 84] **(III/B)**. Internal fixation should be considered for type II odontoid fractures with a predental interval of more than 5mm, and for hangman's fractures with more than 11° of angulation of C2 on C3 [85] **(III/B)**.

Axis fractures

Odontoid fractures

Odontoid fractures are the most common fractures of the axis. They accounted for 59% of C2 fractures in a series of 340 cases by Greene *et al*; the type II fracture pattern was the most common, followed by type III [59]. No guidelines exist for the management of odontoid fractures.

Case series using cervical orthoses have reported satisfactory healing of type I and III fractures [86-88] **(III/B)**, although treatment of type III fractures with an orthosis alone is associated with a 10% incidence of non-union and as high as a 40% incidence of malunion [89] **(III/B)**. Even so, Greene *et al* successfully treated 68 out of 69 patients with type III odontoid fractures in halo immobilization for a mean duration of 12 weeks [59]. In a smaller series by Polin *et al*, 13 patients were all successfully treated in a halo vest [90], while a larger series of 80 patients published by Julien *et al* reported a lower rate of union of 84% [91]. Taken together, there is level III evidence supporting the halo orthosis in the treatment of type III odontoid fractures **(III/B)**.

Treatment of type II fractures in a halo yields an approximately 29% incidence of union, outside of the type IIA fracture pattern identified by Hadley *et al*, which uniformly fails to heal in halo immobilization [92]. Factors influencing failure to heal in a halo include dens displacement of more than 6mm [93] and patient age over 50 years [94] **(III/B)**.

Hangman's fractures

An external orthosis has been reported to be effective in the treatment of hangman's fractures. Three large case series have demonstrated success using halo immobilization [59, 79, 95], while other series have reported success using a cervical collar [96, 97] **(III/B)**.

Subaxial fractures

There is currently no consensus for the treatment of subaxial spine injuries. In 1989, a retrospective review of 124 patients with cervical spine injury by Bucholz and Cheung comparing halo with spinal fusion showed that of 57 patients with subaxial spine injuries, halo failed in 13, nine of whom had locked or perched facets [98]. At around the same time Rockswold *et al* reviewed 140 cases comparing halo immobilization with surgical fusion, and found a higher failure rate with halo immobilization in a subgroup of patients who sustained hyperflexion-ventral subluxation injuries with disruption of the dorsal ligamentous complex (46%) compared with patients with other types of fractures (13%) [99]. This is consistent with a review of 245 cases by Glaser et al, which showed a 30% failure rate with halo immobilization in patients with 'ventral and dorsal spinal column injuries' compared with 12% in other groups [100]. A more recent retrospective outcomes study of 90 isolated unilateral facet fractures found that patients treated non-operatively reported worse outcomes, particularly at longer follow-up, despite having a more benign fracture pattern [101].

In 2008, the Subaxial Injury Classification system was proposed to assign severity scores to different types of subaxial spine injuries, which then aid in determining treatment options [102]. This system takes into account injury morphology, the status of the discoligamentous complex, and the patient's neurological status on presentation. Non-operative treatment is recommended if the total score is less than four. This system has yet to be validated.

Postoperative use of cervical orthoses in arthroplasty versus fusion patients

Anterior cervical discectomy and fusion surgery, used in the treatment of cervical radiculomyelopathy secondary to degenerative disc disease, is a common procedure in the spine surgeon's armamentarium. Patients are often immobilized in an orthosis with activity restrictions for 6-12 weeks to help promote fusion. The choice of whether to use an orthosis is often at the surgeon's discretion. Recently, cervical disc arthroplasty has been introduced as an alternative to fusion, with the purported benefits of preserving motion segments, avoiding adjacent segment degeneration, restoring disc height, avoiding postoperative orthosis, and allowing an earlier return to functional activities.

Specific to the use of a cervical orthosis in the postoperative management of arthroplasty versus fusion patients, early studies consisted of level III case series in which most studies did not require the use of an orthosis following arthroplasty [103-105]. One study used a cervical collar for 4 weeks [105], and another did

not mention the use of orthoses [106]. As more interest accrued, prospective randomized trials were published. These reported a lower rate of orthosis use in arthroplasty patients [107-109], implying that the absence of orthoses may have been a contributing factor in the quicker return-to-work times observed in this treatment group compared with patients who underwent fusion [107]. However, as none of these studies formally addressed the use of an orthosis between treatment arms (in fact, the use of an orthosis was left to the discretion of the surgeon in these studies), conclusions as to whether an orthosis may be excluded in the postoperative management of arthroplasty patients cannot be drawn based on this evidence alone.

Treatment of thoracolumbar fractures

Multiple case series have shown that an external orthosis can be used to treat fractures of the thoracolumbar spine [110-116] (III/B). In fact, prior to the late 1970s, non-operative treatment with recumbency and postural reduction was accepted as the gold standard [117-121]. Custom-fitted body jackets, such as the modified Minerva vest, are used in treating fractures of the upper thoracic spine, while midthoracic and thoracolumbar fractures can be treated with Jewett braces, Milwaukee braces, or bivalve plastic-molded thoracolumbar body jackets [122].

Advantages of an orthosis include pain relief, reduction of intradiscal pressure, and restriction of gross body movements [123-128], while disadvantages include the potential for pressure sores, possible lack of a mechanical stabilizing effect on the lumbar spine, discomfort after bracing, and emotional stress imparted on the patient [122, 129-131]. Some have argued that conservative management results in neurologic deterioration with progressive spinal stenosis, worsening kyphotic deformity, and delayed radiculopathy [132-138].

There is currently insufficient evidence supporting treatment guidelines for thoracolumbar fractures. A retrospective study of 127 patients with acute thoracolumbar burst fractures showed that postural reduction in recumbence followed by bracing in hyperextension for at least 3 months was a safe method of treatment, depending on fracture morphology [139] **(III/B)**. Perhaps the best evidence to date comes from the interim analysis of a multicenter randomized clinical equivalence trial comparing thoracolumbosacral orthosis with no orthosis for the treatment of thoracolumbar AO type A3 burst fractures. This analysis showed equivalence between treatment groups [140] **(Ib/A)**.

Treatment of spinal deformity

Adolescent idiopathic scoliosis

The decision between bracing versus surgery in patients with adolescent idiopathic scoliosis is based on the Cobb measurement, curve pattern, skeletal maturity of the child, cosmetic deformity, and sagittal profile [141]. It is important to determine where the child is in his or her growth spurt, as curves progress during that time [142]. The goals of bracing are to prevent smaller curves (generally <40°) from progressing and correct accompanying cosmetic changes in body form [143-147] **(III/B)**.

Other factors to consider include the curve magnitude and the growth potential of the child (a curve of <20° is less likely to progress and would not require bracing), as well as other 'soft' factors such as parent and sibling heights, their growth spurts, and their age at menarche [141] **(IV/C)**. The ideal candidate for bracing is a child in the active phase of his or her growth spurt, with a curve of 30-39°. In such a patient the chance of curve progression is more than 68%, and a prospective controlled study by Nachemson and Peterson showed the results of bracing are better than the natural progression of the disease [148] **(IIa/B)**. These results were consistent with those from a retrospective review of 1,020 patients with adolescent idiopathic scoliosis treated with the Milwaukee brace by Lonstein and Winter [147] **(III/B)**.

Another factor to consider during bracing is the thoracic sagittal profile of the child. Exacerbation of the naturally occurring thoracic lordosis should be avoided, as this would be ineffective in treating the scoliosis [141, 149] **(IV/C)**. Finally, bracing may be chosen in young or less mature children (Tanner

grade 1 or 2, Risser sign 0, premenarchal) as surgery performed at this early stage is associated with a high chance of the crankshaft phenomenon [150, 151] **(III/B)**. A systematic review published in 2007 of clinical studies comparing rates of surgery following observation or bracing in patients with adolescent idiopathic scoliosis failed to show a clear advantage of either treatment in preventing the need for surgery (pooled rate of surgery, 23% after bracing and 22% after observation) [152].

Adult scoliosis

There is scant evidence for the use of orthoses in the treatment of adult scoliosis. A systematic review of non-surgical treatment revealed two studies [153]: a case report on the use of a lumbosacral orthosis in treating a patient with neurogenic claudication and adult scoliosis [154]; and a follow-up study from the same group involving 29 women who were treated with a lumbosacral orthosis in an attempt to establish 'sagittal realignment' [155]. Given the limited studies available, support is lacking for the use of orthoses in adult scoliosis **(IV/C)**.

Postoperative use of lumbar orthosis in arthroplasty versus fusion patients

Similar to studies looking at orthoses in the postoperative management of cervical fusion patients, several prospective, multicenter, randomized trials have been published comparing surgical outcomes in lumbar arthroplasty versus fusion. Of these, more studies reported the absence of orthosis use in the arthroplasty arm compared with 6 weeks of immobilization in an orthosis in the fusion group [156-158]. As such, there is stronger evidence suggesting that an orthosis is not necessary in the postoperative management of lumbar arthroplasty patients **(Ib/A)**.

Conclusions

The use of orthoses in the management of most spine disorders has been built on a large body of level III data. The evidence-based recommendations for the

Table 1. Summary of evidence-based recommendations for the use of cervical orthoses.

Pathological process	Treatment recommendation	Evidence level/ recommendation
Whiplash injury	Early activity with no orthosis	Ib/A
Atlanto-occipital dislocation	Orthosis alone should be used with caution	III/B
Occipital condyle fractures	Treat with cervical orthoses to prevent development of delayed neurologic deficits	IV/C
Atlantoaxial instability	Cervical orthoses may be used for inflammatory or infectious processes and for atlantoaxial subluxation	III/B
Atlas fractures	Fractures with intact transverse ligament and <7mm lateral mass displacement should be treated in a cervical collar for 3 months and followed with dynamic X-rays	IIIB
	Fractures with >7mm lateral mass displacement should be immobilized in a halo vest for 3 months and followed with dynamic X-rays	III/B
	Isolated fractures with disrupted ligament and bony avulsion (Dickman type II) should be immobilized in a halo vest for 3 months and followed with dynamic X-rays	III/B
Combined C1/C2 fractures	Treatment of C2 fracture drives decision-making for combined fractures. Halo immobilization should be used while waiting for surgical planning	III/B
Axis fractures		
Odontoid fractures		
Type I	Satisfactory healing with cervical orthoses	III/B
Type II	Halo alone yields a 29% union rate, except for with type IIA fractures, which uniformly fail to heal in a halo	III/B
Type III	Use of cervical orthoses alone is be associated with a 10% rate of non-union and 40% rate of malunion	III/B
Hangman's fractures	May be successfully managed with a halo	III/B
Subaxial spine fractures	Higher rates of failure using halo fixation in patients with hyperflexion subluxation injuries with a disrupted dorsal ligamentous complex	III/B
Cervical arthroplasty vs. fusion	Lower rates of orthosis use were observed in the arthroplasty arms of randomized trials, but use of an orthosis was left at the discretion of the surgeon	III/B

Table 2. Summary of evidence-based recommendations for the use of thoracolumbar orthoses.

Pathological process	Treatment recommendation	Evidence level/ recommendation
Acute burst fracture	Equivalence between orthosis versus no orthosis for thoracolumbar AO type A3 burst fractures	Ib/A
Adolescent idiopathic scoliosis	Goals of orthosis include preventing curve progression and correcting accompanying changes in body form	III/B
	Curves of <20° are less likely to progress and do not require bracing	III/B
	Children in the active phase of growth with curves of 30-39° will benefit from bracing	IIb/B
	Bracing may be considered in young, less mature children (Tanner grade 1 or 2, Risser sign 0, premenarchal) to prevent crankshaft phenomenon with early surgery	III/B
Adult scoliosis	Evidence to support the use of an orthosis in adult scoliosis is lacking	IV/C
Lumbar arthroplasty vs. fusion	An orthosis was not required in the postoperative management of arthroplasty patients compared with 6 weeks of immobilization in the fusion arm	Ib/A

use of cervical and thoracolumbar orthoses are summarized in Tables 1 and 2. There is an overall recognition of the need for randomized clinical trials to validate these observations.

Recommendations	Evidence level
◆ The recommended treatment for whiplash injury is early activity with no orthosis.	Ib/A
◆ There is equivalence between an orthosis versus no orthosis in treating patients with thoracolumbar AO type A3 burst fractures.	Ib/A
◆ An orthosis is not required in the postoperative management of lumbar arthroplasty patients.	Ib/A

References

1. Smith GE. The most ancient splints. *BMJ* 1908; 1: 732.

2. Sypert GW. External spinal orthotics. *Neurosurgery* 1987; 20(4): 642-9.

3. Morris JM, Lucas DB. Biomechanics of spinal bracing. *Ariz Med* 1964. 21: 170-6.

4. Wolf JW, Jones HC. Cervical orthoses. In: *The Cervical Spine*. T.C.S. Society, Ed. Philadelphia: Lippincott, 1981; 54-61.

5. Hartman JT, Palumbo F, Hill BJ. Cineradiography of the braced normal cervical spine. A comparative study of five commonly used cervical orthoses. *Clin Orthop Relat Res* 1975; (109): 97-102.

6. Johnson RM, Hart DL, Simmons EF, Ramsby GR, Southwick WO. Cervical orthoses. A study comparing their effectiveness in restricting cervical motion in normal subjects. *J Bone Joint Surg Am* 1977; 59(3): 332-9.

7. Zeleznik R, Chapin W, Hart D, Smith H, Southwick WO, Zito M. Yale cervical orthosis: fabrication. *Phys Ther* 1978; 58(7): 861-4.

8. Anderson PA, Budorick TE, Easton KB, Henley MB, Salciccioli GG. Failure of halo vest to prevent *in vivo* motion in patients with injured cervical spines. *Spine* (Phila Pa 1976) 1991; 16(10 Suppl.): S501-5.

9. Ray A, Iyer RV, King AT. Cerebral abscess as a delayed complication of halo fixation. *Acta Neurochir* (Wien) 2006; 148(9): 1015-6.

10. Spitzer WO, Skovron ML, Salmi LR, *et al*. Scientific monograph of the Quebec Task Force on Whiplash-Associated Disorders: redefining 'whiplash' and its management. *Spine* (Phila Pa 1976) 1995; 20(8 Suppl.): 1S-73.

11. Peeters GG, Verhagen AP, de Bie RA, Oostendorp RA. The efficacy of conservative treatment in patients with whiplash injury: a systematic review of clinical trials. *Spine* (Phila Pa 1976) 2001; 26(4): E64-73.

12. Rosenfeld M, Seferiadis A, Carlsson J, Gunnarsson R. Active intervention in patients with whiplash-associated disorders improves long-term prognosis: a randomized controlled clinical trial. *Spine* (Phila Pa 1976) 2003; 28(22): 2491-8.

13. Schnabel M, Ferrari R, Vassiliou T, Kaluza G. Randomised, controlled outcome study of active mobilisation compared with collar therapy for whiplash injury. *Emerg Med J* 2004; 21(3): 306-10.

14. Powers B, Miller MD, Kramer RS, Martinez S, Gehweiler JA Jr. Traumatic anterior atlanto-occipital dislocation. *Neurosurgery* 1979; 4(1): 12-7.

15. Przybylski GJ, Clyde BL, Fitz CR. Craniocervical junction subarachnoid hemorrhage associated with atlanto-occipital dislocation. *Spine* (Phila Pa 1976) 1996; 21(15): 1761-8.

16. Nischal K, Chumas P, Sparrow O. Prolonged survival after atlanto-occipital dislocation: two case reports and review. *Br J Neurosurg* 1993; 7(6): 677-82.

17. Lee C, Woodring JH, Walsh JW. Carotid and vertebral artery injury in survivors of atlanto-occipital dislocation: case reports and literature review. *J Trauma* 1991; 31(3): 401-7.

18. Kaufman RA, Dunbar JS, Botsford JA, McLaurin RL. Traumatic longitudinal atlanto-occipital distraction injuries in children. *AJNR Am J Neuroradiol* 1982; 3(4): 415-9.

19. Donahue DJ, Muhlbauer MS, Kaufman RA, Warner WC, Sanford RA. Childhood survival of atlantooccipital dislocation: underdiagnosis, recognition, treatment, and review of the literature. *Pediatr Neurosurg* 1994; 21(1): 105-11.

20. Dickman CA, Papadopoulos SM, Sonntag VK, Spetzler RF, Rekate HL, Drabier J. Traumatic occipitoatlantal dislocations. *J Spinal Disord* 1993; 6(4): 300-13.

21. Steinmetz MP, Lechner RM, Anderson JS. Atlantooccipital dislocation in children: presentation, diagnosis, and management. *Neurosurg Focus* 2003; 14(2): ecp1.

22. Farley FA, Graziano G, Hensinger RN. Traumatic atlanto-occipital dislocation in a child. *Spine* (Phila Pa 1976) 1992; 17(12): 1539-41.

23. Evarts CM. Traumatic occipito-atlantal dislocation. *J Bone Joint Surg Am* 1970; 52(8): 1653-60.

24. Garrett M, Consiglieri G, Kakarla UK, Chang SW, Dickman CA. Occipitoatlantal dislocation. *Neurosurgery* 66(3 Suppl.): 48-55.

25. Bell C. Surgical observations. *Middlesex Hosp J* 1817; 4: 469.

26. Bloom AI, Neeman Z, Slasky BS, *et al*. Fracture of the occipital condyles and associated craniocervical ligament injury: incidence, CT imaging and implications. *Clin Radiol* 1997; 52(3): 198-202.

27. Link TM, Schuierer G, Hufendiek A, Horch C, Peters PE. Substantial head trauma: value of routine CT examination of the cervicocranium. *Radiology* 1995; 196(3): 741-5.

28. Lam CH, Stratford J. Bilateral hypoglossal nerve injury with occipital condylar fracture. *Can J Neurol Sci* 1996; 23(2): 145-8.

29. Bozboga M, Unal F, Hepgul K, Izgi N, Turantan MI, Turker K. Fracture of the occipital condyle. Case report. *Spine* (Phila Pa 1976) 1992; 17(9): 1119-21.

30. Desai SS, Coumas JM, Danylevich A, Hayes E, Dunn EJ. Fracture of the occipital condyle: case report and review of the literature. *J Trauma* 1990; 30(2): 240-1.

31. Bolender N, Cromwell LD, Wendling L. Fracture of the occipital condyle. *AJR Am J Roentgenol* 1978; 131(4): 729-31.

32. Castling B, Hicks K. Traumatic isolated unilateral hypoglossal nerve palsy - case report and review of the literature. *Br J Oral Maxillofac Surg* 1995; 33(3): 171-3.

33. Deeb ZL, Rothfus WE, Goldberg AL, Daffner RH. Occult occipital condyle fractures presenting as tumors. *J Comput Tomogr* 1988; 12(4): 261-3.

34. Demisch S, Lindner A, Beck R, Zierz S. The forgotten condyle: delayed hypoglossal nerve palsy caused by fracture of the occipital condyle. *Clin Neurol Neurosurg* 1998; 100(1): 44-5.

35. Noble ER, Smoker WR. The forgotten condyle: the appearance, morphology, and classification of occipital condyle fractures. *AJNR Am J Neuroradiol* 1996; 17(3): 507-13.

36. Orbay T, Aykol S, Seckin Z, Ergun R. Late hypoglossal nerve palsy following fracture of the occipital condyle. *Surg Neurol* 1989; 31(5): 402-4.

37. Paley MD, Wood GA. Traumatic bilateral hypoglossal nerve palsy. *Br J Oral Maxillofac Surg* 1995; 33(4): 239-41.

38. Urculo E, Arrazola M, Arrazola M, Jr., Riu I, Moyua A. Delayed glossopharyngeal and vagus nerve paralysis following occipital condyle fracture. Case report. *J Neurosurg* 1996; 84(3): 522-5.

39. Wasserberg J, Bartlett RJ. Occipital condyle fractures diagnosed by high-definition CT and coronal reconstructions. *Neuroradiology* 1995; 37(5): 370-3.

40. Anderson PA, Montesano PX. Morphology and treatment of occipital condyle fractures. *Spine* (Phila Pa 1976) 1988; 13(7): 731-6.

41. Fielding JW, Hawkins J, Ratzan SA. Management of atlanto-axial instability. *Bull NY Acad Med* 1976; 52(7): 752-60.

42. Wetzel FT, La Rocca H. Grisel's syndrome. *Clin Orthop Relat Res* 1989; (240): 141-52.

43. Semine AA, Ertel AN, Goldberg MJ, Bull MJ. Cervical-spine instability in children with Down syndrome (trisomy 21). *J Bone Joint Surg Am* 1978; 60(5): 649-52.

44. McGraw RW, Rusch RM. Atlanto-axial arthrodesis. *J Bone Joint Surg Br* 1973; 55(3): 482-9.

45. Menezes AH. Decision making. *Childs Nerv Syst* 2008; 24(10): 1147-53.

46. Menezes AH. Congenital and acquired abnormalities of the craniovertebral junction. In: *Neurological Surgery*. Youman J, Ed. Philadelphia: Saunders, 1995; 1035-89.

47. Yamazaki M, Someya Y, Aramomi M, Masaki Y, Okawa A, Koda M. Infection-related atlantoaxial subluxation (Grisel syndrome) in an adult with Down syndrome. *Spine* (Phila Pa 1976) 2008; 33(5): E156-60.

48. Youssef K, Daniel S. Grisel syndrome in adult patients. Report of two cases and review of the literature. *Can J Neurol Sci* 2009; 36(1): 109-13.

49. Lui TN, Lee ST, Wong CW, *et al.* C1-C2 fracture-dislocations in children and adolescents. *J Trauma* 1996; 40(3): 408-11.

50. Vieweg U, Schultheiss R. A review of halo vest treatment of upper cervical spine injuries. *Arch Orthop Trauma Surg* 2001; 121(1-2): 50-5.

51. Rahimi SY, Stevens EA, Yeh DJ, Flannery AM, Choudhri HF, Lee MR. Treatment of atlantoaxial instability in pediatric patients. *Neurosurg Focus* 2003; 15(6): ECP1.

52. Fielding JW, Hawkins RJ. Atlanto-axial rotatory fixation. (Fixed rotatory subluxation of the atlanto-axial joint.) *J Bone Joint Surg Am* 1977; 59(1): 37-44.

53. White AA 3rd, Panjabi MM. *Clinical Biomechanics of the Spine*, 2nd ed. Philadelphia: J.B. Lippincott, 2000; 125-9.

54. Haliasos N, Norris J. Conservative management of a traumatic unilateral rotatory atlantoaxial subluxation in an adult: case report and review. *Injury Extra* 2007; 38: 387-91.

55. Born CT, Mure AJ, Iannacone WM, DeLong WG Jr. Three-dimensional computerized tomographic demonstration of bilateral atlantoaxial rotatory dislocation in an adult: report of a case and review of the literature. *J Orthop Trauma* 1994; 8(1): 67-72.

56. Jones RN. Rotatory dislocation of both atlanto-axial joints. *J Bone Joint Surg Br* 1984; 66(1): 6-7.

57. Moore KR, Frank EH. Traumatic atlantoaxial rotatory subluxation and dislocation. *Spine* (Phila Pa 1976) 1995; 20(17): 1928-30.

58. Robertson PA, Swan HA. Traumatic bilateral rotatory facet dislocation of the atlas on the axis. *Spine* (Phila Pa 1976) 1992; 17(10): 1252-4.

59. Greene KA, Dickman CA, Marciano FF, Drabier JB, Hadley MN, Sonntag VK. Acute axis fractures. Analysis of management and outcome in 340 consecutive cases. *Spine* (Phila Pa 1976) 1997; 22(16): 1843-52.

60. Hadley MN, Zabramski JM, Browner CM, Rekate H, Sonntag VK. Pediatric spinal trauma. Review of 122 cases of spinal cord and vertebral column injuries. *J Neurosurg* 1988; 68(1): 18-24.

61. Arkader A, Hosalkar HS, Drummond DS, Dormans JP. Analysis of halo-orthoses application in children less than three years old. *J Child Orthop* 2007; 1(6): 337-44.

62. Copley LA, Dormans JP, Pepe MD, Tan V, Browne RH. Accuracy and reliability of torque wrenches used for halo application in children. *J Bone Joint Surg Am* 2003; 85-A (11): 2199-204.

63. Sawers A, DiPaola C, Rechtine GR 2nd. Suitability of the noninvasive halo for cervical spine injuries: a retrospective analysis of outcomes. *Spine J* 2009; 9(3): 216-20.

64. Skaggs DL, Lerman LD, Albrektson J, Lerman M, Stewart DG, Tolo VT. Use of a noninvasive halo in children. *Spine* (Phila Pa 1976) 2008; 33(15): 1650-4.

65. Hadley MN, Dickman CA, Browner CM, Sonntag VK. Acute traumatic atlas fractures: management and long term outcome. *Neurosurgery* 1988; 23(1): 31-5.

66. Levine AM, Edwards CC. Fractures of the atlas. *J Bone Joint Surg Am* 1991; 73(5): 680-91.

67. Sherk HH, Nicholson JT. Fractures of the atlas. *J Bone Joint Surg Am* 1970; 52(5): 1017-24.

68. Landells CD, Van Peteghem PK. Fractures of the atlas: classification, treatment and morbidity. *Spine* (Phila Pa 1976) 1988; 13(5): 450-2.

69. Dickman CA, Hadley MN, Browner C, Sonntag VK. Neurosurgical management of acute atlas-axis combination fractures. A review of 25 cases. *J Neurosurg* 1989; 70(1): 45-9.

70. Management of combination fractures of the atlas and axis in adults. *Neurosurgery* 2002; 50(3 Suppl.): S140-7.

71. Jefferson G. Fractures of the atlas vertebra: report of four cases and a review of those previously recorded. *Br J Surg* 1920; 7: 407-22.

72. Gehweiler J, Duff D, Salutario M, Miller MD, Clark M. Fractures of the atlas vertebra. *Skeletal Radiol* 1976; 23: 97-102.

73. Spence KF Jr, Decker S, Sell KW. Bursting atlantal fracture associated with rupture of the transverse ligament. *J Bone Joint Surg Am* 1970; 52(3): 543-9.

74. Dickman CA, Greene KA, Sonntag VK. Injuries involving the transverse atlantal ligament: classification and treatment guidelines based upon experience with 39 injuries. *Neurosurgery* 1996; 38(1): 44-50.

75. Kakarla UK, Chang SW, Theodore N, Sonntag VK. Atlas fractures. *Neurosurgery* 2010; 66(3 Suppl.): 60-7.

76. Fowler JL, Sandhu A, Fraser RD. A review of fractures of the atlas vertebra. *J Spinal Disord* 1990; 3(1): 19-24.

77. Lee TT, Green BA, Petrin DR. Treatment of stable burst fracture of the atlas (Jefferson fracture) with rigid cervical collar. *Spine* (Phila Pa 1976) 1998; 23(18): 1963-7.

78. Ryan MD, Henderson JJ. The epidemiology of fractures and fracture-dislocations of the cervical spine. *Injury* 1992; 23(1): 38-40.

79. Effendi B, Roy D, Cornish B, Dussault RG, Laurin CA. Fractures of the ring of the axis. A classification based on the analysis of 131 cases. *J Bone Joint Surg Br* 1981; 63-B(3): 319-27.

80. Fielding JW, Francis WR Jr, Hawkins RJ, Pepin J, Hensinger R. Traumatic spondylolisthesis of the axis. *Clin Orthop Relat Res* 1989; (239): 47-52.

81. Levine AM, Edwards CC. The management of traumatic spondylolisthesis of the axis. *J Bone Joint Surg Am* 1985; 67(2): 217-26.

82. Muller EJ, Wick M, Muhr G. Traumatic spondylolisthesis of the axis: treatment rationale based on the stability of the different fracture types. *Eur Spine J* 2000; 9(2): 123-8.

83. Segal LS, Grimm JO, Stauffer ES. Non-union of fractures of the atlas. *J Bone Joint Surg Am* 1987; 69(9): 1423-34.

84. Kesterson L, Benzel E, Orrison W, Coleman J. Evaluation and treatment of atlas burst fractures (Jefferson fractures). *J Neurosurg* 1991; 75(2): 213-20.

85. Hadley MN, Walters BC, Grabb PA, *et al*. Isolated fractures of the atlas in adults. *Neurosurgery* 2002; 50(3 Suppl.): S120-4.

86. Anderson LD, D'Alonzo RT. Fractures of the odontoid process of the axis. *J Bone Joint Surg Am* 1974; 56(8): 1663-74.

87. Traynelis VC. Evidence-based management of type II odontoid fractures. *Clin Neurosurg* 1997; 44: 41-9.

88. Chiba K, Fujimura Y, Toyama Y, Fujii E, Nakanishi T, Hirabayashi K. Treatment protocol for fractures of the odontoid process. *J Spinal Disord* 1996; 9(4): 267-76.

89. Clark CR, White AA 3rd. Fractures of the dens. A multicenter study. *J Bone Joint Surg Am* 1985; 67(9): 1340-8.

90. Polin RS, Szabo T, Bogaev CA, Replogle RE, Jane JA. Nonoperative management of types II and III odontoid fractures: the Philadelphia collar versus the halo vest. *Neurosurgery* 1996; 38(3): 450-6; discussion 456-7.

91. Julien TD, Frankel B, Traynelis VC, Ryken TC. Evidence-based analysis of odontoid fracture management. *Neurosurg Focus* 2000; 8(6): e1.

92. Hadley MN, Browner CM, Liu SS, Sonntag VK. New subtype of acute odontoid fractures (type IIA). *Neurosurgery* 1988; 22(1 Pt 1): 67-71.

93. Hadley MN, Browner C, Sonntag VK. Axis fractures: a comprehensive review of management and treatment in 107 cases. *Neurosurgery* 1985; 17(2): 281-90.

94. Lennarson PJ, Mostafavi H, Traynelis VC, Walters BC. Management of type II dens fractures: a case-control study. *Spine* (Phila Pa 1976) 2000; 25(10): 1234-7.

95. Francis WR, Fielding JW, Hawkins RJ, Pepin J, Hensinger R. Traumatic spondylolisthesis of the axis. *J Bone Joint Surg Br* 1981; 63-B(3): 313-8.

96. Grady MS, Howard MA, Jane JA, Persing JA. Use of the Philadelphia collar as an alternative to the halo vest in patients with C-2, C-3 fractures. *Neurosurgery* 1986; 18(2): 151-6.

97. Govender S, Charles RW. Traumatic spondylolisthesis of the axis. *Injury* 1987; 18(5): 333-5.

98. Bucholz RD, Cheung KC. Halo vest versus spinal fusion for cervical injury: evidence from an outcome study. *J Neurosurg* 1989; 70(6): 884-92.

99. Rockswold GL, Bergman TA, Ford SE. Halo immobilization and surgical fusion: relative indications and effectiveness in the treatment of 140 cervical spine injuries. *J Trauma* 1990; 30(7): 893-8.

100. Glaser JA, Whitehill R, Stamp WG, Jane JA. Complications associated with the halo-vest. A review of 245 cases. *J Neurosurg* 1986; 65(6): 762-9.

101. Dvorak MF, Fisher CG, Aarabi B, *et al*. Clinical outcomes of 90 isolated unilateral facet fractures, subluxations, and dislocations treated surgically and nonoperatively. *Spine* (Phila Pa 1976) 2007; 32(26): 3007-13.

102. Patel AA, Dailey A, Brodke DS, *et al*. Subaxial cervical spine trauma classification: the Subaxial Injury Classification system and case examples. *Neurosurg Focus* 2008; 25(5): E8.

103. Wigfield CC, Gill SS, Nelson RJ, Metcalf NH, Robertson JT. The new Frenchay artificial cervical joint: results from a two-year pilot study. *Spine* (Phila Pa 1976) 2002; 27(22): 2446-52.

104. Pimenta L, McAfee PC, Cappuccino A, Bellera FP, Link HD. Clinical experience with the new artificial cervical PCM (Cervitech) disc. *Spine J* 2004; 4(6 Suppl.): 315-21S.

105. Bertagnoli R, Yue JJ, Pfeiffer F, *et al*. Early results after ProDisc-C cervical disc replacement. *J Neurosurg Spine* 2005; 2(4): 403-10.

106. Shim CS, Lee SH, Park HJ, Kang HS, Hwang JH. Early clinical and radiologic outcomes of cervical arthroplasty with Bryan Cervical Disc prosthesis. *J Spinal Disord Tech* 2006; 19(7): 465-70.

107. Steinmetz MP, Patel R, Traynelis V, Resnick DK, Anderson PA. Cervical disc arthroplasty compared with fusion in a workers' compensation population. *Neurosurgery* 2008; 63(4): 741-7.

108. Garrido BJ, Taha TA, Sasso RC. Clinical outcomes of Bryan cervical disc arthroplasty. A prospective, randomized, controlled, single site trial with 48-month follow-up. *J Spinal Disord Tech* 2010; 23(6): 367-71.

109. Sasso RC, Smucker JD, Hacker RJ, Heller JG. Clinical outcomes of BRYAN cervical disc arthroplasty: a prospective, randomized, controlled, multicenter trial with 24-month follow-up. *J Spinal Disord Tech* 2007; 20(7): 481-91.

110. Blauth M, Bastian L, Knop C, Lange U, Tusch G. [Inter-observer reliability in the classification of thoraco-lumbar spinal injuries.] *Orthopade* 1999; 28(8): 662-81.

111. Dai LD. Low lumbar spinal fractures: management options. *Injury* 2002; 33(7): 579-82.

112. Dick W. [Internal fixation of the thoracic and lumbar vertebrae.] *Aktuelle Probl Chir Orthop* 1984; 28: 1-125.

113. Hartman MB, Chrin AM, Rechtine GR. Non-operative treatment of thoracolumbar fractures. *Paraplegia* 1995; 33(2): 73-6.

114. Panjabi MM, Oxland TR, Kifune M, Arand M, Wen L, Chen A. Validity of the three-column theory of thoracolumbar fractures. A biomechanic investigation. *Spine (Phila Pa 1976)* 1995; 20(10): 1122-7.

115. Rohlmann A, Bergmann G, Graichen F, Neff G. Braces do not reduce loads on internal spinal fixation devices. *Clin Biomech (Bristol, Avon)* 1999; 14(2): 97-102.

116. White AA, Panjabi MM. *Clinical Biomechanics of the Spine*, 2nd ed. Philadelphia: JB Lippincott, 1990.

117. Bedbrook GM. Treatment of thoracolumbar dislocation and fractures with paraplegia. *Clin Orthop Relat Res* 1975; 112: 27-43.

118. Gertzbein SD, Court-Brown CM, Marks P, *et al*. The neurological outcome following surgery for spinal fractures. *Spine (Phila Pa 1976)* 1988; 13(6): 641-4.

119. Jacobs RR, Asher MA, Snider RK. Thoracolumbar spinal injuries. A comparative study of recumbent and operative treatment in 100 patients. *Spine (Phila Pa 1976)* 1980; 5(5): 463-77.

120. Watson-Jones R. *Fractures and Joint Injuries*. Baltimore: Williams and Wilkins, 1960.

121. Weinstein JN, Collalto P, Lehmann TR. Thoracolumbar 'burst' fractures treated conservatively: a long-term follow-up. *Spine (Phila Pa 1976)* 1988; 13(1): 33-8.

122. Benzel EC, Larson SJ. Postoperative stabilization of the posttraumatic thoracic and lumbar spine: a review of concepts and orthotic techniques. *J Spinal Disord* 1989; 2(1): 47-51.

123. Cantor JB, Lebwohl NH, Garvey T, Eismont FJ. Nonoperative management of stable thoracolumbar burst fractures with early ambulation and bracing. *Spine (Phila Pa 1976)* 1993; 18(8): 971-6.

124. Chow GH, Nelson BJ, Gebhard JS, Brugman JL, Brown CW, Donaldson DH. Functional outcome of thoracolumbar burst fractures managed with hyperextension casting or bracing and early mobilization. *Spine (Phila Pa 1976)* 1996; 21(18): 2170-5.

125. Melchiorre PJ. Acute hospitalization and discharge outcome of neurologically intact trauma patients sustaining thoracolumbar vertebral fractures managed conservatively with thoracolumbosacral orthoses and physical therapy. *Arch Phys Med Rehabil* 1999; 80(2): 221-4.

126. Liu YJ, Chang MC, Wang ST, Yu WK, Liu CL, Chen TH. Flexion-distraction injury of the thoracolumbar spine. *Injury* 2003; 34(12): 920-3.

127. Tropiano P, Huang RC, Louis CA, Poitout DG, Louis RP. Functional and radiographic outcome of thoracolumbar and lumbar burst fractures managed by closed orthopaedic reduction and casting. *Spine (Phila Pa 1976)* 2003; 28(21): 2459-65.

128. Pfeifer M, Begerow B, Minne HW. Effects of a new spinal orthosis on posture, trunk strength, and quality of life in women with postmenopausal osteoporosis: a randomized trial. *Am J Phys Med Rehabil* 2004; 83(3): 177-86.

129. Axelsson P, Johnsson R, Stromqvist B. Effect of lumbar orthosis on intervertebral mobility. A roentgen stereophotogrammetric analysis. *Spine (Phila Pa 1976)* 1992; 17(6): 678-81.

130. Tezer M, Erturer RE, Ozturk C, Ozturk I, Kuzgun U. Conservative treatment of fractures of the thoracolumbar spine. *Int Orthop* 2005; 29(2): 78-82.

131. Matsunaga S, Hayashi K, Naruo T, Nozoe S, Komiya S. Psychologic management of brace therapy for patients with idiopathic scoliosis. *Spine (Phila Pa 1976)* 2005; 30(5): 547-50.

132. Bedbrook GM. Fracture dislocations of the spine with and without paralysis. A case for conservative and against operative techniques. In: *Controversies in Orthopaedic Surgery*. Leach RE, Hoaglund FT, Riseborough EJ, Eds. Philadelphia: WB Saunders Company, 1982; 423.

133. Denis F. The three column spine and its significance in the classification of acute thoracolumbar spinal injuries. *Spine (Phila Pa 1976)* 1983; 8(8): 817-31.

134. Jacobs RR, Nordwall A, Nachemson A. Reduction, stability, and strength provided by internal fixation systems for thoracolumbar spinal injuries. *Clin Orthop Relat Res* 1982; 171: 300-8.

135. Johnsson R, Herrlin K, Hagglund G, Stromqvist B. Spinal canal remodeling after thoracolumbar fractures with intraspinal bone fragments. 17 cases followed 1-4 years. *Acta Orthop Scand* 1991; 62(2): 125-7.

136. McAfee PC, Bohlman HH, Yuan HA. Anterior decompression of traumatic thoracolumbar fractures with incomplete neurological deficit using a retroperitoneal approach. *J Bone Joint Surg Am* 1985; 67(1): 89-104.

137. McEvoy RD, Bradford DS. The management of burst fractures of the thoracic and lumbar spine. Experience in 53 patients. *Spine (Phila Pa 1976)* 1985; 10(7): 631-7.

138. Whitesides TE Jr. Traumatic kyphosis of the thoracolumbar spine. *Clin Orthop Relat Res* 1977(128): 78-92.

139. Dai LY, Jiang LS, Jiang SD. Conservative treatment of thoracolumbar burst fractures: a long-term follow-up results with special reference to the load sharing classification. *Spine (Phila Pa 1976)* 2008; 33(23): 2536-44.

140. Bailey CS, Dvorak MF, Thomas KC, *et al*. Comparison of thoracolumbosacral orthosis and no orthosis for the treatment of thoracolumbar burst fractures: interim analysis of a multicenter randomized clinical equivalence trial. *J Neurosurg Spine* 2009; 11(3): 295-303.

141. Lonstein JE. Scoliosis: surgical versus nonsurgical treatment. *Clin Orthop Relat Res* 2006; 443: 248-59.

142. Duval-Beaupere G. Pathogenic relationship between scoliosis and growth. In: *Scoliosis and Growth*. Zorab PA, Ed. Edinburgh: Churchill Livingstone, 1971; 58-64.

143. Carr WA, Moe JH, Winter RB, Lonstein JE. Treatment of idiopathic scoliosis in the Milwaukee brace. *J Bone Joint Surg Am* 1980; 62(4): 599-612.

144. Emans JB, Kaelin A, Bancel P, Hall JE, Miller ME. The Boston bracing system for idiopathic scoliosis. Follow-up results in 295 patients. *Spine (Phila Pa 1976)* 1986; 11(8): 792-801.

145. Keiser R, Shufflebarger HL. The Milwaukee brace in idiopathic scoliosis: evaluation of 123 completed cases. *Clin Orthop Relat Res* 1976; 118: 19-24.

146. Lonstein JE, Winter RB. Adolescent idiopathic scoliosis. Nonoperative treatment. *Orthop Clin North Am* 1988; 19(2): 239-46.

147. Lonstein JE, Winter RB. The Milwaukee brace for the treatment of adolescent idiopathic scoliosis. A review of one thousand and twenty patients. *J Bone Joint Surg Am* 1994; 76(8): 1207-21.

148. Nachemson AL, Peterson LE. Effectiveness of treatment with a brace in girls who have adolescent idiopathic scoliosis. A prospective, controlled study based on data from the Brace Study of the Scoliosis Research Society. *J Bone Joint Surg Am* 1995; 77(6): 815-22.

149. Deacon P, Flood BM, Dickson RA. Idiopathic scoliosis in three dimensions. A radiographic and morphometric analysis. *J Bone Joint Surg Br* 1984; 66(4): 509-12.

150. Dubousset J, Herring JA, Shufflebarger H. The crankshaft phenomenon. *J Pediatr Orthop* 1989; 9(5): 541-50.

151. Roberto RF, Lonstein JE, Winter RB, Denis F. Curve progression in Risser stage 0 or 1 patients after posterior spinal fusion for idiopathic scoliosis. *J Pediatr Orthop* 1997; 17(6): 718-25.

152. Dolan LA, Weinstein SL. Surgical rates after observation and bracing for adolescent idiopathic scoliosis: an evidence-based review. *Spine* (Phila Pa 1976) 2007; 32(19 Suppl.): S91-100.

153. Everett CR, Patel RK. A systematic literature review of nonsurgical treatment in adult scoliosis. *Spine* (Phila Pa 1976) 2007; 32(19 Suppl.): S130-4.

154. Weiss HR, Dallmayer R. Brace treatment of spinal claudication in an adult with lumbar scoliosis - a case report. *Stud Health Technol Inform* 2006; 123: 586-9.

155. Weiss HR, Dallmayer R, Stephan C. First results of pain treatment in scoliosis patients using a sagittal realignment brace. *Stud Health Technol Inform* 2006; 123: 582-5.

156. Zigler JE, Burd TA, Vialle EN, Sachs BL, Rashbaum RF, Ohnmeiss DD. Lumbar spine arthroplasty: early results using the ProDisc II: a prospective randomized trial of arthroplasty versus fusion. *J Spinal Disord Tech* 2003; 16(4): 352-61.

157. Berg S, Tullberg T, Branth B, Olerud C, Tropp H. Total disc replacement compared to lumbar fusion: a randomised controlled trial with 2-year follow-up. *Eur Spine J* 2009; 18(10): 1512-9.

158. Geisler FH, Blumenthal SL, Guyer RD, *et al.* Neurological complications of lumbar artificial disc replacement and comparison of clinical results with those related to lumbar arthrodesis in the literature: results of a multicenter, prospective, randomized investigational device exemption study of Charite intervertebral disc. Invited submission from the Joint Section Meeting on Disorders of the Spine and Peripheral Nerves, March 2004. *J Neurosurg Spine* 2004; 1(2): 143-54.

Chapter 9

Osteoporotic vertebral compression fractures

Robert G Whitmore MD, Chief Resident of Neurosurgery 1, 2
Zoher Ghogawala MD FACS, Director 2; Chairman,
Department of Neurosurgery 3, Associate Professor of Neurosurgery 4
Richard Schlenk MD, Neurosurgery Program Director 5

1 DEPARTMENT OF NEUROSURGERY, HOSPITAL OF THE UNIVERSITY OF PENNSYLVANIA,
PHILADELPHIA, PENNSYLVANIA, USA
2 WALLACE CLINICAL TRIALS CENTER, GREENWICH, CONNECTICUT, USA
3 LAHEY CLINIC MEDICAL CENTER, BURLINGTON, MASSACHUSETTS, USA
4 TUFTS UNIVERSITY SCHOOL OF MEDICINE, BOSTON, MASSACHUSETTS, USA
5 CLEVELAND CLINIC FOUNDATION, CLEVELAND, OHIO, USA

Introduction

Osteoporosis is a systemic skeletal disease characterized by low bone mass and microarchitectural deterioration of bone tissue, with a consequent increase in bone fragility and susceptibility to fractures. Osteoporotic vertebral compression fractures are common, with more than 547,000 estimated to have occurred in 2005 [1] and more than 150,000 hospitalizations per year [2]. Perhaps more than 200,000 cases per year are refractory to non-operative care [3].

Long-term consequences of vertebral compression fractures include impaired mobility and function, pulmonary disorders, and increased mortality [4, 5]. Decreased activity, depression, lowered self-esteem, anxiety, diminished social roles, and increased dependence are secondary consequences of vertebral fractures in the elderly [6]. In one study, the mortality rate 5 years after a clinically symptomatic osteoporotic vertebral compression fracture was 15%

greater than expected [7]. The financial costs associated with all osteoporotic fractures in the USA exceed $20 billion per year [8].

This chapter reviews the clinical presentation, evaluative methods, and treatment options for patients who suffer from osteoporotic vertebral compression fractures.

Methodology

A National Library of Medicine computerized literature search was performed from 1966 to 2010 using each of the following headings separately to build a wide database of articles: 'osteoporotic vertebral compression fractures,' 'vertebroplasty,' and 'kyphoplasty.' The titles of the articles were carefully reviewed and those indicative of the management of osteoporotic vertebral compression fractures were preferentially selected. Abstracts pertaining specifically to 'vertebroplasty' and 'kyphoplasty' were further targeted. The references obtained from selected papers were reviewed for possible inclusion.

Clinical manifestations

Symptoms and sequelae

Two-thirds of osteoporotic vertebral compression fractures are asymptomatic and are diagnosed as an incidental finding on an X-ray [9]. It has been estimated that only 30% of compression fractures are actually diagnosed [10]. The most common presenting complaint is a sudden onset of new pain in the region affected. Thoracic fractures may present with symptoms that radiate ventrally if exiting roots are compressed. This is seen infrequently with lumbar compression fractures. Pain is often precipitated with normal daily activities, such as sudden bending, lifting, or coughing. The pain is usually aggravated by movement or sitting, and patients may complain of difficulty sleeping due to paraspinal muscle spasms. These symptoms may gradually improve over 4-6 weeks, as new bone forms and the fracture heals [11].

Although symptoms improve with time in most patients, some experience persistent severe back pain and ensuing chronic symptoms. A focal kyphotic deformity may develop at the site of the compression fracture. Kyphosis can beget further kyphosis and lead to global sagittal imbalance and a cosmetically displeasing 'dowager's hump.' Severe deformities result in diminished abdominal space and a protuberant abdomen, often causing loss of appetite. Neck pain may develop as a result of kyphosis, due to the patient extending his or her neck. Decreased lung capacity and restrictive respiratory problems may also develop, increasing the chances of pneumonia [12]. However, this is rare unless a severe degree of kyphosis develops. A height loss of more than 6cm warrants spine radiographs as the likelihood of a vertebral compression fracture is greatly increased [13].

A compression fracture can become a severely debilitating injury. Patients may require greater pain control, remain bedridden with increased risks of deep venous thrombosis and pulmonary embolism, and become nutritionally depleted, predisposing them to additional fractures. Of patients who experience an incidental compression fracture, more than 19% will have an additional fracture in the subsequent year. The presence of multiple fractures upon initial presentation increases the additional fracture incidence to 24% [14]. The presence of prevalent vertebral compression fractures is also a strong predictor of incidental hip fractures [15]. In tests of physical performance, such as lifting, walking downstairs, or bending, patients with vertebral fractures demonstrate significant decline [16] and report fears of falling and experiencing more fractures [17, 18].

Evaluation

Back pain in the elderly is common, with a high prevalence of osteoarthritis as the etiology. Fracture pain upon presentation to the clinician must be distinguished from other degenerative causes. The onset and duration of pain are also useful in diagnosing vertebral compression fractures. A patient with an acute compression fracture will often have point tenderness upon palpation of the spinous process at the fractured level, and movement or ambulation will usually worsen the pain.

Lower extremity weakness, loss of balance, incontinence, or other neurologic findings suggestive of spinal cord compression are less characteristic of vertebral compression fractures. Finally, a careful history of risk factors for malignancy and infection is also required. Recent weight loss, past history of malignancy, night sweats, or unexplained fever are pertinent details that may reveal the underlying etiology of the back pain. Any known sources of infection (e.g., endocarditis) must raise suspicion for osteomyelitis and vertebral collapse.

Physical examination and laboratory studies

The physical examination begins with careful observation of the patient's posture. Kyphotic deformity is a common finding, particularly with multiple compression fractures. A detailed neurologic examination is necessary to rule out spinal cord compression or radiculopathy. Increased pain when the patient flexes and extends may also suggest the

Chapter 9

presence of a compression fracture. In rare cases, kyphosis from compression fractures may lead to compromised pulmonary function.

If the suspicion for infection or malignancy is high, targeted laboratory studies can help with diagnosis. A complete blood cell count with differential, erythrocyte sedimentation rate, or C-reactive protein level will help diagnose infection. In middle-aged or older men, prostate-specific antigen testing may be useful for detecting occult malignancy. Similarly, the urine or serum may be tested for Bence-Jones proteins or other signs of multiple myeloma.

Imaging

Initial imaging should consist of anteroposterior and lateral radiographs of the thoracic and lumbar spine, allowing easy identification of ventral vertebral wedging, biconcave deformities, and loss of vertebral height (Figure 1) [19]. Comparison to prior radiographs is particularly helpful for distinguishing acute from chronic fractures. If the age of the fracture is uncertain, or if malignancy, infection, or spinal cord compression is suspected, MRI is required to determine the chronicity and potential etiology of the pathological fracture. On T2-weighted and specifically short T1 inversion recovery (STIR) sequences, which suppress the fat signal, unhealed fractures will show as a hyperintense signal in the affected vertebral body. Conversely, T1-weighted sequences will demonstrate decreased intensity. Post-contrast MRI imaging is useful if malignancy or infection is suspected.

A CT scan in conjunction with a nuclear medicine bone scan can be helpful in determining which levels are acute in patients for whom MRI is contraindicated

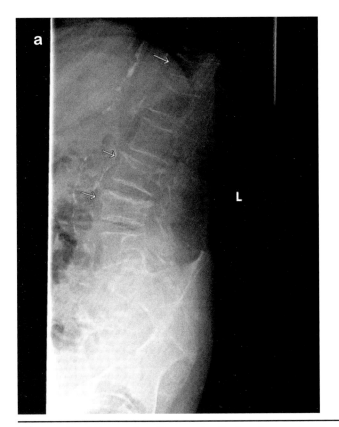 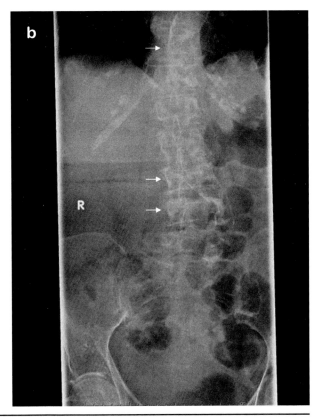

Figure 1. a) Lateral radiograph of a lumbar spine demonstrating multiple compression fractures (arrows), identified by biconcave deformities and loss of vertebral height. b) Anteroposterior radiograph of a lumbar spine again demonstrating multiple compression fractures.

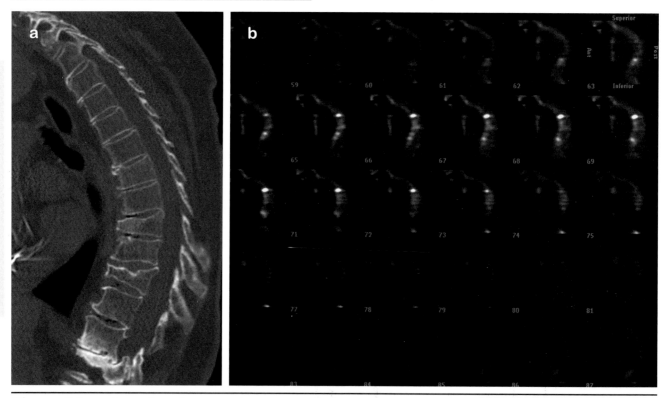

Figure 2. In patients for whom MRI is contraindicated, a CT scan in conjunction with a nuclear medicine bone scan is helpful for identifying acute compression fractures. a) In this sagittal image of the thoracic spine, multiple compression fractures may be appreciated at the apex of the kyphosis. b) Sagittal images from a technetium-99m bone scan demonstrate increased uptake, consistent with a metabolically active acute fracture.

(Figure 2). CT will demonstrate the presence of vertebral fracture and technetium-99m, used in a bone scan, will collect in areas of bone that are metabolically active, such as an acute fracture. For fractures of more than 3-4 months old in an elderly patient, bone scintigraphy (a bone scan) may be more accurate in diagnosis than MRI [20] **(III/B)**. As confirmation of osteoporosis, dual-energy X-ray absorptiometry of the spine will give a quantitative assessment of bone density. Dual-energy X-ray absorptiometry is also helpful for predicting the likelihood of future compression fractures and guiding the appropriate medical management.

Management

Conservative therapy

The initial management goals are to reduce pain and improve mobility. A secondary goal is to prevent further compression fractures. Patients may benefit from non-steroidal anti-inflammatory drugs (NSAIDs) and low-dose opioid medications. Controversy still exists over the use of NSAIDs in the setting of an acute fracture. A pooled meta-analysis of 11 studies suggests there is an association between NSAID use and bone non-union for patients after spinal fusion surgery and repair of long-bone fractures. However, when only higher-quality studies were included in the analysis, the association between NSAID use and bone non-union could no longer be identified [21] **(IIb/B)**.

Several randomized controlled trials (RCTs) have shown that calcitonin reduces pain from osteoporotic compression fractures at as early as a week, and the effects last approximately 4 weeks [22] **(Ia/A)**. However, calcitonin provides less increase in bone mineral density than bisphosphonates and may thus be used in conjunction with other agents. Pamidronate has also been shown to reduce acute pain from osteoporotic compression fractures, although the effect is less pronounced than with calcitonin [19, 23] **(Ib/A)**. For patients suffering from muscle spasm, non-benzodiazepine muscle relaxants may provide some relief, although these medications can have significant side effects in the elderly. Non-benzodiazepine muscle relaxants include metaxalone and cyclobenzaprine, which are thought to act centrally, although the precise mechanism is unclear.

Early mobilization is important to decrease the likelihood of complications such as pressure ulcers, pneumonia, and deep venous thrombosis. The use of physical therapy in combination with a supportive brace has been shown to decrease pain and improve function [24, 25] **(Ib/A)**. The various types of supportive back braces have not been studied, and some clinicians avoid bracing due to concerns about muscle atrophy [26].

Although conservative therapy will fail in approximately 25% of patients [19], continued use of bisphosphonates decreases the chance of additional vertebral fractures by more than 50% in the following 2 years [27, 28] **(Ib/A)**. Similarly, use of recombinant human parathyroid hormone in postmenopausal women with osteoporosis reduces the risk for new vertebral fractures [29] **(Ib/A)**. Calcium supplementation, smoking cessation, and alcohol moderation are important lifestyle modifications for preventing further compression fractures.

Vertebroplasty and kyphoplasty (Table 1)

In both percutaneous vertebral augmentation procedures, polymethylmethacrylate (PMMA) cement is typically injected into the fractured and collapsed vertebral body with the primary goals of pain relief and improved functional capacity. A further goal of kyphoplasty is to improve spinal alignment and potentially prevent development of a kyphotic or scoliotic deformity. In recent years, these procedures have been performed at a rapidly increasing rate by a variety of different specialists. Vertebroplasty rates among Medicare enrollees doubled from 2001 to 2005, increasing by 32% from 2001 to 2002 alone [30].

Current indications for vertebroplasty and kyphoplasty include an acute, painful, unhealed compression fracture, either from osteoporosis, neoplasm, or trauma. There are relatively few contraindications, which include recent infection, uncorrected bleeding disorder, inability to tolerate sedation, and fracture-related compromise of the spinal canal. A fractured dorsal cortex of the vertebral body is a relative contraindication, as it is associated with an increased risk of cement leakage into the spinal canal [31] **(III/B)**. Severe loss of vertebral body height will render needle placement technically difficult and make fluoroscopic visualization for guidance challenging. In these cases, a preprocedure CT scan is particularly helpful for delineating the bony anatomy.

Risks and side effects

Although both vertebroplasty and kyphoplasty are considered generally safe and well tolerated in elderly populations, there are some documented risks and complications. One of the most common complications associated with these procedures is rib fracture, with an incidence as high as 3% [32, 33] **(III/B)**. Another common complication, although often clinically silent, is cement leakage beyond the confines of the vertebral body. The reported incidence of cement leakage is widely variable, from as high as 66% to as low as 1% in experienced hands [32-35] **(III/B)**. Depending on the location and volume of cement leaked, the patient may experience no symptoms or persistent pain, radiculopathy, and even irreversible paraparesis, despite cement evacuation [36, 37]. There is also a small risk that cement leaked into perivertebral veins may embolize to the lungs and behave as a symptomatic pulmonary embolism [34, 38] **(III/B)**.

Another potential concern of vertebroplasty and kyphoplasty is whether these procedures predispose adjacent vertebral levels to fracture. Trout *et al* performed a retrospective review of 432 patients who had undergone vertebroplasty. They reported a new fracture in 20% of patients, and found that the new fracture was more likely to occur in a shorter time period and at the level adjacent to the treated level [39] **(III/B)**. The same authors speculated that abnormal biomechanical forces are generated by the injection of

Table 1. Summary of studies involving vertebroplasty or kyphoplasty for the treatment of vertebral compression fractures. *Continued overleaf.*

Reference	Description	Results	Conclusions	Evidence class/recommendation
Klazen et al, 2010 [44]	202 patients with acute vertebral compression fractures randomized to VP or conservative therapy	Pain relief, measured by VAS, was significantly better at 1 month and 1 year in patients treated with VP	VP offers better pain relief than conservative therapy for patients with acute osteoporotic vertebral compression fractures	Ib/A
Klazen et al, 2010 [41]	202 patients with acute vertebral compression fractures randomized to VP or conservative therapy to assess the incidence of new vertebral compression fractures in patients treated with VP	Incidence of new vertebral compression fractures was not different after VP compared with conservative therapy at a mean of 11.4 months of follow-up	VP is not a risk factor for new vertebral compression fractures	Ib/A
Rousing et al, 2010 [46]	50 patients with acute or subacute osteoporotic vertebral fractures randomized to VP or conservative therapy	Pain relief, measured by VAS, was significantly better immediately after the procedures in the VP group compared with conservative therapy, but there was no difference between groups at 3- and 12-month follow-up	VP offers better immediate pain relief than conservative therapy for patients with acute/subacute vertebral compression fractures, but this difference is not maintained over follow-up	Ib/A
Kallmes et al, 2009 [57]	131 patients with subacute or chronic vertebral compression fractures randomized to VP or sham procedure, followed for 1 month	At 1 month, there was no difference in pain relief or disability between the two groups, although both groups experienced improvements in pain and function from baseline	VP does not provide benefit over a sham procedure for pain relief and improved function in patients with subacute or chronic compression fractures	Ib/A
Buchbinder et al, 2009 [58]	78 patients with subacute or chronic vertebral compression fractures randomized to VP or sham procedure, followed for 6 months	At all timepoints, there was no difference in pain relief or function between the VP group or the control group	VP does not provide benefit over a sham procedure for pain relief and improved function in patients with subacute or chronic compression fractures	Ib/A
Voormolen et al, 2007 [45]	34 patients with subacute or chronic vertebral compression fractures randomized to either VP or conservative therapy	VP patients had significantly better pain relief and used fewer analgesics 1 day after treatment compared with conservative therapy; function and mobility were significantly better in the VP group 2 weeks after treatment	VP provides better pain relief and improved mobility and function compared with conservative therapy in the short term	Ib/A

Table 1. Summary of studies involving vertebroplasty or kyphoplasty for the treatment of vertebral compression fractures. *Continued.*

Reference	Description	Results	Conclusions	Evidence class/recommendation
Diamond *et al*, 2003 [11]	79 patients with acute vertebral compression fractures divided into cohorts receiving either VP or conservative therapy, followed for a mean of 215 days	There were significantly greater improvements in pain and physical functioning compared with conservative therapy 24 hours after VP, but outcomes were no different at 6 and 12 months	VP offers better immediate pain relief than conservative therapy for patients with acute vertebral compression fractures, but this difference is not maintained over follow-up	IIa/B
Wardlaw *et al*, 2009 [42]	300 patients with acute vertebral compression fractures randomized to KP or conservative therapy, followed for 1 year	Pain and physical function, measured by SF-36 PCS, was significantly better with KP group compared with conservative therapy	KP offers better pain relief and improved physical function than conservative therapy for acute vertebral compression fractures	Ib/A
Kumar *et al*, 2010 [65]	52 patients with vertebral compression fractures who were treated with either VP or KP and assessed to 42 weeks' follow-up for pain, function, and quality of life	Both procedures were associated with significant improvements in pain, function, and quality of life compared with baseline. KP was associated with more significant improvements than VP and these were maintained over long-term follow-up	KP may offer more significant benefits of pain relief, improved function, and quality of life than VP for osteoporotic compression fractures	IIa/B
Grafe *et al*, 2005 [55]	60 patients with chronic osteoporotic compression fractures treated with KP or conservative treatment and followed for 1 year	Pain scores improved significantly more in the KP group than the control group. There were significantly fewer new compression fractures in the KP group	KP offers greater pain relief and may lead to fewer additional compression fractures compared with conservative therapy	IIa/B

KP = kyphoplasty; PCS = physical component summary; SF = Short Form; VAS = Visual Analogue Scale; VP = vertebroplasty

cement into the vertebral body, and vertebral endplate fractures are an indicator of these stresses [40].

However, the development of adjacent and remote fractures occurs in nearly one out of five patients after an incidental fracture without vertebral augmentation [14]. More definite evidence now suggests that vertebroplasty is not a risk factor for new primary osteoporotic compression fractures. Klazen *et al* conducted a multicenter RCT comparing vertebroplasty with conservative therapy in 202 patients [41]. After a mean follow-up of 11.4 months, they found no higher fracture risk for adjacent-versus-distant vertebrae in the vertebroplasty group **(Ib/A)**. The only risk factor for new compression fractures from primary osteoporosis was the number of compression fractures at baseline. Other well-designed trials have also reached the same conclusion [42] **(Ib/A)**.

In patients with secondary causes of osteoporosis, however, including hyperthyroidism, hypercortisolism, hyperparathyroidism, alcohol abuse, and immobilization, the adjacent fracture rate may be as high as 49% over 11 months [43] **(III/B)**. Clinicians must carefully follow these patients after cement augmentation, as further intervention is often required.

Efficacy of percutaneous vertebroplasty

The current evidence regarding the efficacy of vertebroplasty and kyphoplasty is conflicting. An RCT published in 2010 evaluated the use of percutaneous vertebroplasty versus conservative therapy in patients with acute osteoporotic compression fractures [44]. A total of 202 patients with vertebral compression fractures of less than 6 weeks old were randomized to either treatment. Pain relief, as measured on a Visual Analogue Scale (VAS), was significantly better in patients treated with vertebroplasty at 1 month and 1 year post-procedure **(Ib/A)**.

An RCT comparing percutaneous vertebroplasty with optimal pain management found that the patients who received vertebroplasty had significantly better pain relief 1 day after the procedure compared with those who received conservative therapy. This difference was also noted at 2 weeks post-procedure, but was less significant. Patients who received vertebroplasty also made better progress in mobility, function, and stature than the control group [45] **(Ib/A)**. However, it is worth noting that the patients included in this study had pain refractory to optimal medical therapy for between 6 weeks and 6 months. In a similar study, 49 patients with acute or semi-acute compression fractures were randomized to either percutaneous vertebroplasty or conservative treatment. Pain scores were significantly better in the group receiving vertebroplasty immediately after the procedure, but this difference was lost at 3- and 12-month follow-up [46] **(Ib/A)**.

A prospective, non-randomized study comparing percutaneous vertebroplasty with conservative therapy was conducted on 79 patients with acute vertebral fractures and a 1- to 6-week history of pain. The study reported a 53% reduction in pain scores and a 29% improvement in physical functioning in patients 24 hours after percutaneous vertebroplasty [11] **(IIa/B)**. Patients treated with conservative therapy reported no change in pain scores or physical functioning. The average length of hospital stay was reduced from 15 to 9 days in the group treated with

vertebroplasty. However, clinical outcomes were similar in each group at 6 weeks and 6-12 months. Therefore, the current evidence suggests a short-term benefit with percutaneous vertebroplasty for acute vertebral compression fracture.

Very few long-term studies have been conducted on percutaneous vertebroplasty. In one study, 13 patients were followed for 5 years after percutaneous vertebroplasty. Pain reduction was stable out to 5 years and there was no radiographic evidence of further collapse of the treated vertebrae, although new fractures were diagnosed in three patients [47] **(III/B)**. Another study that followed patients treated with percutaneous vertebroplasty for 2 years found stable reductions in pain and no progression of vertebral deformity [48] **(III/B)**.

Efficacy of kyphoplasty

Several observational studies support similar benefits of kyphoplasty. In one, 78 patients underwent kyphoplasty and were followed for a minimum of 12 months with the Short Form (SF)-36, VAS, and Oswestry Disability Index. Significant improvements were seen on all functional outcome measures both in the immediate postoperative period and at 1 year follow-up [49] **(III/B)**. Another retrospective study of 117 patients found that pain scores, ambulation ability, and the need for prescription pain medications improved significantly after kyphoplasty and remained unchanged or improved at 2-year follow-up [50] **(III/B)**. Phillips *et al* reported that 29 patients with osteoporotic compression fractures who underwent kyphoplasty experienced significant pain relief 1 week after the procedure, which persisted at 1-year follow-up [51] **(III/B)**. In addition, the authors noted an average of 14.2° sagittal alignment correction after the procedure.

Crandall *et al* studied the response of acute and chronic vertebral compression fractures to kyphoplasty [52]. Acute fractures were defined as less than 10 weeks old, and chronic fractures as more than 4 months old. At 2 weeks post-procedure, 90% of acute and 87% of chronic fractures were associated with pain relief **(IIb/B)**. Acute fractures were significantly more reducible, with restoration of

89% of normal vertebral height obtained in 60% of acute fractures, but only 26% of chronic fractures. Several studies have also demonstrated that kyphoplasty for a vertebral compression fracture will significantly reduce the associated deformity, restoring body height and segmental kyphosis [51, 53] **(III/B)**. However, most kyphosis correction by kyphoplasty is limited to the vertebral body treated, and only in multilevel procedures is the sagittal realignment clinically significant [54].

Wardlaw *et al* performed a multicenter RCT to evaluate kyphoplasty versus conservative treatment for acute vertebral compression fractures [42]. A total of 300 patients were assigned to kyphoplasty or non-surgical care, and the primary outcome was the change from baseline to 1 month in the SF-36 physical component summary. Mean SF-36 physical component summary scores were more significantly improved at 1 month in the kyphoplasty group (7.2 points) than in the non-surgical group (2.0 points) **(Ib/A)**. The frequency of adverse events did not differ between groups. Grafe *et al* found similar results in a cohort study of 60 patients receiving either kyphoplasty or conservative treatment for chronic osteoporotic compression fractures [55]. Pain score improvements were significantly greater in patients who received kyphoplasty than in the control group **(IIa/B)**. Interestingly, there were significantly fewer new compression fractures in the kyphoplasty group compared with the control group.

Meta-analysis

In a study published in 2009, McGirt *et al* reviewed all articles published between 1980 and 2008 for outcomes after vertebroplasty or kyphoplasty for vertebral compression fractures [56]. A total of 74 studies assessing outcomes of vertebroplasty were included but, of these, only one reported level I evidence and three were level II. Likewise, 35 studies on kyphoplasty were included, of which only two provided level II evidence. McGirt *et al* reported that there is evidence that vertebroplasty offers superior pain control in the first 2 weeks after intervention compared with optimal medical therapy [56] **(Ib/A)**. The evidence suggests that vertebroplasty improves functional outcomes of patients, and that benefits in

both pain relief and physical function persist out to 2 years after the procedure. Similarly, there is evidence that kyphoplasty offers better pain relief and improved physical function compared with optimal medical therapy at 6 months post-procedure **(IIb/B)**.

Recent controversy

However, much of the controversy surrounding vertebroplasty and kyphoplasty for vertebral compression fractures comes from two recent, independent RCTs. Kallmes *et al* randomly assigned 131 patients to either vertebroplasty or a sham procedure in which 0.25% bupivacaine was injected into the periosteum of the pedicles of the affected vertebra [57]. Initial recruitment into the study was slow and the inclusion criteria were liberalized so that patients had pain of at least 3/10 and fractures were less than 1 year old. Primary outcome measures were the modified Roland-Morris Disability Questionnaire and a pain scale at 1 month. At 1 month, there was no significant difference in either outcome measure between the two groups, although both vertebroplasty and sham patients had significantly improved pain and function at 1 month compared with baseline **(Ib/A)**. A second trial by Buchbinder *et al* randomized 78 patients with osteoporotic vertebral compression fractures to either percutaneous vertebroplasty or a sham intervention, in which the pedicle of the collapsed body was probed with a needle, but no cement injected [58]. Inclusion criteria similarly allowed fractures up to 1 year old. The primary endpoint was the overall pain score at 3 months after the procedure. There was no significant difference between groups in the primary outcome measure at 3 months, although both groups showed reductions in pain compared with baseline **(Ib/A)**.

Since these two articles were published in the *New England Journal of Medicine*, there have been several criticisms of the study designs and conclusions [59]. The studies included patients who had had pain for 1 year or less and more than 60% of patients had experienced pain for greater than 6 weeks before the intervention. Since the majority of vertebral compression fractures would be expected to heal in a few months, it is unclear if the studies were testing the efficacy of vertebroplasty for acute or chronic fractures. Kallmes *et al* did not require an MRI/bone scan to determine chronicity of the fracture [57]. No clear correlation was demonstrated between the patient's pain location, severity of pain, imaging findings, and pain on physical examination in either study. Furthermore, the 'sham' procedure in which local anesthetic was injected into the periosteum may have actually treated facet arthritis or other sources of back pain separate from the vertebral compression fracture. Therefore, the sham treatment may have represented an actual intervention rather than a placebo. The amount of pain relief in these studies was measured on a 10-point scale, and in Buchbinder *et al* the studies were powered to detect a change of 2.5 on that scale [58]. Critics note that the minimum clinically important difference on a 10-point pain scale may be actually 1.5; therefore, the study was not sensitive enough to detect differences between the control group and vertebroplasty group [60]. In both the Buchbinder *et al* and Kallmes *et al* studies, difficulties were faced in subject enrollment [57, 58]. In the study by Kallmes *et al*, out of more than 1,800 patients screened, only 431 were identified as eligible and 131 (30%) were enrolled. In this scenario, it is very likely that a selection bias may have compromised the results of the trials.

Vertebroplasty or kyphoplasty for pathologic compression fractures from malignancy

Fewer reports have addressed the efficacy of vertebroplasty or kyphoplasty for pathologic compression fractures from malignancy. In one prospective cohort study of 65 patients with metastatic compression fractures, pain measured by VAS and function measured by the Oswestry Disability Index were significantly improved after kyphoplasty, and this improvement was sustained at 2-year follow-up [61] **(IIb/B)**. Balloon kyphoplasty was associated with a 12% rate of cement leakage and an 8% rate of additional vertebral fracture in this study population. Some groups have advocated for the more aggressive use of vertebroplasty for malignant fractures, even in patients with epidural tumor involvement and spinal cord compression. Saliou *et al* treated 51 terminally ill patients with malignant vertebral compression fractures and epidural extension with percutaneous vertebroplasty.

At 1 year, 92% of patients reported adequate pain relief from the procedure and only one patient experienced worsened neurologic symptoms [62] **(III/B)**. Another group reported combining percutaneous vertebroplasty for metastatic compression fractures with interstitial implantation of ^{125}I seeds. The Karnofsky Performance Scores and VAS pain scores were improved in the group implanted with ^{125}I seeds compared with vertebroplasty alone, although there was no difference in tumor progression [63] **(Ib/A)**. A literature review from 2009 strongly recommended the use of vertebral augmentation for pain relief and improving functional outcome in patients with metastatic vertebral compression fractures, despite only moderate evidence in the literature [64].

Vertebroplasty versus kyphoplasty

At this time, only two studies have compared vertebroplasty versus kyphoplasty for osteoporotic compression fractures. Kumar *et al* prospectively studied 28 patients who received vertebroplasty and 24 patients who received kyphoplasty for 42 weeks of follow-up [65]. Both vertebroplasty and kyphoplasty were found to be effective in improving pain, functional disability, and quality of life. However, kyphoplasty demonstrated a 15% greater amount of pain relief over vertebroplasty, which was significantly different and durable to the last follow-up. Similarly, kyphoplasty showed significantly greater functional improvements and higher quality of life than vertebroplasty **(IIa/B)**.

This study is limited by its non-randomized design and small cohort size. However, it does suggest that an RCT comparing the two techniques would be useful for guiding practice. In addition, a rigorous cost analysis must be performed to determine if kyphoplasty is a cost-effective intervention. Lee *et al* performed a meta-analysis of the complications of vertebroplasty and kyphoplasty [66]. The analysis included 121 reports published prior to 2006. Vertebroplasty was found to have a significantly increased rate of procedure-related complications compared with kyphoplasty. Vertebroplasty also had a significantly higher rate of symptomatic and asymptomatic cement leakage compared with kyphoplasty (p<0.05) **(IIb/B)**. This study is limited by its meta-analytic design, and only 24% of the papers reviewed collected complications in a prospective fashion.

Surgical management

Regardless of the underlying etiology of the vertebral compression fracture, neurologic decline from bony retropulsion or canal compromise warrants operative management. The various surgical approaches and indications are beyond the scope of this chapter, and are dependent on the individual characteristics of each case.

Conclusions

Vertebral compression fractures are a common cause of back pain and debilitation in the elderly and traumatic populations. Due to the frail health of these populations, a vertebral compression fracture may lead to poor outcomes as immobility, poor nutrition, and chronic pain cause further complications. Most vertebral compression fractures heal spontaneously over a few months with conservative management. However, a large body of evidence supports the use of vertebroplasty and kyphoplasty for pain relief and improved functional outcomes in patients with vertebral compression fractures. At this time, it is not clear if one procedure has improved outcomes over the other, and an RCT may be necessary to answer this question.

Chapter 9

Recommendations	Evidence level
◆ Percutaneous vertebroplasty offers better pain relief and improved functional outcomes over conservative therapy for acute vertebral compression fractures.	Ia/A
◆ Kyphoplasty offers better pain relief and improved functional outcomes over conservative therapy for acute vertebral compression fractures.	Ib/A
◆ Percutaneous vertebroplasty is not a risk factor for new vertebral compression fractures.	Ib/A
◆ Percutaneous vertebroplasty offers better pain relief and improved functional outcomes over conservative therapy for subacute or chronic vertebral compression fractures, but these benefits are not maintained after 2 weeks.	Ib/A

References

1. National Osteoporosis Foundation. America's Bone Health: The State of Osteoporosis and Low Bone Mass in Our Nation. 2005. Available from http://www.nof.org/sites/default/files/pdfs/PressRoomKit.pdf. Accessed August 23, 2010.

2. Riggs BL, Meltons LJ 3rd. The worldwide problem of osteoporosis: insights afforded by epidemiology. *Bone* 1995; 17(5 Suppl.): 505S-11.

3. Cooper C, Atkinson EJ, O'Fallon WM, Melton LJ 3rd. Incidence of clinically diagnosed vertebral fractures: a population-based study in Rochester, Minnesota, 1985-1989. *J Bone Miner Res* 1992; 7(2): 221-7.

4. Silverman SL. The clinical consequences of vertebral compression fracture. *Bone* 1992; 13(Suppl. 2): S27-31.

5. Schlaich C, Minne HW, Bruckner T, *et al*. Reduced pulmonary function in patients with spinal osteoporotic fractures. *Osteoporos Int* 1998; 8(3): 261-7.

6. Gold DT. The clinical impact of vertebral fractures: quality of life in women with osteoporosis. *Bone* 1996; 18(3 Suppl.): 185S-9.

7. Cooper C, Atkinson EJ, Jacobsen SJ, O'Fallon WM, Melton LJ 3rd. Population-based study of survival after osteoporotic fractures. *Am J Epidemiol* 1993; 137: 1001-5.

8. Ray NF, Chan JK, Thamer M, Melton LJ 3rd. Medical expenditures for the treatment of osteoporotic fractures in the United States in 1995: report from the National Osteoporosis Foundation. *J Bone Miner Res* 1997; 12: 24-35.

9. Vogt TM, Ross PD, Palermo L, et al. Vertebral fracture prevalence among women screened for the Fracture Intervention Trial and a simple clinical tool to screen for undiagnosed vertebral fractures. Fracture Intervention Trial Research Group. Mayo Clin Proc 2000; 75: 888-96.

10. Cooper C, Melton LJ. Vertebral fractures. BMJ 1992; 304: 793-4.

11. Diamond TH, Champion B, Clark WA. Management of acute osteoporotic vertebral fractures: a nonrandomized trial comparing percutaneous vertebroplasty with conservative therapy. Am J Med 2003; 114: 257-65.

12. Schlaich C, Minne HW, Bruckner T, et al. Reduced pulmonary function in patients with spinal osteoporotic fractures. Osteoporos Int 1998; 8: 261-7.

13. Siminoski K, Warshawski RS, Jen H, Lee K. The accuracy of historical height loss for the detection of vertebral fractures in postmenopausal women. Osteoporos Int 2006; 17: 290-6.

14. Lindsay R, Silverman SL, Cooper C, et al. Risk of new vertebral fracture in the year following a fracture. JAMA 2001; 285: 320-3.

15. Ismail AA, Cockerill W, Cooper C, et al. Prevalent vertebral deformity predicts incident hip though not distal forearm fracture: results from the European Prospective Osteoporosis Study. Osteoporos Int 2001; 12: 85-90

16. Greendale GA, DeAmicis TA, Bucur A, et al. A prospective study of the effect of fracture on measured physical performance: results from the MacArthur Study - MAC. J Am Geriatr Soc 2000; 48: 546-9.

17. Cook DJ, Guyatt GH, Adachi JD, et al. Quality of life issues in women with vertebral fractures due to osteoporosis. Arthritis Rheum 1993; 36: 750-6.

18. Papaioannou A, Watts NB, Kendler DL, Yuen CK, Adachi JD, Ferko N. Diagnosis and management of vertebral fractures in elderly adults. Am J Med 2002; 113: 220-8.

19. Agulnek AN, O'Leary KJ, Edwards BJ. Acute vertebral fracture. J Hosp Med 2009; 4: E20-4.

20. Masala S, Schillaci O, Massari F, et al. MRI and bone scan imaging in the preoperative evaluation of painful vertebral fractures treated with vertebroplasty and kyphoplasty. In Vivo 2005; 19: 1055-60

21. Dodwell ER, Latorre JG, Parisini E, et al. NSAID exposure and risk of nonunion: a meta-analysis of case-control and cohort studies. Calcif Tissue Int 2010; 87: 193-202.

22. Knopp JA, Diner BM, Blitz M, Lyritis GP, Rowe BH. Calcitonin for treating acute pain of osteoporotic vertebral compression fractures: a systematic review of randomized, controlled trials. Osteoporos Int 2005; 16: 1281-90.

23. Armingeat T, Brondino R, Pham T, Legre V, Lafforgue P. Intravenous pamidronate for pain relief in recent osteoporotic vertebral compression fracture: a randomized double-blind controlled study. Osteoporos Int 2006; 17: 1659-65.

24. Stadhouder A, Buskens E, Vergroesen DA, Fidler MW, de Nies F, Oner FC. Nonoperative treatment of thoracic and lumbar spine fractures: a prospective randomized study of different treatment options. J Orthop Trauma 2009; 23: 588-94.

25. Malmros B, Mortensen L, Jensen MB, Charles P. Positive effects of physiotherapy on chronic pain and performance in osteoporosis. Osteoporos Int 1998; 8: 215-21.

26. Tamayo-Orozco J, Arzac-Palumbo P, Peon-Vidales H, Mota-Bolfeta R, Fuentes F. Vertebral fractures associated with osteoporosis: patient management. Am J Med 1997; 103: 44-8S; discussion 8-50S.

27. Harris ST, Watts NB, Genant HK, et al. Effects of risedronate treatment on vertebral and nonvertebral fractures in women with postmenopausal osteoporosis: a randomized controlled trial. Vertebral Efficacy With Risedronate Therapy (VERT) Study Group. JAMA 1999; 282: 1344-52.

28. Matsumoto T, Hagino H, Shiraki M, et al. Effect of daily oral minodronate on vertebral fractures in Japanese postmenopausal women with established osteoporosis: a randomized placebo-controlled double-blind study. Osteoporos Int 2009; 20: 1429-37.

29. Greenspan SL, Bone HG, Ettinger MP, et al. Effect of recombinant human parathyroid hormone (1-84) on vertebral fracture and bone mineral density in postmenopausal women with osteoporosis: a randomized trial. Ann Intern Med 2007; 146: 326-39.

30. Gray DT, Hollingworth W, Onwudiwe N, Deyo RA, Jarvik JG. Thoracic and lumbar vertebroplasties performed in US Medicare enrollees, 2001-2005. JAMA 2007; 298: 1760-2.

31. Weill A, Chiras J, Simon JM, Rose M, Sola-Martinez T, Enkaoua E. Spinal metastases: indications for and results of percutaneous injection of acrylic surgical cement. Radiology 1996; 199: 241-7.

32. Hodler J, Peck D, Gilula LA. Midterm outcome after vertebroplasty: predictive value of technical and patient-related factors. Radiology 2003; 227: 662-8.

33. Evans AJ, Jensen ME, Kip KE, et al. Vertebral compression fractures: pain reduction and improvement in functional mobility after percutaneous polymethylmethacrylate vertebroplasty retrospective report of 245 cases. Radiology 2003; 226: 366-72.

34. Venmans A, Klazen CA, Lohle PN, et al. Percutaneous vertebroplasty and pulmonary cement embolism: results from VERTOS II. AJNR Am J Neuroradiol 2010; 31(8): 1451-3.

35. Vasconcelos C, Gailloud P, Beauchamp NJ, Heck DV, Murphy KJ. Is percutaneous vertebroplasty without pretreatment venography safe? Evaluation of 205 consecutives procedures. AJNR Am J Neuroradiol 2002; 23: 913-17.

36. Cosar M, Sasani M, Oktenoglu T, et al. The major complications of transpedicular vertebroplasty. J Neurosurg Spine 2009; 11: 607-13.

37. Shapiro S, Abel T, Purvines S. Surgical removal of epidural and intradural polymethylmethacrylate extravasation complicating percutaneous vertebroplasty for an osteoporotic lumbar compression fracture. Case report. J Neurosurg 2003; 98: 90-2.

38. Padovani B, Kasriel O, Brunner P, Peretti-Viton P. Pulmonary embolism caused by acrylic cement: a rare complication of percutaneous vertebroplasty. AJNR Am J Neuroradiol 1999; 20: 375-7.

39. Trout AT, Kallmes DF, Kaufmann TJ. New fractures after vertebroplasty: adjacent fractures occur significantly sooner. AJNR Am J Neuroradiol 2006; 27: 217-23.

40. Trout AT, Kallmes DF, Layton KF, Thielen KR, Hentz JG. Vertebral endplate fractures: an indicator of the abnormal forces generated in the spine after vertebroplasty. *J Bone Miner Res* 2006; 21: 1797-802.

41. Klazen CA, Venmans A, de Vries J, *et al.* Percutaneous vertebroplasty is not a risk factor for new osteoporotic compression fractures: results from VERTOS II. *AJNR Am J Neuroradiol* 2010; 31(8): 1447-50.

42. Wardlaw D, Cummings SR, Van Meirhaeghe J, *et al.* Efficacy and safety of balloon kyphoplasty compared with non-surgical care for vertebral compression fracture (FREE): a randomised controlled trial. *Lancet* 2009; 373: 1016-24.

43. Harrop JS, Prpa B, Reinhardt MK, Lieberman I. Primary and secondary osteoporosis' incidence of subsequent vertebral compression fractures after kyphoplasty. *Spine* (Phila Pa 1976) 2004; 29: 2120-5.

44. Klazen CA, Lohle PN, de Vries J, *et al.* Vertebroplasty versus conservative treatment in acute osteoporotic vertebral compression fractures (VERTOS II): an open-label randomised trial. *Lancet* 2010; 376(9746): 1085-92.

45. Voormolen MH, Mali WP, Lohle PN, *et al.* Percutaneous vertebroplasty compared with optimal pain medication treatment: short-term clinical outcome of patients with subacute or chronic painful osteoporotic vertebral compression fractures. The VERTOS study. *AJNR Am J Neuroradiol* 2007; 28: 555-60.

46. Rousing R, Hansen KL, Andersen MO, Jespersen SM, Thomsen K, Lauritsen JM. Twelve-months follow-up in forty-nine patients with acute/semiacute osteoporotic vertebral fractures treated conservatively or with percutaneous vertebroplasty: a clinical randomized study. *Spine* (Phila Pa 1976) 2010; 35: 478-82.

47. Perez-Higueras A, Alvarez L, Rossi RE, Quinones D, Al-Assir I. Percutaneous vertebroplasty: long-term clinical and radiological outcome. *Neuroradiology* 2002; 44: 950-4.

48. Grados F, Depriester C, Cayrolle G, Hardy N, Deramond H, Fardellone P. Long-term observations of vertebral osteoporotic fractures treated by percutaneous vertebroplasty. *Rheumatology* (Oxford) 2000; 39: 1410-4.

49. Coumans JV, Reinhardt MK, Lieberman IH. Kyphoplasty for vertebral compression fractures: 1-year clinical outcomes from a prospective study. *J Neurosurg* 2003; 99: 44-50.

50. Ledlie JT, Renfro MB. Kyphoplasty treatment of vertebral fractures: 2-year outcomes show sustained benefits. *Spine* (Phila Pa 1976) 2006; 31: 57-64.

51. Phillips FM, Ho E, Campbell-Hupp M, McNally T, Todd Wetzel F, Gupta P. Early radiographic and clinical results of balloon kyphoplasty for the treatment of osteoporotic vertebral compression fractures. *Spine* (Phila Pa 1976) 2003; 28: 2260-5; discussion 5-7.

52. Crandall D, Slaughter D, Hankins PJ, Moore C, Jerman J. Acute versus chronic vertebral compression fractures treated with kyphoplasty: early results. *Spine J* 2004; 4: 418-24.

53. Gaitanis IN, Carandang G, Phillips FM, *et al.* Restoring geometric and loading alignment of the thoracic spine with a vertebral compression fracture: effects of balloon (bone tamp) inflation and spinal extension. *Spine J* 2005; 5: 45-54.

54. Pradhan BB, Bae HW, Kropf MA, Patel VV, Delamarter RB. Kyphoplasty reduction of osteoporotic vertebral compression fractures: correction of local kyphosis versus overall sagittal alignment. *Spine* (Phila Pa 1976) 2006; 31: 435-41.

55. Grafe IA, Da Fonseca K, Hillmeier J, *et al.* Reduction of pain and fracture incidence after kyphoplasty: 1-year outcomes of a prospective controlled trial of patients with primary osteoporosis. *Osteoporos Int* 2005; 16: 2005-12.

56. McGirt MJ, Parker SL, Wolinsky JP, Witham TF, Bydon A, Gokaslan ZL. Vertebroplasty and kyphoplasty for the treatment of vertebral compression fractures: an evidenced-based review of the literature. *Spine J* 2009; 9: 501-8.

57. Kallmes DF, Comstock BA, Heagerty PJ, *et al.* A randomized trial of vertebroplasty for osteoporotic spinal fractures. *N Engl J Med* 2009; 361: 569-79.

58. Buchbinder R, Osborne RH, Ebeling PR, *et al.* A randomized trial of vertebroplasty for painful osteoporotic vertebral fractures. *N Engl J Med* 2009; 361: 557-68.

59. Fisher CG, Vaccaro AR, Thomas KC, *et al.* Evidence-based recommendations for spine surgery. *Spine* (Phila Pa 1976) 2010; 35: E678-86.

60. Grotle M, Brox JI, Vollestad NK. Concurrent comparison of responsiveness in pain and functional status measurements used for patients with low back pain. *Spine* (Phila Pa 1976) 2004; 29: E492-501.

61. Pflugmacher R, Taylor R, Agarwal A, *et al.* Balloon kyphoplasty in the treatment of metastatic disease of the spine: a 2-year prospective evaluation. *Eur Spine J* 2008; 17: 1042-8.

62. Saliou G, Kocheida el M, Lehmann P, *et al.* Percutaneous vertebroplasty for pain management in malignant fractures of the spine with epidural involvement. *Radiology* 2010; 254: 882-90.

63. Yang Z, Yang D, Xie L, *et al.* Treatment of metastatic spinal tumors by percutaneous vertebroplasty versus percutaneous vertebroplasty combined with interstitial implantation of 125I seeds. *Acta Radiol* 2009; 50: 1142-8.

64. Mendel E, Bourekas E, Gerszten P, Golan JD. Percutaneous techniques in the treatment of spine tumors: what are the diagnostic and therapeutic indications and outcomes? *Spine* (Phila Pa 1976) 2009; 34: S93-100.

65. Kumar K, Nguyen R., Bishop S. A comparative analysis of the results of vertebroplasty and kyphoplasty in osteoporotic vertebral compression fractures. *Neurosurgery* 2010; 67: 171-88.

66. Lee MJ, Dumonski M, Cahill P, Stanley T, Park D, Singh K. Percutaneous treatment of vertebral compression fractures: a meta-analysis of complications. *Spine* (Phila Pa 1976) 2009; 34: 1228-32.

Osteoporotic vertebral compression fractures

Chapter 10

Metastatic tumors of the spine

Ran Harel MD

Faculty, Spine Surgery and Spine Radiosurgery 1

Lilyana Angelov MD

Head Section of Spine Tumors and Staff Neurosurgeon 2

1 THE DEPARTMENT OF NEUROSURGERY AND SPINE SURGERY
THE TALPIOT MEDICAL LEADERSHIP PROGRAM, SHEBA MEDICAL CENTER, ISRAEL
2 CENTER FOR SPINE HEALTH, CLEVELAND CLINIC, CLEVELAND, OHIO, USA
BRAIN TUMOR AND NEUROONCOLOGY CENTER, CLEVELAND CLINIC, CLEVELAND, OHIO, USA

Introduction

Cancer incidence and prevalence are rising as our population ages and treatment options continue to improve [1, 2]. However, a rising prevalence of cancer patients is expected to increase the incidence of spine metastases, the most commonly occurring site of skeletal secondary tumors [3]. Spine metastases are currently reported in as many as 50% of cancer patients [4, 5] and result in devastating sequelae in 5-14% [6, 7]. The vast majority of spinal metastases occur in patients with breast, lung, prostate, and renal carcinoma, reflecting both the prevalence of these cancer types and their predilection to bone [3, 8, 9]. Overall, 95% of spinal metastases primarily involve the vertebral body of the spinal column and may expand into the epidural space [3]. Clinically, the thoracic spine is involved in 70% of metastases to the spine [8-10], while classic autopsy studies demonstrate the lumbar spine is more commonly affected [3]. Intradural metastases are far less common: 0.8-3.9% are extramedullary and only 0.5% of spine metastases are found in the intradural intramedullary compartment [11, 12].

Signs and symptoms

Up to 10% of cancer patients present with spinal metastases as the initial finding [8, 9, 13]. Pain is the most common manifestation, occurring in 90% of these patients [8, 14, 15]. Spinal tumor pain can present as local pain exaggerated by palpation or percussion. It can also be radicular in nature, implying compression or invasion of the nerve roots, or mechanical pain that is relieved by rest, provoked by movement and warranting spinal instability precautions [8, 13, 16, 17]. Night pain or pain when recumbent is a classic feature of spine malignancy, and is believed to result from lengthening of the spine, distension of the spinal epidural venous plexus, and unmasking the pain due to low levels of endogenous corticosteroids [18]. Every cancer patient should be regularly evaluated with specific questions addressing these symptoms and their presence. A complaint of back pain is a red flag that should prompt further investigation.

Motor dysfunction is the second most common finding in metastatic spine patients at presentation, ranging from 35% to 75% [3]. Patients usually complain of extremity heaviness and the physical examination is positive for motor deficits. Sensory deficits often accompany the motor ones, and sphincter control is frequently preserved at the initial stages of the disease [3, 13, 18].

Methodology

For this review, a comprehensive literature search was performed using the PubMed electronic database (1950-May 2010). The text strings used for the search were combinations of the following: 'spine metastases,' 'spine metastasis,' 'radiation,' 'chemotherapy,' 'bisphosphonates,' 'isotopes, surgery,' 'decompression,' 'stabilization,' 'fusion,' 'vertebroplasty,' 'kyphoplasty,' 'radiosurgery.'

Only English-written papers were evaluated. Hematologic malignancy studies were excluded. Both authors determined the level of evidence and grade of each citation.

Treatment overview

Historically, patients suffering from spinal metastases are reported to have median overall survival of 7 months, ranging from 3 to 16 months [18-21], while those with epidural spread have a median survival of 3-6 months [18, 22]. This short life expectancy, along with the presence of a systemic primary and associated comorbidities, supports a more palliative treatment approach in these patients rather than a curative regimen. However, with advanced cancer treatment options and care, patient survival appears to be increasing overall. Thus, treating these lesions or associated symptoms appropriately and effectively to prevent undesired sequelae [1, 13] and maintain a patient's quality of life becomes essential.

Steroids

Corticosteroids are used routinely for the treatment of spine tumors, especially when spinal cord compression occurs. Steroids reduce edema in the spinal cord and have been shown to reduce the size of hematogenous tumors and occasionally of breast cancer [8, 18].

Sorensen et al conducted a randomized trial on the effects of high-dose steroids for metastatic epidural spinal cord compression (MESCC) prior to radiotherapy compared with radiotherapy alone [23]. The initial dose was 96mg intravenous dexamethasone followed by 3 days of 96mg oral dexamethasone and 10 days of tapering. A statistically significant difference was shown in ambulation rates at 3 and 6 months, with no effect on survival. These data led to a recommendation to use steroids with conventionally fractionated radiation therapy (Ib/A).

Vecht et al conducted a randomized trial on MESCC patients, comparing a 10mg dexamethasone loading dose with a 100mg loading dose followed by 16mg oral dexamethasone [24]. No statistical difference between treatment regimens was observed. Although the study group was small, the authors concluded that as the higher dose had no added benefit, the smaller dose is recommended (Ib/A). Similarly, a Cochrane review examining steroid dosing showed no benefit with higher doses in terms of ambulatory rate, but a significant elevation in steroid-related adverse events [25] (Ia/A).

In contrast, Maranzano et al have challenged the need to prescribe steroids in all MESCC patients [26]. They treated patients with metastatic disease and MESCC, a short expected survival time, and no neurologic deficit at presentation or radiculopathy only with radiation alone. All patients demonstrated stable or improved neurologic status and 85% had improved pain scores. The authors concluded that patients with no neurologic deficits harboring radiosensitive tumors can undergo spine radiation without concurrent steroids (III/B). There is sufficient grade A evidence to justify the use of steroids for spinal cord compression patients with neurologic deficits; however, the higher dose is related to an increased risk of adverse events and is hence not recommended. Evidence for the treatment of neurologically intact patients is lacking.

Radiation therapy

Before radiation therapy became available, surgical decompression in the form of a laminectomy was the only treatment option for patients with metastatic cord compression. Spinal radiotherapy was introduced in the 1950s and several large retrospective studies, comparing it with laminectomy, failed to show a benefit of surgical decompression [25, 27-29] **(III/B)**.

Young *et al* conducted a small prospective randomized trial comparing laminectomy and radiation to radiation alone, with no significant difference between the two groups [30] **(Ib/A)**. As a result, for many years, conventional radiation alone for patients with metastatic spine tumors was considered the standard of care. Radiation therapy has never been compared with supportive therapy alone in a randomized trial, nor has it been compared with surgery with no adjuvant radiation [7, 18, 25]. The benefits of radiation for spinal metastases have been repeatedly confirmed in large-scale retrospective studies showing improved or retained function [18, 22, 31-34] **(III/B)**. Gerszten *et al* performed a systematic review of the literature regarding conventional radiation therapy for spine metastases in which they included 49 papers, three of which were randomized and four prospective [35]. The post-radiation ambulatory rate was 60-80%, pain control was achieved in 50-70% of patients, and local control was achieved in 61-89% (mean 77%) **(Ia/A)**.

However, despite the general acknowledgement that radiotherapy has a major role in the treatment of spine metastatic disease, the daily dose and fraction number are not agreed upon. While patients are usually treated with 30Gy divided over 10 fractions in the USA, patients in Europe are treated with shorter protocols and a higher fraction dose [18, 36, 37]. A randomized prospective trial on behalf of the Bone Pain Trial Working Party compared single-fraction 8Gy radiation therapy versus 20Gy in five fractions and 30Gy in 10 fractions in 765 patients. Equivalent results in terms of survival, pain control, pathologic fractures, spinal cord compression, and side effects were seen in all three groups; however, the low-dose group was found to have an increased risk for re-treatment [38] **(Ib/A)**. Rades *et al* retrospectively evaluated 1,304 patients treated with five different radiation regimens [39]. They found no statistical difference between the groups in survival, pain control, and side effects. However, they again found a significantly higher recurrence rate with the low-dose protocols after 1 year of follow-up. The authors concluded that patients with a short estimated survival

time should be treated with one 8Gy fraction, while those with better prognosis should receive 10 fractions of 3Gy **(III/B)**.

In contrast, Maranzano *et al* prospectively compared a single 8Gy dose with a split course of three fractions of 5Gy followed by five fractions of 3Gy in 276 patients with short life expectancy [40]. No statistical difference was noted and the authors recommended the single-fraction protocol **(Ib/A)**. A study conducted by the same group comparing single 8Gy dosing to two fractions of 8Gy also showed no difference [41] **(Ib/A)**.

A Cochrane review included 10 randomized prospective studies questioning the preferred treatment regimen [42]. Pain control was equivalent in the low-dose short protocols and the high-dose long protocol, while pathologic fractures and re-treatment rates were significantly elevated in the short protocol arm **(Ia/A)**. A meta-analysis conducted by Chow *et al* encompassed 16 randomized trials examining the optimal dosing regimen [37]. As previously shown, the hypofractionated regimens demonstrated the same results with regard to pain control and tumor control, but were associated with significantly increased re-treatment rates **(Ia/A)**.

Conventional radiation therapy delivered in either long or short protocols for spinal metastases is supported by high-level evidence **(Ia/A)**, widely acceptable, and strongly recommended. The evidence supports the use of short protocols for patients with an unfavorable prognosis and short expected survival **(Ia/A)**.

Systemic therapies

Chemotherapy

The long-term control of metastases, including those in the spine, often entails systemic chemotherapy. Chemotherapy can be administered as monotherapy or involve a combination of agents. The treatment of choice largely depends on the histology of the tumor and its chemosensitivity or receptor status rather than the specific location of a given metastasis [43, 44]. Typically, hormonal drugs are used for prostate and breast spine metastases, and cytotoxic agents for most other cancers and when hormonal therapy begins to fail in patients who were initially treated with it. The literature has abundant reports of chemotherapy for systemic disease but data are lacking on treatments specific to spine metastases, resulting in a low level of evidence for chemotherapy **(IV/C)**.

Bisphosphonates

Bisphosphonates are a group of drugs that bind to the surface of the bone, impairing osteoclast-mediated bone resorption and reducing tumor-associated osteolysis. They are used as co-analgesics in patients with moderate and severe bone pain and can reduce the frequency of skeletal-related events such as pathologic fractures, hypercalcemia, and spinal cord compression, or the need for surgery or radiation therapy [18, 45-47]. Multiple randomized prospective trials have demonstrated a statistically significant decrease in fracture rate or skeletal events with bisphosphonates relative to placebo [48-50] **(Ib/A)**. Machado *et al* conducted a meta-analysis of 18 randomized studies comparing various bisphosphonate generics with placebo [51]. All of the drugs resulted in lower rates of skeletal events when compared with placebo, but no agent showed superior results over the others. The drugs had no effect on survival **(Ia/A)**. With respect to the specific impact of bisphosphonates on the spinal column rather than the entire skeleton, there is a paucity of data; however, there is a high level of evidence that bisphosphonates reduce skeletal events and hence should be considered in these patients.

Radioisotopes

Systemically administered drugs can also act as local radiation therapy to the spine. Radioisotopes such as strontium-89 or rhenium-186 can be injected intravenously and are characterized by their affinity to osteoblastic bone. Multiple studies, although not specifically limited to the spine, have shown benefit in terms of pain reduction in the treatment of multiple bone metastases. Finlay *et al* and Bauman *et al* have reviewed the prospective randomized trials for bone metastases radioisotope treatment [52, 53]. Both reviews concluded there is a significant pain reduction associated with the treatment. However, severe side effects, including irreversible bone marrow suppression, limit the use of these isotopes to patients with multiple synchronous painful metastases and good marrow function, where no further treatment modalities are available **(Ia/A)**. Radioisotopes may occasionally be considered in a very select subgroup of patients for the management of diffuse bony spinal metastases.

History: surgical approaches

The first reported surgical decompression for a spinal tumor was described in the literature as early as 1895, in an era before radiotherapy [54]. Decompressing the spinal cord via a dorsal approach laminectomy relieves the pressure on the spinal cord and potentially reverses neurologic deficits. However, most metastases to the spinal column involve the ventral elements, causing dorsal shift of the spinal cord. Decompressive laminectomy allows further displacement of the cord, thus increasing the risk of neurologic injury related to mechanical damage as well as cord vascular insufficiency. Furthermore, removal of the dorsal elements in vertebrae where the tumor has already resulted in ventral compromise creates potential instability [9, 55] **(IV/C)**. The location of the tumor within the vertebra, the spine region involved, local kyphosis or lordosis, and the position of the instantaneous axis of rotation all play a role in determining the risk for a pathologic fracture [56-58]. Surgical decompression without instrumentation, whether performed via the ventral or dorsal approach, can cause further instability to the metastatic spine [9, 59] **(IV/C)**. It is not surprising then that after the introduction of radiotherapy and the publication of large studies comparing surgery against radiation therapy, surgical decompression was widely abandoned [25, 28-30] **(Ib/A)**.

Surgeons, however, continued to operate on patients with spinal metastases who presented with progressive neurologic deterioration after radiation therapy. In 1983, Constans *et al* published a series describing a single institutional experience with 600 patients with metastatic spine disease and progressive neurologic deterioration, where most patients had undergone decompressive laminectomy followed by irradiation [60]. The reported neurologic outcome after further decompression was consistent, with 44% of patients experiencing improvement and stable disease in 41% **(III/B)**. In 1984, Harrington described his experience with 52 patients suffering from ventrally compressing spinal metastases [59]. Harrington used ventral or lateral approaches, with decompression of the cord followed by polymethylmethacrylate (PMMA) to replace the vertebra ventrally, and dorsal instrumentation with Harrington rods **(III/B)**.

A paradigm shift

Since then, advances in surgical techniques and new and improved spinal instrumentation have led to a shift in the paradigm for spinal metastases treatment [6, 61, 62]. Siegal and Siegal prospectively compared radiation therapy combined with corticosteroids versus surgical decompression and fusion in patients in whom radiation therapy had failed, those with radioresistant tumors, or patients with unknown pathology [63]. Despite surgically treating an unfavorable group, the ambulation rate was higher in the operative group **(IIb/B)**. A meta-analysis comparing combined surgery and radiation results in the new surgical era versus conventional radiation alone demonstrated that surgical patients were more likely to remain ambulatory or regain ambulation [34] **(III/B)**. This study included 24 surgical papers and four radiation papers. All except one were non-randomized, had no control group, and investigated prospective or retrospective cohorts **(III/B)**.

In 2005, Patchell et al published a randomized multicenter trial comparing surgery and radiation with radiation alone for the treatment of MESCC [7]. This study showed a clear benefit for surgical management in terms of maintaining and regaining ambulation, and lower utilization of corticosteroids and analgesics. The authors concluded that surgical intervention should be the first line of treatment for these patients **(Ib/A)**. Further analysis of the data showed surgery to be

cost-effective as the treatment of ambulatory patients is less expensive [64] **(IIa/B)**.

Study criticisms

These studies changed the treatment algorithms in many centers, but their conclusions are controversial. Criticism of Patchell's study centers on potential patient-selection biases. Specifically, this multicenter study took longer than 10 years to recruit 101 patients, and the radiation-only group was found to have a poorer than expected outcome when compared with other radiation-alone studies [65, 66]. This has led some to conclude that this study suggests surgery should be reserved for good-prognosis patients with relatively radioresistant tumors **(IV/C)**. A Cochrane review published in 2008 comparing decompressive surgery with radiation therapy cited only Patchell's study [7], and concluded that decompressive surgery should be used in the first line for ambulatory patients with long expected survival and radioresistant histologies [25] **(Ia/A)**.

Methods of surgical resection

Surgical resection can be performed with various methods [6, 67-69]:

* *En bloc* resection (the removal of the tumor in one piece with wide excisional margins), a technique usually utilized for primary bone tumors.
* Debulking piecemeal resection (removal of the tumor in small pieces with no significant margins), utilized for patients with a good performance status and anticipated survival of longer than 3 months.
* Palliative surgery (partial/limited resection of the tumor to relieve cord compression).

Ibrahim et al prospectively examined the impact of resection modality on survival and function in patients with metastatic spine tumors [6]. Patients selected for tumor excision were younger and had better neurologic scores and more limited disease than those stratified to the palliative surgery group. As

Chapter 10

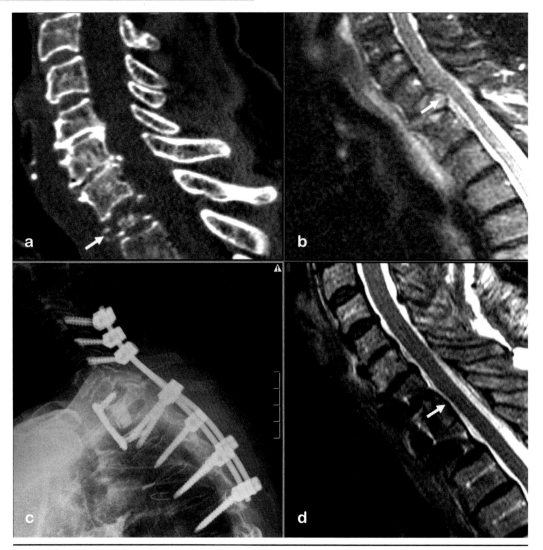

Figure 1. A 67-year-old woman previously diagnosed with breast carcinoma presented with back and neck pain, bilateral arm pain, and left arm weakness. a) CT demonstrated a T1 compression fracture with canal compromise (arrow). b) MRI demonstrated canal compromise and cord compression (arrow). c) The patient underwent a T1 corpectomy and instrumentation with a polymethylmethacrylate graft and ventral plate, as well as dorsal instrumentation and fusion with screws and rods. d) The postoperative T2-weighted MRI demonstrates cerebrospinal fluid around the spinal cord (arrow), indicative of a decompressed cord.

might be expected, the palliative group did significantly worse in terms of survival and neurologic function, but since this was the high-risk group, the authors could only conclude that excisional surgery is a viable option for spine metastases **(IIb/B)**.

The subaxial cervical spine can be approached by either a ventral or dorsal approach, or with a combined approach [9, 67, 68, 70-72] **(III/B)**. Ventral thoracic tumors can be resected via thoracotomy, a retropleural lateral approach, or dorsolateral approach, and various methods have been developed for approaching and fusing the spine utilizing these approaches [9, 13, 68, 73] **(III/B)**. Lumbar ventral lesions can be approached via a retroperitoneal or transabdominal approach, or via a dorsal transpedicular approach [9, 10, 13, 73, 74] **(III/B)**. Polly *et al* reviewed the literature looking for the optimal approach to tackle the spine [75]. They reviewed 32 papers. There was no level I evidence, one level II study, five level III studies, and 26 level IV studies. Their conclusion was that the level of evidence was low and only recommended approaching T2-T5 by a dorsal or dorsolateral approach, while no recommendations could be drawn concerning other levels (Figure 1) **(III/B)**.

In summary, recent level I evidence suggests that surgical decompression can be beneficial for the treatment of patients with spinal metastases, although some limitations may restrict the application of this strategy to all patients. Sufficient evidence justifies a surgical approach for expected long-term survivors, patients with radioresistant histologies, and those in whom radiation therapy fails. Recommendations regarding the resection extent and preferred approach are not uniformly agreed upon, and are not supported by a high level of evidence.

Novel approaches

As the prevalence of surgery for spinal metastases is rising, new techniques are being utilized to ease the procedure for both surgeon and patient.

Embolization

Resection of spine metastases has been reported to be associated with extensive blood loss during the procedure, especially in very vascular tumors such as renal cell carcinoma [76, 77]. Preoperative angiography can show the tumor vascular supply, while embolization by means of injecting particles, coils, or Onyx can reduce blood flow in the tumor [78, 79]. Embolization has been shown to reduce extensive blood loss; however, some cases cannot be embolized effectively, mainly because of anatomic variation and where the tumor is supplied by the artery of Adamkiewicz [80]. Surgery should be

performed within 48 hours of embolization and the surgical and anesthesia teams should be aware that successful embolization does not preclude excessive blood loss [76-80] **(IV/C)**.

Mendel *et al* have reviewed the literature regarding preoperative embolization for spinal tumors [81]. Ten retrospective papers were included and analyzed, reporting more than 50% reduction in operative blood loss and a 4% rate of embolization-related neurologic complications **(III/B)**. Despite a lack of evidence, embolization for tumors that are anticipated to be vascular is widely accepted.

Minimally invasive surgery

Percutaneous procedures

Metastatic spine patients often suffer from comorbidities, malnourishment, a diminished immune system, considerable pain, and limited survival duration. Thoracic and lumbar ventral or combined approaches often involve organ mobilization and high operative bleeding risk, and are painful. Recent advances in visualization solutions have enabled the development of minimally invasive approaches for the treatment of spinal metastases.

Rosenthal *et al* have described the use of a thoracic endoscope for ventral thoracic corpectomies [82]. Huang *et al* retrospectively compared patients with metastatic tumors operated on by open thoracotomy to those operated on by thoracoscopy [83]. They reported equivalent results in surgical blood loss and operative time, outcomes at 1 and 2 years, neurologic improvement, and complications, but significantly shorter stays in the intensive care unit for patients in the thoracoscopy group **(III/B)**.

An endoscope can also be utilized in thoracic corpectomy via a unilateral dorsolateral approach for better visualization and resection of the contralateral side [84] **(III/B)**. Mini-abdominal approaches have been described to expose L2-S1 levels, and laparoscopic retroperitoneal approaches for the exposure of the thoracolumbar region [85]. However, these approaches are not widely used for metastatic disease **(IV/C)**.

Percutaneous pedicle screws have been introduced for fixation of the spine, either as an augmentation of a ventral approach or as a stand-alone procedure. Internal fixation using a dorsal minimal approach results in potentially better outcomes in terms of instability-related pain and fewer adverse events [86] **(III/B)**.

Vertebral augmentation

Pathologic fractures often occur in patients with metastatic involvement of the spine, causing pain, deformity, and occasionally neurologic compromise. Vertebroplasty is a percutaneous minimally invasive procedure performed by inserting a needle through the pedicle to the vertebral body and filling the fractured body with PMMA [87-89]. Kyphoplasty was introduced in the late 1990s and involves passing a balloon through a cannula and inflating it in the vertebral body in order to potentially restore vertebral height and to create a cavity in the vertebral body which will be filled by PMMA [88, 90].

Mendel *et al* reviewed the literature regarding vertebroplasty or kyphoplasty for spinal tumors [81]. Six level II papers and 22 level III papers were found. Both methods have resulted in substantial pain reduction, although radiologic and symptomatic cement leakage was higher in the vertebroplasty group. The authors recommended vertebral augmentation techniques in general for metastatic spine lesions, although no specific recommendation could be made regarding which of the two is superior **(IIb/B)**.

A meta-analysis comparing the procedures in non-pathologic fractures showed excellent pain control in both groups, with higher rates of cement leakage in the vertebroplasty group [91] **(IIa/B)**. Hentschel *et al* challenged the contraindications for vertebroplasty or kyphoplasty in metastatic patients and concluded that in this population, these procedures can be performed even in the presence of significant vertebral body collapse, epidural disease, and a fractured dorsal vertebral body, although the incidence of adverse events is higher [92] **(III/B)**.

Image guidance

Tumors tend to envelop the anatomic structures and distort them, making localization challenging. The use of anatomic landmarks alone for hardware placement is nearly impossible at times. Navigation systems are surgical adjuncts relaying preoperative or intraoperative imaging designed to assist the surgeon in the localization of three-dimensional structures. Use of navigation systems can potentially shorten the surgical time, reduce skin incision size and soft tissue resection, and result in higher tumor resection rates and more accurate hardware placement [93, 94] **(III/B)**.

As minimally invasive surgery is a technology-derived medical field, it is constantly advancing while the evidence lags behind. Moderate evidence supports the use of vertebral augmentation for painful pathologic vertebral fractures. Other procedures should be pursued based on the surgeon's experience and preference.

Stereotactic radiosurgery

Stereotactic radiosurgery (SRS) was developed and defined by the Swedish neurosurgeon Lars Leksell in 1951. At that time, Leksell sought to deliver high-dose photon energy to an intended target, while a steep fall-off dose gradient protected the adjacent brain [95]. The cranial anatomy is fixed in relation to the skull and can be immobilized relative to a reference frame. In contrast, movement is one of the spine's functions and temporary fixation is not a viable option. However, technological advancements in appropriate patient immobilization [96-98], radiation targeting, and precision delivery with image-guided radiation therapy [96, 99-101] and intensity-modulated radiation therapy [102, 103] have made extracranial radiosurgery feasible in recent years.

The most common indication for spine radiosurgery is pain. Typically, 70-90% of all patients treated present with localized tumor-related pain. Other indications for the procedure include:

◆ Initial tumor treatment, often for radioresistant histologies.

- Treatment after surgery for residual tumor (Figure 2).
- Local tumor progression after other treatment modalities such as surgery, conventional radiation, and chemotherapy have failed.

Several retrospective and prospective cohorts have reported that SRS results in a high rate of pain relief, with 85-92% of patients experiencing pain relief within a few days to weeks of treatment [99, 104-108] **(III/B)**. Spine radiosurgery allows for the delivery of 'ablative' radiation doses with minimal side effects and results in local control rates of 77-94% [105, 109-113] **(III/B)**. These studies included patients with tumors considered to be more radioresistant, such as colon or renal cell carcinoma [104-106, 114-117].

Gerszten *et al* reported a single-institution result for patients with spinal metastases treated by radiosurgery [106]. They reported 90% and 88% radiographic local tumor control for primary treated tumors and progressive tumors following conventional radiation, respectively. Long-term pain improvement was 86%, and 85% of patients presenting with neurologic deficit improved **(III/B)**.

Renal cell carcinoma is considered to be a radioresistant tumor, but the reported local control with SRS is 87.5% [105] **(III/B)**. In our series of 108 patients (154 treated targets), we prospectively evaluated the impact of treatment with spine radiosurgery on pain and quality of life. Pain scores were improved over baseline in 77% of patients

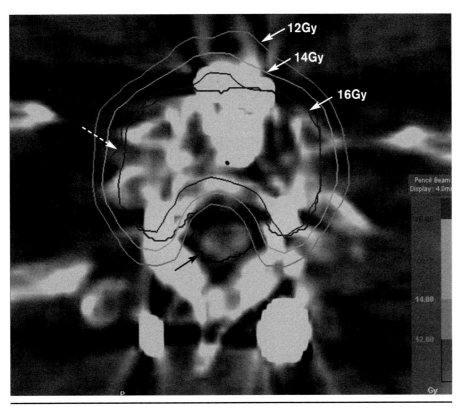

Figure 2. Postoperatively, the patient was treated with adjuvant stereotactic radiosurgery. The dotted white arrow indicates the ouline of the target region (clinical target volume) and the black arrow indicates the spinal cord. The other white arrows indicate the 16Gy prescription isodose line, the 14Gy isodose line, and the 12Gy dose fall-off region from the targeted tumor. At last follow-up (12 months), the patient had no evidence of tumor progression.

(p<0.001) as early as 1 week post-treatment, and at 12 months post-treatment 89% of patients had continued pain improvement (p<0.008) over baseline. Independent quality of life functional scores were also significantly improved relative to baseline at as early as 1 month post-treatment [107] **(III/B)**. The long-term local control rate was 87% (R Harel, L Angelov, unpublished data).

A review of the literature by Gerszten *et al* identified 29 SRS studies, all containing low-quality evidence [35]

(III/B). Pain reduction was reported in 85-100% of patients, neurologic recovery occurred in 57-92% of patients, and the local control rate was 75-100%. The authors compared these results with their review results of the literature regarding conventional radiation for spine metastases, and concluded that radiosurgery is superior in terms of pain control, local control, and neurologic function. The authors recommended treating patients with oligometastatic disease or radioresistant histologies with radiosurgery rather than conventional radiation **(III/B)**.

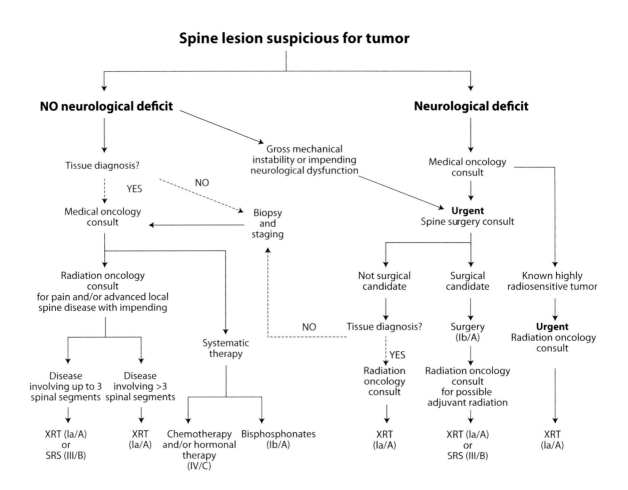

Figure 3. Proposed treatment algorithm for patients with spine lesions suspicious for a metastatic tumor. The presence or absence of neurologic deficits, tissue confirmation, and multidisciplinary integration are key features in the appropriate and effective management of these patients.

Rock et al reported on 18 patients treated with spine surgery followed by SRS, and concluded that radiosurgery for residual disease is an effective treatment for pain control and neurologic stabilization or improvement [115] **(III/B)**. In another series from our own institution by Harel et al, surgical patients receiving adjuvant SRS experienced no instrumentation failures and a 50% fusion rate at 6 months as compared with adjuvant conventional radiation therapy, where there was a 43% rate of instrument failure and a fusion rate of only 17% [118]. Gerszten et al reported the results of combined percutaneous vertebral augmentation techniques with SRS for painful pathologic fractures [119]. Eleven patients were enrolled in this retrospective study, which reported 100% pain relief and 100% local tumor control **(III/B)**.

As with any relatively new treatment modality, a high level of evidence for SRS is scarce and current recommendations are based on level III evidence. Definite treatment recommendations with SRS can be made for radioresistant spine metastases and tumors recurring after conventional radiation. SRS following surgery has a potential benefit in limiting radiation to the surrounding tissue, hence possibly reducing wound complications and increasing the fusion rate. Primary treatment of metastases probably results in better pain control and local control compared with conventional radiation.

Treatment algorithm

Guidelines for treating spinal metastases are not available, and treatment regimens vary widely according to the availability of treatment modalities, geographic variations dependent on health insurance coverage, medical costs, personnel, and religious beliefs. Treatment algorithms have been previously suggested [20, 120] **(IV/C)**. According to our experience and current evidence, we propose an algorithm outlining a general approach to spinal metastases. We

believe this algorithm could be implemented in any institution with spine surgery and irradiation capabilities (Figure 3). The proposed algorithm primarily delineates the treatment regimen according to the patient's neurologic status at presentation and outlines the specialty consultation and treatment recommended for a particular patient condition **(IV/C)**.

Conclusions

A high level of evidence supports the treatment of spinal metastases with the following modalities:

* Corticosteroids.
* Conventional radiation.
* Direct surgical decompression for radioresistant tumors or anticipated long-term survivors.
* Bisphosphonates.
* Vertebral augmentation for painful pathologic fractures.

Moderate and low-level evidence supports the following treatments:

* Direct surgical decompression for progressive disease following conventional radiation.
* Preoperative embolization for vascular metastases.
* Spine SRS for patients with radioresistant tumors, oligometastatic disease, and tumor progression.

There is no or very-low-quality evidence to support the following:

* Minimally invasive surgery for metastatic disease.
* Spinal SRS as primary treatment for radiosensitive histology.
* Recommendations regarding the choice of surgical approach or extent of resection.

Recommendations	Evidence level
◆ Metastatic spinal cord compression with neurologic deficits should be treated with corticosteroids.	Ia/A
◆ High-dose steroids for metastatic cord compression are associated with an increased complication rate and are not associated with better outcomes.	Ia/A
◆ Conventional radiation is effective for the treatment of spine metastases in terms of pain reduction, local control, and ambulatory rate.	Ia/A
◆ Short radiation therapy protocols are equivalent to long protocols in terms of pain control, but are associated with higher rates of pathologic fractures and re-treatment.	Ia/A
◆ Bisphosphonates reduce the rate of skeletal events but have no effect on survival.	Ia/A
◆ Radioisotope treatment is associated with significant pain reduction and severe adverse events.	Ia/A
◆ Direct surgical decompression as a primary treatment is more effective than radiation in patients with radioresistant tumors, oligometastatic disease, or long expected survival.	Ia/A
◆ Direct surgical decompression is beneficial for patients in whom radiation treatment has failed and those without a histologic diagnosis.	III/B
◆ No specific surgical approach or extent of resection has shown superior results.	III/B
◆ Preoperative embolization for vascular tumors reduces operative blood loss by more than 50% and is associated with a 4% rate of neurologic complications.	III/B
◆ Vertebral augmentation significantly reduces pathologic fracture-related pain.	Ib/A
◆ Vertebroplasty and kyphoplasty are equivalent in terms of pain control.	Ib/A
◆ Spine SRS is associated with better pain control and an improved local control rate when compared with conventional radiation.	III/B
◆ Spine SRS is beneficial for lesion progression following conventional radiation.	III/B

References

1. Winstead ER. After treatment: the needs of cancer survivors. *NCI Cancer Bulletin* 2005; 2(43): 1-2.
2. Hayat MJ, Howlader N, Reichman ME, Edwards BK. Cancer statistics, trends, and multiple primary cancer analyses from the Surveillance, Epidemiology, and End Results (SEER) Program. *Oncologist* 2007; 12(1): 20-37.
3. Jacobs WB, Perrin RG. Evaluation and treatment of spinal metastases: an overview. *Neurosurg Focus* 2001; 11(6): e10.
4. Wong DA, Fornasier VL, MacNab I. Spinal metastases: the obvious, the occult, and the impostors. *Spine* (Phila Pa 1976) 1990; 15(1): 1-4.
5. Heidecke V, Rainov NG, Burkert W. Results and outcome of neurosurgical treatment for extradural metastases in the cervical spine. *Acta Neurochir* (Wien) 2003; 145(10): 873-80; discussion 880-1.
6. Ibrahim A, Crockard A, Antonietti P, *et al.* Does spinal surgery improve the quality of life for those with extradural (spinal) osseous metastases? An international multicenter prospective observational study of 223 patients. Invited submission from the Joint Section Meeting on Disorders of the Spine and Peripheral Nerves, March 2007. *J Neurosurg Spine* 2008; 8(3): 271-8.
7. Patchell RA, Tibbs PA, Regine WF, *et al.* Direct decompressive surgical resection in the treatment of spinal cord compression caused by metastatic cancer: a randomised trial. *Lancet* 2005; 366(9486): 643-8.

8. Camins MB, Jenkins AL, Singhal A, Perrin RG. Tumors of the vertebral axis: benign, primary malignant, and metastatic tumors. In: *Youmans Neurological Surgery,* 5th ed. Winn RH, Youmans JR, Eds. Philadelphia: WB Saunders Company, 2004: 4835-68.

9. Steinmetz MP, Mekhail A, Benzel EC. Management of metastatic tumors of the spine: strategies and operative indications. *Neurosurg Focus* 2001; 11(6): e2.

10. Holman PJ, Suki D, McCutcheon I, Wolinsky JP, Rhines LD, Gokaslan ZL. Surgical management of metastatic disease of the lumbar spine: experience with 139 patients. *J Neurosurg Spine* 2005; 2(5): 550-63.

11. Schick U, Marquardt G, Lorenz R. Intradural and extradural spinal metastases. *Neurosurg Rev* 2001; 24(1): 1-5; discussion 6-7.

12. Perrin RG, Livingston KE, Aarabi B. Intradural extramedullary spinal metastasis. A report of 10 cases. *J Neurosurg* 1982; 56(6): 835-7.

13. Witham TF, Khavkin YA, Gallia GL, Wolinsky JP, Gokaslan ZL. Surgery insight: current management of epidural spinal cord compression from metastatic spine disease. *Nat Clin Pract Neurol* 2006; 2(2): 87-94.

14. Helweg-Larsen S, Sorensen PS. Symptoms and signs in metastatic spinal cord compression: a study of progression from first symptom until diagnosis in 153 patients. *Eur J Cancer* 1994; 30A(3): 396-8.

15. Perrin RG, Larsen BH, Rohde K, *et al*. Intradural extramedullary spinal cord compression. Occurrence, symptoms, clinical presentations and prognosis in 398 patients with spinal cord compression. *Acta Neurochir* (Wien) 1990; 107(1-2): 37-43.

16. Cardoso ER, Ashamalla H, Weng L, *et al*. Percutaneous tumor curettage and interstitial delivery of samarium-153 coupled with kyphoplasty for treatment of vertebral metastases. *J Neurosurg Spine* 2009; 10(4): 336-42.

17. Yang Z, Yang D, Xie L, *et al*. Treatment of metastatic spinal tumors by percutaneous vertebroplasty versus percutaneous vertebroplasty combined with interstitial implantation of 125I seeds. *Acta Radiol* 2009; 50(10): 1142-8.

18. Cole JS, Patchell RA. Metastatic epidural spinal cord compression. *Lancet Neurol* 2008; 7(5): 459-66.

19. Bartels RH, Feuth T, van der Maazen R, *et al*. Development of a model with which to predict the life expectancy of patients with spinal epidural metastasis. *Cancer* 2007; 110(9): 2042-9.

20. Bartels RH, van der Linden YM, van der Graaf WT. Spinal extradural metastasis: review of current treatment options. *CA Cancer J Clin* 2008; 58(4): 245-59.

21. van der Linden YM, Dijkstra SP, Vonk EJ, Marijnen CA, Leer JW. Prediction of survival in patients with metastases in the spinal column: results based on a randomized trial of radiotherapy. *Cancer* 2005; 103(2): 320-8.

22. Loblaw DA, Laperriere NJ, Mackillop WJ. A population-based study of malignant spinal cord compression in Ontario. *Clin Oncol* (R Coll Radiol) 2003; 15(4): 211-7.

23. Sorensen S, Helweg-Larsen S, Mouridsen H, Hansen HH. Effect of high-dose dexamethasone in carcinomatous metastatic spinal cord compression treated with radiotherapy: a randomised trial. *Eur J Cancer* 1994; 30A(1): 22-7.

24. Vecht CJ, Haaxma-Reiche H, van Putten WL, de Visser M, Vries EP, Twijnstra A. Initial bolus of conventional versus high-dose dexamethasone in metastatic spinal cord compression. *Neurology* 1989; 39(9): 1255-7.

25. George R, Jeba J, Ramkumar G, Chacko AG, Leng M, Tharyan P. Interventions for the treatment of metastatic extradural spinal cord compression in adults. *Cochrane Database Syst Rev* 2008; 4: CD006716.

26. Maranzano E, Latini P, Beneventi S, *et al*. Radiotherapy without steroids in selected metastatic spinal cord compression patients. A Phase II trial. *Am J Clin Oncol* 1996; 19(2): 179-83.

27. Stark RJ, Henson RA, Evans SJ. Spinal metastases. A retrospective survey from a general hospital. *Brain* 1982; 105(Pt 1): 189-213.

28. Sherman RM, Waddell JP. Laminectomy for metastatic epidural spinal cord tumors. Posterior stabilization, radiotherapy, and preoperative assessment. *Clin Orthop Relat Res* 1986; 207: 55-63.

29. Hirabayashi H, Ebara S, Kinoshita T, *et al*. Clinical outcome and survival after palliative surgery for spinal metastases: palliative surgery in spinal metastases. *Cancer* 2003; 97(2): 476-84.

30. Young RF, Post EM, King GA. Treatment of spinal epidural metastases. Randomized prospective comparison of laminectomy and radiotherapy. *J Neurosurg* 1980; 53(6): 741-8.

31. Helweg-Larsen S, Sorensen PS, Kreiner S. Prognostic factors in metastatic spinal cord compression: a prospective study using multivariate analysis of variables influencing survival and gait function in 153 patients. *Int J Radiat Oncol Biol Phys* 2000; 46(5): 1163-9.

32. Maranzano E, Latini P. Effectiveness of radiation therapy without surgery in metastatic spinal cord compression: final results from a prospective trial. *Int J Radiat Oncol Biol Phys* 1995; 32(4): 959-67.

33. Helweg-Larsen S. Clinical outcome in metastatic spinal cord compression. A prospective study of 153 patients. *Acta Neurol Scand* 1996; 94(4): 269-75.

34. Klimo P Jr, Thompson CJ, Kestle JR, Schmidt MH. A meta-analysis of surgery versus conventional radiotherapy for the treatment of metastatic spinal epidural disease. *Neuro Oncol* 2005; 7(1): 64-76.

35. Gerszten PC, Mendel E, Yamada Y. Radiotherapy and radiosurgery for metastatic spine disease: what are the options, indications, and outcomes? *Spine* (Phila Pa 1976) 2009; 34(22 Suppl.): S78-92.

36. Loblaw DA, Laperriere NJ. Emergency treatment of malignant extradural spinal cord compression: an evidence-based guideline. *J Clin Oncol* 1998; 16(4): 1613-24.

37. Chow E, Harris K, Fan G, Tsao M, Sze WM. Palliative radiotherapy trials for bone metastases: a systematic review. *J Clin Oncol* 2007; 25(11): 1423-36.

38. Rades D, Stalpers LJ, Veninga T, *et al*. 8 Gy single fraction radiotherapy for the treatment of five radiation schedules and

prognostic factors for metastatic skeletal pain: randomised comparison with a multifraction schedule over 12 months of patient follow-up. Bone Pain Trial Working Party. *Radiother Oncol* 1999; 52(15): 3366-75.

39. Rades D, Stalpers LJ, Veninga T, *et al*. Evaluation of five radiation schedules and prognostic factors for metastatic spinal cord compression. *J Clin Oncol* 2005; 23(15): 3366-75.

40. Maranzano E, Bellavita R, Rossi R, *et al*. Short-course versus split-course radiotherapy in metastatic spinal cord compression: results of a Phase III, randomized, multicenter trial. *J Clin Oncol* 2005; 23(15): 3358-65.

41. Maranzano E, Trippa F, Casale M, *et al*. 8 Gy single-dose radiotherapy is effective in metastatic spinal cord compression: results of a Phase III randomized multicentre Italian trial. *Radiother Oncol* 2009; 93(2): 174-9.

42. Sze WM, Shelley M, Held I, Mason M. Palliation of metastatic bone pain: single fraction versus multifraction radiotherapy - a systematic review of the randomised trials. *Cochrane Database Syst Rev* 2004; 2: CD004721.

43. Landreneau FE, Landreneau RJ, Keenan RJ, Ferson PF. Diagnosis and management of spinal metastases from breast cancer. *J Neurooncol* 1995; 23(2): 121-34.

44. Mercadante S, Fulfaro F. Management of painful bone metastases. *Curr Opin Oncol* 2007; 19(4): 308-14.

45. Costa L, Major PP. Effect of bisphosphonates on pain and quality of life in patients with bone metastases. *Nat Clin Pract Oncol* 2009; 6(3): 163-74.

46. Berenson JR, Rajdev L, Broder M. Managing bone complications of solid tumors. *Cancer Biol Ther* 2006; 5(9): 1086-9.

47. Heun JM, Jatoi A. Osseous metastases: drugs that enhance bone integrity and prevent adverse skeletal events. *Expert Opin Pharmacother* 2009; 10(5): 723-6.

48. Rosen LS, Gordon D, Tchekmedyian S, *et al*. Zoledronic acid versus placebo in the treatment of skeletal metastases in patients with lung cancer and other solid tumors: a Phase III, double-blind, randomized trial - the Zoledronic Acid Lung Cancer and Other Solid Tumors Study Group. *J Clin Oncol* 2003; 21(16): 3150-7.

49. Saad F, Gleason DM, Murray R, *et al*. A randomized, placebo-controlled trial of zoledronic acid in patients with hormone-refractory metastatic prostate carcinoma. *J Natl Cancer Inst* 2002; 94(19): 1458-68.

50. Theriault RL, Lipton A, Hortobagyi GN, *et al*. Pamidronate reduces skeletal morbidity in women with advanced breast cancer and lytic bone lesions: a randomized, placebo-controlled trial. Protocol 18 Aredia Breast Cancer Study Group. *J Clin Oncol* 1999; 17(3): 846-54.

51. Machado M, Cruz LS, Tannus G, Fonseca M. Efficacy of clodronate, pamidronate, and zoledronate in reducing morbidity and mortality in cancer patients with bone metastasis: a meta-analysis of randomized clinical trials. *Clin Ther* 2009; 31(5): 962-79.

52. Finlay IG, Mason MD, Shelley M. Radioisotopes for the palliation of metastatic bone cancer: a systematic review. *Lancet Oncol* 2005; 6(6): 392-400.

53. Bauman G, Charette M, Reid R, Sathya J. Radiopharmaceuticals for the palliation of painful bone metastasis - a systemic review. *Radiother Oncol* 2005; 75(3): 258-70.

54. Muller GP. III. Laminectomy for injury and tumor of the spinal cord: with a report of six cases. *Ann Surg* 1911; 53(6): 754-63.

55. Witham TF, Khavkin YA, Gallia GL, Wolinsky JP, Gokaslan ZL. Spinal metastases with neurological manifestations. Review of epidural spinal cord compression from metastatic spine disease. *Nat Clin Pract Neurol* 2006; 59(2): 87-94; quiz 116.

56. Tschirhart CE, Finkelstein JA, Whyne CM. Biomechanics of vertebral level, geometry, and transcortical tumors in the metastatic spine. *J Biomech* 2007; 40(1): 46-54.

57. Krishnaney AA, Steinmetz MP, Benzel EC. Biomechanics of metastatic spine cancer. *Neurosurg Clin N Am* 2004; 15(4): 375-80.

58. Dimar JR 2nd, Voor MJ, Zhang YM, Glassman SD. A human cadaver model for determination of pathologic fracture threshold resulting from tumorous destruction of the vertebral body. *Spine* (Phila Pa 1976) 1998; 23(11): 1209-14.

59. Harrington KD. Anterior cord decompression and spinal stabilization for patients with metastatic lesions of the spine. *J Neurosurg* 1984; 61(1): 107-17.

60. Constans JP, de Divitiis E, Donzelli R, Spaziante R, Meder JF, Haye C. Spinal metastases with neurological manifestations. Review of 600 cases. *J Neurosurg* 1983; 59(1): 111-8.

61. Patil CG, Patil TS, Lad SP, Boakye M. Complications and outcomes after spinal cord tumor resection in the United States from 1993 to 2002. *Spinal Cord* 2008; 46(5): 375-9.

62. Tomita K, Kawahara N, Kobayashi T, Yoshida A, Murakami H, Akamaru T. Surgical strategy for spinal metastases. *Spine* (Phila Pa 1976) 2001; 26(3): 298-306.

63. Siegal T, Siegal T. Surgical decompression of anterior and posterior malignant epidural tumors compressing the spinal cord: a prospective study. *Neurosurgery* 1985; 17(3): 424-32.

64. Thomas KC, Nosyk B, Fisher CG, *et al*. Cost-effectiveness of surgery plus radiotherapy versus radiotherapy alone for metastatic epidural spinal cord compression. *Int J Radiat Oncol Biol Phys* 2006; 66(4): 1212-8.

65. van den Bent MJ. Surgical resection improves outcome in metastatic epidural spinal cord compression. *Lancet* 2005; 366(9486): 609-10.

66. Maranzano E, Trippa F. Be careful in getting cost-effectiveness conclusions from a debatable trial! *Int J Radiat Oncol Biol Phys* 2007; 68(1): 314; author reply 314-5.

67. Vrionis FD, Small J. Surgical management of metastatic spinal neoplasms. *Neurosurg Focus* 2003; 15(5): E12.

68. Mazel C, Balabaud L, Bennis S, Hansen S. Cervical and thoracic spine tumor management: surgical indications, techniques, and outcomes. *Orthop Clin North Am* 2009; 40(1): 75-92, vi-vii.

69. Chi JH, Sciubba DM, Rhines LD, Gokaslan ZL. Surgery for primary vertebral tumors: *en bloc* versus intralesional resection. *Neurosurg Clin N Am* 2008; 19(1): 111-7.

70. Fehlings MG, David KS, Vialle L, Vialle E, Setzer M, Vrionis FD. Decision making in the surgical treatment of cervical spine metastases. *Spine* (Phila Pa 1976) 2009; 34(22 Suppl.): S108-17.

71. Jonsson B, Jonsson H Jr, Karlstrom G, Sjostrom L. Surgery of cervical spine metastases: a retrospective study. *Eur Spine J* 1994; 3(2): 76-83.

72. Liu JK, Apfelbaum RI, Chiles BW 3rd, Schmidt MH. Cervical spinal metastasis: anterior reconstruction and stabilization techniques after tumor resection. *Neurosurg Focus* 2003; 15(5): E2.

73. Di Martino A, Vincenzi B, Denaro L, *et al*. 'Internal bracing' surgery in the management of solid tumor metastases of the thoracic and lumbar spine. *Oncol Rep* 2009; 21(2): 431-5.

74. Alamin T, Mayle R. Lumbar tumor resections and management. *Orthop Clin North Am* 2009; 40(1): 93-104, vii.

75. Polly DW Jr, Chou D, Sembrano JN, Ledonio CG, Tomita K. An analysis of decision making and treatment in thoracolumbar metastases. *Spine* (Phila Pa 1976) 2009; 34(22 Suppl.): S118-27.

76. Sundaresan N, Choi IS, Hughes JE, Sachdev VP, Berenstein A. Treatment of spinal metastases from kidney cancer by presurgical embolization and resection. *J Neurosurg* 1990; 73(4): 548-54.

77. Berkefeld J, Scale D, Kirchner J, Heinrich T, Kollath J. Hypervascular spinal tumors: influence of the embolization technique on perioperative hemorrhage. *AJNR Am J Neuroradiol* 1999; 20(5): 757-63.

78. Rehak S, Krajina A, Ungermann L, *et al*. The role of embolization in radical surgery of renal cell carcinoma spinal metastases. *Acta Neurochir* (Wien) 2008; 150(11): 1177-81.

79. Gore P, Theodore N, Brasiliense L, *et al*. The utility of Onyx for preoperative embolization of cranial and spinal tumors. *Neurosurgery* 2008; 62(6): 1204-11; discussion 1211-2.

80. Guzman R, Dubach-Schwizer S, Heini P, *et al*. Preoperative transarterial embolization of vertebral metastases. *Eur Spine J* 2005; 14(3): 263-8.

81. Mendel E, Bourekas E, Gerszten P, Golan JD. Percutaneous techniques in the treatment of spine tumors: what are the diagnostic and therapeutic indications and outcomes? *Spine* (Phila Pa 1976) 2009; 34(22 Suppl.): S93-100.

82. Rosenthal D, Marquardt G, Lorenz R, Nichtweiss M. Anterior decompression and stabilization using a microsurgical endoscopic technique for metastatic tumors of the thoracic spine. *J Neurosurg* 1996; 84(4): 565-72.

83. Huang TJ, Hsu RW, Li YY, Cheng CC. Minimal access spinal surgery (MASS) in treating thoracic spine metastasis. *Spine* (Phila Pa 1976) 2006; 31(16): 1860-3.

84. McLain RF. Spinal cord decompression: an endoscopically assisted approach for metastatic tumors. *Spinal Cord* 2001; 39(9): 482-7.

85. Ofluoglu O. Minimally invasive management of spinal metastases. *Orthop Clin North Am* 2009; 40(1): 155-68, viii.

86. Logroscino CA, Proietti L, Tamburrelli FC. Minimally invasive spine stabilisation with long implants. *Eur Spine J* 2009; 18(Suppl. 1): 75-81.

87. Alvarez L, Perez-Higueras A, Quinones D, Calvo E, Rossi RE. Vertebroplasty in the treatment of vertebral tumors: postprocedural outcome and quality of life. *Eur Spine J* 2003; 12(4): 356-60.

88. Chi JH, Gokaslan ZL. Vertebroplasty and kyphoplasty for spinal metastases. *Curr Opin Support Palliat Care* 2008; 2(1): 9-13.

89. Pilitsis JG, Rengachary SS. The role of vertebroplasty in metastatic spinal disease. *Neurosurg Focus* 2001; 11(6): e9.

90. Khanna AJ, Neubauer P, Togawa D, Kay Reinhardt M, Lieberman IH. Kyphoplasty and vertebroplasty for the treatment of spinal metastases. *Support Cancer Ther* 2005; 3(1): 21-5.

91. Eck JC, Nachtigall D, Humphreys SC, Hodges SD. Comparison of vertebroplasty and balloon kyphoplasty for treatment of vertebral compression fractures: a meta-analysis of the literature. *Spine J* 2008; 8(3): 488-97.

92. Hentschel SJ, Burton AW, Fourney DR, Rhines LD, Mendel E. Percutaneous vertebroplasty and kyphoplasty performed at a cancer center: refuting proposed contraindications. *J Neurosurg Spine* 2005; 2(4): 436-40.

93. Haberland N, Ebmeier K, Hliscs R, *et al*. Neuronavigation in surgery of intracranial and spinal tumors. *J Cancer Res Clin Oncol* 2000; 126(9): 529-41.

94. Kalfas IH. Image-guided spinal navigation: application to spinal metastases. *Neurosurg Focus* 2001; 11(6): e5.

95. Barnett GH, Linskey ME, Adler JR, *et al*. Stereotactic radiosurgery - an organized neurosurgery-sanctioned definition. *J Neurosurg* 2007; 106(1): 1-5.

96. Yenice KM, Lovelock DM, Hunt MA, *et al*. CT image-guided intensity-modulated therapy for paraspinal tumors using stereotactic immobilization. *Int J Radiat Oncol Biol Phys* 2003; 55(3): 583-93.

97. Wulf J, Hadinger U, Oppitz U, Olshausen B, Flentje M. Stereotactic radiotherapy of extracranial targets: CT-simulation and accuracy of treatment in the stereotactic body frame. *Radiother Oncol* 2000; 57(2): 225-36.

98. Lohr F, Debus J, Frank C, *et al*. Noninvasive patient fixation for extracranial stereotactic radiotherapy. *Int J Radiat Oncol Biol Phys* 1999; 45(2): 521-7.

99. Ryu S, Fang Yin F, Rock J, *et al*. Image-guided and intensity-modulated radiosurgery for patients with spinal metastasis. *Cancer* 2003; 97(8): 2013-8.

100. Ryu SI, Chang SD, Kim DH, *et al*. Image-guided hypo-fractionated stereotactic radiosurgery to spinal lesions. *Neurosurgery* 2001; 49(4): 838-46.

101. Murphy MJ, Chang S, Gibbs I, Le QT, Martin D, Kim D. Image-guided radiosurgery in the treatment of spinal metastases. *Neurosurg Focus* 2001; 11(6): e6.

102. Das IJ, Cheng CW, Chopra KL, Mitra RK, Srivastava SP, Glatstein E. Intensity-modulated radiation therapy dose prescription, recording, and delivery: patterns of variability among institutions and treatment planning systems. *J Natl Cancer Inst* 2008; 100(5): 300-7.

103. Yu CX, Amies CJ, Svatos M. Planning and delivery of intensity-modulated radiation therapy. *Med Phys* 2008; 35(12): 5233-41.

104. Ryu S, Rock J, Rosenblum M, Kim JH. Patterns of failure after single-dose radiosurgery for spinal metastasis. *J Neurosurg* 2004; 101(Suppl. 3): 402-5.

105. Gerszten PC, Burton SA, Ozhasoglu C, *et al*. Stereotactic radiosurgery for spinal metastases from renal cell carcinoma. *J Neurosurg Spine* 2005; 3(4): 288-95.

106. Gerszten PC, Burton SA, Ozhasoglu C, Welch WC. Radiosurgery for spinal metastases: clinical experience in 500 cases from a single institution. *Spine* (Phila Pa 1976) 2007; 32(2): 193-9.

107. Angelov L. Stereotactic spine radiosurgery (SRS) for pain and tumor control in patients with spinal metastases from renal cell carcinoma: a prospective study. *Int J Radiation Oncol Biol Physics* 2009; 75(3): s112-3.

108. Amdur RJ, Bennett J, Olivier K, *et al*. A prospective, Phase II study demonstrating the potential value and limitation of radiosurgery for spine metastases. *Am J Clin Oncol* 2009; 32(5): 515-20.

109. Rock JP, Ryu S, Yin FF, Schreiber F, Abdulhak M. The evolving role of stereotactic radiosurgery and stereotactic radiation therapy for patients with spine tumors. *J Neurooncol* 2004; 69(1-3): 319-34.

110. Rock JP, Ryu S, Yin FF. Novalis radiosurgery for metastatic spine tumors. *Neurosurg Clin N Am* 2004; 15(4): 503-9.

111. Gerszten PC, Lunsford LD, Rutigliano MJ, Kondziolka D, Flickinger JC, Martinez AJ. Single-stage stereotactic diagnosis and radiosurgery: feasibility and cost implications. *J Image Guid Surg* 1995; 1(3): 141-50.

112. Gerszten PC, Welch WC. Cyberknife radiosurgery for metastatic spine tumors. *Neurosurg Clin N Am* 2004; 15(4): 491-501.

113. Gerszten PC, Burton SA, Welch WC, *et al*. Single-fraction radiosurgery for the treatment of spinal breast metastases. *Cancer* 2005; 104(10): 2244-54.

114. Chang EL, Shiu AS, Mendel E, *et al*. Phase I/II study of stereotactic body radiotherapy for spinal metastasis and its pattern of failure. *J Neurosurg Spine* 2007; 7(2): 151-60.

115. Rock JP, Ryu S, Shukairy MS, *et al*. Postoperative radiosurgery for malignant spinal tumors. *Neurosurgery* 2006; 58(5): 891-8.

116. Sahgal A, Chou D, Ames C, *et al*. Image-guided robotic stereotactic body radiotherapy for benign spinal tumors: the University of California San Francisco preliminary experience. *Technol Cancer Res Treat* 2007; 6(6): 595-604.

117. Yamada Y, Lovelock DM, Yenice KM, *et al*. Multifractionated image-guided and stereotactic intensity-modulated radiotherapy of paraspinal tumors: a preliminary report. *Int J Radiat Oncol Biol Phys* 2005; 62(1): 53-61.

118. Harel R, Chao S, Krishnaney A, *et al*. Spine instrumentation failure after spine tumor resection and radiation: comparing conventional radiotherapy with stereotactic radiosurgery outcomes. *World Neurosurg* 2010; 74(4-5): 517-22.

119. Gerszten PC, Monaco EA 3rd. Complete percutaneous treatment of vertebral body tumors causing spinal canal compromise using a transpedicular cavitation, cement augmentation, and radiosurgical technique. *Neurosurg Focus* 2009; 27(6): E9.

120. Cappuccio M, Gasbarrini A, Van Urk P, Bandiera S, Boriani S. Spinal metastasis: a retrospective study validating the treatment algorithm. *Eur Rev Med Pharmacol Sci* 2008; 12(3): 155-60.

Chapter 11

Motion-preservation strategies for the cervical spine

Jau-Ching Wu MD, Attending Surgeon 1, 2
Cheerag D Upadhyaya MD, Fellow, Spine Surgery 3
Praveen V Mummaneni MD, Associate Professor and Vice Chairman 3

1 DEPARTMENT OF NEUROSURGERY, NEUROLOGICAL INSTITUTE,
TAIPEI VETERANS GENERAL HOSPITAL, TAIWAN
2 SCHOOL OF MEDICINE, NATIONAL YANG-MING UNIVERSITY, TAIWAN
3 DEPARTMENT OF NEUROLOGICAL SURGERY, UNIVERSITY OF CALIFORNIA,
SAN FRANCISCO, CALIFORNIA, USA

Introduction

Anterior cervical discectomy and fusion (ACDF) has become the standard of care in the surgical treatment of cervical radiculopathy and myelopathy. One-level ACDF (with allograft and plating) has been demonstrated to have a 95% fusion rate and high patient satisfaction [1] **(III/B)**. Diminished range of cervical motion with an estimated loss of 7° of flexion/extension for each level of fusion is an inherent limitation of ACDF [2]. Cervical disc replacement technology has been developed with the goal of preserving motion while offering the same level of patient satisfaction. Furthermore, cervical arthroplasty may theoretically decrease the incidence of adjacent segment degeneration. Currently, cervical arthroplasty offers a treatment option for symptomatic cervical radiculopathy or myelopathy in selected patients.

Methodology

A systemic review of articles identified from a search of PubMed, the Cochrane Collaboration database, and the National Guideline Clearinghouse database from 1 October 2000 through 1 October 2011 was performed. Inclusion criteria were US Food and Drug Administration trials comparing cervical artificial disc replacement with ACDF, with a mean follow-up of more than 4 years. Exclusion criteria were non-Food and Drug Administration trials and studies with a follow-up of less than 4 years. The bibliographies were screened and the full text was reviewed for the final inclusion.

Background

Adjacent-level disease

Adjacent segment degeneration rostral and caudal to the level of fusion remains a clinical concern. In a biomechanical study, experimentally simulated C5-C6 fusion was associated with increased intradiscal pressures at both the superior and inferior adjacent segments [3]. Hilibrand et al conducted a study with 374 patients who had a total of 409 ACDF operations. Repeated surgical intervention was required in 2.9%

of patients per year for symptomatic adjacent segment disease [4] **(III/B)**. Furthermore, the authors predicted that 10 years after ACDF, 26% of patients would develop adjacent segment disease.

Goffin *et al* followed 180 patients after ACDF for more than 60 months, and found that adjacent segment degeneration occurred in 92% of patients [5] **(III/B)**. In addition, the severity of deterioration correlated with the time since surgery. No difference was found in the incidence of adjacent segment degeneration between patients undergoing ACDF for trauma versus degenerative disease [5]. This last finding suggests that adjacent segment degeneration is less likely to be secondary to natural history, but rather a consequence of altered cervical biomechanics after fusion. The natural history and actual incidence of adjacent segment disease remains uncertain [6-9].

Development of cervical disc replacement

Maintenance of cervical motion and the theoretical risk of adjacent segment degeneration drove the development of cervical arthroplasty as an alternative to spinal fusion after anterior cervical discectomy. Development of the artificial cervical disc began in the early 1990s in Europe. In 1998, Cummins *et al* reported on 20 patients implanted with an early model of an artificial cervical disc [10] **(III/B)**. Over the last decade, this model has evolved into the currently available PRESTIGE ST Cervical Disc System (Medtronic, Memphis, TN, USA) [6].

Prospective randomized trials for cervical arthroplasty

Three prospective randomized multicenter trials comparing artificial discs with ACDF in patients treated for single-level cervical degenerative disc disease have been published (Table 1) [2, 11-13]. Each of these US Food and Drug Administration Investigational Device Exception studies used a non-inferiority design with 1:1 randomization and a reported follow-up duration of up to 24 months.

Enrollment and demographics

The PRESTIGE ST trial enrolled 276 investigational (arthroplasty) patients and 265 control (ACDF) patients [2]. The Bryan (Medtronic) trial enrolled 242 investigational and 221 control patients [12]. Finally, the ProDisc-C (Synthes Spine, Westchester, PA, USA) trial recruited 103 investigational and 106 control patients [13]. All studies reported 24 months of follow-up. Age, sex, and working status were similar between the investigational and control groups in all three trials.

Functional outcomes

The Neck Disability Index (NDI), Short Form-36 (SF-36), and a Visual Analogue Scale (VAS) of neck and arm pain were used as outcome measurements in all three trials. Measurements were obtained pretreatment as well as at multiple post-treatment time points.

Neck Disability Index

NDI scores improved at all follow-up time points in all three trials in both investigational and control groups, implying that both cervical arthroplasty and ACDF are effective treatments for cervical degenerative disc disease. In the PRESTIGE ST trial, the NDI scores improved markedly at 12 and 24 months [2]. Patients in the investigational group had a mean improvement in NDI score of at least 2 points greater than the control group. The difference in NDI score significantly favored the investigational group at 1.5 months and 3 months of follow-up **(Ib/A)**. Furthermore, the percentage of patients experiencing more than 15 points of improvement from baseline was greater in the investigational group at each point in the follow-up.

Statistically significant reductions in NDI scores were noted in the investigational and control groups in the Bryan study at all follow-up time points [12]. In addition, significantly greater improvements in NDI scores were found in the investigational arm at all intervals. The NDI success rate – the proportion of

Table 1. Prospective randomized trials for cervical arthroplasty. *Continued overleaf.*

Author	Description	n	Device	Results	Conclusions	Evidence level/ recommendation
Mummaneni *et al*, 2007 [2]	541 patients (32 centers), prospective, randomized One-level arthroplasty (n=276) vs. one-level ACDF (n=265) Follow-up to 24 months	541	PRESTIGE ST	At 12 and 24 months: 2-point greater improvement in the NDI score, higher rate of neurologic success, lower rate of revision surgery and supplemental fixation, greater mean improvement in SF-36, and relief of neck pain in the investigational group Patients returned to work 16 days sooner, and the rate of adjacent-segment reoperation was significantly lower in the investigational group The cervical disc implant maintained segmental sagittal angular motion averaging >7° No cases of implant failure or migration in the investigational group	PRESTIGE ST maintained physiological segmental motion at 24 months after implantation and was associated with improved neurologic success and clinical outcomes, and a reduced rate of secondary surgeries compared with ACDF	Ib/A
Heller *et al*, 2009 [12]	Prospective, randomized, multicenter study One-level arthroplasty (n=242) vs. one-level ACDF (n=221) Follow-up to 24 months	463	Bryan	Analysis of 12- and 24-month data showed improvement in all clinical outcome measures for both groups; however, 24 months after surgery, the investigational group had a statistically greater improvement in the primary outcome variables: NDI score and overall success The rate of implant-related serious adverse events was 1.7% in the investigational group and 3.2% in the control group There was no statistical difference between the two groups with regard to the rate of secondary surgical procedures performed subsequent to the index procedure Patients who received the artificial cervical disc returned to work nearly 2 weeks earlier than fusion patients (p=0.015)	Two-year follow-up results indicate that cervical disc arthroplasty is a viable alternative to anterior cervical discectomy and fusion in patients with persistently symptomatic, single-level cervical disc disease	Ib/A

Chapter 11

Table 1. Prospective randomized trials for cervical arthroplasty. *Continued.*

Author	Description	n	Device	Results	Conclusions	Evidence level/recommendation
Murrey *et al*, 2009 [13]	Prospective, randomized, multicenter study (13 centers) ProDisc-C (n=103) vs. ACDF (n=106) Follow-up to 24 months	209	ProDisc-C	NDI, SF-36, VAS neck pain, and VAS arm were statistically lower at all follow-up time points compared with preoperative levels, but were not different between treatments Neurologic success also showed no difference At 24 months postoperatively, 84.4% of ProDisc-C patients achieved ≥4° of motion or maintained motion relative to preoperative baseline levels In the 24-month postoperative period, 8.5% of fusion patients needed reoperation, revision, or supplemental fixation vs. 1.8% of ProDisc-C patients (p=0.033). At 24 months, 89.9% of ProDisc-C patients were not on strong narcotics or muscle relaxants vs. 81.5% of fusion patients (statistically significant)	ProDisc-C is a safe and effective surgical treatment for patients with disabling cervical radiculopathy because of single-level disease By all primary and secondary measures evaluated, clinical outcomes after ProDisc-C implantation were either equivalent or superior to those after fusion	Ib/A

ACDF = anterior cervical discectomy and fusion; NDI = Neck Disability Index; SF = Short Form; VAS = Visual Analogue Scale

patients with more than 15 points of improvement – was statistically higher in the investigational group at all points of follow-up **(Ib/A)**.

Both the investigational and control groups in the ProDisc-C study exhibited significant improvements in NDI scores at all points of follow-up [13]. The ProDisc-C group had a statistically significant greater improvement in NDI score at 3 months of follow-up, but the difference was no longer statistically significant at 24 months of follow-up. In addition, the NDI success rate was not statistically significant at 24 months **(Ib/A)**.

In summary, at 24 months of follow-up, the Bryan study demonstrated a significantly greater improvement in NDI scores in the investigational arm [12]. The

PRESTIGE-ST and ProDisc-C trials did not demonstrate significant differences in NDI scores between the investigational and control groups at 24 months of follow-up **(Ib/A)**.

Short Form-36

In all three trials and at all points of follow-up, SF-36 scores were significantly improved versus baseline in both the investigational and control groups. The PRESTIGE ST trial did not demonstrate a statistically significant difference between the investigational and control groups in either the physical component summary (PCS) or mental component summary (MCS) measures at 12 and 24 months [2]. In the Bryan study, both the PCS and MCS measures were

Chapter 11

significantly improved at 1.5 and 12 months of follow-up, but this difference was lost at 24 months [12]. Similarly, there was a statistically significant improvement in SF-36 scores in the ProDisc-C group at 1.5 and 3 months of follow-up, but this difference was lost at 24 months [13] **(Ib/A)**.

Visual Analogue Scale

VAS neck pain improved significantly compared with baseline in both the investigational and control groups in all three trials. In the Bryan study, there was a significant improvement in VAS neck pain in the investigational group versus the control group at all follow-up time points. The PRESTIGE ST study demonstrated a statistically significant difference between the groups at 12 months, but significance was lost at 24 months. The ProDisc-C study also statistically favored the investigational arm at 3 months, but this difference was lost at all subsequent points of follow-up.

VAS arm pain also improved significantly compared with baseline in both the investigational and control groups in all three trials. The Bryan study demonstrated a statistically significant difference between the investigational and control groups at 12 months of follow-up. Otherwise, there were no statistically significant differences in VAS arm pain between the groups in the trials [2, 12, 13] **(Ib/A)**.

Adverse events

Adverse events were defined as events associated with the implant or its implantation, including both medical and surgical complications. There were no significant differences in the rate of adverse events between the investigational and control groups in any of the three trials **(Ib/A)**.

Secondary surgical procedures

All trials recorded secondary surgical procedures. These surgeries included revision operations, hardware removal, supplemental fixations, and reoperations. A revision surgery was defined as any

procedure in which the original implant was adjusted or modified.

In the PRESTIGE ST trial, 1.9% of patients in the control group and no patients in the investigation arm had undergone revision at 2 years. Supplemental fixation occurred in 3.4% of patients in the control group and none in the arthroplasty group. The difference in both revision and supplemental fixation was statistically significant. Three percent of control patients experienced graft failure or migration, while there were no cases of hardware failure or migration in the arthroplasty group. Implant removal was necessary in 3.4% of patients in the control group and 1.8% in the investigational group (not statistically significant). Arthroplasty removal was due to persistent postoperative radiculopathy and revised with an ACDF [2] **(Ib/A)**.

In the Bryan study, secondary surgical procedures were performed in 3.6% of ACDF patients (three removals, one reoperation, and four supplemental fixations) and 2.5% of arthroplasty patients (three removals, two reoperations, and one revision). There was no significant difference between the control and investigational groups [12] **(Ib/A)**.

The ProDisc-C study demonstrated an 8.5% rate of secondary surgical procedures in the control group (five revisions, one reoperation, and three supplemental fixations) compared with 1.9% in the arthroplasty group (two removals). This difference was significantly different, favoring the arthroplasty group [13] **(Ib/A)**.

Adjacent-level disease

Adjacent-level disease is defined as degeneration of the intervertebral discs adjacent to the index level. It varies in severity from an asymptomatic radiographic finding to severe radiculopathy with neurologic deficit. In the three trials, adjacent-level disease was defined as requiring further surgical intervention at adjacent levels.

The PRESTIGE ST study noted 11 additional operations for 12 levels of adjacent-level disease in nine patients in the ACDF group. Three patients in the arthroplasty group underwent three operations for

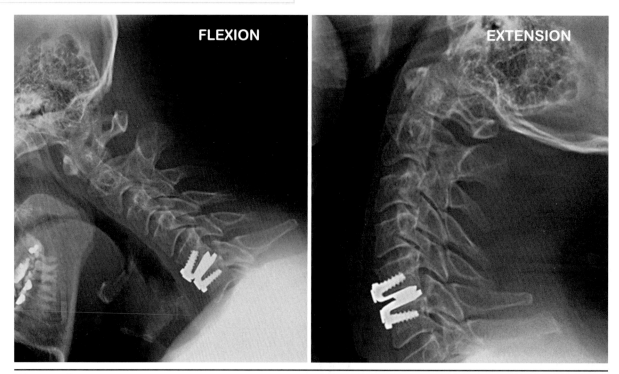

Figure 1. Flexion and extension with the PRESTIGE ST Cervical Disc System.

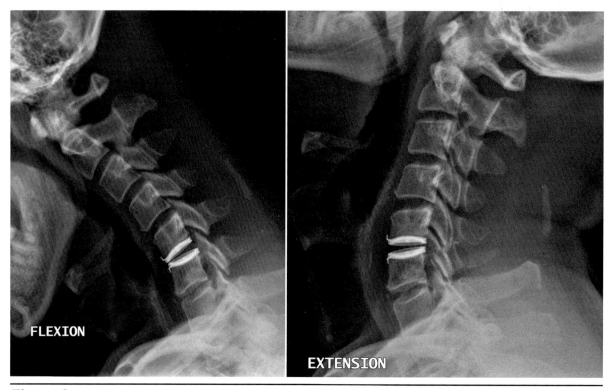

Figure 2. Flexion and extension with Bryan cervical disc arthroplasty.

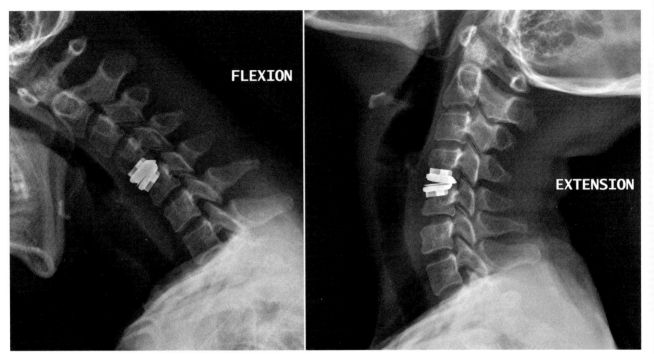

Figure 3. Flexion and extension with ProDisc-C.

three levels. This difference was significantly different at 24 months [2] **(Ib/A)**. In the ProDisc-C group, one additional surgery was performed for adjacent-level disease in the ACDF group, but none in the arthroplasty group [13] **(Ib/A)**.

The incidence of adjacent-level disease was relatively small in these clinical trials. Furthermore, 24 months of follow-up is insufficient to determine if arthroplasty will significantly decrease the incidence of adjacent-level disease. Follow-up studies with greater time spans will be necessary to better resolve this important issue.

Radiographic outcomes

Plain radiographic studies were obtained preoperatively, intraoperatively, and postoperatively for comparison in the clinical studies. Neutral and dynamic lateral flexion-extension radiographs were used to evaluate the segmental motion of the cervical spine as well as device function (Figures 1-3).

In the PRESTIGE ST study, there were no cases of implant failure, migration, or subsidence in the study

group, and one case of ectopic ossification. The investigational group demonstrated a mean angular motion of 7.55° preoperatively and 7.59° at 12 and 24 months postoperatively. Cervical arthroplasty successfully maintained physiological segmental motion at the index level [2] **(Ib/A)**. A fusion rate of 97.5% was observed in the control group at 24 months **(Ib/A)**.

In the Bryan study, the mean range of motion in the arthroplasty group was 6.5° preoperatively and 8.1° ± 4.8° postoperatively at 24 months of follow-up. The ACDF group had a fusion rate of 94.3%. Again, cervical arthroplasty successfully maintained segmental motion after 24 months [12] **(Ib/A)**.

In the ProDisc-C study, the average range of motion in the arthroplasty group was 9.36° at 24 months. Overall, 84.4% of arthroplasty patients maintained segmental motion [13] **(Ib/A)**. Three arthroplasty patients (2.9%) developed ectopic ossification and consequently autofused the index segment. The centers that routinely utilized non-steroidal anti-inflammatory medications had a minimal incidence of ectopic ossification.

Conclusions

The best currently available evidence in the literature suggests that both cervical arthroplasty and ACDF are safe and effective for treating single-level degenerative disc disease at 24 months of follow-up **(Ib/A)**. Further investigation with longer follow-up will be necessary to determine if arthroplasty decreases adjacent-level disease.

Recommendations	Evidence level
◆ At 24 months of follow-up, both cervical arthroplasty and ACDF demonstrated similarly excellent clinical results for the treatment of one-level cervical degenerative disc disease.	Ib/A
◆ Cervical arthroplasty preserves the range of motion at the index level at 24-month follow-up in over 90% of patients.	Ib/A
◆ The effect of cervical arthroplasty on adjacent level disease remains uncertain at 24-month follow-up.	Ib/A

References

1. Mummaneni PV, Haid RW. The future in the care of the cervical spine: interbody fusion and arthroplasty. Invited submission from the Joint Section Meeting on Disorders of the Spine and Peripheral Nerves, March 2004. *J Neurosurg Spine* 2004; 1(2): 155-9.

2. Mummaneni PV, Burkus JK, Haid RW, Traynelis VC, Zdeblick TA. Clinical and radiographic analysis of cervical disc arthroplasty compared with allograft fusion: a randomized controlled clinical trial. *J Neurosurg Spine* 2007; 6(3): 198-209.

3. Eck JC, Humphreys SC, Lim TH, *et al*. Biomechanical study on the effect of cervical spine fusion on adjacent-level intradiscal pressure and segmental motion. *Spine* (Phila Pa 1976) 2002; 27(22): 2431-4.

4. Hilibrand AS, Carlson GD, Palumbo MA, Jones PK, Bohlman HH. Radiculopathy and myelopathy at segments adjacent to the site of a previous anterior cervical arthrodesis. *J Bone Joint Surg Am* 1999; 81(4): 519-28.

5. Goffin J, Geusens E, Vantomme N, *et al*. Long-term follow-up after interbody fusion of the cervical spine. *J Spinal Disord Tech* 2004; 17(2): 79-85.

6. DiAngelo DJ, Roberston JT, Metcalf NH, McVay BJ, Davis RC. Biomechanical testing of an artificial cervical joint and an anterior cervical plate. *J Spinal Disord Tech* 2003; 16(4): 314-23.

7. Dohler JR, Kahn MR, Hughes SP. Instability of the cervical spine after anterior interbody fusion. A study on its incidence and clinical significance in 21 patients. *Arch Orthop Trauma Surg* 1985; 104(4): 247-50.

8. Rihn JA, Lawrence J, Gates C, Harris E, Hilibrand AS. Adjacent segment disease after cervical spine fusion. *Instr Course Lect* 2009; 58: 747-56.

9. Javedan SP, Dickman CA. Cause of adjacent-segment disease after spinal fusion. *Lancet* 1999; 354(9178): 530-1.

10. Cummins BH, Robertson JT, Gill SS. Surgical experience with an implanted artificial cervical joint. *J Neurosurg* 1998; 88(6): 943-8.

11. Mummaneni PV, Robinson JC, Haid RW Jr. Cervical arthroplasty with the PRESTIGE LP cervical disc. *Neurosurgery* 2007; 60(4 Suppl. 2): 310-14; discussion 314-15.

12. Heller JG, Sasso RC, Papadopoulos SM, *et al*. Comparison of Bryan cervical disc arthroplasty with anterior cervical decompression and fusion: clinical and radiographic results of a randomized, controlled, clinical trial. *Spine* (Phila Pa 1976) 2009; 34(2): 101-7.

13. Murrey D, Janssen M, Delamarter R, *et al*. Results of the prospective, randomized, controlled multicenter Food and Drug Administration investigational device exemption study of the ProDisc-C total disc replacement versus anterior discectomy and fusion for the treatment of 1-level symptomatic cervical disc disease. *Spine J* 2009; 9(4): 275-86.

Introduction

Functional neurosurgery

Kenneth P Vives MD, Associate Professor;
Chief of Stereotactic and Functional Neurosurgery
Dennis D Spencer MD, Harvey and Kate Cushing Professor of
Neurosurgery; Chairman, Department of Neurosurgery

DEPARTMENT OF NEUROSURGERY, YALE UNIVERSITY, NEW HAVEN, CONNECTICUT, USA

The evolution of functional neurosurgery is very similar to that of other aspects of neurosurgery. A combination of pure serendipity and thoughtful experimentation has resulted in the set of procedures available to functional neurosurgeons today. The early pioneers of this field were often both courageous and fiercely intuitively intelligent as they applied keen observation of patients and their syndromes to the development of novel procedures to affect and enhance the function of the brain and positively impact patient's lives. Some of these procedures have evolved and been looked at through the lens of evidence-based medicine. Many have not.

The following chapters provide a necessary pause for reflection upon the procedures that these early pioneers made available to us. Many of the diseases that functional neurosurgeons treat are chronic and not immediately life-threatening. This heightens the need to ensure that the treatments being provided are safe and effective. Specifically in areas of the treatment of epilepsy, movement disorders, and psychiatric disorders, we hope to provide an overview of the rationale for the surgical treatments that are currently offered to patients and a needed critique of the evidence utilized to do so.

The surgical treatment of epilepsy is usefully divided into the treatment of temporal and extratemporal epilepsy, and then into the treatment of patients with identifiable anatomic lesions and those without. These boundaries are recognized as artificial, with significant overlap; however, the quality and amount of published evidence for the use of these treatments divides itself along these lines. Temporal lobectomy, lesionectomy, and extratemporal lobar resections are resective techniques that deserve consideration. Functional hemispherectomy, callosotomy, and multiple subpial transections can be utilized to modify the spread of seizures. We also briefly survey the use of newer therapies based upon electrical stimulation to ameliorate seizures.

Deep brain stimulation (DBS) represents one area where government regulation has helped medicine focus on obtaining quality information in order to ensure a technique is safe and effective. A natural modernization of the lesioning techniques utilized by early pioneers, DBS holds the promise of reversibility and tunability. These features can be incredibly useful in the treatment of conditions such as Parkinson's disease, where the natural history predicts that therapy will need to change as the patient's disease advances. In the process of bringing devices to market for DBS, a significant amount of evidence has been accumulated to demonstrate the technique's effectiveness for Parkinson's disease and essential tremor. Ongoing trials and humanitarian device exemptions will hopefully provide similar evidence for the use of DBS as treatment for dystonia, obsessive compulsive disorder, and depression. Beyond these initial conditions, there may well be limitless other indications for the use of DBS to modify and enhance the function of the human brain.

In some of these areas the evidence is substantial; in others, it is lacking. For some of the procedures currently in use, it is recognized that the double-blind randomized controlled trial that would definitively establish the procedure as being safe and effective will never be performed. Often, the patients are too few and too heterogeneous. Likewise, their treatments are often heterogeneous and change over time. The diseases and their medical treatments are also moving targets, and the needed length of time for useful outcomes' studies is prohibitive. However, it remains useful to critically look at the evidence that exists in the hope that we can glean a light to help lead us forward in an evidence-based manner.

Chapter 12

Temporal lobectomy for mesial temporal sclerosis

Alexander M Papanastassiou MD

Assistant Professor of Neurosurgery 1

Kenneth P Vives MD

Associate Professor; Chief of Stereotactic and Functional Neurosurgery 2

Dennis D Spencer MD, Harvey and Kate Cushing Professor of Neurosurgery;

Chairman, Department of Neurosurgery 2

1 UNIVERSITY OF TEXAS HEALTH SCIENCE CENTER, SAN ANTONIO, TEXAS, USA
2 DEPARTMENT OF NEUROSURGERY, YALE UNIVERSITY,
NEW HAVEN, CONNECTICUT, USA

Introduction

Epilepsy has a prevalence of approximately five per 1,000 people worldwide and is refractory to medical treatment in approximately one-third of patients [1, 2]. Mesial temporal sclerosis (MTS) is a common cause of temporal lobe epilepsy, and is amenable to surgical therapy. Figure 1 shows right-sided MTS in a coronal slice of a T2-weighted image of the brain. If preoperative evaluation of the patient using seizure semiology, ictal EEG, MRI findings, and functional imaging gives concordant data then surgery without invasive recording is indicated. A variety of approaches have been developed for treating MTS, often in the context of the broader category of temporal lobe epilepsy (TLE). This chapter reviews the evidence supporting the various operations.

Methodology

A National Library of Medicine computerized PubMed/MEDLINE literature search from January 1966 through February 2010 was performed with the

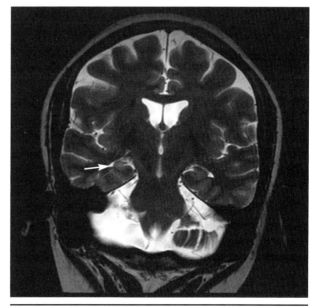

Figure 1. Right-sided mesial temporal sclerosis in a coronal slice of a T2-weighted image of the brain. The right hippocampus (arrow) is atrophic with an increased T2 signal.

medical subject heading 'epilepsy, temporal lobe/surgery,' resulting in 2,252 abstracts for review. The titles of the abstracts were reviewed, and articles on the subject of temporal lobectomy for MTS were included. The bibliographies of selected papers were reviewed to identify related articles. The Cochrane database was searched without identifying additional articles.

Standard temporal lobectomy

There is one study providing class I evidence supporting standard temporal lobectomy in comparison with best medical management for patients with MTS [3] (Ib/A). This study is summarized and commented upon in detail because it is the highest quality study regarding the surgical management of MTS, resulting in a grade A recommendation for this procedure.

At 1 year, 58% of patients with medically refractory TLE undergoing a standard temporal lobe resection were seizure-free, compared with 8% of patients undergoing continued medical therapy (Ib/A). Complications in the surgical group included one patient with a small thalamic infarct resulting in sensory abnormalities in the left thigh; one patient with wound infection; and two patients with a decline in verbal memory that interfered with their occupations. There was one death in the medical group, consistent with expected mortality in medically refractory epilepsy.

This study included 80 patients with TLE. Eligible patients were aged at least 16 years and had had seizures with strong temporal lobe semiology for more than 1 year. The seizures had to have occurred monthly, on average, during the year prior to randomization, despite treatment with two or more anticonvulsant drugs, one of which was phenytoin, carbamazepine, or valproic acid. Exclusion criteria included brain lesions that required urgent surgery; evidence on MRI of extratemporal lesions capable of producing the patient's seizures or of bilateral, and equally severe, epileptogenic lesions in the temporal lobe; focal extratemporal spikes or slowing on scalp-recorded EEG; progressive central nervous system disorders; active psychosis; pseudoseizures; a full-scale IQ of less than 70; and previous surgery for epilepsy.

Because patients were selected based on their semiology rather than MRI criteria, this study addressed temporal lobe epilepsy rather than MTS in particular. Nonetheless, of the study population, 71.3% showed MTS on MRI, while 16.3% had normal MRIs and 12.5% were lesional. Of the 40 patients randomly assigned to surgery, six patients had recordings from subdural electrodes to lateralize and localize the region of onset, and four patients (10%) did not undergo surgery. One patient declined surgery, two were not deemed eligible for surgery because the results of the EEG, MRI, and neuropsychological tests were non-concordant, and one did not have seizures during inpatient investigations. Therefore, of the 40 patients assigned to surgery, 30 were presumed to have TLE due to MTS and underwent a temporal lobe resection, although pathological confirmation was not reported. The outcome results were not stratified by pathological substrate, and were consistent with expected rates of seizure freedom in an unselected group of TLE patients including both mesial TLE (MTLE) and non-lesional cases.

The operation used in the study was a standard temporal lobectomy performed by three surgeons. The lateral neocortical resection included 4.0-4.5cm on the dominant side and 6.0-6.5cm on the non-dominant side. The superior temporal gyrus (STG) was resected on both sides. The medial resection included the amygdala and most commonly 4cm of hippocampus, but sometimes a minimum of 1.0-3.0cm of hippocampus. A total of 24 patients had operations on the left side of the temporal lobe, and 12 had operations on the right side.

A standard protocol was used for neuropsychological outcomes but not reported in detail. Patients with poor memory function bilaterally or on the side opposite that of the origin of the seizure underwent bilateral intracarotid amobarbital sodium tests. Patients with adequate memory on the side of the origin of the seizure and poor memory function on the contralateral side did not have surgery. In our experience, dominant-sided resections can only be performed safely in patients with verbal memory scores that are two standard deviations below normal and with adequate (≥2/10) non-dominant support of memory on intracarotid amobarbital testing. A resection of the medial structures on the dominant side in a patient will otherwise lead to a clinically significant decline in verbal memory scores. It is not known if application of this decision-making approach would have prevented resections in the two patients in this study who experienced a significant decline in verbal memory scores.

The proportion of patients with various extents of medial resection was not reported, so no conclusions can be drawn on the importance of resection of the medial structures. Depending on the number of patients undergoing medial resections of 1.0-3.0cm of hippocampus, it is possible that this variation contributed to the somewhat lower rate of seizure freedom than may be expected in this population.

The above findings are strongly supported by the prospective Multicenter Study of Epilepsy Surgery [4]. Among patients who had undergone mesial temporal resections, 77% of 312 patients were seizure-free for a 1-year period during initial follow-up (1-5 years), and 68% of 297 patients were seizure-free for a 2-year period during long-term follow-up (2-7.3 years). The higher rates of seizure freedom may be due to different patient characteristics, such as the proportion of MTLE patients in each study, or differences in the surgical approach, although the medial temporal resection in the Multicenter Study was not standardized.

Extent of medial resection

Based on depth electrode recordings from medial temporal structures and historical evidence regarding the pathology of MTS, in the late 1970s and early 1980s surgeons began to perform radical resection of medial temporal lobe structures, including the amygdala, hippocampus, and parahippocampus while sparing the lateral temporal neocortex, except for the pole. However, epilepsy surgeons still debate the optimal extent of medial resection for treating MTS.

Supporting radical resection of the medial temporal lobe structures is one prospective, double-blind,

randomized controlled trial [5] **(Ib/A)**. In this study, 70 patients with MTLE defined by intracranial subdural strip electrode recordings were randomized to partial hippocampectomy to the anterior margin of the cerebral peduncle or total hippocampectomy to the superior colliculus. Lateral neocortical resection included the STG, middle temporal gyrus, and inferior temporal gyrus 4.5cm from the temporal pole for both dominant and non-dominant surgeries. Partial hippocampectomy led to freedom from seizures and auras in 38.2% of patients, while total hippocampectomy was associated with freedom from seizures and auras in 69.4% of patients (p=0.009). No difference in neuropsychological outcome between the groups was detected **(Ib/A)**.

This study strongly supports complete resection of the medial temporal structures **(Ib/A)**. One limiting factor is that patients who had only auras were not separated from those with complex partial seizures or generalized seizures. Another criticism raised by some is the lack of confirmation of resection with postoperative MRI. In some studies, intended resection varies from actual resection [6].

A prior prospective non-randomized study of temporal lobectomy in TLE patients along with a follow-up study by the same group support the importance of the extent of resection in medial temporal regions in particular. Both medial and lateral components of resections were variable and had been tailored based on seizure-onset and functional data [6]. Additional recent studies also support this finding [7, 8] **(III/B)**.

Results from prior non-randomized, retrospective studies may be interpreted as showing similar or decreased rates of seizure freedom with variable or partial resection of the medial structures [9] **(III/B)**. However, this evidence is of lower quality than the randomized controlled trial by Wyler *et al* [5] and does not alter our interpretation of the data – that complete resection of the mesial structures is preferable in standard resections.

Electrocorticography (ECoG) has also been used to determine how much of the hippocampus should be resected. In a prospective series, 140 consecutive TLE patients underwent ECoG-guided hippocampal resection. The class I seizure outcomes experienced by this group, measured as 0-1 seizures including auras, was independent of extent of resection [10] **(IIb/B)**. In this group, 38 patients underwent a resection of less than 2.5cm of the hippocampus measured from the uncal recess; of these, 66-69% had class I outcomes, compared with 68% of the 102 patients who underwent resection of 2.5cm or more. In an earlier series of 14 patients who underwent this approach, verbal memory decline was related to the lateral but not the medial extent of the resection [11]. Similar results using ECoG to guide medial resection have been obtained in retrospective case series [12]. These studies show similar rates of seizure freedom to the studies of standard temporal lobectomy in TLE patients described above. The results of McKhann *et al* cannot be compared directly with the randomized controlled trial of Wyler *et al* described above because McKhann *et al* employed ECoG to guide hippocampal resection, and included all TLE patients rather than MTLE patients alone [10]. In contrast, Wyler *et al* randomly assigned MTLE patients to partial or complete hippocampal resection [5]. Although the level of evidence supporting ECoG-guided resection of medial structures is lower than that supporting complete resection of medial structures, the similar rates of success in obtaining seizure freedom using an ECoG-guided approach make this another option for the treatment of TLE.

If complete resection of the medial temporal lobe structures is critical for curing MTS then MTLE patients who have undergone a partial hippocampectomy should achieve seizure freedom with completion of the hippocampectomy at rates similar to MTLE patients undergoing first-time complete hippocampectomy. Studies have not addressed this question specifically, but a review of retrospective case series showed approximate rates of seizure freedom of 30-57% in this setting [13] **(III/B)**. The somewhat lower rate of seizure freedom after resection of residual structures appears to be due to the presence of neocortical, contralateral medial temporal, or other seizure-onset regions in some patients.

Some retrospective case series advocate for sparing of the amygdala [14], amygdala resection with minimal hippocampal resection [15], or isolated lateral neocortical resection [16] **(III/B)**. Interpretation of these studies specifically with regard to MTLE is not possible because patient populations with TLE were studied. In addition, the lateral neocortical resection series has been found to have significant resection of medial structures [17]. Rates of seizure freedom are likely not as high with these approaches as with other approaches to temporal lobectomy. However, these studies show that substantial rates of seizure control can be achieved even with these operations **(III/B)**.

Standard temporal lobectomy with sparing of the superior temporal gyrus

Many surgeons have spared the STG when performing a standard or modified temporal lobectomy due to the presence in the STG of sites critical for naming, as determined by stimulation mapping [18]. Approximately 18% of patients undergoing a standard temporal lobectomy on the left language-dominant side may be expected to harbor such sites in the STG [19].

One small (n=30) prospective randomized study compared naming outcomes in left-sided language-dominant TLE patients who underwent left-sided standard temporal lobectomy with or without resection of the STG [20]. Naming outcomes were measured by the Boston Naming Test and the Visual Naming subtest of the Multilingual Aphasia Examination; no difference in naming outcome or seizure freedom was found based on resection type **(Ib/A)**. Sixty percent of patients who underwent STG resection and 55% of those with STG preservation were seizure-free.

One concern with this study is the small sample size, with 16 patients in the STG resection group and 14 in the STG preservation group. The authors estimate that two to four patients who underwent STG resection would be expected to harbor language-stimulation sites in the STG. No trend was observed in this regard. Of the study population, six patients had unilateral hippocampal atrophy with concordant data, while 21 patients were found to have mesial onset and three patients had medial and lateral onset with invasive recording. This evidence does not establish equivalence between the two procedures, and leaves open the option to perform either operation.

Anteromedial temporal lobe resection

Resection of 3cm of the anterior temporal pole with sparing of the STG and radical *en bloc* resection of the medial temporal lobe structures (Figure 2) began in the late 1970s [21]. This procedure has shown similar rates of seizure freedom compared with standard temporal lobectomy in prospective studies [4, 22, 23] **(IIb/B)**.

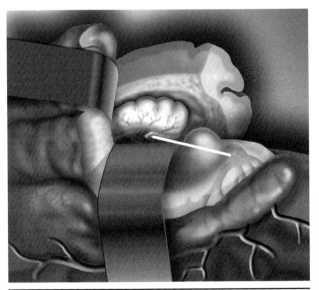

Figure 2. Amygdala resection during anteromedial temporal lobe resection. The medial temporal pole is resected subpially from the anterior to expose the middle cerebral artery. The velum terminale, the union of the taenia of the fimbria fornix and the stria terminalis at the origin of the choroid plexus, is located in the temporal horn. The amygdala is resected inferior to a line between the velum terminale and the genu of the middle cerebral artery at the junction between the M1 and M2 segments, shown in white. Resecting inferior to this line prevents entry into the basal ganglia and crus cerebri.

Selective amygdalohippocampectomy

One small (n=28) prospective randomized trial comparing anterior temporal lobectomy (ATL) with selective amygdalohippocampectomy (SAH) in MTLE patients has been published in abstract form only [24]. The rates of seizure freedom were similar in the ATL (67%) and SAH (69%) groups. Recall on two out of three variables of the Rey Auditory Verbal Learning Test was significantly better after SAH. Performance on the Boston Naming Test and Wechsler Memory Scale-Revised Logical Memory and Visual Reproduction subtests did not vary with surgical procedure. The details of the operations were not included, and the magnitude and clinical significance of the difference measured is uncertain.

In contrast to these findings, a prospective non-randomized two-center comparison of temporal pole resection with amygdalohippocampectomy (TPR+) and transsylvian TS-SAH in 97 MTLE patients showed that verbal memory outcome was worse after left-sided operation, especially in patients who underwent TS-SAH [23] **(IIa/B)**. Figural memory outcome was worse after right-sided operation, preferentially for TPR+. Only patients who were seizure-free were studied.

Across studies, seizure-free outcomes after anteromedial temporal resection, ATL, and SAH are comparable **(III/B)**. Several retrospective studies have shown somewhat better neuropsychological outcomes after selective procedures [25-32], while others have shown no difference [17, 33-36] **(III/B)**. Given the lack of high-quality evidence and conflicting results among the available studies, there does not appear to be a clear indication for one of these procedures over another.

Comparison of the transcortical and transsylvian SAH approaches has been made in a prospective randomized study of 80 patients with MRI-diagnosed MTS [37]. Rates of seizure freedom were not significantly different, with 76.9% of patients who underwent transcortical SAH (MTG-SAH) and 73.2% of TS-SAH patients free from seizures **(Ib/A)**. In this series, all patients showed improved attention, and patients with left-sided procedures of either type experienced an improvement in working memory and

Chapter 12

a decline in verbal memory. Patients who underwent MTG-SAH but not TS-SAH experienced an improvement in verbal fluency. No selection for surgery based on preoperative verbal memory performance was described. Taken together, these results indicate little difference between surgical approaches, and either procedure seems appropriate **(Ib/A)**.

Conclusions

Standard temporal lobectomy for MTS is superior to best medical therapy in medically refractory temporal lobe epilepsy, as demonstrated in one level I study. Level I evidence favors standard temporal lobectomy with complete resection of medial structures over partial resection of medial structures, and standard temporal lobectomy with sparing of the STG was equivalent to standard temporal lobectomy with resection of the STG in a small randomized study. Surgeries supported by strong level II evidence include anteromedial temporal lobe resection, tailored temporal lobectomy with medial resection tailored by ECoG, and SAH. Although approaches have been developed to remove the medial temporal structures with little or no removal of the lateral structures, there is no consensus on whether this leads to improved neuropsychological outcomes. Rates of seizure freedom are comparable across most of the surgical approaches described, although systematic comparisons are not always available.

Recommendations	Evidence level
◆ The evidence suggests that effective treatments for MTS include the following:	
• standard temporal lobectomy;	Ib/A
• standard temporal lobectomy with complete resection of medial structures;	Ib/A
• standard temporal lobectomy with sparing of the STG;	Ib/A
• anteromedial temporal lobe resection;	IIb/B
• tailored temporal lobectomy with medial resection tailored by ECoG;	IIb/B
• selective amygdalohippocampectomy.	IIa/B

References

1. Hauser WA, Annegers JF, Kurland LT. Prevalence of epilepsy in Rochester, Minnesota: 1940-1980. *Epilepsia* 1991; 32: 429-45.

2. Kwan P, Brodie MJ. Early identification of refractory epilepsy. *N Engl J Med* 2000; 342: 314-9.

3. Wiebe S, Blume WT, Girvin JP, Eliasziw M. A randomized, controlled trial of surgery for temporal-lobe epilepsy. *N Engl J Med* 2001; 345: 311-8.

4. Spencer SS, Berg AT, Vickrey BG, *et al.* Initial outcomes in the Multicenter Study of Epilepsy Surgery. *Neurology* 2003; 61: 1680-5.

5. Wyler AR, Hermann BP, Somes G. Extent of medial temporal resection on outcome from anterior temporal lobectomy: a randomized prospective study. *Neurosurgery* 1995; 37: 982-90.

6. Awad IA, Katz A, Hahn JF, Kong AK, Ahl J, Lüders H. Extent of resection in temporal lobectomy for epilepsy. I. Interobserver analysis and correlation with seizure outcome. *Epilepsia* 1989; 30: 756-62.

7. Bonilha L, Kobayashi E, Mattos JP, Honorato DC, Li LM, Cendes F. Value of extent of hippocampal resection in the surgical treatment of temporal lobe epilepsy. *Arq Neuropsiquiatr* 2004; 62: 15-20.

8. Bonilha L, Yasuda CL, Rorden C, *et al.* Does resection of the medial temporal lobe improve the outcome of temporal lobe epilepsy surgery? *Epilepsia* 2007; 48: 571-8.

9. Jack CR, Sharbrough FW, Marsh WR. Use of MR imaging for quantitative evaluation of resection for temporal lobe epilepsy. *Radiology* 1988; 169: 463-8.

10. McKhann GM, Schoenfeld-McNeill J, Born DE, Haglund MM, Ojemann GA. Intraoperative hippocampal electrocorticography to predict the extent of hippocampal

resection in temporal lobe epilepsy surgery. *J Neurosurg* 2000; 93: 44-52.

11. Ojemann GA, Dodrill CB. Verbal memory deficits after left temporal lobectomy for epilepsy. Mechanism and intraoperative prediction. *J Neurosurg* 1985; 62: 101-7.

12. Son EI, Howard MA, Ojemann GA, Lettich E. Comparing the extent of hippocampal removal to the outcome in terms of seizure control. *Stereotact Funct Neurosurg* 1994; 62: 232-7.

13. Wyler AR, Hermann BP, Richey ET. Results of reoperation for failed epilepsy surgery. *J Neurosurg* 1989; 71: 815-9.

14. Goldring S, Edwards I, Harding GW, Bernardo KL. Results of anterior temporal lobectomy that spares the amygdala in patients with complex partial seizures. *J Neurosurg* 1992; 77: 185-93.

15. Feindel W, Rasmussen T. Temporal lobectomy with amygdalectomy and minimal hippocampal resection: review of 100 cases. *Can J Neurol Sci* 1991; 18(Suppl. 1): 603-5.

16. Hardiman O, Burke T, Phillips J, *et al.* Microdysgenesis in resected temporal neocortex: incidence and clinical significance in focal epilepsy. *Neurology* 1988; 38: 1041-7.

17. Jones-Gotman M, Zatorre RJ, Olivier A, *et al.* Learning and retention of words and designs following excision from medial or lateral temporal-lobe structures. *Neuropsychologia* 1997; 35: 963-73.

18. Hermann BP, Wyler AR, Somes G, Clement L. Dysnomia after left anterior temporal lobectomy without functional mapping: frequency and correlates. *Neurosurgery* 1994; 35: 52-6.

19. Ojemann G, Ojemann J, Lettich E, Berger M. Cortical language localization in left, dominant hemisphere. An electrical stimulation mapping investigation in 117 patients. *J Neurosurg* 1989; 71: 316-26.

20. Hermann B, Davies K, Foley K, Bell B. Visual confrontation naming outcome after standard left anterior temporal lobectomy with sparing versus resection of the superior temporal gyrus: a randomized prospective clinical trial. *Epilepsia* 1999; 40: 1070-6.

21. Spencer DD, Spencer SS, Mattson RH, Williamson PD, Novelly RA. Access to the posterior medial temporal lobe structures in the surgical treatment of temporal lobe epilepsy. *Neurosurgery* 1984; 15: 667-71.

22. Spencer SS, Berg AT, Vickrey BG, *et al.* Predicting long-term seizure outcome after resective epilepsy surgery: the multicenter study. *Neurology* 2005; 65: 912-8.

23. Helmstaedter C, Richter S, Röske S, Oltmanns F, Schramm J, Lehmann TN. Differential effects of temporal pole resection with amygdalohippocampectomy versus selective amygdalohippocampectomy on material-specific memory in patients with mesial temporal lobe epilepsy. *Epilepsia* 2008; 49: 88-97.

24. Hadar EJ, Bingaman W, Foldvary N, Chelune G, Comair Y. A prospective analysis of outcome after amygdalohippocampectomy and anterior temporal lobectomy for refractory epilepsy. Congress of Neurological Surgeons meeting, San Diego, 2001.

25. Renowden SA, Matkovic Z, Adams CB, *et al.* Selective amygdalohippocampectomy for hippocampal sclerosis: postoperative MR appearance. *AJNR Am J Neuroradiol* 1995; 16: 1855-61.

26. Helmstaedter C, Elger CE, Hufnagel A, Zentner J, Schramm J. Different effects of left anterior temporal lobectomy, selective amygdalohippocampectomy, and temporal cortical lesionectomy on verbal learning, memory, and recognition. *J Epilepsy* 1996; 9: 39-45.

27. Pauli E, Pickel S, Schulemann H, Buchfelder M, Stefan H. Neuropsychologic findings depending on the type of the resection in temporal lobe epilepsy. *Adv Neurol* 1999; 81: 371-7.

28. Clusmann H, Schramm J, Kral T, *et al.* Prognostic factors and outcome after different types of resection for temporal lobe epilepsy. *J Neurosurg* 2002; 97: 1131-41.

29. Helmstaedter C, Reuber M, Elger CC. Interaction of cognitive aging and memory deficits related to epilepsy surgery. *Ann Neurol* 2002; 52: 89-94.

30. Morino M, Uda T, Naito K, *et al.* Comparison of neuropsychological outcomes after selective amygdalohippocampectomy versus anterior temporal lobectomy. *Epilepsy Behav* 2006; 9: 95-100.

31. Paglioli E, Palmini A, Portuguez M, *et al.* Seizure and memory outcome following temporal lobe surgery: selective compared with nonselective approaches for hippocampal sclerosis. *J Neurosurg* 2006; 104: 70-8.

32. Tanriverdi T, Olivier A. Cognitive changes after unilateral cortico-amygdalohippocampectomy unilateral selective-amygdalohippocampectomy mesial temporal lobe epilepsy. *Turk Neurosurg* 2007; 17: 91-9.

33. Goldstein LH, Polkey CE. Behavioural memory after temporal lobectomy or amygdalo-hippocampectomy. *Br J Clin Psychol* 1992; 31: 75-81.

34. Goldstein LH, Polkey CE. Short-term cognitive changes after unilateral temporal lobectomy or unilateral amygdalo-hippocampectomy for the relief of temporal lobe epilepsy. *J Neurol Neurosurg Psychiatry* 1993; 56: 135-40.

35. Wolf RL, Ivnik RJ, Hirschorn KA, Sharbrough FW, Cascino GD, Marsh WR. Neurocognitive efficiency following left temporal lobectomy: standard versus limited resection. *J Neurosurg* 1993; 79: 76-83.

36. Hader WJ, Pillay N, Myles ST, Partlo L, Wiebe S. The benefit of selective over standard surgical resections in the treatment of intractable temporal lobe epilepsy. *Epilepsia* 2005; 46: 253-60.

37. Lutz MT, Clusmann H, Elger CE, Schramm J, Helmstaedter C. Neuropsychological outcome after selective amygdalohippocampectomy with transsylvian versus transcortical approach: a randomized prospective clinical trial of surgery for temporal lobe epilepsy. *Epilepsia* 2004; 45: 809-16.

Chapter 12

Temporal lobectomy for mesial temporal sclerosis

Chapter 13

Surgical outcomes in non-lesional epilepsy

Juan Torres-Reveron MD PhD, Resident in Neurosurgery

Kenneth P Vives MD, Associate Professor;

Chief of Stereotactic and Functional Neurosurgery

Dennis D Spencer MD, Harvey and Kate Cushing Professor of

Neurosurgery; Chairman, Department of Neurosurgery

DEPARTMENT OF NEUROSURGERY, YALE UNIVERSITY, NEW HAVEN, CONNECTICUT, USA

Introduction

Epilepsy is one of the most common neurologic diseases and carries a significant financial and disability burden [1]. For many years, the mainstays of therapy have been the identification of seizure semiology and pharmacologic treatment to either eliminate seizures or decrease their frequency, thereby improving the patient's quality of life. Despite new pharmacologic interventions and an array of antiepileptic agents, many patients continue to experience daily seizures that prevent them from working and require them to adjust their lives to accommodate their seizure frequency and pattern.

During the last 20 years, significant advances in identification of seizure foci [2, 3] and surgical technique [4] have improved the outcome of epilepsy surgery, particularly for seizures of temporal origin associated with a clear lesion visible by MRI or mesial temporal lobe sclerosis (MTLS). Furthermore, a randomized controlled trial has provided evidence that surgery is superior to prolonged medical therapy in achieving seizure freedom [5]. In this trial, patients in the medical group were placed on a waiting list of 1 year for epilepsy monitoring, while those in the surgical group were admitted to the epilepsy monitoring unit within 48 hours of randomization. Patients were followed for 1 year and their seizures were documented. Outcomes were evaluated at the 1-year time point. The surgical patients had a significantly better quality of life and 58% were free of seizures impairing awareness, compared with only 8% in the medical group **(Ib/A)**. Even with large numbers of studies indicating that surgery provides excellent seizure control, and in many cases seizure freedom, as well as documenting the low morbidity and mortality of the procedures [6-8], surgical intervention remains a 'last resort' therapy for epilepsy management.

Patient selection is critical for the success of epilepsy surgery. Although most patients will have an identifiable lesion on MRI (lesional patients), 20-40% of presurgical patients have a negative MRI (non-lesional patients) [9-12]. This group is particularly challenging as surgical decisions are based on seizure semiology, localization during intracranial studies, and adjunct imaging (i.e., positron emission tomography [PET], single photon emission computed tomography [SPECT]), which may not have the spatial resolution to identify the seizure foci. Furthermore, evaluation of surgery outcomes is complicated as some patients with negative MRI scans have been found to have histopathologic lesions [13-21]. Our review of the literature found that non-lesional patients have worse outcomes than lesional patients in terms of both seizure freedom and seizure control. In patients where a histopathologic lesion was identified, even though the MRI was negative, the outcome was better than for patients in whom no pathological lesion was present. Finally, correlation of EEG with other imaging modalities also improved the outcomes in this patient population.

Methodology

A Medline search was conducted using the terms 'epilepsy surgery,' 'non-lesional epilepsy surgery,' 'MRI negative epilepsy surgery,' and 'MRI negative epilepsy.' Studies were selected from 2000 to the present, as any differences in MRI technology should be minimized in this period. Most studies were not dedicated to non-lesional patients, but were rather retrospective studies in which a proportion of patients had a negative MRI. Where possible, non-lesional or MRI-negative patients were extracted from the data if their outcomes were reported separately. Pathological findings were documented if reported. The citations in each report were examined to extract previous studies.

We concentrated on Engel class I outcomes for each study, as there are differences between the Engel and International League Against Epilepsy classifications in the other outcome subdivisions.

It is important to note that the classification of MRI-negative epilepsy has undergone a shift over the years as the awareness of MTLS as a pathological entity has improved. Some of the studies included cases of MTLS as 'non-lesional' patients, but most found other pathologies in the patients not related to sclerosis.

Level of evidence

There is only one randomized controlled trial in epilepsy surgery [5] **(Ib/A)**. All of the other studies presented are from either retrospective or prospective

non-randomized evaluations of surgical cases or meta-analyses of case reports **(III/B)**.

The presence of a lesion is predictive of good outcome after surgery

A meta-analysis by Téllez-Zenteno *et al* published in 2010 evaluated epilepsy surgery studies since 1995 and compared the rates of seizure freedom in lesional and non-lesional patients [22]. The data set incorporated 40 studies and included both temporal and extratemporal cases, as well as adult and pediatric populations. Seizure-freedom rates in patients with at least 1-year of follow-up were extracted from the studies. Histopathology was used in some studies to identify lesional patients.

Table 1 shows adapted data from the study [22]. It is evident that, regardless of the anatomic location, the presence of a lesion on MRI is predictive of seizure freedom after surgery (46% of non-lesional patients vs. 70% of lesional patients). Furthermore, surgery in extratemporal non-lesional cases is associated with the lowest rates of seizure freedom. Interestingly, the finding of a histopathologic lesion, even in patients with an initially negative MRI, also carries a good

Table 1. Results of epilepsy surgery in lesional and non-lesional patients, evaluated using MRI. *Adapted from Téllez-Zenteno et al, 2010* [22].

Surgery	Lesional		Non-lesional	
	n	% Seizure-free (95% CI)	n	% Seizure-free (95% CI)
Temporal and extratemporal	965	70 (68-73)	398	46 (41-51)
Temporal lobe	514	75 (79-89)	226	51 (45-57)
Extratemporal lobe	225	60 (54-66)	124	35 (27-42)

CI = confidence interval

prognosis for seizure freedom (39% for non-lesional patients vs. 67% for lesional patients) **(III/B)**. However, the usefulness of histopathology as a prognostic factor is limited, as it does not provide *a priori* information to discuss the possible outcomes with the patient during the surgical decision process.

Summary of surgical studies during the last 10 years

The advent of improved imaging techniques has not changed the surgical prognosis for non-lesional epilepsy patients. Examining the studies reported during the last 10 years (Table 2) shows that the proportion of MRI-negative patients in the different studies has remained stable at 26% [13-15, 17, 18, 21, 23-39]. This is in line with previous reports [9-12]. Of those patients who underwent surgical resection, only 37% were able to achieve class I Engel outcomes.

The most common pathology in non-lesional patients was cortical dysplasia (14 out of 23 studies) followed by gliosis (seven out of 23 studies). Other non-specific abnormalities were encountered in several studies. MTLS was included in four of the studies.

Engel class I outcomes were experienced by more than 50% of patients in five out of the eight pediatric studies reviewed. There is no indication that surgical technique or postoperative management was different in any of the studies. Brain tumors were the most common pathology in MRI-positive pediatric patients, while gliosis, MTLS, and non-specific findings were common in those without MRI lesions [38]. Paolicchi *et al* found that completeness of resection of the presumptive seizure foci was associated with better outcomes [39] **(III/B)**. However, it is important to note that this can be limited by functional areas during extratemporal resections. The presence of a dipole cluster in the area of resection on magnetoencephalography (MEG) evaluation was also associated with improved seizure-freedom outcomes [30] **(III/B)**. Patients who did not achieve seizure freedom had either scatter or bilateral MEG dipoles in that study, suggesting that MEG may play a larger role in the future evaluation of these patients to improve outcomes.

A meta-analysis of extratemporal lobe epilepsy in pediatric patients indicates that outcomes are poor in patients without a lesion [24] **(III/B)**. Postoperative seizure outcome was associated with seizure type and pathological findings. There was a marginally significant association with age and surgical outcome. The authors suggest that older children may do better than younger ones, presumably due to the difficulty in finding a seizure focus in the younger population. Furthermore, in contrast to the adult population, in pediatric patients seizures can improve with brain development. Therefore, the decision for surgery has to be weighed appropriately.

In the adult group, the factors affecting outcome were similar to those in the pediatric population. Cukiert *et al* achieved excellent postoperative outcomes in a small group of patients by resecting widely around the seizure focus [17] **(III/B)**.

Different techniques have been used to improve the identification of seizure foci, including intracranial EEG [26], stereoelectroencephalography (SEEG), PET, and subtraction ictal SPECT data correlated with MRI (SISCOM). McGonigal *et al* found no difference in detecting a lesion in MRI-positive or -negative patients using SEEG, and 65% of patients achieved class I Engel outcomes in that study [21] **(III/B)**. Abnormalities in SPECT and SISCOM data, absence of contralateral interictal discharges, and subtle MRI findings were also associated with good outcomes [28]. Cortical dysplasia may appear as a normal MRI but is associated with a positive PET scan in 75-90% of patients, and surgical resection is effective in eliminating seizures in 80% of cases [40] **(III/B)**. Therefore, the use of PET for localization in non-lesional patients may acquire a larger role.

Furthermore, the presence of a high-frequency epileptiform oscillation in the seizure focus during intracranial EEG studies has been correlated with improved seizure freedom [26] **(III/B)**. Some researchers advocate extensive coverage using subdural electrodes [17], while others suggest that intracranial studies should be avoided in patients where other modalities suggest multifocality [18] **(III/B)**.

Chapter 13

Table 2. Summary of studies with non-lesional patients as evaluated by MRI (MRI-negative). *Continued overleaf.*

Study	Study design	Patients, n			
		Total	MRI-negative	Surgical treatment (MRI-negative)	Class I Engel outcome (%)
Lowe *et al*, 2010 [23]	Retrospective	76	76	76	51 (67)
Ansari *et al*, 2010 [24]	Meta-analysis, pediatric	95	36	Unknown	14 (39)[a]
Seo *et al*, 2009 [25]	Retrospective, pediatric	27	27	27	18 (67)
Wetjen *et al*, 2009 [26]	Retrospective	51	51	31	14 (50)
Bien *et al*, 2009 [27]	Retrospective	1200	190	29	11 (38)
Bell *et al*, 2009 [28]	Retrospective	272	44	44	24 (60)
Jayakar *et al*, 2008 [29]	Retrospective, pediatric	101	101	101	44 (44)
McGonigal *et al*, 2007 [21]	Retrospective, prospective	100	43	43	13 (65)
Ramachandran *et al*, 2007 [30]	Retrospective, pediatric	61	14	14	7 (50)
Alarcón *et al*, 2006 [13]	Retrospective, prospective	241	41	41	9 (47)
Lee *et al*, 2005 [15]	Retrospective	89	89	89	42 (47)
Sindou *et al*, 2006 [31]	Retrospective	100	13	13	8 (60)
Carne *et al*, 2004 [32]	Retrospective	60	30	20	16 (80)
Chapman *et al*, 2005 [14]	Retrospective	823	24	24	9 (37)

Table 2. Summary of studies with non-lesional patients as evaluated by MRI (MRI-negative). *Continued.*

Study	Study design	Patients, n			
		Total	MRI-negative	Surgical treatment (MRI-negative)	Class I Engel outcome (%)
Sinclair et al, 2004 [33]	Retrospective, pediatric	35	4	4	1 (25)
Stavem et al, 2004 [34]	Retrospective	63	29	29	9 (31)
Sinclair et al, 2003 [35]	Retrospective, pediatric	42	8	8	4 (50)
Hong et al, 2002 [36]	Retrospective	41	41	41	16 (39)
Siegel et al, 2001 [18]	Retrospective	115	43	31	15 (48)
Cukiert et al, 2001 [17]	Retrospective	16	10	10	9 (90)
Kral et al, 2001 [37]	Retrospective, pediatric	32	5	5	1 (20)
Sinclair et al, 2001 [38]	Retrospective, pediatric	42	9	9	5 (56)
Paolicchi et al, 2001 [39]	Retrospective, pediatric	75	35	35	18 (51)

[a] = based on MRI

Algorithm for evaluation of non-concordant preoperative data

We have previously published an algorithm for the evaluation of potential epilepsy surgery patients [41]. At our institution, patients undergo phase I and II evaluations (Figure 1) during the surgical decision-making process. For those patients in whom preoperative data localize seizure foci with certainty, invasive monitoring is not needed. These patients are treated according to the location of the seizures (temporal vs. extratemporal) and the extent of the abnormality (focal vs. hemispheric). Patients who have developmental anomalies or where preoperative evaluations are discordant or indeterminate are scheduled for invasive monitoring.

Surgery is not performed in patients where preoperative data along with the invasive evaluation suggest a bitemporal diffuse localization or in patients who have multifocal or unlocalized seizures by intracranial EEG. Corpus callosotomy is reserved for patients with multifocal or unlocalized seizures who may benefit from seizure reduction, with the understanding that seizure freedom will not be achieved.

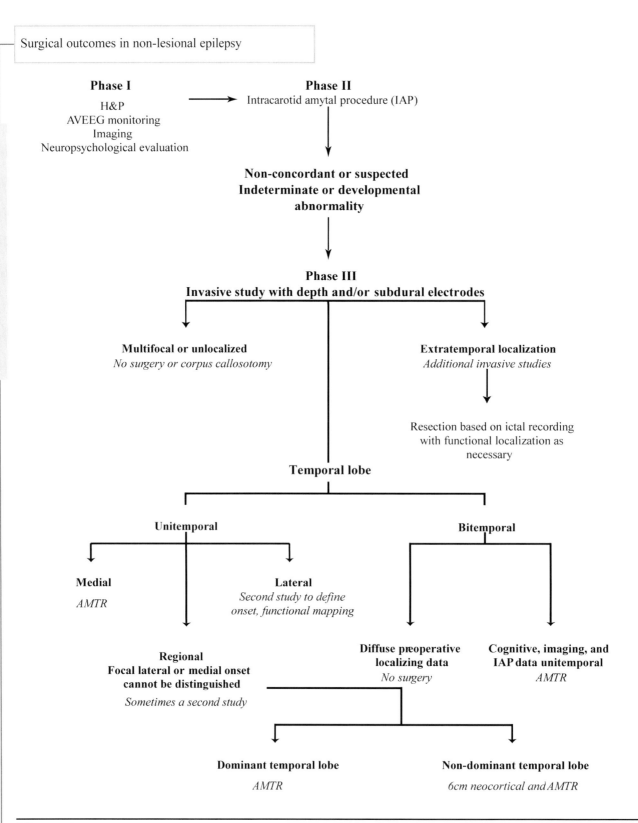

Figure 1. Algorithm for evaluation of epilepsy patients with non-concordant preoperative data. Patients with discordant preoperative data are usually candidates for subdural electrode placement. The type of resection procedure that the patient undergoes depends on the hemispheric location and focality of the lesion. AMTR = anteromesial temporal resection; AVEEG = audio-visual EEG; H&P = history and physical examination; IAP = intracarotid amytal procedure.

Multiple invasive studies may be indicated in patients with extratemporal localization (survey study followed by a more directed study with denser coverage). Following seizure localization, these data are correlated with functional imaging and mapping data to determine the available area for resection.

Conclusions

Despite advances in imaging and the advent of new modalities, the rate of seizure freedom in non-lesional epilepsy patients has not improved significantly over the last decade, and remains below the rate achieved for patients in whom a lesion is evident.

Although there is no significant correlation between the duration of epilepsy symptoms and outcomes from surgery, there is a tendency for better outcomes with shorter duration of disease [23] **(III/B)**. It is clear that, for carefully selected patients, epilepsy surgery is beneficial. It remains to be determined whether earlier surgery improves outcomes.

Recommendations	Evidence level
◆ In MRI-negative patients, correlated positive findings with other imaging modalities and finding of a histopathologic lesion leads to improved outcomes following surgery for non-lesional epilepsy.	III/B
◆ Non-lesional patients with temporal onset of seizures have better outcomes than those with extratemporal locations.	III/B
◆ Cortical dysplasia is one of the most common histopathologic findings in MRI-negative patients and responds well to resection.	III/B
◆ Patients without lesions may need multiple invasive studies for better delineation of the seizure foci and improvement in outcomes.	III/B

References

1. de Boer HM, Mula M, Sander JW. The global burden and stigma of epilepsy. *Epilepsy Behav* 2008; 12: 540-6.
2. Duncan JS. Imaging and epilepsy. *Brain* 1997; 120: 339-77.
3. Craven I, Kotsarini C, Hoggard N. Recent advances in imaging epilepsy. *Postgrad Med J* 2010; 86: 552-9.
4. Wyler AR. Recent advances in epilepsy surgery: temporal lobectomy and multiple subpial transections. *Neurosurgery* 1997; 41: 1294-302.
5. Wiebe S, Blume WT, Girvin JP, Eliasziw M. A randomized, controlled trial of surgery for temporal-lobe epilepsy. *N Engl J Med* 2001; 345: 311-8.
6. Tanriverdi T, Ajlan A, Poulin N, Olivier A. Morbidity in epilepsy surgery: an experience based on 2,449 epilepsy surgery procedures from a single institution. *J Neurosurg* 2009; 110: 1111-23.
7. Salanova V, Markand O, Worth R. Temporal lobe epilepsy surgery: outcome, complications and late mortality in 215 patients. *Epilepsia* 2002; 43: 170-4.
8. McClelland S 3rd, Guo H, Okuyemi KS. Population-based analysis of morbidity and mortality following surgery for intractable temporal lobe epilepsy in the United States. *Arch Neurol* 2011; 68: 725-9.
9. Cascino GD, O'Brien TJ. Resection for epilepsy in the setting of a nonlocalizing MRI. In: *Treatment of Epilepsy*. Wyllie E, Ed. Philadelphia: Lippincott Williams and Williams, 2001; 1135-45.
10. Engel J Jr. Outcome with respect to seizures. In: *Surgical Treatment of the Epilepsies*. Engel J Jr, Ed. New York: Raven Press, 1987; 553-71.
11. Spencer S, Sperling M, Shewmon D. Intracranial electrodes. In: *Epilepsy: A Comprehensive Textbook*. Engel J Jr, Pedley T, Eds. Philadelphia: Lippincott-Raven Publishers, 1997; 1719-47.
12. Berg AT, Vickrey BG, Langfitt JT, *et al*. The multicenter study of epilepsy surgery: recruitment and selection for surgery. *Epilepsia* 2003; 44: 1425-33.
13. Alarcón G, Valentin A, Watt C, *et al*. Is it worth pursuing surgery for epilepsy in patients with normal neuroimaging? *J Neurol Neurosurg Psychiatry* 2006; 77: 474-80.

14. Chapman K, Wyllie E, Najm I, *et al.* Seizure outcome after epilepsy surgery in patients with normal preoperative MRI. *J Neurol Neurosurg Psychiatry* 2005; 76: 710-13.

15. Lee SK, Lee SY, Kim KK, Hong KS, Lee DS, Chung CK. Surgical outcome and prognostic factors of cryptogenic neocortical epilepsy. *Ann Neurol* 2005; 58: 525-32.

16. Sylaja PN, Radhakrishnan K, Kesavadas C, Sarma PS. Seizure outcome after anterior temporal lobectomy and its predictors in patients with apparent temporal lobe epilepsy and normal MRI. *Epilepsia* 2004; 45: 803-8.

17. Cukiert A, Buratini JA, Machado E, *et al.* Results of surgery in patients with refractory extratemporal epilepsy with normal or nonlocalizing magnetic resonance findings investigated with subdural grids. *Epilepsia* 2001; 42: 889-94.

18. Siegel AM, Jobst BC, Thadani VM, *et al.* Medically intractable, localization-related epilepsy with normal MRI: presurgical evaluation and surgical outcome in 43 patients. *Epilepsia* 2001; 42: 883-8.

19. Holmes MD, Born DE, Kutsy RL, Wilensky AJ, Ojemann GA, Ojemann LM. Outcome after surgery in patients with refractory temporal lobe epilepsy and normal MRI. *Seizure* 2000; 9: 407-11.

20. Scott CA, Fish DR, Smith SJ, *et al.* Presurgical evaluation of patients with epilepsy and normal MRI: role of scalp video-EEG telemetry. *J Neurol Neurosurg Psychiatry* 1999; 66: 69-71.

21. McGonigal A, Bartolomei F, Régis J, *et al.* Stereoelectroencephalography in presurgical assessment of MRI-negative epilepsy. *Brain* 2007; 130: 3169-83.

22. Téllez-Zenteno JF, Hernández Ronquillo L, Moien-Afshari F, Wiebe S. Surgical outcomes in lesional and non-lesional epilepsy: a systematic review and meta-analysis. *Epilepsy Res* 2010; 89: 310-8.

23. Lowe NM, Eldridge P, Varma T, Wiechmann UC. The duration of temporal lobe epilepsy and seizure outcome after epilepsy surgery. *Seizure* 2010; 19: 261-3.

24. Ansari SF, Maher CO, Tubbs RS, Terry CL, Cohen-Gadol AA. Surgery for extratemporal nonlesional epilepsy in children: a meta-analysis. *Childs Nerv Syst* 2010; 26: 945-51.

25. Seo JH, Noh BH, Lee JS, *et al.* Outcome of surgical treatment in non-lesional intractable childhood epilepsy. *Seizure* 2009; 18: 625-9.

26. Wetjen NM, Marsh WR, Meyer FB, *et al.* Intracranial electroencephalography seizure onset patterns and surgical outcomes in nonlesional extratemporal epilepsy. *J Neurosurg* 2009; 110: 1147-52.

27. Bien CG, Szinay M, Wagner J, Clusmann H, Becker AJ, Urbach H. Characteristics and surgical outcomes of patients with refractory magnetic resonance imaging-negative epilepsies. *Arch Neurol* 2009; 66: 1491-9.

28. Bell ML, Rao S, So EL, *et al.* Epilepsy surgery outcomes in temporal lobe epilepsy with a normal MRI. *Epilepsia* 2009; 50: 2053-60.

29. Jayakar P, Dunoyer C, Dean P, *et al.* Epilepsy surgery in patients with normal or nonfocal MRI scans: integrative strategies offer long-term seizure relief. *Epilepsia* 2008; 49: 758-64.

30. Ramachandran Nair R, Otsubo H, Shroff MM, *et al.* MEG predicts outcome following surgery for intractable epilepsy in children with normal or nonfocal MRI findings. *Epilepsia* 2007; 48: 149-57.

31. Sindou M, Guenot M, Isnard J, Ryvlin P, Fischer C, Mauguière F. Temporo-mesial epilepsy surgery: outcome and complications in 100 consecutive adult patients. *Acta Neurochir* (Wien) 2006; 148: 39-45.

32. Carne RP, O'Brien TJ, Kilpatrick CJ, *et al.* MRI-negative PET-positive temporal lobe epilepsy: a distinct surgically remediable syndrome. *Brain* 2004; 127: 2276-85.

33. Sinclair DB, Aronyk K, Snyder T, *et al.* Extratemporal resection for childhood epilepsy. *Pediatr Neurol* 2004; 30: 177-85.

34. Stavem K, Bjørnæs H, Langmoen IA. Predictors of seizure outcome after temporal lobectomy for intractable epilepsy. *Acta Neurol Scand* 2004; 109: 244-9.

35. Sinclair DB, Aronyk K, Snyder T, *et al.* Pediatric temporal lobectomy for epilepsy. *Pediatr Neurosurg* 2003; 38: 195-205.

36. Hong, KS, Lee SK, Kim JY, Lee DS, Chung CK. Pre-surgical evaluation and surgical outcome of 41 patients with non-lesional neocortical epilepsy. *Seizure* 2002; 11: 184-92.

37. Kral T, Kuczaty S, Blümcke I, *et al.* Postsurgical outcome of children and adolescents with medically refractory frontal lobe epilepsies. *Child's Nerv Syst* 2001; 17: 595-601.

38. Sinclair DB, Wheatley M, Aronyk K, *et al.* Pathology and neuroimaging in pediatric temporal lobectomy for intractable epilepsy. *Pediatr Neurosurg* 2001; 35: 239-46.

39. Paolicchi JM, Jayakar P, Dean P, *et al.* Predictors of outcome in pediatric epilepsy surgery. *Neurology* 2000; 54: 642-7.

40. Lerner JT, Salamon N, Hauptman JS, *et al.* Assessment and surgical outcomes for mild type I and severe type II cortical dysplasia: a critical review and the UCLA experience. *Epilepsia* 2009; 50: 1310-35.

41. Vives KP, Al-Rodham N, Spencer DD. Use of magnetic resonance imaging in surgical strategies for epilepsy. In: *Neuroimaging in Epilepsy: Principles and Practice.* Cascino GD, Jack CR, Eds. Massachusetts: Butterworth-Heinemann, 1996; 235-59.

Chapter 14

Neuromodulation procedures for movement disorders

Kenneth P Vives MD

Associate Professor; Chief of Stereotactic
and Functional Neurosurgery

DEPARTMENT OF NEUROSURGERY, YALE UNIVERSITY, NEW HAVEN, CONNECTICUT, USA

Introduction

Neurosurgical treatment of movement disorders has evolved considerably over the last two decades, from the use of lesioning as the predominant means of surgical treatment to the current use of deep brain stimulation (DBS) in developed countries. The use of stimulators requires continued, intermittent interaction with the neurologist and infrequent visits back to the implanting surgeon for replacement batteries. This chapter examines the evidence available to support the use of these stimulators for the treatment of Parkinson's disease (PD), essential tremor (ET), and dystonia.

When analyzing the evidence available for DBS, it is critical to understand how treatment comparisons were made. Some studies only compare patients with their own baseline, preoperative condition. Other studies attempt to compare patients with the stimulator on versus the stimulator off. The length of time that the stimulator is off prior to evaluation varies greatly between studies. There is emerging evidence that stimulation in some PD and dystonia patients can have long-lasting effects through network modification and these effects may only occur over time. This seems to be much less the case in patients where

stimulators are implanted in the ventral intermediate thalamic nucleus (VIM) for ET, but this has not been systematically studied. It is possible that these types of effects also take time to 'wash out' after stimulation is discontinued. This phenomenon may make it more difficult to see treatment effects if the stimulation is terminated too close to the time of evaluation. In PD, this is made even more complicated by patients' expected daily fluctuations from levodopa therapy. This necessitates repeated evaluations during 'on-medication' and 'off-medication' times – thus adding to the complexity of these studies.

When ascertaining the level of evidence and recommendation, it is important to note that these only pertain to the population studied. By and large, the studies referenced in this chapter have assessed the clinical utility of DBS in medically refractory patients who, even with optimal medical therapy, were experiencing significant disease-related symptoms. Some of the studies revealed significant findings in secondary endpoints, as opposed to the primary endpoint for which the trial was designed. Attention is drawn to these factors and they are taken into account when ascertaining the strength of the evidence and the level of recommendation.

Methodology

A National Library of Medicine computerized literature search was performed of publications from 1966 to 2011 using each of the following headings separately to build a wide database of articles: 'deep brain stimulation' and 'DBS.' These headings were then limited to human case series, trials, and meta-analyses and then carefully screened for relevance. The bibliographies of these articles were reviewed for other possible inclusions.

Parkinson's disease

Deep brain stimulation of the subthalamic nucleus

The subthalamic nucleus (STN) remains the preferred target for DBS among movement disorders surgeons because of its compact size and reliable clinical outcome. The predominant measure of outcome in initial publications was improvement in the motor section (part 3) of the Unified Parkinson's Disease Rating Scale (UPDRS). Early case series revealed that at 12 months, patients experienced an average rating improvement of 50%. Other symptoms also improved, including tremor (80%), rigidity (60%), bradykinesia (55%), and dyskinesia (80-90%) [1, 2]. Following these initial publications, many additional case series and a few randomized controlled trials were published.

In August 2006, Deuschl *et al* published the results of a 156-patient, randomized-pairs trial comparing bilateral STN DBS with medication alone [3]. The primary endpoints were the Parkinson's Disease Questionnaire (PDQ)-39 and the UPDRS-III. At 6 months, 50 of the 78 pairs demonstrated a greater improvement with DBS compared with medication alone on the PDQ-39, with a mean increased score of 9.5. On the UPDRS-III, 55 out of 78 pairs had a mean increase of 19.5. Significant differences between the treatments were also reported for mobility, activities of daily living (ADLs), emotional well-being, stigma, and bodily discomfort **(Ib/A)**.

Schüpbach *et al* reported on a small group of 20 patients with earlier-stage PD [4]. This randomized controlled study assessed patients at 6, 12, and 18 months. Quality of life (QoL) was improved by 24% in surgical patients versus 0% in the non-surgical group. Significant improvements were seen in the surgical group in the severity of motor symptoms in the 'off' state, the degree of levodopa-related symptoms, and the amount of levodopa taken, while declines were seen for each of these in the medication-only group **(Ib/A)**.

The CSP-468 Study Group published its results in 2009. The group randomized 255 advanced PD patients to surgery versus best medical therapy [5]. The surgery was either targeted at the STN (n=60) or the globus pallidus interna (GPi, n=61). Later analysis showed only minor differences between the groups. The primary outcome measure was the amount of time spent in the 'on' state without troubling dyskinesia. Those patients who underwent surgery gained a mean of 4.6 hours per day of 'on' time without troubling dyskinesia compared with 0 hours per day for patients who received best medical therapy. Motor function and summary QoL scores also improved significantly in the surgery group **(Ib/A)**.

In June 2010, Williams *et al* published the results of a UK-based, open-label randomized trial comparing surgery plus best medical therapy with best medical therapy alone [6]. The study randomized 366 patients with advanced PD for whom medical therapy was failing. All the patients in the surgery group who underwent surgery (n=178) were given DBS and in 174 the target was the STN. The primary endpoint was functional status as assessed by the PDQ-39. At 1-year follow-up, the mean improvement in PDQ-39 summary score compared with baseline was 5 points in the surgery group and 0.3 points in the best medical therapy group **(Ib/A)**. Significant differences were also observed in the mobility, ADL, and bodily discomfort domains. A smaller comparative case series of 25 patients comparing STN DBS with subcutaneous apomorphine infusion also confirmed the superiority of DBS in reducing dyskinesia duration and severity compared with this specific medical therapy [7] **(IIa/B)**.

The strongest evidence for this treatment arguably comes from a meta-analysis published by Kleiner-Fisman *et al* in 2008 [8] **(Ia/A)**. The authors selected 34 studies out of 680 relevant publications for inclusion in the analysis. Patients who underwent surgery in the stimulation 'on' and medication 'off' state compared with those who received the preoperative medication 'off' state experienced an estimated decrease of 50% in the UPDRS-II (ADL) score and 52% in the UPDRS-III (motor) score. The average reduction in levodopa following surgery was 55.9%, the average reduction in dyskinesia following surgery was 69.1%, and the average reduction in daily 'off' periods was 68.2%. Importantly, the average improvement in QoL using PDQ-39 was 34.5±15.3%. This is arguably level I data. However, not all of the papers in the review were of the same quality and many of the studies were not blinded or randomized.

Based upon the above literature, treatment of advanced PD patients with DBS in the STN would likely merit a recommendation of grade A, based upon the consistent finding in the level Ib trials and the one possible level Ia publication.

The globus pallidus interna versus the subthalamic nucleus

In 1999, Burchiel et al compared GPi with STN electrode placement [9]. In this small study, 10 patients were randomized to receive bilateral GPi or STN electrode implants. One GPi patient was not utilized in the follow-up. The rest of the patients, whether 'on' or 'off' medication, were evaluated preoperatively and then postoperatively at 10 days and 3, 6, and 12 months by evaluators blinded to the site of implantation. At 12 months, there was no significant difference between the groups in the 'off' or 'on' medication state in the UPDRS motor score, with 39% and 44% improvements over baseline in the 'off' medication state in each respective electrode placement group and approximately 20% for both in the 'on' medication state (Ib/A). At 12 months there was a statistically significant difference in bradykinesia scores for patients in the 'on' medication state, with the GPi site being more effective. They also found greater medication reductions in the STN-implanted group than in the GPi-implanted group, although both groups experienced reductions in medication-induced dyskinesias.

Anderson et al followed up on this study in 2005 by enrolling 15 additional patients and performing further analysis [10]. They again found no significant difference between the electrode placement groups in the UPDRS motor scores 'off' or 'on' medication (Ib/A), and reported that only 'off' medication scores were significantly changed from baseline. Although there was a trend toward greater medication reductions in the STN group compared with the GPi group, this was no longer significant.

A multicenter study of 69 PD patients with electrodes implanted in the STN (n=49) or the GPi (n=20) looked at the 3-4-year outcomes [11]. There was no randomization and no blinding and the study was hampered by a high attrition rate for its late data point. However, the study confirmed significant improvements over baseline for patients in the 'off' medication state in both electrode placement groups. Patients in the 'on' medication state in both electrode placement groups also showed a significant worsening over time in motor UPDRS, ADLs, and gait. Patients implanted in the STN, but not the GPi, experienced a decline in speech and postural stability when in the 'on' medication state (IIa/B).

Okun et al looked at 52 subjects randomized to unilateral STN or GPi DBS in a prospective blinded trial designed to study mood and cognition [12]. There were no significant differences in mood and cognition between patients with electrodes implanted in the STN or the GPi in the optimal DBS state (Ib/A). A worsening of letter verbal fluency was seen in STN-implanted patients, even with the stimulator off, suggesting a surgical rather than a stimulation-induced effect. The same group published an additional paper on QoL outcomes using the PDQ-39 [13]. This study included 42 patients and compared QoL for stimulators implanted in the GPi versus the STN. In addition to the above findings, on average, all patients experienced an improvement in QoL after surgery. However, there was a statistically significant difference in that GPi patients improved more than STN patients (38% vs. 14%, respectively). GPi-implanted patients experienced statistically significant improvements on the mobility, ADLs, stigma, and social support subscales while STN-implanted patients did not. In regression analyses, only changes in depression independently predicted changes in overall QoL, while decreased verbal fluency may have contributed to the lesser improvement seen in the STN-implanted patients **(Ib/A)**.

Moro *et al* published their multicenter prospective series comparing outcomes at 5-6 years' follow-up in patients with bilateral STN or GPi electrode implants [14]. The implantation site was not randomized. The STN-implanted patients (n=49) and the GPi-implanted patients (n=20) had statistically improved motor scores in the stimulator 'on' state compared with the stimulator 'off' state and compared with baseline. In addition, medication reductions were greater in the STN-implanted patients than in the GPi-implanted patients, while adverse events were also greater in the STN patients **(IIa/B)**.

The most definitive paper to date on this topic was published by the CSP-468 study group [15]. PD patients (n=229) were randomized to receive either bilateral STN or GPi DBS. The evaluators were blinded to the site of implantation and assessments were performed with the patients off medication and with the stimulator on. At 24 months, there was no significant difference between the groups on the UPDRS motor score. The study confirmed that STN-implanted patients, on average, had greater reductions in the amount of dopaminergic medications necessary. The other most notable finding of the study was that the depression scores of STN-implanted patients worsened, while those of GPi-implanted patients improved. There was no significant difference in adverse events. The study group concluded that non-motor functions, such as depression, may need to be considered when selecting a surgical site. Letters to the editor discussing this research pointed out that the differences in medication regimens between the groups were not controlled for and may have contributed to the differences in depressive symptoms experienced by the patients **(Ib/A)**.

The above-listed studies contribute to an overall recommendation of grade A that the STN and GPi sites for DBS electrodes provide equivalent outcomes for motor scores on the UPDRS. There were a number of other, not as consistent, findings in secondary endpoints in these trials, including that greater reductions in medications may be seen in

STN-implanted patients versus GPi-implanted patients. STN-implanted patients may have more difficulties with speech and verbal fluency, worse depression, and inferior QoL outcomes compared with GPi-implanted patients.

Gait

In 2010, St George *et al* published a meta-regression of long-term studies of PD patients with DBS electrodes implanted in the STN or GPi to look at the issues of postural instability and gait disturbance [16]. They included 11 publications with follow-up times of at least 3 years, and an overall mean follow-up time of 4.5 years. Using a random-effects meta-regression, they found that overall postural instability and gait disturbance in patients in the 'off' medication state improved immediately after surgery, but gradually deteriorated over time. In the 'on' medication state, there was a significant difference between GPi- and STN-implanted patients, although both groups initially improved after implantation. On average, within 2 years, STN-implanted patients declined back to their preoperative level of functioning, while no such decline was observed in the GPi-implanted patients **(IIb/B)**. The limitations of this study, stated in the article, were fewer long-term GPi studies and a relatively high overall attrition rate of 11%.

To address the difficulties associated with treating patients with levodopa-resistant gait disorder, investigators have been studying the effects of adding DBS electrodes targeting the pedunculopontine nucleus (PPN). Following initial reports by Mazzone *et al* and Plaha *et al* [17, 18], Stefani *et al* published a paper on a series of six patients in 2007 [19]. They demonstrated that patients off medication achieved a lower UPDRS-III rating at 3 months using PPN stimulation alone compared with STN stimulation alone or STN and PPN stimulation. When looking specifically at those components of the UPDRS-III that measure axial stability, no significant difference was found between STN, PPN, or STN and PPN stimulation. The combined-stimulation group showed a greater improvement in ADLs, although the statistical significance of this was not adequately discussed **(IIa/B)**.

In 2010, Moro *et al* published their results in another six patients [20]. They performed DBS with unilateral electrode placement in the PPN. After a period of optimization over 3 months, they performed a double-blinded comparison at 3 and 12 months. UPDRS-II and III were measured in the medication 'on' and 'off' states, with primary endpoints of the falling, freezing, gait, and balance subscores. The randomization was only for a 1-week period prior to assessment with the stimulator on or off. At 3 and 12 months, there were no statistically significant differences between total scores or subscores, but the scores were significantly improved compared with baseline. This small study was likely underpowered to see differences **(IIa/B)**.

Ferraye *et al* also studied a group of six PD patients with continued gait issues who had previously been implanted bilaterally in the STN and then had bilateral PPN electrodes added in a double-blinded fashion with stimulation on or off [21]. As a group, objective freezing improved with stimulation when patients were in the 'off' medication state, and was unchanged when patients were in the 'on' medication state **(IIa/B)**. These two studies are both small and have their flaws. Further study is needed to ascertain whether stimulation of the PPN should routinely be used for PD patients with refractory gait disorders.

Essential tremor

The use of DBS for movement disorders grew directly from the observation of tremor suppression during VIM mapping during thalamotomies for PD and ET. Benabid *et al* initially used DBS stimulation in patients requiring additional control after having undergone a unilateral lesion [22]. This was then expanded to patients with other types of tremor [23, 24]. In the latter paper, 177 patients, 20 of whom carried the diagnosis of ET, were implanted with a total of 36 electrodes. Patients were evaluated in a non-blinded fashion using a 5-point scale at 3 months and last follow-up (≥6 months). At 3 months, 75% of patients had scores of 3 or 4 (complete disappearance of tremor or reappearance of only slight tremor on rare occasions) and 61.1% maintained this at last follow-

up **(III/B)**. Following these initial case series, other case series confirmed the benefits and safety of this treatment [25-31]. It should be noted that a systematic review of DBS for ET was published by Flora *et al* in 2010 [32]. This publication nicely details the evidence from numerous studies and concludes that DBS may be considered a safe and effective treatment for medically refractory ET patients. Specific examples of some of the studies that brought the authors to that conclusion are detailed below. The reader is referred to the original paper for further in-depth discussion **(III/B)**.

Long-term outcomes have been reported by Rehncrona *et al* in 19 ET patients [33]. Seventeen patients underwent unilateral implantation, one patient underwent bilateral implantation, and one patient underwent staged bilateral implantation. At 2 years and at most recent follow-up (6-7 years) patients were randomized to have the stimulator turned on or off for 4 hours prior to evaluation. Both patients and evaluators were blinded. Patients with stimulation on, as a group, experienced a statistically significant decrease in upper-extremity and postural tremor compared with both baseline and the stimulation off state at both 2 years and 6-7 years. All but three patients continued to have decreased tremor at the 6-7 year evaluation. Decreases in lower-extremity tremor were significant at 2 years, but did not reach statistical significance at 6-7 years **(Ib/A)**.

In 2006, Pahwa *et al* reported VIM DBS outcomes in 26 ET patients enrolled in a 5-year study [34]. In this unblinded study, 13 out of 16 unilaterally implanted patients experienced overall benefit in investigator-ascertained global scales. There was a statistically significant 46% improvement in overall tremor rating compared with baseline, 75% reduction in tremor rating in the targeted limb, 51% improvement in ADLs, 57% improvement in drawing scores, and 44% improvement in pouring scores. In the seven patients with bilateral implantation, the overall tremor reduction increased to 78% compared with baseline (statistically significant). Although there were different reductions between left-limb-targeted and right-limb-targeted tremor, no statistical comparisons were reported **(III/B)**.

Most recently, in 2010, Zhang *et al* reported on 34 patients who had undergone unilateral or bilateral DBS electrode placement in the VIM [35]. Unfortunately, there was substantial patient attrition over time, with only 12 patients available for follow-up in 2008. The average follow-up time was 56.9 months. There was a statistically significant improvement in patients' overall tremor scores compared with baseline. Visual Analogue Scale scoring of tremor and handwriting showed significant improvements compared with baseline of 80.4% and 69.7%, respectively. There was a gradual increase in stimulation parameters over time, and the overall hardware complication rate was 23.5% **(III/B)**.

Overall, based upon the above studies, DBS in the VIM can be recommended with a grade of A for patients with medically refractory tremor.

Dystonia

In a systematic review of the diagnosis and treatment of primary dystonia, Albanese *et al* examined one class Ib study and nine class II or III studies, and concluded that patients with primary (familial or sporadic) generalized or segmental dystonia or those with complex cervical dystonia were the best candidates for DBS [36]. They stated that DBS should be considered a good second-line option in patients with primary dystonia who have failed medication or botulinum toxin treatment. They also emphasized that there are additional surgical options, such as selective peripheral denervation and intrathecal baclofen, for patients with cervical dystonia. Furthermore, patients with secondary dystonia did not experience pronounced improvements and further experience with DBS in these patients is needed. The most important of these studies is discussed in further detail below **(IIb/B)**.

Coubes *et al* studied seven patients with early-onset primary dystonia (DYT1) (six children and one adult) who underwent DBS with bilateral GPi electrode placement at their most recent follow-up (all >1 year) [37]. Compared with their own baseline, patients improved by an average of 90.3% on the Burke-Fahn-Marsden Dystonia Rating Scale (BFMDRS). The same group later published the results of a 2-year follow-up of 31 primary generalized dystonia patients with and without DYT1 mutations [38]. These patients experienced improvements over baseline of 79% and 65% in the clinical and functional BFMDRS. No difference was seen in patients with DYT1 mutations compared with those without **(III/B)**.

Vidailhet *et al* studied 22 patients with primary dystonia (DYT1) in a prospective multicenter study [39]. Patients were studied at 3, 6, and 12 months after bilateral implantation of DBS electrodes into the GPi in the presence and absence of neurostimulation. A number of scales were used and patients and investigators were blinded at the time of scoring. Patients randomized to the group with stimulation 'off' had their stimulators turned off 10 hours prior to scoring. Using the BFMDRS, patients experienced statistically significant improvement at 3 months, which was maintained with a mean decrease of 51% out to 12 months. Patients experienced better outcomes with stimulation 'on' compared with stimulation 'off'. Although the majority of patients had substantial improvement, four patients had limited improvement or worsening, despite adequate anatomic placement. Patients' global disability scores and general health and physical functioning scores on the Short Form-36 (SF-36) questionnaire were also significantly improved following surgery, while there was no change in scores for cognitive functioning or depression. Five adverse events occurred, none with permanent sequelae. In 2007, the group published a prospective 3-year follow-up of the same patient group [40]. Intent-to-treat analysis showed that the motor improvements observed at 12 months were maintained at 3 years (51% and 58%, respectively), as were the improvements on the SF-36. Cognition and mood remained stable **(Ib/A)**.

Kupsch *et al* published a series of 40 patients with primary generalized or segmental dystonia implanted with DBS electrodes in the GPi [41]. These patients were randomly assigned to either stimulation or sham stimulation for 3 months. The primary endpoint was change from baseline on the BFMDRS (0-120 points). Patients and evaluators were blinded as to the state of the stimulator. There was a statistically significant greater improvement in scores in the stimulation group compared with the sham stimulation group (-15.8 vs. -1.4). In the open-label extension, patients who had been randomized to sham stimulation achieved similar results to the stimulation group once they received the treatment. At 6 months, the group showed significant improvements in all movement symptoms except speech and swallowing. In this group, there were no significant differences between the five patients with the *DYT1* mutation and the 13 patients with primary generalized dystonia without the mutation. The most common adverse event was dysarthria, experienced by 12% of patients, which resolved with reprogramming in all but one patient **(Ib/A)**.

Several studies have been conducted specifically of DBS for primary cervical dystonia. In a pilot study, Ostrem *et al* prospectively studied nine patients with primary cervical dystonia who had electrodes implanted bilaterally in the STN [42]. Using the Toronto Western Spasmodic Torticollis Scale (TWSTRS) as the primary measure of outcome, patients experienced a significant decrease in score over baseline (approximately 63% by my calculation). QoL also improved. There were no serious adverse events, although some patients reported depressive symptoms and three had marked weight gain **(III/B)**. In contrast, Cacciola *et al* studied 10 patients with electrodes implanted bilaterally in the GPi [43]. At a mean follow-up of 16.9 months, patients experienced a significant improvement in the TWSTRS of 68.1% – in the same range as that experienced by patients with electrodes implanted in the STN **(III/B)**. Kiss *et al* performed a single-blinded multicenter study of 10 patients with DBS electrodes implanted in the GPi for cervical dystonia [44]. They also demonstrated a significant improvement in the TWSTRS over baseline at 6 and 12 months' follow-up **(III/B)**. Hung *et al* reported similar findings in 10 patients in a non-blinded trial [45] **(III/B)**.

Currently, the US Food and Drug Administration has approved the use of DBS for chronic refractory primary dystonia under the auspices of a humanitarian device exemption for patients aged 7 years or older. Individual institutional review board approval is required and Medtronic continues to collect data on safety and efficacy. This approval was granted in 2003.

The above studies contribute to a recommendation of grade A for the use of DBS in primary generalized dystonia and grade B for its use in cervical dystonia. There are far less data to support the routine use of DBS for dystonias other than primary generalized or for spasmodic torticollis, although some patients with these diagnoses were mixed into other trials. In non-systematic reviews, Ostrem *et al* and Aziz *et al* have both examined the evidence and surgical options for patients with segmental, secondary, and focal dystonias (in addition to primary generalized dystonia and cervical dystonia) [46, 47]. The studies reviewed for these less common dystonias had few patients and many were heterogeneous with respect to diagnoses and outcome. These disorders require further systematic study before recommendations can be made regarding the routine use of DBS for these conditions [48] **(IV/C)**.

Conclusions

In contrast to many other areas of neurosurgery, substantial evidence in the literature facilitates prediction of the outcome of DBS in select patient populations. Unfortunately, none of these treatments has been shown to be disease-modifying. Particularly in PD, treatments that can alter the course of the disease need to be sought and validated. In addition, better outcome measures and biomarkers for disease progression will potentially strengthen our ability to detect differences in outcomes.

Recommendations	Evidence level
◆ In medically refractory patients with PD, DBS to the STN is superior to best medical therapy for motor outcome.	Ib/A
◆ In PD patients, there is no difference in motor outcome between placement in the STN or GPi.	Ib/A
◆ PD patients implanted in the STN can experience greater reductions in medications than GPi patients.	IIa/B
◆ PD patients implanted in the GPi experience improvement in depression scores, while patients implanted in the STN experience worsening.	Ib/A
◆ Gait is better preserved over time in PD patients implanted in the GPi compared with the STN.	IIb/B
◆ DBS placed in the VIM is safe and effective for the treatment of refractory ET.	Ib/A
◆ DBS placed in the GPi is effective in the treatment of primary generalized dystonia.	Ib/A
◆ DBS is effective in the treatment of refractory primary cervical dystonia.	IIb/B

References

1. Benabid AL, Pollak P, Gross C, et al. Acute and long-term effects of subthalamic nucleus stimulation in Parkinson's disease. Stereotact Funct Neurosurg 1994; 62: 76-84.

2. Limousin P, Krack P, Pollak P, et al. Electrical stimulation of the subthalamic nucleus in advanced Parkinson's disease. N Engl J Med 1998; 339: 1105-11.

3. Deuschl G, Schade-Brittinger C, Krack P, et al. A randomized trial of deep-brain stimulation for Parkinson's disease. N Engl J Med 2006; 355: 896-908.

4. Schüpbach WM, Maltête D, Houeto JL, et al. Neurosurgery at an earlier stage of Parkinson disease: a randomized, controlled trial. Neurology 2007; 68: 267-71.

5. Weaver FM, Follett K, Stern M, et al. Bilateral deep brain stimulation vs. best medical therapy for patients with advanced Parkinson disease: a randomized controlled trial. JAMA 2009; 301: 63-73.

6. Williams A, Gill S, Varma T, et al. Deep brain stimulation plus best medical therapy versus best medical therapy alone for advanced Parkinson's disease (PD SURG trial): a randomised, open-label trial. Lancet Neurol 2010; 9: 581-91.

7. Antonini A, Isaias IU, Rodolfi G, et al. A 5-year prospective assessment of advanced Parkinson disease patients treated with subcutaneous apomorphine infusion or deep brain stimulation. J Neurol 2011; 258: 579-85.

8. Kleiner-Fisman G, Herzog J, Fisman DN, et al. Subthalamic nucleus deep brain stimulation: summary and meta-analysis of outcomes. Mov Disord 2006; 21(Suppl. 14): S290-304.

9. Burchiel KJ, Anderson VC, Favre J, Hammerstad JP. Comparison of pallidal and subthalamic nucleus deep brain stimulation for advanced Parkinson's disease: results of a randomized, blinded pilot study. Neurosurgery 1999; 45: 1375-82.

10. Anderson VC, Burchiel KJ, Hogarth P, Favre J, Hammerstad JP. Pallidal vs. subthalamic nucleus deep brain stimulation in Parkinson disease. Arch Neurol 2005; 62: 554-60.

11. Rodriguez-Oroz MC, Obeso JA, Lang AE, et al. Bilateral deep brain stimulation in Parkinson's disease: a multicentre study with 4 years follow-up. Brain 2005; 128: 2240-9.

12. Okun MS, Fernandez HH, Wu SS, et al. Cognition and mood in Parkinson's disease in subthalamic nucleus versus globus pallidus interna deep brain stimulation: the COMPARE trial. Ann Neurol 2009; 65: 586-95.

13. Zahodne LB, Okun MS, Foote KD, et al. Greater improvement in quality of life following unilateral deep brain stimulation surgery in the globus pallidus as compared to the subthalamic nucleus. J Neurol 2009; 256: 1321-9.

14. Moro E, Lozano AM, Pollak P, et al. Long-term results of a multicenter study on subthalamic and pallidal stimulation in Parkinson's disease. Mov Disord 2010; 25: 578-86.

15. Follett KA, Weaver FM, Stern M, et al. Pallidal versus subthalamic deep-brain stimulation for Parkinson's disease. N Engl J Med 2010; 362: 2077-91.

16. St George RJ, Nutt JG, Burchiel KJ, Horak FB. A meta-regression of the long-term effects of deep brain stimulation on balance and gait in PD. Neurology 2010; 75: 1292-9.

17. Mazzone P, Lozano A, Stanzione P, et al. Implantation of human pedunculopontine nucleus: a safe and clinically relevant target in Parkinson's disease. Neuroreport 2005; 16: 1877-81.

18. Plaha P, Gill SS. Bilateral deep brain stimulation of the pedunculopontine nucleus for Parkinson's disease. Neuroreport 2005; 16: 1883-7.

19. Stefani A, Lozano AM, Peppe A, et al. Bilateral deep brain stimulation of the pedunculopontine and subthalamic nuclei in severe Parkinson's disease. Brain 2007; 130: 1596-607.

20. Moro E, Hamani C, Poon YY, *et al*. Unilateral pedunculopontine stimulation improves falls in Parkinson's disease. *Brain* 2010; 133: 215-24.

21. Ferraye MU, Debû B, Fraix V, *et al*. Effects of pedunculopontine nucleus area stimulation on gait disorders in Parkinson's disease. *Brain* 2010; 133: 205-14.

22. Benabid AL, Pollak P, Gervason C, *et al*. Long-term suppression of tremor by chronic stimulation of the ventral intermediate thalamic nucleus. *Lancet* 1991; 337: 403-6.

23. Benabid AL, Pollak P, Gao D, *et al*. Chronic electrical stimulation of the ventralis intermedius nucleus of the thalamus as a treatment of movement disorders. *J Neurosurg* 1996; 84: 203-14.

24. Pollak P, Benabid AL, Gervason CL, Hoffmann D, Seigneuret E, Perret J. Long-term effects of chronic stimulation of the ventral intermediate thalamic nucleus in different types of tremor. *Adv Neurol* 1993; 60: 408-13.

25. Fields JA, Tröster AI, Woods SP, *et al*. Neuropsychological and quality of life outcomes 12 months after unilateral thalamic stimulation for essential tremor. *J Neurol Neurosurg Psychiatry* 2003; 74: 305-11.

26. Hariz GM, Lindberg M, Bergenheim AT. Impact of thalamic deep brain stimulation on disability and health-related quality of life in patients with essential tremor. *J Neurol Neurosurg Psychiatry* 2002; 72: 47-52.

27. Koller W, Pahwa R, Busenbark K, *et al*. High-frequency unilateral thalamic stimulation in the treatment of essential and parkinsonian tremor. *Ann Neurol* 1997; 42: 292-9.

28. Lee JY, Kondziolka D. Thalamic deep brain stimulation for management of essential tremor. *J Neurosurg* 2005; 103: 400-3.

29. Limousin P, Speelman JD, Gielen F, Janssens M. Multicentre European study of thalamic stimulation in parkinsonian and essential tremor. *J Neurol Neurosurg Psychiatry* 1999; 66: 289-96.

30. Ondo W, Jankovic J, Schwartz K, Almaguer M, Simpson RK. Unilateral thalamic deep brain stimulation for refractory essential tremor and Parkinson's disease tremor. *Neurology* 1998; 5: 1063-9.

31. Pahwa R, Lyons KL, Wilkinson SB, *et al*. Bilateral thalamic stimulation for the treatment of essential tremor. *Neurology* 1999; 53: 1447-50.

32. Flora ED, Perera CL, Cameron AL, Maddern GJ. Deep brain stimulation for essential tremor: a systematic review. *Mov Disord* 2010; 25: 1550-9.

33. Rehncrona S, Johnels B, Widner H, Törnqvist AL, Hariz M, Sydow O. Long-term efficacy of thalamic deep brain stimulation for tremor: double-blind assessments. *Mov Disord* 2003; 18: 163-70.

34. Pahwa R, Lyons KE, Wilkinson SB, *et al*. Long-term evaluation of deep brain stimulation of the thalamus. *J Neurosurg* 2006; 104: 506-12.

35. Zhang K, Bhatia S, Oh MY, Cohen D, Angle C, Whiting D. Long-term results of thalamic deep brain stimulation for essential tremor. *J Neurosurg* 2010; 112: 1271-6.

36. Albanese A, Barnes MP, Bhatia KP, *et al*. A systematic review on the diagnosis and treatment of primary (idiopathic) dystonia and dystonia plus syndromes: report of an EFNS/MDS-ES Task Force. *Eur J Neurol* 2006; 13: 433-44.

37. Coubes P, Roubertie A, Vayssiere N, Hemm S, Echenne B. Treatment of DYT1-generalised dystonia by stimulation of the internal globus pallidus. *Lancet* 2000; 355: 2220-1.

38. Coubes P, Cif L, El Fertit H, *et al*. Electrical stimulation of the globus pallidus internus in patients with primary generalized dystonia: long-term results. *J Neurosurg* 2004; 101: 189-94.

39. Vidailhet M, Vercueil L, Houeto JL, *et al*. Bilateral deep-brain stimulation of the globus pallidus in primary generalized dystonia. *N Engl J Med* 2005; 352: 459-67.

40. Vidailhet M, Vercueil L, Houeto JL, *et al*. Bilateral, pallidal, deep-brain stimulation in primary generalised dystonia: a prospective 3-year follow-up study. *Lancet Neurol* 2007; 6: 223-9.

41. Kupsch A, Benecke R, Müller J, *et al*. Pallidal deep-brain stimulation in primary generalized or segmental dystonia. *N Engl J Med* 2006; 355: 1978-90.

42. Ostrem JL, Racine CA, Glass GA, *et al*. Subthalamic nucleus deep brain stimulation in primary cervical dystonia. *Neurology* 2011; 76: 870-8.

43. Cacciola F, Farah JO, Eldridge PR, Byrne P, Varma TK. Bilateral deep brain stimulation for cervical dystonia: long-term outcome in a series of 10 patients. *Neurosurgery* 2010; 67: 957-63.

44. Kiss ZH, Doig-Beyaert K, Eliasziw M, Tsui J, Haffenden A, Suchowersky O. The Canadian multicentre study of deep brain stimulation for cervical dystonia. *Brain* 2007; 130: 2879-86.

45. Hung SW, Hamani C, Lozano AM, *et al*. Long-term outcome of bilateral pallidal deep brain stimulation for primary cervical dystonia. *Neurology* 2007; 68: 457-9.

46. Ostrem JL, Starr PA. Treatment of dystonia with deep brain stimulation. *Neurotherapeutics* 2008; 5: 320-30.

47. Aziz TZ, Green AL. Dystonia: a surgeon's perspective. *Parkinsonism Relat Disord* 2009; 15(Suppl. 3): S75-80.

48. Eltahawy HA, Saint-Cyr J, Giladi N, Lang AE, Lozano AM. Primary dystonia is more responsive than secondary dystonia to pallidal interventions: outcome after pallidotomy or pallidal deep brain stimulation. *Neurosurgery* 2004; 54: 613-9.

Chapter 14

Chapter 14

Chapter 15

Neuromodulation procedures for medical and psychiatric conditions

Matthew K Mian BSE, Medical Student

Sameer A Sheth MD PhD, Chief Resident in Neurosurgery

Emad N Eskandar MD, Associate Professor,
Director of Stereotactic and Functional Neurosurgery

DEPARTMENT OF NEUROSURGERY, MASSACHUSETTS GENERAL HOSPITAL, HARVARD MEDICAL SCHOOL, BOSTON, MASSACHUSETTS, USA

Introduction

Neuromodulation can be defined as the deliberate manipulation of the nervous system to produce a change in its behavior. The vast majority of neuromodulatory procedures in current practice rely on the creation of a precise lesion or the delivery of targeted electrical stimulation. Although the history of these techniques encompasses at least half a century, this chapter focuses on the subset of procedures still in current use that have been (or are being) investigated for efficacy.

Methodology

A PubMed computerized literature search was conducted for each of the neuromodulatory procedures discussed. Priority was given to articles based on the highest available level of evidence for each procedure or indication (e.g., recommendations for dorsal spinal cord stimulation were based on level I – rather than level II or III – studies). In all cases, bibliographies of selected papers were carefully reviewed to identify other pertinent articles.

Pain alleviation

Despite a vast literature on neuromodulation for alleviating chronic pain conditions, there exists a paucity of class I data. Table 1 offers a summary of studies supporting three applications of central nervous system electrical stimulation to chronic pain disorders [1-16]. Owing to a dearth of class I or II data regarding peripheral neuromodulation for pain [17, 18], we omit discussion of these procedures here.

Spinal cord stimulation

Dorsal column spinal cord stimulation (SCS) has been evaluated in randomized trials for both complex regional pain syndrome type I (CRPS-I; i.e., reflex sympathetic dystrophy) and intractable low back pain following surgery (i.e., failed back surgery syndrome).

In 2000, Kemler *et al* reported on a trial in which CRPS-I patients were randomized to either SCS plus physical therapy (n=36) or physical therapy alone (n=18) [1]. Patients randomized to SCS underwent a test stimulation period, following which patients without a clinical response were explanted. Test

Table 1. Studies of neuromodulation for the treatment of select chronic pain conditions. *Continued overleaf.*

Study	Study design	n	Conclusions
SCS for CRPS-I			
Kemler et al, 2000 [1]	RCT	54	Addition of SCS to physical therapy reduces pain and improves health-related quality of life more than physical therapy alone (Ib/A) but is not accompanied by functional improvement
Taylor et al, 2006 [2]	MA (25 case series)	-	An average of 67% of CRPS-I patients experience VAS pain score reductions of ≥50% with SCS
SCS for failed back surgery syndrome			
North et al, 2005 [3]	RCT	50	SCS is superior to reoperation in achieving VAS pain score reductions of >50% among patients with persistent low back pain following surgery (Ib/A)
Taylor et al, 2005 [4]	MA (72 case series)	-	67% of patients implanted with an SCS system for either failed back surgery syndrome or chronic back and leg pain experienced VAS pain score reductions of ≥50%
Kumar et al, 2007 [5]	RCT	100	SCS is superior to medical management in achieving VAS pain score reductions of ≥50% for persistent radicular pain following surgery for disc herniation (Ib/A)

Motor cortex stimulation for trigeminal neuropathic pain				
			Long-term response, % [a]	Follow-up, months
Meyerson et al, 1993 [6]	CS	5	100	8-28
Herregodts et al, 1995 [7]	CS	5	80	4-23
Katayama et al, 1994 [8]	CS	3	66	4
Ebel et al, 1996 [9]	CS	7	43	6-24
Nguyen et al, 1997, 1999, 2000 [10-12]	CS	12	83	27

Chapter 15

Table 1. Studies of neuromodulation for the treatment of select chronic pain conditions. *Continued.*

Study	Study design	n	Conclusions	
			Motor cortex stimulation for trigeminal neuropathic pain	
			Long-term response, % [a]	**Follow-up, months**
Brown and Pilitsis, 2005 [13]	CS	10	60	10
Pirotte *et al*, 2005 [14]	CS	6	83	6-60
Rasche *et al*, 2006 [15]	CS	10	50	12-120
Lefaucheur *et al*, 2009 [16]	CS	6	33	9-12

CRPS-I = complex regional pain syndrome type I; CS = case series; MA = meta-analysis; RCT = randomized controlled trial; SCS = spinal cord stimulation; VAS = Visual Analogue Scale; [a] = defined as a ≥50% reduction in VAS pain score with respect to the preoperative baseline

stimulation was successful in 24 of the implanted patients (67%), and in an intent-to-treat analysis, the SCS group demonstrated a greater mean reduction in Visual Analogue Scale (VAS) pain score versus the physical therapy group after 6 months (2.4cm decrease vs. 0.2cm increase; p<0.001). However, there was no difference in functional status between the two groups **(Ib/A)**. In a subsequent meta-analysis, Taylor *et al* concluded that an average of 67% of CRPS-I patients experience VAS pain score reductions of 50% or more with SCS [2].

Data have also supported the use of SCS in patients with failed back surgery syndrome. North *et al* described a prospective trial with a cross-over component in which patients with persistent or recurrent radicular pain following lumbosacral spine surgery were randomized to either SCS (n=24) or reoperation (n=26) [3]. Patients assigned initially to SCS were less likely to cross over (5/24 vs. 14/26 patients, p=0.02) and they required fewer opiate analgesics (p<0.025) **(Ib/A)**. Further work has suggested that 67% of failed back surgery syndrome patients experience VAS pain score reductions of at least 50% [4]. Finally, Kumar *et al* randomized patients

with persistent radicular pain following lumbar disc herniation surgery to SCS plus medical management (n=52) or medical management alone (n=48) [5]. Patients receiving SCS were significantly more likely to experience a VAS pain score reduction of 50% or more (48% vs. 9% of patients, p<0.001) **(Ib/A)**.

Motor cortex stimulation

Although motor cortex stimulation (MCS) lacks randomized trials to endorse its use, case series in the past two decades have documented its efficacy when applied specifically to patients with trigeminal neuropathic pain [6-16] **(III/B)**. Most studies of MCS for trigeminal neuropathic pain report that 60-80% of patients experience VAS pain score reductions of at least 50%. However, case series investigating this technique are typically small (often <10 patients), and there may be a bias toward reporting only series with positive outcomes. Prospective trials of MCS for trigeminal neuropathic pain will thus be critical to verifying its efficacy.

Epilepsy

Vagus nerve stimulation

Chronic, intermittent vagus nerve stimulation (VNS) is a safe and effective adjunctive therapy for patients with medically refractory epilepsy who are not ideal candidates for resective surgery. The basis for US Food and Drug Administration approval of VNS in 1997 included data from a pair of double-blind randomized controlled trials of patients with partial-onset seizures.

The first study randomized 114 subjects to one of two protocols of intermittent stimulation: therapeutic high-frequency stimulation ('high') and a control consisting of stimulation at a presumed sub-therapeutic frequency ('low') [19]. After 14 weeks, the high-stimulation group achieved a significant reduction in seizure frequency relative to those receiving low stimulation (24.5% vs. 6.1%; p=0.01). In addition, more patients in the high-stimulation group achieved a 50% or greater reduction in seizure frequency (31% vs. 13%; p=0.02) **(Ib/A)**.

The second study enrolled 199 patients with complex partial or secondarily generalized seizures, randomizing them to either high- (n=94) or low-frequency (n=102) stimulation (the same paradigm as the first study) [20]. In the 3 months after implantation, the high-stimulation group had a greater average reduction in total seizure frequency (28% vs. 15%; p=0.04), as well as greater improvements in global evaluation scores compared with the low-stimulation group **(Ib/A)**.

A pair of open-label extension studies subsequently assigned all participants of these previous two studies to high-frequency stimulation and followed them prospectively for 12 months [21, 22]. Both studies suggested that the VNS-associated reduction in seizures increases with time, with patients sustaining median reductions in seizure frequency of 32% and 45% by the end of the 12-month period [21, 22] **(III/B)**.

Deep brain stimulation of the anterior nuclei of the thalamus

Investigators have evaluated deep brain stimulation (DBS) of the anterior nuclei of the thalamus (ANT) for patients with pharmacoresistant partial-onset seizures who have either failed or are not candidates for resective surgery. The rationale for stimulating the ANT involves several lines of evidence:

* The ANT – by virtue of their anatomic connections – are positioned to maintain and transmit propagating seizures.
* High-frequency stimulation of the ANT desynchronizes cortical activity at distant sites [23-25].
* High-frequency stimulation of the ANT raises seizure thresholds in an animal model of epilepsy [26].

Indeed, a series of small studies in humans have suggested that ANT DBS can be clinically effective [25, 27-30].

In 2010, the Stimulation of the ANT for Epilepsy (SANTE) Study Group reported on the results of a multicenter, double-blind randomized trial of ANT DBS in patients with medically refractory partial seizures [31]. Patients were implanted with bilateral ANT electrodes and randomized to either active (n=54) or sham (n=55) stimulation. In the final month of the 3-month blinded phase of the trial, the active-stimulation group had a 29% greater reduction in estimated seizure frequency than the sham-stimulation group (p=0.002), with unadjusted respective median declines of 40.4% and 14.5% in the two treatment arms, respectively **(Ib/A)**. The blinded phase was followed by an open-label extension in which all patients received active stimulation. After 2 years, there was a median reduction in seizure frequency of 56%, with 54% of patients experiencing declines of at least 50% **(III/B)**.

Psychiatric conditions

History

Surgical interventions for psychiatric conditions were first attempted in the late 1930s, prior to the widespread adoption of stereotactic surgical

Table 2. Studies of lesioning as a treatment for psychiatric conditions. *Continued overleaf.*

Study	Study design	n	Responders, %
Anterior capsulotomy for OCD			
Lippitz et al, 1999 [41]	CS	19[a] 10[b]	47[c] 70[c]
Christensen et al, 2002 [62]	CS	2[a]	100[c]
Oliver et al, 2003 [45]	CS	15[a]	53[d]
Liu et al, 2008 [44]	CS	35[a]	86[c]
Rück et al, 2008 [43]	CS	25[a,b]	48[e]
Lopes et al, 2009 [46]	CS	5[b]	60[e]
Csigó et al, 2010 [42]	CC	5[a]	NA
Cingulotomy for MDD			
Ballantine et al, 1967 [39]	CS	26	77[f]
Ballantine et al, 1987 [47]	CS	83	41[g]
Spangler et al, 1996 [50]	CS	10	60[h]
Steele et al, 2008 [49]	CS	8	25[i]
Shields et al, 2008 [48]	CS	33	33[j]

Chapter 15

Table 2. Studies of lesioning as a treatment for psychiatric conditions. *Continued overleaf.*

Study	Study design	n	Responders, %
Cingulotomy for OCD			
Ballantine et al, 1987 [47]	CS	32	25[g]
Jenike et al, 1991 [54]	CS	35	25-30
Baer et al, 2005 [51]	CS	18	5
Spangler et al, 1996 [50]	CS	15	27[g]
Dougherty et al, 2002 [52]	CS	44	32[e]
Richter et al, 2004 [53]	CS	15	27[e]
Subcaudate tractotomy for MDD[k]			
Ström-Olsen et al, 1971 [56]	CS	75	41
Goktepe et al, 1975 [55]	CS	78	68
Hodgkiss et al, 1995 [57]	CS	185	34
Subcaudate tractotomy for OCD[k]			
Ström-Olsen et al, 1971 [56]	CS	20	50
Goktepe et al, 1975 [55]	CS	18	50
Hodgkiss et al, 1995 [57]	CS	15	33
Limbic leucotomy for MDD and bipolar disorder			
Mitchell-Heggs et al, 1976 [59]	CS	9	56[k]
Kelly et al, 1973 [58]	CS	5	40[k]
Cho et al, 2008 [60]	CS	16	69

Table 2. Studies of lesioning as a treatment for psychiatric conditions. *Continued.*

Study	Study design	n	Responders, %
Limbic leucotomy for OCD			
Mitchell-Heggs et al, 1976 [59]	CS	27	67[k]
Kelly et al, 1973 [58]	CS	17	41[k]
Hay et al, 1993 [61]	CC	26	38

CC = case-control; CS = case series; MDD = major depressive disorder; NA = not assessed; OCD = obsessive-compulsive disorder; Y-BOCS = Yale-Brown Obsessive-Compulsive Scale; [a] = surgical capsulotomy; [b] = gamma capsulotomy

Responder defined as: decrease in the Y-BOCS of [c] = $\geq 50\%$, [d] = $\geq 33\%$, [e] = $\geq 35\%$; [f] = significantly improved'; [g] = authors' level 5 (normal without other treatment) and 4 (normal with pharmacological or behavioral treatment) [47]; [h] = score of 1-2 on the Clinical Global Improvement Scale and 3-5 on the Current, Global, Psychiatric-Social Status Scale [50]; [i] = decrease in the Hamilton Depressive Scale of $\geq 50\%$; [j] = decrease in the Beck Depression Inventory of $\geq 35\%$; [k] = authors' level I (completely recovered) or II (mild residual symptoms) [56, 59]

techniques in humans [32]. An early pioneer in this field, Egas Moniz, developed the prefrontal leucotomy (later termed lobotomy) for severe affective and psychotic disorders, an accomplishment that earned him the 1949 Nobel Prize in Physiology or Medicine. However, increasingly indiscriminate application of this procedure and recognition of its side-effect burden [33], as well as the development of neuroleptics such as chlorpromazine [34], contributed to the decline in use of prefrontal leucotomy over the following decade.

The careful application of stereotactic techniques to neurosurgery, first introduced in humans in 1947, heralded the modern stereotactic era. The initial report by Spiegel et al actually mentions a psychiatric condition as the primary indication for early stereotactic studies: lesioning the medial nucleus of the thalamus to 'reduce the emotional reactivity by a procedure much less drastic than frontal lobotomy' [35]. Shortly thereafter, Leksell and Talairach et al developed anterior capsulotomy, disrupting the fiber connections between the orbitofrontal cortex and the thalamus [36, 37]. Knight targeted the connections between prefrontal cortex and the cingulate, amygdala, and other limbic structures with

subcaudate tractotomy [38], and Ballantine et al ablated the dorsal anterior cingulate cortex itself with cingulotomy [39]. Limbic leucotomy, a combination of cingulotomy and subcaudate tractotomy, was developed by Kelly et al to disrupt both connective pathways [40]. The significantly improved side-effect profile of these precise ablative procedures compared with that of frontal lobotomy, along with increasing awareness of severe neuroleptic side effects such as tardive dyskinesia, fueled a resurgence of interest in psychiatric neurosurgery. These four lesion-based approaches are still in use today, and provided the groundwork for recent trials of DBS for psychiatric conditions.

Lesions for psychiatric conditions

Anterior capsulotomy, cingulotomy, subcaudate tractotomy, and limbic leucotomy have been applied for the treatment of several psychiatric disorders in patients refractory to pharmacological and behavioral therapy, most notably major depressive disorder (MDD) and obsessive-compulsive disorder (OCD) (Table 2) [39, 41-62]. Response metrics have varied across studies, but many have employed the Yale-Brown Obsessive-Compulsive Scale (Y-BOCS) [63] to measure OCD severity and the Beck Depression Inventory [64] and/or Hamilton Depression Scale (HAM-D) [65] to measure MDD severity. The existing literature for surgical treatment of both disorders consists primarily of case series, with very few prospective controlled trials comparing one intervention with another or with best medical therapy.

By targeting fibers coursing through the anterior limb of the internal capsule, anterior capsulotomy disrupts connections between the orbitofrontal cortex and the caudate and medial thalamic nuclei. The lesion can be produced by either thermocoagulation, provided by a surgically directed radiofrequency probe, or radiosurgery with collimated gamma rays. Case series with at least five patients employing either surgical capsulotomy or gamma capsulotomy for the treatment of severe OCD report response rates of 47-86% [41-46] **(III/B)**. This heterogeneity is likely the result of several factors, including variations in patient selection, surgical technique, response metric, and follow-up duration, and similarly exists in studies employing other ablative procedures. One recent non-randomized controlled study compared outcomes of capsulotomy with best non-surgical treatment in 10 patients with severe OCD [42]. Five patients underwent capsulotomy along with intensive long-term rehabilitation (consisting of pharmacotherapy and behavioral therapy), while five patients matched for age, gender, and symptom severity participated in rehabilitation alone. At 6 months, the Y-BOCS scores of the five surgical patients were reduced by 48%, whereas those of the matched non-surgical patients were reduced by 19% (p<0.05), demonstrating the benefit of capsulotomy over best conventional therapy for the treatment of refractory OCD [42] **(IIa/B)**.

Whitty *et al* developed anterior cingulectomy – resection of 4cm of the dorsal anterior cingulate via open craniotomy – in an effort to increase the precision of frontal lobotomy [66]. Stereotactic cingulotomy, introduced in the 1960s, was a refinement of the procedure that reduced complications [39]. Case series investigating the efficacy of cingulotomy for MDD have reported response rates varying from 25% to 77% [39, 47-50] **(III/B)**, while

response rates for cingulotomy for OCD vary from 25% to 56% [47, 50-54] **(III/B)**. Although not compared systematically, several studies have suggested that patients with MDD tend to enjoy a better response to cingulotomy than those with OCD [33, 47, 67] **(IV/C)**. One small non-blinded trial randomized four patients with severe OCD to either anterior capsulotomy or cingulotomy, and assessed the postoperative results with several psychiatric and cognitive metrics [68]. Reductions in Comprehensive Psychopathological Rating Scale [69] scores for the capsulotomy patients were 95% and 39% for the psychiatric and cognitive metrics, respectively, while those for cingulotomy patients were 88% and 43%. The authors stated that these results suggest better efficacy for capsulotomy than cingulotomy in controlling obsessive symptoms **(IIb/B)**, but recognized the limitation of the small sample size [68].

Subcaudate tractotomy consists of placing a stereotactic lesion in the substantia innominata of the ventromedial frontal lobes inferior to the caudate nucleus, in an effort to disrupt frontolimbic connections. This procedure has been performed as a treatment for both MDD and OCD. Response rates range from 34% to 68% in the case series literature [55-57, 70, 71] **(III/B)**.

By disrupting frontolimbic connections traversing both the cingulate region and the anterior limb of the internal capsule, limbic leucotomy was designed to provide better efficacy than either subcaudate tractotomy or anterior cingulotomy alone [40]. The few existing series employing limbic leucotomy for major affective disorders (including MDD and bipolar disorder) or OCD have reported response rates comparable with those from other procedures, ranging from 38% to 69% [58-60] **(III/B)**. One study compared the results of surgery in 26 OCD patients (17 receiving limbic leucotomy, six receiving cingulotomy, and three receiving subcaudate tractotomy) with a retrospectively matched non-surgical group of 10 patients [61]. With a 10-year mean follow-up, 38% of surgical patients showed significant improvement compared with none of the non-surgical patients, suggesting a beneficial effect attributable to surgery **(IIa/B)**.

When considering these results, it is important to keep in mind the severity and refractoriness of the psychiatric illnesses being treated. The approximately 35-65% response rate observed in these case series, in addition to the positive results from the few case-control studies and the single small randomized study, represent evidence for an important treatment option for these desperate patients, despite the lack of Ia/A data. Nevertheless, future studies can certainly provide higher-quality evidence by including a randomized, double-blind non-surgical group. Such a design would be particularly amenable to 'non-invasive' radiosurgical procedures such as gamma capsulotomy, but could also be suited to open surgical procedures employing sham surgery such as a partial-thickness burr hole [72]. Whether such studies are performed will likely depend upon ethical considerations and the question of whether true equipoise still exists regarding the efficacy of ablative surgery for otherwise intractable psychiatric disorders.

Vagus nerve stimulation for depression

The application of VNS to treatment-resistant depression emerged from the observation of improved mood in epilepsy patients treated with VNS [20, 73]. Table 3 gives a summary of studies in this area [74-81]. The initial US-based multisite open-label pilot trial showed a response rate (≥50% reduction in HAM-D score) of 40% in the first 30 patients [74], which reduced to 31%

Chapter 15

Table 3. Studies examining vagus nerve stimulation as a treatment for depression.

Study	Study design	n	Responders, %[a]
Rush *et al*, 2000 [74]	CS	30	40
Sackeim *et al*, 2001 [75]	CS	59	31
Marangell *et al*, 2002 [76]	CS	59	44
Nahas *et al*, 2005 [77]	CS	59	42
Rush *et al*, 2005 [80]	CS	205	27
George *et al*, 2005 [81]	CC	205	27
Schlaepfer *et al*, 2008 [78]	CS	74	53
Bajbouj *et al*, 2010 [79]	CS	49	53

CC = case-control; CS = case series; [a] = responder defined as a decrease in the Hamilton Depressive Scale of ≥50%

Chapter 15

Table 4. Studies of DBS as a treatment for psychiatric conditions.

Study	Study design	n	Responders, %
ALIC or VC/VS DBS for OCD[a]			
Nuttin et al, 1999 [83]	CS	4	NA
Nuttin et al, 2003 [84]	BC	6	75
Abelson et al, 2005 [85]	BC	4	25
Greenberg et al, 2006 [90]	CS	8	50
Goodman et al, 2010 [87]	BC	6	67
Greenberg et al, 2010 [88]	BC	26	62
Huff et al, 2010 [86]	BC	10	10
STN DBS for OCD[b]			
Mallet et al, 2008 [89]	BC	16	75
Subgenual cingulate DBS for MDD[c]			
Mayberg et al, 2005 [91]	CS	6	67
Lozano et al, 2008 [92]	CS	20	60
VC/VS DBS for MDD[c]			
Malone et al, 2009 [93]	CS	15	53
Schlaepfer et al, 2008 [94]	BC	3	NA

ALIC = anterior limbs of the internal capsules; BC = blinded, sham-controlled trial; CS = case series; DBS = deep brain stimulation; MDD = major depressive disorder; NA = not assessed; OCD = obsessive-compulsive disorder; STN = subthalamic nucleus; VC = ventral capsule; VS = ventral striatum; Y-BOCS = Yale-Brown Obsessive-Compulsive Scale

Responder defined as: decrease in the Y-BOCS of [a] = ≥35%; [b] = ≥25%; [c] = decrease in the Hamilton Depressive Scale of ≥50%

following the addition of the next 29 patients at the 3-month follow-up [75] **(III/B)**. Within the same 59-patient cohort, the response rate increased to 44% at the 1-year follow-up [76] and stabilized at 42% at 2 years [77] **(III/B)**. A similar European multisite open-label study with 74 patients reported a 3-month response rate of 37%, increasing to 53% at 1 year [78] and stabilizing at 53% at 2 years [79] **(III/B)**.

Given the success of the US pilot study, the same group implemented a randomized, blinded, sham-controlled acute-phase trial in which 235 patients were randomized to 10 weeks of either VNS or sham treatment. This trial failed to meet its primary endpoint, with a response rate of only 15% in the VNS group compared with 10% in the sham group (p=0.25) [82]. In the subsequent open phase, all patients received VNS for 1 year, with an overall response rate of 27% [80] **(III/B)**.

A cohort of 124 patients similar in demographics and psychiatric and treatment histories who underwent best non-surgical treatment was compared with the VNS-treated group. The response rate among the non-surgical patients was 13%, significantly less than the 27% rate in the VNS-treated group (p=0.01) [81] **(IIa/B)**.

Deep brain stimulation for psychiatric conditions

The promising results and minimal complications associated with lesion-based psychiatric surgery over four decades, coupled with the successful application of DBS to movement disorders, motivated the investigation of DBS for psychiatric conditions. Besides the reversible nature of electrical stimulation compared with lesioning, DBS offers the advantage of facilitating randomized double-blind placebo-controlled trials. As with ablative surgery, the psychiatric disorders investigated most commonly with DBS are OCD and MDD (Table 4) [83-94].

Obsessive-compulsive disorder

Nuttin *et al* reported the first attempt of psychiatric surgery with DBS, in which leads were placed into the anterior limbs of the internal capsules (ALIC) in four patients with intractable OCD [83]. This target was chosen based on the success of anterior capsulotomy as a treatment for this disorder. In this descriptive study, three of the four patients achieved some form of beneficial response. The same group reported their experience with six patients implanted with DBS electrodes, four of whom were assessed using a double-blind random cross-over design of 'on' and 'off' stimulation periods with 21 months of follow-up [84]. During the stimulation 'on' phase, three patients (75%) responded to therapy, as defined by a 35% or greater reduction in Y-BOCS score, demonstrating the beneficial effect of ALIC DBS [84] **(Ib/A)**. Another small trial of ALIC DBS with four OCD patients adopted a similar double-blind randomized design of 'on' and 'off' stimulation, with one responder (25%) [85] **(Ib/A)**. A double-blind sham-controlled cross-over study of unilateral ALIC DBS in 10 OCD patients found only a 10% response rate, demonstrating the necessity for bilateral stimulation [86] **(III/B)**.

Building on the experience gained with anterior capsulotomy, in which outcomes were improved with more ventral lesions, many DBS studies have adopted a ventral target within the ALIC, termed the ventral capsule/ventral striatum (VC/VS) [87]. In a randomized, staggered-onset, double-blind study of VC/VS DBS in six OCD patients, four patients (67%) responded significantly with a 12-month follow-up [87] **(Ib/A)**. Greenberg *et al* pooled results from four centers performing VC/VS DBS for OCD [88]. Two of the sites adopted double-blind 'on'/'off' stimulation designs (accounting for 16 patients), whereas the other two sites were open label. These pooled results showed that 16 patients (62%) responded with Y-BOCS reductions of at least 35%, providing the best evidence to date for the utility of VC/VS DBS for intractable OCD [88] **(Ib/A)**.

One well-designed study investigated the anteromedial subthalamic nucleus (STN) as a target for DBS in patients with OCD [89]. Sixteen OCD patients were studied in a multicenter, double-blind, sham-controlled cross-over investigation of anteromedial STN DBS. This choice of target was motivated by observations of reduction in OCD severity in Parkinson's disease patients treated with STN DBS [95, 96]. The response rate was 75%, although these authors used the less stringent criterion of a 25% or more reduction in Y-BOCS score. This study demonstrates the efficacy of modulating OCD symptoms by stimulating the limbic STN **(Ib/A)**.

In addition to these controlled trials, a handful of small trials or series have investigated the efficacy of DBS for OCD targeting the ventral ALIC [90, 97-101], STN [95], ventral caudate nucleus [102, 103], and inferior thalamic peduncle [104, 105], with positive results **(III/B)**.

Major depressive disorder

The first studies of DBS for MDD targeted the subgenual cingulate, based on the finding that this region appeared to be involved in modulating negative mood states such as acute sadness and longstanding depression [106]. Mayberg *et al* implanted six patients with treatment-resistant depression with DBS electrodes in the subgenual cingulate, of whom four met the stringent response criterion of at least 50% reduction in HAM-D [91] **(III/B)**. The same group reported their findings in an additional 14 patients, for a total of 20 patients, targeting the same region for DBS in each patient [92]. The same criterion for responder status was achieved by 12 patients (60%) [92] **(III/B)**.

Other groups have targeted the VC/VS, based on anterior capsulotomy results and observations of

reduced depressive symptoms in OCD patients treated with VC/VS DBS. Malone *et al* studied 15 patients with severe depression in an open-label series [93]. Again defining response as at least a 50% reduction in HAM-D score, they reported eight responders (53%) **(III/B)**. Another small study of three patients targeted the nucleus accumbens, a constituent of the ventral striatum [94]. These authors added a period of double-blinded sham stimulation to the postoperative design, and noted significant decreases (p=0.02) in mean HAM-D scores during the blinded stimulation 'on' phase **(IIa/B)**.

Two case reports of inferior thalamic peduncle stimulation for MDD have also reported positive results [104, 107] **(III/B)**.

Conclusions

The last several decades have witnessed the growth of neuromodulation into a distinct and mature neurosurgical discipline. Although movement disorders such as Parkinson's disease remain the most common indication for central nervous system neuromodulation, clinical studies now support the use of targeted electrical stimulation or lesioning for epilepsy, chronic pain syndromes, depression, and OCD. In addition, experimental neuromodulatory strategies are currently in development for indications ranging from cluster headaches to obesity and dementia. Indeed, this is an exciting era in the field of neuromodulation. In the coming years, basic and translational research will continue to inform our understanding of central nervous system circuitry and rationalize the strategies by which we target that circuitry in the treatment of human disease.

Recommendations	Evidence level

- Dorsal column SCS can benefit patients with CRPS-I and is superior to physical therapy alone. — Ib/A
- Dorsal column SCS plus medical management is superior to medical management alone for reducing pain in patients with failed back surgery syndrome. — Ib/A
- MCS can provide relief to patients with intractable trigeminal neuropathic pain. — III/B
- VNS is an effective adjunctive therapy for reducing seizure frequency among patients with pharmacoresistant partial-onset epilepsy who are not candidates for resective surgery. — Ib/A
- Bilateral ANT DBS reduces seizure frequency in patients with medically refractory partial seizures. — Ib/A
- Ablative procedures for MDD and OCD, including anterior capsulotomy, cingulotomy, subcaudate tractotomy, and limbic leucotomy, can provide meaningful benefit for treatment-refractory patients. — III/B
- Anterior capsulotomy is superior to cingulotomy for the treatment of patients with refractory OCD. — IIb/B
- Cingulotomy provides more benefit to patients with refractory MDD than to those with OCD. — IV/C
- ALIC, VC/VS, and STN DBS provide significant benefit to patients with refractory OCD. — Ib/A
- Bilateral ALIC DBS is superior to unilateral (right) ALIC DBS for refractory OCD. — III/B
- Subgenual cingulate and VC/VS DBS provide significant benefit to patients with refractory MDD. — III/B, IIa/B
- VNS can provide meaningful benefit to some patients with treatment-resistant depression. — III/B

Chapter 15

References

1. Kemler MA, Barendse GA, van Kleef M, *et al.* Spinal cord stimulation in patients with chronic reflex sympathetic dystrophy. *N Engl J Med* 2000; 343: 618-24.

2. Taylor RS, Van Buyten J-P, Buchser E. Spinal cord stimulation for complex regional pain syndrome: a systematic review of the clinical and cost-effectiveness literature and assessment of prognostic factors. *Eur J Pain* 2006; 10: 91-101.

3. North RB, Kidd DH, Farrokhi F, Piantadosi SA. Spinal cord stimulation versus repeated lumbosacral spine surgery for chronic pain: a randomized, controlled trial. *Neurosurgery* 2005; 56: 98-106.

4. Taylor RS, Van Buyten J-P, Buchser E. Spinal cord stimulation for chronic back and leg pain and failed back surgery syndrome: a systematic review and analysis of prognostic factors. *Spine* 2005; 30: 152-60.

5. Kumar K, Taylor RS, Jacques L, *et al.* Spinal cord stimulation versus conventional medical management for neuropathic pain: a multicentre randomised controlled trial in patients with failed back surgery syndrome. *Pain* 2007; 132: 179-88.

6. Meyerson BA, Lindblom U, Linderoth B, Lind G, Herregodts P. Motor cortex stimulation as treatment of trigeminal neuropathic pain. *Acta Neurochir Suppl* (Wien) 1993; 58: 150-3.

7. Herregodts P, Stadnik T, De Ridder F, D'Haens J. Cortical stimulation for central neuropathic pain: 3-D surface MRI for easy determination of the motor cortex. *Acta Neurochir Suppl* (Wien) 1995; 64: 132-5.

8. Katayama Y, Tsubokawa T, Yamamoto T. Chronic motor cortex stimulation for central deafferentation pain: experience with bulbar pain secondary to Wallenberg syndrome. *Stereotact Funct Neurosurg* 1994; 62: 295-9.

9. Ebel H, Rust D, Tronnier V, Böker D, Kunze S. Chronic precentral stimulation in trigeminal neuropathic pain. *Acta Neurochir* (Wien) 1996; 138: 1300-6.

10. Nguyen JP, Keravel Y, Feve A, et al. Treatment of deafferentation pain by chronic stimulation of the motor cortex: report of a series of 20 cases. Acta Neurochir Suppl (Wien) 1997; 68: 54-60.

11. Nguyen JP, Lefaucher JP, Le Guerinel C, et al. Motor cortex stimulation in the treatment of central and neuropathic pain. Arch Med Res 2000; 31: 263-5.

12. Nguyen JP, Lefaucheur JP, Decq P, et al. Chronic motor cortex stimulation in the treatment of central and neuropathic pain. Correlations between clinical, electrophysiological and anatomical data. Pain 1999; 82: 245-51.

13. Brown JA, Pilitsis JG. Motor cortex stimulation for central and neuropathic facial pain: a prospective study of 10 patients and observations of enhanced sensory and motor function during stimulation. Neurosurgery 2005; 56: 290-7.

14. Pirotte B, Voordecker P, Neugroschl C, et al. Combination of functional magnetic resonance imaging-guided neuronavigation and intraoperative cortical brain mapping improves targeting of motor cortex stimulation in neuropathic pain. Neurosurgery 2005; 56: 344-59.

15. Rasche D, Ruppolt M, Stippich C, Unterberg A, Tronnier VM. Motor cortex stimulation for long-term relief of chronic neuropathic pain: a 10-year experience. Pain 2006; 121: 43-52.

16. Lefaucheur JP, Drouot X, Cunin P, et al. Motor cortex stimulation for the treatment of refractory peripheral neuropathic pain. Brain 2009; 132: 1463-71.

17. Bittar RG, Teddy PJ. Peripheral neuromodulation for pain. J Clin Neurosci 2009; 16: 1259-61.

18. Cruccu G, Aziz TZ, Garcia-Larrea L, et al. EFNS guidelines on neurostimulation therapy for neuropathic pain. Eur J Neurol 2007; 14: 952-70.

19. The Vagus Nerve Stimulation Study Group. A randomized controlled trial of chronic vagus nerve stimulation for treatment of medically intractable seizures. Neurology 1995; 45: 224-30.

20. Handforth A, DeGiorgio CM, Schachter SC, et al. Vagus nerve stimulation therapy for partial-onset seizures: a randomized active-control trial. Neurology 1998; 51: 48-55.

21. Salinsky MC, Uthman BM, Ristanovic RK, Wernicke JF, Tarver WB. Vagus nerve stimulation for the treatment of medically intractable seizures. Results of a 1-year open-extension trial. Vagus Nerve Stimulation Study Group. Arch Neurol 1996; 53: 1176-80.

22. DeGiorgio CM, Schachter SC, Handforth A, et al. Prospective long-term study of vagus nerve stimulation for the treatment of refractory seizures. Epilepsia 2000; 41: 1195-200.

23. Monnier M, Kalberer M, Krupp P. Functional antagonism between diffuse reticular and intralaminary recruiting projections in the medial thalamus. Exp Neurol 1960; 2: 271-89.

24. Steriade M, Jones EG, McCormick D. Thalamus: Functional Organization Influencing Neurotransmission in the Lateral Geniculate Nucleus. Philadelphia: Elsevier, 1997.

25. Kerrigan JF, Litt B, Fisher RS, et al. Electrical stimulation of the anterior nucleus of the thalamus for the treatment of intractable epilepsy. Epilepsia 2004; 45: 346-54.

26. Mirski MA, Rossell LA, Terry JB, Fisher RS. Anticonvulsant effect of anterior thalamic high frequency electrical stimulation in the rat. Epilepsy Res 1997; 28: 89-100.

27. Hodaie M, Wennberg RA, Dostrovsky JO, Lozano AM. Chronic anterior thalamus stimulation for intractable epilepsy. Epilepsia 2002; 43: 603-8.

28. Lee KJ, Jang KS, Shon YM. Chronic deep brain stimulation of subthalamic and anterior thalamic nuclei for controlling refractory partial epilepsy. Acta Neurochir Suppl 2006; 99: 87-91.

29. Lim SN, Lee ST, Tsai YT, et al. Electrical stimulation of the anterior nucleus of the thalamus for intractable epilepsy: a long-term follow-up study. Epilepsia 2007; 48: 342-7.

30. Osorio I, Overman J, Giftakis J, Wilkinson SB. High frequency thalamic stimulation for inoperable mesial temporal epilepsy. Epilepsia 2007; 48: 1561-71.

31. Fisher R, Salanova V, Witt T, et al. Electrical stimulation of the anterior nucleus of thalamus for treatment of refractory epilepsy. Epilepsia 2010; 51: 899-908.

32. Moniz E. Prefrontal leucotomy in the treatment of mental disorders. Am J Psychiatry 1937; 93: 1379-85.

33. Binder DK, Iskandar BJ. Modern neurosurgery for psychiatric disorders. Neurosurgery 2000; 47: 9-21.

34. Pipard J. Leucotomy in Britain today. J Ment Sci 1962; 108: 249-55.

35. Spiegel EA, Wycis HT, Marks M, Lee AJ. Stereotaxic apparatus for operations on the human brain. Science 1947; 106: 349-50.

36. Leksell L. The stereotaxic method and radiosurgery of the brain. Acta Chir Scand 1951; 102: 316-19.

37. Talairach J, Hecaen H, David M. Lobotomie préfrontal limitée par électrocoagulation des fibres thalamo-frontales à leur émergence du bras antérieur de la capsule interne. In: Congress Neurologique International, Paris, 1949: 1412.

38. Knight G. Stereotactic tractotomy in the surgical treatment of mental illness. J Neurol Neurosurg Psychiatry 1965; 28: 304-10.

39. Ballantine HT Jr, Cassidy WL, Flanagan NB, Marino R Jr. Stereotaxic anterior cingulotomy for neuropsychiatric illness and intractable pain. J Neurosurg 1967; 26: 488-95.

40. Kelly D, Richardson A, Mitchell-Heggs N. Stereotactic limbic leucotomy: neurophysiological aspects and operative technique. Br J Psychiatry 1973; 123: 133-40.

41. Lippitz BE, Mindus P, Meyerson BA, Kihlström L, Lindquist C. Lesion topography and outcome after thermocapsulotomy or gamma knife capsulotomy for obsessive-compulsive disorder: relevance of the right hemisphere. Neurosurgery 1999; 44: 452-8.

42. Csigó K, Harsányi A, Demeter G, Rajkai C, Németh A, Racsmány M. Long-term follow-up of patients with obsessive-compulsive disorder treated by anterior capsulotomy: a neuropsychological study. J Affect Disord 2010: 126: 198-205.

43. Rück C, Karlsson A, Steele JD, et al. Capsulotomy for obsessive-compulsive disorder: long-term follow-up of 25 patients. Arch Gen Psychiatry 2008; 65: 914-21.

44. Liu K, Zhang H, Liu C, et al. Stereotactic treatment of refractory obsessive compulsive disorder by bilateral

capsulotomy with 3 years follow-up. *J Clin Neurosci* 2008; 15: 622-9.

45. Oliver B, Gascón J, Aparicio A, *et al*. Bilateral anterior capsulotomy for refractory obsessive-compulsive disorders. *Stereotact Funct Neurosurg* 2003; 81: 90-5.

46. Lopes AC, Greenberg BD, Norén G, *et al*. Treatment of resistant obsessive-compulsive disorder with ventral capsular/ventral striatal gamma capsulotomy: a pilot prospective study. *J Neuropsychiatry Clin Neurosci* 2009; 21: 381-92.

47. Ballantine HT Jr, Bouckoms AJ, Thomas EK, Giriunas IE. Treatment of psychiatric illness by stereotactic cingulotomy. *Biol Psychiatry* 1987; 22: 807-19.

48. Shields DC, Asaad W, Eskandar EN, *et al*. Prospective assessment of stereotactic ablative surgery for intractable major depression. *Biol Psychiatry* 2008; 64: 449-54.

49. Steele JD, Christmas D, Eljamel MS, Matthews K. Anterior cingulotomy for major depression: clinical outcome and relationship to lesion characteristics. *Biol Psychiatry* 2008; 63: 670-7.

50. Spangler WJ, Cosgrove GR, Ballantine HT Jr, *et al*. Magnetic resonance image-guided stereotactic cingulotomy for intractable psychiatric disease. *Neurosurgery* 1996; 38: 1071-6.

51. Baer L, Rauch SL, Ballantine HT Jr, *et al*. Cingulotomy for intractable obsessive-compulsive disorder. Prospective long-term follow-up of 18 patients. *Arch Gen Psychiatry* 1995; 52: 384-92.

52. Dougherty DD, Baer L, Cosgrove GR, *et al*. Prospective long-term follow-up of 44 patients who received cingulotomy for treatment-refractory obsessive-compulsive disorder. *Am J Psychiatry* 2002; 159: 269-75.

53. Richter EO, Davis KD, Hamani C, Hutchison WD, Dostrovsky JO, Lozano AM. Cingulotomy for psychiatric disease: microelectrode guidance, a callosal reference system for documenting lesion location, and clinical results. *Neurosurgery* 2004; 54: 622-8.

54. Jenike MA, Baer L, Ballantine T, *et al*. Cingulotomy for refractory obsessive-compulsive disorder. A long-term follow-up of 33 patients. *Arch Gen Psychiatry* 1991; 48: 548-55.

55. Goktepe EO, Young LB, Bridges PK. A further review of the results of sterotactic subcaudate tractotomy. *Br J Psychiatry* 1975; 126: 270-80.

56. Ström-Olsen R, Carlisle S. Bi-frontal stereotactic tractotomy. A follow-up study of its effects on 210 patients. *Br J Psychiatry* 1971; 118: 141-54.

57. Hodgkiss AD, Malizia AL, Bartlett JR, Bridges PK. Outcome after the psychosurgical operation of stereotactic subcaudate tractotomy, 1979-1991. *J Neuropsychiatry Clin Neurosci* 1995; 7: 230-4.

58. Kelly D, Richardson A, Mitchell-Heggs N, Greenup J, Chen C, Hafner RJ. Stereotactic limbic leucotomy: a preliminary report on forty patients. *Br J Psychiatry* 1973; 123: 141-8.

59. Mitchell-Heggs N, Kelly D, Richardson A. Stereotactic limbic leucotomy - a follow-up at 16 months. *Br J Psychiatry* 1976; 128: 226-40.

60. Cho DY, Lee WY, Chen CC. Limbic leukotomy for intractable major affective disorders: a 7-year follow-up study using nine

comprehensive psychiatric test evaluations. *J Clin Neurosci* 2008; 15: 138-42.

61. Hay P, Sachdev P, Cumming S, *et al*. Treatment of obsessive-compulsive disorder by psychosurgery. *Acta Psychiatr Scand* 1993; 87: 197-207.

62. Christensen DD, Laitinen LV, Schmidt LJ, Hariz MI. Anterior capsulotomy for treatment of refractory obsessive-compulsive disorder: results in a young and an old patient. *Stereotact Funct Neurosurg* 2002; 79: 234-44.

63. Goodman WK, Price LH, Rasmussen SA, *et al*. The Yale-Brown Obsessive Compulsive Scale. I. Development, use, and reliability. *Arch Gen Psychiatry* 1989; 46: 1006-11.

64. Beck AT, Ward CH, Mendelson M, Mock J, Erbaugh J. An inventory for measuring depression. *Arch Gen Psychiatry* 1961; 4: 561-71.

65. Hamilton M. A rating scale for depression. *J Neurol Neurosurg Psychiatry* 1960; 23: 56-62.

66. Whitty CW, Duffield JE, Tov PM, Cairns H. Anterior cingulectomy in the treatment of mental disease. *Lancet* 1952; 1: 475-81.

67. Leiphart JW, Valone FH 3rd. Stereotactic lesions for the treatment of psychiatric disorders. *J Neurosurg* 2010; 113: 1204-11.

68. Fodstad H, Strandman E, Karlsson B, West KA. Treatment of chronic obsessive compulsive states with stereotactic anterior capsulotomy or cingulotomy. *Acta Neurochir* (Wien) 1982; 62: 1-23.

69. Asberg M, Montgomery SA, Perris C, Schalling D, Sedvall G. A comprehensive psychopathological rating scale. *Acta Psychiatr Scand Suppl* 1978; 271: 5-27.

70. Poynton AM, Kartsounis LD, Bridges PK. A prospective clinical study of stereotactic subcaudate tractotomy. *Psychol Med* 1995; 25: 763-70.

71. Woerdeman PA, Willems PW, Noordmans HJ, Berkelbach van der Sprenkel JW, van Rijen PC. Frameless stereotactic subcaudate tractotomy for intractable obsessive-compulsive disorder. *Acta Neurochir* (Wien) 2006; 148: 633-7.

72. Horng SH, Miller FG. Placebo-controlled procedural trials for neurological conditions. *Neurotherapeutics* 2007; 4: 531-6.

73. Daban C, Martinez-Aran A, Cruz N, Vieta E. Safety and efficacy of vagus nerve stimulation in treatment-resistant depression. A systematic review. *J Affect Disord* 2008; 110: 1-15.

74. Rush AJ, George MS, Sackeim HA, *et al*. Vagus nerve stimulation (VNS) for treatment-resistant depressions: a multicenter study. *Biol Psychiatry* 2000; 47: 276-86.

75. Sackeim HA, Rush AJ, George MS, *et al*. Vagus nerve stimulation (VNS) for treatment-resistant depression: efficacy, side effects, and predictors of outcome. *Neuropsychopharmacology* 2001; 25: 713-28.

76. Marangell LB, Rush AJ, George MS, *et al*. Vagus nerve stimulation (VNS) for major depressive episodes: one-year outcomes. *Biol Psychiatry* 2002; 51: 280-7.

77. Nahas Z, Marangell LB, Husain MM, *et al*. Two-year outcome of vagus nerve stimulation (VNS) for treatment of major depressive episodes. *J Clin Psychiatry* 2005; 66: 1097-104.

78. Schlaepfer TE, Frick C, Zobel A, *et al*. Vagus nerve stimulation for depression: efficacy and safety in a European study. *Psychol Med* 2008; 38: 651-61.

79. Bajbouj M, Merkl A, Schlaepfer TE, et al. Two-year outcome of vagus nerve stimulation in treatment-resistant depression. J Clin Psychopharmacol 2010; 30: 273-81.

80. Rush AJ, Sackeim HA, Marangell LB, et al. Effects of 12 months of vagus nerve stimulation in treatment-resistant depression: a naturalistic study. Biol Psychiatry 2005; 58: 355-63.

81. George MS, Rush AJ, Marangell LB, et al. A one-year comparison of vagus nerve stimulation with treatment as usual for treatment-resistant depression. Biol Psychiatry 2005; 58: 364-73.

82. Rush AJ, Marangell LB, Sackeim HA, et al. Vagus nerve stimulation for treatment-resistant depression: a randomized, controlled acute phase trial. Biol Psychiatry 2005; 58: 347-54.

83. Nuttin B, Cosyns P, Demeulemeester H, Gybels J, Meyerson B. Electrical stimulation in anterior limbs of internal capsules in patients with obsessive-compulsive disorder. Lancet 1999; 354: 1526.

84. Nuttin BJ, Gabriëls LA, Cosyns PR, et al. Long-term electrical capsular stimulation in patients with obsessive-compulsive disorder. Neurosurgery 2003; 52: 1263-72.

85. Abelson JL, Curtis GC, Sagher O, et al. Deep brain stimulation for refractory obsessive-compulsive disorder. Biol Psychiatry 2005; 57: 510-6.

86. Huff W, Lenartz D, Schormann M, et al. Unilateral deep brain stimulation of the nucleus accumbens in patients with treatment-resistant obsessive-compulsive disorder: outcomes after one year. Clin Neurol Neurosurg 2010; 112: 137-43.

87. Goodman WK, Foote KD, Greenberg BD, et al. Deep brain stimulation for intractable obsessive compulsive disorder: pilot study using a blinded, staggered-onset design. Biol Psychiatry 2010; 67: 535-42.

88. Greenberg BD, Gabriels LA, Malone DA Jr, et al. Deep brain stimulation of the ventral internal capsule/ventral striatum for obsessive-compulsive disorder: worldwide experience. Mol Psychiatry 2010; 15: 64-79.

89. Mallet L, Polosan M, Jaafari N, et al. Subthalamic nucleus stimulation in severe obsessive-compulsive disorder. N Engl J Med 2008; 359: 2121-34.

90. Greenberg BD, Malone DA, Friehs GM, et al. Three-year outcomes in deep brain stimulation for highly resistant obsessive-compulsive disorder. Neuropsychopharmacology 2006; 31: 2384-93.

91. Mayberg HS, Lozano AM, Voon V, et al. Deep brain stimulation for treatment-resistant depression. Neuron 2005; 45: 651-60.

92. Lozano AM, Mayberg HS, Giacobbe P, Hamani C, Craddock RC, Kennedy SH. Subcallosal cingulate gyrus deep brain stimulation for treatment-resistant depression. Biol Psychiatry 2008; 64: 461-7.

93. Malone DA Jr, Dougherty DD, Rezai AR, et al. Deep brain stimulation of the ventral capsule/ventral striatum for treatment-resistant depression. Biol Psychiatry 2009; 65: 267-75.

94. Schlaepfer TE, Cohen MX, Frick C, et al. Deep brain stimulation to reward circuitry alleviates anhedonia in refractory major depression. Neuropsychopharmacology 2008; 33: 368-77.

95. Mallet L, Mesnage V, Houeto JL, et al. Compulsions, Parkinson's disease, and stimulation. Lancet 2002; 360: 1302-4.

96. Fontaine D, Mattei V, Borg M, et al. Effect of subthalamic nucleus stimulation on obsessive-compulsive disorder in a patient with Parkinson disease. Case report. J Neurosurg 2004; 100: 1084-6.

97. Franzini A, Messina G, Gambini O, et al. Deep-brain stimulation of the nucleus accumbens in obsessive compulsive disorder: clinical, surgical and electrophysiological considerations in two consecutive patients. Neurol Sci 2010; 31: 353-9.

98. Gabriëls L, Cosyns P, Nuttin B, Demeulemeester H, Gybels J. Deep brain stimulation for treatment-refractory obsessive-compulsive disorder: psychopathological and neuropsychological outcome in three cases. Acta Psychiatr Scand 2003; 107: 275-82.

99. Anderson D, Ahmed A. Treatment of patients with intractable obsessive-compulsive disorder with anterior capsular stimulation. Case report. J Neurosurg 2003; 98: 1104-8.

100. Sturm V, Lenartz D, Koulousakis A, et al. The nucleus accumbens: a target for deep brain stimulation in obsessive-compulsive- and anxiety-disorders. J Chem Neuroanat 2003; 26: 293-9.

101. Plewnia C, Schober F, Rilk A, et al. Sustained improvement of obsessive-compulsive disorder by deep brain stimulation in a woman with residual schizophrenia. Int J Neuropsychopharmacol 2008; 11: 1181-3.

102. Aouizerate B, Cuny E, Bardinet E, et al. Distinct striatal targets in treating obsessive-compulsive disorder and major depression. J Neurosurg 2009; 111: 775-9.

103. Aouizerate B, Cuny E, Martin-Guehl C, et al. Deep brain stimulation of the ventral caudate nucleus in the treatment of obsessive-compulsive disorder and major depression. Case report. J Neurosurg 2004; 101: 682-6.

104. Jiménez F, Velasco F, Salín-Pascual R, et al. Neuromodulation of the inferior thalamic peduncle for major depression and obsessive compulsive disorder. Acta Neurochir Suppl 2007; 97: 393-8.

105. Jiménez-Ponce F, Velasco-Campos F, Castro-Farfán G, et al. Preliminary study in patients with obsessive-compulsive disorder treated with electrical stimulation in the inferior thalamic peduncle. Neurosurgery 2009; 65: 203-9.

106. Mayberg HS, Liotti M, Brannan SK, et al. Reciprocal limbic-cortical function and negative mood: converging PET findings in depression and normal sadness. Am J Psychiatry 1999; 156: 675-82.

107. Jiménez F, Velasco F, Salin-Pascual R, et al. A patient with a resistant major depression disorder treated with deep brain stimulation in the inferior thalamic peduncle. Neurosurgery 2005; 57: 585-93.

Chapter 16

Stimulation of the central nervous system for chronic pain

Ryder Gwinn MD

Director of Epilepsy and Functional Neurosurgery

SWEDISH MEDICAL CENTER, SWEDISH NEUROSCIENCE INSTITUTE, SEATTLE, WASHINGTON, USA

Introduction

Chronic pain places a massive burden on the physical and mental well-being of people throughout the world. It is estimated that almost one-third of the population in the USA and the UK live with chronic pain [1, 2]. Back pain accounted for 16-25% of the overall pain prevalence in these studies, and the incidence of chronic pain was found to increase with age. The social and economic impact of chronic pain is difficult to measure, but it is clearly associated with poor socioeconomic status. In a recent European study, 19% of respondents had lost their job as a result of their chronic pain, while 13% had changed their job [3]. The same study found that 21% of patients were diagnosed with depression as a result of their pain [3]. Because of the pervasive nature of the problem, the personal and societal burden inflicted by chronic pain, and the incomplete success achieved by pharmacological and psychological interventions, more attention is being given to therapies that involve stimulation of the nervous system.

Stimulation of the nervous system for the treatment of chronic pain has been performed in some form for thousands of years. Magnetic bracelets for headaches and arthritis are reported to have been used as early as 9000 BC [4], while the use of electric torpedo fish for the treatment of headaches and gout was described in Rome around 46 AD [5]. The relatively recent advent of chronically implanted stimulators has now made it possible to electrically interact with the nervous system at every level from the skin to deep brain nuclei. This has opened therapeutic windows in the treatment of chronic pain that were not previously available, to the point that the field of pain medicine is undergoing a rapid transformation. For decades, therapies for chronic pain have been centered on pharmacology and psychology; now, there is a rapid shift in favor of interventional procedures and, in particular, the use of neurostimulators. Many factors contribute to this shift, including the limited success in treating chronic pain with medications, the rapid miniaturization and increasing sophistication of electrodes and pulse generators, and economic factors favoring interventional therapies in general. Device manufacturers are rapidly advancing the capabilities of these neurostimulators, while simultaneously promoting their use in larger numbers of patients. Although there is fairly extensive literature advocating the use of neurostimulation for the treatment of chronic pain, clarification of its mechanisms of action and the validation of its efficacy has lagged behind its explosive adaptation.

This chapter explores the evidence available to support the use of neurostimulation in the treatment of chronic pain, focusing on the most commonly used and rapidly advancing modality – spinal cord stimulation (SCS). It also briefly reviews the literature supporting the use of deep brain and cortical stimulation for pain, although objective data validating the efficacy of these techniques are lacking.

Methodology

A National Library of Medicine computerized literature search was performed of publications from 1966 to 2010 using the headings 'pain' and 'neuromodulation' to create a master database of articles. From this database, abstracts were individually reviewed and a sub-search was performed using the keywords 'randomized' and 'evidence-based.' The identified abstracts were all reviewed for possible relevance, and appropriate papers were obtained. The bibliographies of many papers were also reviewed to further obtain relevant studies.

Spinal cord stimulation

After the gate theory of pain was proposed by Melzack and Wall in 1965 [6], a neurosurgeon, Norman Shealy, tested the theory experimentally by stimulating the dorsal columns of cats. He implanted the first human spinal cord stimulator in March 1967 [7]. The first six patients were reported at the Harvey Cushing Society in 1969, and Avery Laboratories began to market dorsal column stimulators in 1972. The technique quickly went out of favor because of technical limitations such as oxidizing electrodes and surgical complications such as cerebrospinal fluid leaks, epidural hematomas, and fibrosis associated with the subdural placement of electrodes.

Gradually, over the next two decades, advances in technology led to a slow resurgence in the use of SCS to control chronic pain. The first major advance was the use of advanced cardiac pacemaker technology to provide fully implantable pulse generators with integrated batteries [8]. Prior to this, commercially available implanted systems were electrodes passively activated by radiofrequency impulses generated externally. The second major technological development was the advent of percutaneous leads inserted into the epidural space by use of needles, making the technique significantly less invasive.

Today, spinal cord stimulators are approved by the US Food and Drug Administration (FDA) for the treatment of chronic intractable pain of the back or limbs. The most common application is in the treatment of failed back surgery syndrome (FBSS), sometimes known as post-laminectomy syndrome. Other chronic pain syndromes commonly treated with SCS include complex regional pain syndrome types I and II (CRPS-I and -II), post-herpetic neuralgia, ischemic peripheral vascular disease, interstitial cystitis, occipital neuralgia, and atypical trigeminal neuralgia.

A body of literature supports the use of SCS in the treatment of all these conditions. A Medline search for 'spinal cord stimulation' and 'pain' yielded 3,891 results as of October 2010. Unfortunately, nearly all of this literature is observational in nature, with a scarcity of studies comparing test groups with controls. The lack of class I evidence demonstrating the efficacy of SCS has hampered its acceptance by the neurosurgical and general medical communities, although practitioners within the field have been very enthusiastic about results seen in their chronic pain patients. Fortunately, over the past 10-15 years, individuals in the field have recognized the need for better science to determine if outcomes really justify the risk to the patient and the costs associated with SCS. Blinded trials have not yet been performed because of the manner in which the therapy is currently delivered. Because the FDA-approved SCS devices induce a paresthesia, and this paresthesia is necessary to provide pain relief, it is impossible to deliver sham stimulation without the patient knowing. Prospective randomized trials have been performed comparing SCS with other treatment modalities for patients with CRPS and FBSS. These indications account for the vast majority of SCS implants today.

Complex regional pain syndrome

CRPS is a condition in which neuropathic pain results from an injury to the arms or legs. It is frequently associated with burning pain, temperature changes, color changes, sweating, and swelling. When the original injury is associated with tissue damage but no known nerve damage, it is known as CRPS-I. When there is associated nerve injury, it is known as CRPS-II. This syndrome was previously known as reflex sympathetic dystrophy (RSD), and was one of the earliest indications for SCS. Initial reports suggested a high degree of pain control with SCS [9-12]. Because of the expense and potential complications associated with the therapy, Kemler *et al* conducted a prospective randomized trial of SCS in the setting of RSD, publishing the results in the *New England Journal of Medicine* in 2000 [13]. Patients who had at least a 6-month history of RSD were randomly assigned to SCS plus physical therapy (n=36) or physical therapy alone (n=18).

Test stimulation was successful in 24 of 36 patients, and these 24 were eventually implanted with electrodes for SCS. At 6 months' follow-up, Visual Analogue Scale pain scores were at least 50% lower in 18 of the 24 patients implanted, and the mean score was decreased by 3.6 in the 24 implanted patients versus an increase of 0.2 in the control group (p<0.001). Significant improvements were also seen in health-related quality of life in the implanted patients. Complications occurred in six of the implanted patients (25%), largely due to unsatisfactory electrode positioning (five patients). Overall, improvements were seen in both the pain scores and quality of life measurements of implanted patients who had failed all other forms of therapy for RSD **(Ib/A)**.

CRPS is completely neuropathic in origin, and as such is ideally suited for treatment with neurostimulation. SCS remains an effective, yet underutilized, treatment option for patients with refractory CRPS.

Failed back surgery syndrome

Lumbosacral spine surgery is undergone by more than 200,000 patients each year, and approximately 40% of these patients experience persistent or recurrent pain [14]. This represents the most common cause of chronic neuropathic pain [15]. These patients frequently undergo further decompressive surgery, fusion, and interventional pain procedures such as rhizotomies or nerve root injections, and are often given chronic opiate therapy orally or intrathecally. SCS is now being recognized as a safe and potentially superior alternative to these treatments in patients with chronic leg and back pain for whom surgery has failed. Numerous articles have been published outlining the potential benefits of SCS in treating FBSS [16-18].

No trial investigating SCS for FBSS contained randomized treatment groups until North *et al* compared SCS with reoperation in patients who had failed lumbosacral spine surgery [19]. In this trial, a series of 99 patients with chronic lumbosacral pain (leg pain worse than back pain) were offered randomization to SCS or reoperation. Patients could not have any instability or disabling neurological deficit, but were considered to be surgical candidates with radicular pain and concordant imaging findings. Thirty patients were randomized to each group; 24 patients underwent a trial of SCS and 26 underwent surgery (Figure 1) [19]. Patients were allowed to cross over to surgery immediately if they failed the SCS trial, and to SCS after 6 months if they failed reoperation. Endpoints included cross-over from one randomized procedure to the other, success at last follow-up, and improvement in daily activities, neurological status, and medication use. Success was defined as at least 50% pain relief and patient agreement that they would repeat the treatment again for the result obtained.

SCS was superior to reoperation at 2 years' follow-up, with 12% of patients in the reoperation group achieving success compared with 47% of patients in the SCS group. Many more patients crossed over from surgery to SCS (14/26 patients) than in the other direction (5/24 patients). None of the patients who crossed over from SCS to surgery achieved success. Of those who crossed from surgery to SCS, 43% achieved success. The results of this randomized

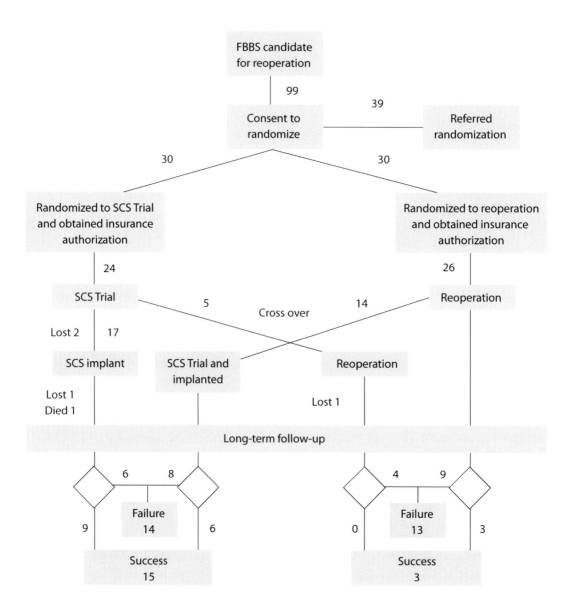

Figure 1. Flow chart showing study design and outcomes for a randomized trial of SCS versus reoperation. Patients could elect to cross over from one procedure to the other if the results of the procedure that they were randomized to were unsatisfactory. FBSS = failed back surgery syndrome; SCS = spinal cord stimulation. *Reproduced with permission from the Congress of Neurological Surgeons and Wolters Kluwer Health, © 2005. North RB, et al [19].*

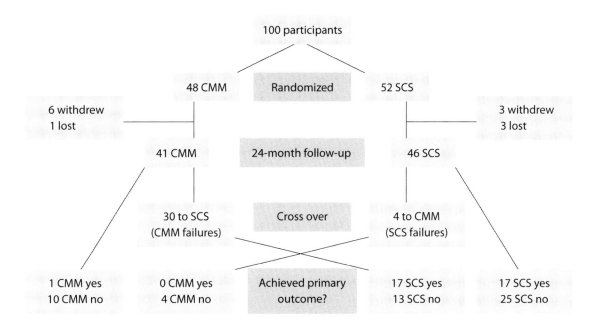

Figure 2. Patient flow and primary outcome at 2 years' follow-up for patients enrolled in the PROCESS study comparing spinal cord stimulation (SCS) with conventional medical management (CMM). Primary outcome was met in 34 of 72 (47%) patients receiving SCS, and in one of 15 (7%) patients receiving CMM.

Reproduced with permission from the Congress of Neurological Surgeons and Wolters Kluwer Health, © 2008. Kumar K, et al [21].

study provide the first clear evidence that SCS is more efficacious than reoperation for patients with FBSS, otherwise known as post-laminectomy syndrome **(Ib/A)**.

Although this study was randomized, the efficacy of the comparison group (reoperation) was itself under scrutiny. A true randomized controlled trial comparing SCS with best medical management was not completed until 2007, with the Prospective Randomized Controlled Multicenter Trial of the Effectiveness of Spinal Cord Stimulation (PROCESS) study [20]. This multicenter trial randomized 100 patients with FBSS to either a trial of SCS with

potential permanent implantation or continued treatment of their back and leg pain with conventional medical management (CMM). CMM included use of medications, nerve blocks, epidural injections, and/or physical therapy. The primary outcome was the proportion of patients achieving 50% or better improvement in leg pain at 6 months' follow-up. Patients were allowed to cross over to the other therapy after 6 months if they did not achieve the primary outcome. The 2-year outcomes were reported in 2008 [21].

Patient flow and primary outcome at 2 years' follow-up are shown in Figure 2. Leg pain was improved by 50% or more in 48% of SCS patients at 6 months' follow-up, but in only 9% of patients receiving CMM. At 2 years' follow-up, most CMM patients had crossed over to SCS therapy, and 47% of patients receiving SCS were continuing to receive significant relief from their leg pain. Secondary outcome measures such as quality of life and disability were significantly improved at the 2-year follow-up compared with baseline for patients receiving SCS; interestingly, however, scores for back pain were not significantly improved **(Ib/A)**.

The PROCESS study was able to convincingly show that SCS is superior to CMM in patients with FBSS, while the study conducted by North *et al* suggests SCS is superior to reoperation in these patients when it comes to controlling leg pain **(Ib/A)**. Unfortunately, more than 30% of SCS patients in the PROCESS study required surgical revision of their stimulators during the course of the trial. In addition, most patients with FBSS have some component of back pain, which was not shown to be significantly improved in either of these studies.

Significant changes in SCS technology have taken place since these two studies were conducted, which may increase the effectiveness of the therapy today. Spinal cord stimulators implanted for these trials employed four contacts, while current systems can control up to 16 epidural contacts. This may allow for improved flexibility of programming, and greater ability to achieve control of both leg and back pain. A prospective randomized trial comparing SCS with reoperation with this newer technology is currently underway.

Intracranial stimulation for pain

Intracranial targets have been identified that may provide relief from chronic pain when stimulated. These targets include the motor cortex, the sensory thalamus (the ventral posterolateral nucleus and the ventral posteromedial nucleus), periaqueductal gray matter, and periventricular gray matter. Success in stimulating intracranial targets for treating pain has been reported since 1954 [22], and more than 80 papers have now been published on the topic. There

is currently no FDA-approved treatment for chronic pain using intracranial neurostimulation. However, currently approved deep brain and SCS systems may be employed to stimulate intracranial structures for pain in an off-label fashion.

Cortical stimulation

Motor cortex stimulation has been studied for the treatment of neuropathic pain syndromes, including atypical facial pain, and central pain syndromes such as post-stroke pain. Most of these case series report good results in the short term for both neuropathic facial pain and post-stroke pain [23-27] **(III/B)**. A prospective study of 10 patients combined with a retrospective review reported 50% or better control of neuropathic facial pain with motor cortex stimulation in 29 of 38 patients (76%) [28] **(III/B)**.

More recently, trials of motor cortex stimulation with double-blind protocols have been reported [29, 30]. In the study by Velasco *et al*, patients with unilateral neuropathic pain were implanted with electrodes over the motor cortex after undergoing a successful trial (8/11 patients) [30]. Etiology of pain included postherpetic neuralgia, thalamic infarct, brachial plexus trauma, and cervical root avulsion. At day 60 or 90 post-implant, the stimulators were turned off for 30 days in a randomized and double-blind fashion. In eight implanted patients, pain was significantly reduced from baseline with stimulation and significantly increased when the stimulation was turned off. Pain was reduced from 40% to 86% in all patients at 1 year of follow-up. Positioning of the electrode over the motor cortex serving the affected area of the body appeared to be critical to success, and patients with complete deafferentation of the painful areas did not fare as well. This study, while small in size, represents the best evidence yet that motor cortex stimulation is effective in relieving chronic neuropathic pain **(Ib/A)**. Randomized, blinded, controlled trials with larger enrollment and longer follow-up times will be required to provide the best level of clinical evidence and most reliable recommendation for the use of motor cortex stimulation in treating chronic neuropathic pain.

Deep brain stimulation

Stimulation of deep brain structures for the treatment of pain was first reported in 1954, and studies have suggested that targets may be specific to certain types of pain. A meta-analysis of 13 series was conducted in 2010, evaluating the long-term outcomes of 1,114 patients treated with deep brain stimulation for chronic pain [31]. The overall success rate for pain control was 50% (561/1,114 patients), with a range of 19-79%. The success rate for neuropathic pain was 42% (296/711 patients), while 61% of patients with nociceptive pain achieved long-term success (272/443 patients). Success rates did fall somewhat as follow-up intervals increased. Ventral posterolateral nucleus stimulation was fairly successful when used for neuropathic pain (228/409 patients, 56%), but not at all helpful when used for nociceptive pain (0/51 patients). Conversely, periventricular gray matter stimulation was somewhat unsuccessful in the treatment of neuropathic pain (35/155 patients, 23%), but relatively good at relieving nociceptive pain (172/291 patients, 59%) **(III/B)**.

In the reviewed studies, deep brain stimulation appeared to be most effective for pain resulting from cervical or brachial plexus avulsion, peripheral neuropathy, or failed low back surgery syndrome. Contrasting with the results of motor cortex stimulation, deep brain stimulation was much less effective for the treatment of thalamic pain or pain from spinal cord injury **(III/B)**.

A randomized, double-blind, cross-over study has examined the effect of unilateral hypothalamic stimulation for chronic cluster headache [32]. This study of 11 patients in Europe did not meet its endpoint during the blinded phase, although six patients did respond to chronic stimulation over the year-long open-label phase of the study.

Conclusions

Treatment of chronic pain was one of the earliest clinical applications for the emerging field of neurostimulation, yet its efficacy remains largely unproven. Stimulation of the spinal cord for the treatment of trunk and limb pain has now become widely adopted, and two randomized controlled trials have demonstrated its superiority over medical management or repeat surgery in controlling chronic post-laminectomy pain. Other forms of central nervous system stimulation for chronic pain are not FDA approved and are infrequently performed, and studies do not clearly demonstrate their efficacy. There are, nevertheless, some promising results, especially in the use of motor cortex stimulation to control chronic unilateral neuropathic pain.

Given the prevalence of chronic pain in our society and the incredible psychological, social, and economical toll it takes, better treatments need to be aggressively pursued. Neuromodulation technology is rapidly becoming more complex, sophisticated, and miniaturized, and our ability to apply the technology to solve specific clinical problems is improving. High-quality studies will be increasingly relied upon to justify the adoption of these techniques in the general population as an aging society is asked to spend an increasing proportion of health care dollars on complex and expensive ways to alleviate suffering.

Chapter 16

Chapter 16

Recommendations	Evidence level
◆ SCS is approved by the FDA for the treatment of chronic intractable pain of the trunk and/or limbs.	-
◆ SCS is more effective than reoperation as a treatment for chronic leg pain in patients who continue to have pain after an initial surgery.	Ib/A
◆ SCS is more effective than conservative medical management as a treatment for patients who continue to have pain after an initial surgery.	Ib/A
◆ Intracranial neurostimulation for the treatment of chronic pain is not approved by the FDA.	-
◆ Cortical stimulation can be effective as a treatment for chronic neuropathic pain.	Ib/A
◆ Deep brain stimulation of the periaqueductal gray matter or periventricular gray matter can reduce levels of nociceptive pain.	III/B
◆ Deep brain stimulation of the sensory thalamus can relieve chronic neuropathic pain.	III/B

References

1. Johannes CB, Le TK, Zhou X, Johnston JA, Dworkin RH. The prevalence of chronic pain in United States adults: results of an internet-based survey. *J Pain* 2010; 11: 1230-9.

2. Simpson EL, Duenas A, Holmes MW, Papaioannou D, Chilcott J. Spinal cord stimulation for chronic pain of neuropathic or ischaemic origin: systematic review and economic evaluation. *Health Technol Assess* 2009; 13: iii, ix-x, 1-154.

3. Breivik H, Collett B, Ventafridda V, Cohen R, Gallacher D. Survey of chronic pain in Europe: prevalence, impact on daily life, and treatment. *Eur J Pain* 2006; 10: 287-333.

4. Schechter DC. Origins of electrotherapy. I. *NY State J Med* 1971; 71: 997-1008.

5. Kellaway P. The part played by electric fish in the early history of bioelectricity and electrotherapy. *Bull Hist Med* 1946; 20: 112-32.

6. Melzack R, Wall PD. Pain mechanisms: a new theory. *Science* 1965; 150: 971-9.

7. Shealy CN, Mortimer JT, Reswick JB. Electrical inhibition of pain by stimulation of the dorsal columns: preliminary clinical report. *Anesth Analg* 1967; 46: 489-91.

8. Lazorthes Y, Siegfried J, Upton ARM. A brief historical review of biostimulation. In: *Neurostimulation: An Overview.* Lazorthes Y, Upton ARM, Eds. Mt. Krisco, New York: Futura Publishing Company, 1985; 5-10.

9. Barolat G, Schwartzman R, Woo R. Epidural spinal cord stimulation in the management of reflex sympathetic dystrophy. *Stereotact Funct Neurosurg* 1989; 53: 29-39.

10. Robaina FJ, Rodriguez JL, de Vera JA, Martin MA. Transcutaneous electrical nerve stimulation and spinal cord stimulation for pain relief in reflex sympathetic dystrophy. *Stereotact Funct Neurosurg* 1989; 52: 53-62.

11. Kumar K, Nath RK, Toth C. Spinal cord stimulation is effective in the management of reflex sympathetic dystrophy. *Neurosurgery* 1997; 40: 503-8.

12. Kemler MA, Barendse GA, Van Kleef M, Van Den Wildenberg FA, Weber WE. Electrical spinal cord stimulation in reflex sympathetic dystrophy: retrospective analysis of 23 patients. *J Neurosurg* 1999; 90: 79-83.

13. Kemler MA, Barendse GA, van Kleef M, *et al.* Spinal cord stimulation in patients with chronic reflex sympathetic dystrophy. *N Engl J Med* 2000; 343: 618-24.

14. Wilkinson H. *The Failed Back Syndrome: Etiology And Therapy*, 2nd ed. Philadelphia: Harper & Row; 1991.

15. Dworkin RH, Backonja M, Rowbotham MC, *et al.* Advances in neuropathic pain: diagnosis, mechanisms, and treatment recommendations. *Arch Neurol* 2003; 60: 1524-34.

16. Turner JA, Loeser JD, Deyo RA, Sanders SB. Spinal cord stimulation for patients with failed back surgery syndrome or complex regional pain syndrome: a systematic review of effectiveness and complications. *Pain* 2004; 108: 137-47.

17. Taylor RS, Van Buyten JP, Buchser E. Spinal cord stimulation for chronic back and leg pain and failed back surgery syndrome: a systematic review and analysis of prognostic factors. *Spine* (Phila Pa 1976) 2005; 30: 152-60.

18. Kumar K, Hunter G, Demeria D. Spinal cord stimulation in treatment of chronic benign pain: challenges in treatment planning and present status, a 22-year experience. *Neurosurgery* 2006; 58: 481-96.

19. North RB, Kidd DH, Farrokhi F, Piantadosi SA. Spinal cord stimulation versus repeated lumbosacral spine surgery for chronic pain: a randomized, controlled trial. *Neurosurgery* 2005; 56: 98-106.

20. Kumar K, Taylor RS, Jacques L, *et al.* Spinal cord stimulation versus conventional medical management for neuropathic pain: a multicentre randomised controlled trial in patients with failed back surgery syndrome. *Pain* 2007; 132: 179-88.

21. Kumar K, Taylor RS, Jacques L, *et al*. The effects of spinal cord stimulation in neuropathic pain are sustained: a 24-month follow-up of the prospective randomized controlled multicenter trial of the effectiveness of spinal cord stimulation. *Neurosurgery* 2008; 63: 762-70.

22. Heath R. *Schizophrenia: A Multidisciplinary Approach to Mind-Brain Relationships*. Cambridge: Harvard University Press, 1954.

23. Ebel H, Rust D, Tronnier V, Böker D, Kunze S. Chronic precentral stimulation in trigeminal neuropathic pain. *Acta Neurochir* (Wien) 1996; 138: 1300-6.

24. Meyerson BA, Lindblom U, Linderoth B, Lind G, Herregodts P. Motor cortex stimulation as treatment of trigeminal neuropathic pain. *Acta Neurochir Suppl* 1993; 58: 150-3.

25. Nguyen JP, Keravel Y, Feve A, *et al*. Treatment of deafferentation pain by chronic stimulation of the motor cortex: report of a series of 20 cases. *Acta Neurochir Suppl* 1997; 68: 54-60.

26. Nguyen JP, Lefaucher JP, Le Guerinel C, *et al*. Motor cortex stimulation in the treatment of central and neuropathic pain. *Arch Med Res* 2000; 31: 263-5.

27. Nguyen JP, Lefaucheur JP, Decq P, *et al*. Chronic motor cortex stimulation in the treatment of central and neuropathic pain. Correlations between clinical, electrophysiological and anatomical data. *Pain* 1999; 82: 245-51.

28. Brown JA, Pilitsis JG. Motor cortex stimulation for central and neuropathic facial pain: a prospective study of 10 patients and observations of enhanced sensory and motor function during stimulation. *Neurosurgery* 2005; 56: 290-7.

29. Nguyen JP, Velasco F, Brugières P, *et al*. Treatment of chronic neuropathic pain by motor cortex stimulation: results of a bicentric controlled crossover trial. *Brain Stimul* 2008; 1: 89-96.

30. Velasco F, Argüelles C, Carrillo-Ruiz JD, *et al*. Efficacy of motor cortex stimulation in the treatment of neuropathic pain: a randomized double-blind trial. *J Neurosurg* 2008; 108: 698-706.

31. Levy R, Deer TR, Henderson J. Intracranial neurostimulation for pain control: a review. *Pain Physician* 2010; 13: 157-65.

32. Fontaine D, Lazorthes Y, Mertens P, *et al*. Safety and efficacy of deep brain stimulation in refractory cluster headache: a randomized placebo-controlled double-blind trial followed by a 1-year open extension. *J Headache Pain* 2010; 11: 23-31.

Chapter 16

Stimulation of the central nervous system for chronic pain

Introduction

Tumors

Fred G Barker II MD

Associate Professor of Neurosurgery

HARVARD MEDICAL SCHOOL, MASSACHUSETTS GENERAL HOSPITAL,
BOSTON, MASSACHUSETTS, USA

The five chapters in this section of *The Evidence for Neurosurgery* discuss some of the most common neuro-oncological questions that neurosurgeons are called on to answer. These questions address whether resection is of benefit in high- and low-grade malignant gliomas; whether surgery or radiosurgery is preferred for vestibular schwannomas; and a variety of scenarios in the care of patients with brain metastases and pituitary tumors. Some general considerations about brain tumor clinical research design and interpretation [1] may help readers of these chapters assess the trustworthiness of the evidence they present, and help in bringing patients to see clinical decisions the way we do before they choose a treatment for themselves.

General considerations

Endpoints

First, are the endpoints used appropriate for the clinical question? For studies on glioblastoma, survival from the date of diagnosis or surgery is a very appropriate endpoint, since the disease itself is rapidly fatal and causes nearly all deaths in this patient cohort. But survival would be a very poor endpoint for

a comparison between surgery and radiosurgery for acoustic neuroma, because in developed countries death attributable to acoustic neuroma (or its treatment) is now very rare.

To clinicians, it seems obvious that preservation of facial nerve function and hearing, relief of balance complaints, headache after surgery, and overall quality of life are more important endpoints to examine in making any decision about treating acoustic neuromas. Evidence presented in Chapter 20 suggests that radiosurgery is superior to surgery for eligible patients on many of these scores; yet many patients with small acoustic neuromas continue to choose surgery. While there are many reasons a patient might rationally reach this decision, sometimes this seems to reflect a patient's focus on the infrequent but serious events that can follow radiosurgery for acoustics: transformation to a malignant tumor or occurrence of a second tumor, or surgery for tumor progression after radiation treatment, which might cause facial palsy. This tendency to weight strongly those consequences of a decision that are rare, but have dire personal results, is one of the best known ways in which real human decision-making is often 'irrational.'

This decision-making style is not the simple linear projection of likely outcomes that we consider rational. Treating physicians can sometimes downplay this decision-making style by either redirecting the patient's attention to the far more common experiences of those who undergo surgery or radiosurgery; or, in this specific case, by pointing out that surgical removal is, rarely, followed by death – about as often, or perhaps more often, as they might encounter the most serious adverse consequences of radiosurgery.

Bias

Second, much of the evidence summarized in these chapters is based on non-randomized treatment comparisons. In brain tumor studies, the largest threat to the validity of these comparisons is often the lack of eligibility of all patients for the two treatments being compared. For example, many non-randomized studies have compared survival after different degrees of surgical resection for malignant glioma. In one recent review on this topic, only one of 38 studies examined stated explicitly that all patients were eligible for total resection [2]. To the degree that resectability is an important prognostic factor for survival in malignant gliomas – independent of the degree of resection actually achieved – studies that use this design will have an intrinsic bias in favor of resection, which cannot be adjusted away using ordinary statistics. Unfortunately, such biases are very common in the neurosurgical oncology evidence base.

Treatment harm

Third, neurosurgical oncology studies often fail to account adequately for the harm done by treatment. Again, studies of the extent of resection in malignant glioma afford a good example. A common setting for these studies is the retrospective analysis of patients who enroll after surgery in a prospective clinical trial of some new radiation or chemotherapy treatment. Such cohorts offer an attractive and affordable way to study outcomes in large numbers of patients who receive relatively uniform treatment after surgery. What is hidden in the design is that such protocols nearly always have a minimum performance status necessary for enrollment, and sometimes other restrictions such as a maximum age. This means that patients who are neurologically injured by surgical resection may not be able to enroll in the protocol and will hence not be included in the study – nor will patients who undergo biopsy because of unresectability, and who have poor performance status because of their tumors. The sum of the effects of these biases is obviously difficult to judge, and even the numbers of patients who are excluded on these bases will be impossible for the investigators to define.

Studies of radiosurgery for any indication are limited by the maximum tumor size the investigators are willing to treat, so historical control cohorts must be carefully constructed to match treated patients in the size and proximity of tumors to critical structures such as the optic chiasm. Comparisons between cohorts treated with different radiosurgery doses are often similarly confounded because treatment dose is tightly correlated with tumor size.

Conclusions

Any surgeon who reads these chapters will immediately notice that very few randomized clinical trials (RCTs) exist that answer the important questions. To some extent, the relative rarity of brain tumors (which are far less common than neurotrauma or degenerative spine disease) makes such trials difficult to design and complete. More likely, though, the attitudes of surgeons and patients are at least as important a barrier to surgical RCTs in this area.

We are accustomed to think of a brain tumor as a serious illness in which decisive action needs to be taken at the start of treatment, and that the consequences of a misstep are so severe that we are bound to 'do our best' for our patients even when we are less than sure that our treatments are really effective. The same could be said about cancer in children, yet the culture of pediatric oncology is strongly oriented toward RCTs. In the USA, more than 70% of pediatric cancer patients enter cooperative group clinical trials – far higher than the trial participation of adult cancer patients, which is typically less than 5% [3]. Perhaps this difference in medical culture helps to explain why progress in curing and alleviating pediatric cancer has been so much greater than for adult cancer over the last 50 years. Before we simply accept the 'evidence' summarized in this section we should ask ourselves why, as a profession, we have so few secure foundations to build our practice on, and when we plan to do something about it.

References

1. Barker FG. Brain tumor outcome studies: design and analysis. In: *Youmans' Neurological Surgery*. Winn HR, Ed. Elsevier, in press.
2. Barker FG. Comment. *Neurosurgery* 2008; 62: 765-6. [Regarding Sanai N, Berger MS. Glioma extent of resection and its impact on patient outcome. *Neurosurgery* 2008; 62: 753-64.]
3. Bleyer WA, Tejeda HA, Murphy SB, Brawley OW, Smith MA Ungerleider RS. Equal participation of minority patients in U.S. national pediatric cancer clinical trials. *J Pediatr Hematol Oncol* 1997; 19(5): 423-7.

Introduction

Tumors

Chapter 17

Brain metastases

Sanjay Patra MD

Chief Resident, Neurosurgery

Steven N Kalkanis MD

Co-Director, Hermelin Brain Tumor Center; Vice-Chair for Operations

DEPARTMENT OF NEUROSURGERY, HENRY FORD HEALTH SYSTEM, DETROIT, MICHIGAN, USA

Introduction

The 2008 American Cancer Society Registry data show that approximately 1.4 million Americans are diagnosed with cancer every year. Because about 40% of these individuals will go on to develop brain metastases (Figure 1), the incidence of these secondary brain tumors is about four to five times that of primary brain tumors [1, 2]. This entity has become one of the neurosurgeon's most commonly encountered neoplastic lesions.

Treatment of these tumors is complex because both tumor- and patient-specific parameters impact decision-making. The past two decades have seen a large increase in treatment options, resulting in longer life expectancy and better quality of life to a point where metastatic lesions to the brain are no longer the major cause of mortality in this patient group. Thus, a paradigm shift has occurred in how aggressively patients with metastatic tumors are treated. Whole-brain radiation therapy (WBRT), which was the mainstay of metastatic brain tumor therapy until the mid-1990s, has now been supplemented with more aggressive local control measures including surgical resection and stereotactic radiosurgery (SRS) [3-5]. Treatment of metastatic brain tumors can span the full spectrum of medical care providers, including neurosurgeons, medical oncologists, radiation oncologists, neuro-oncologists, and neurologists. Given the myriad treatment options and the multiple providers utilizing them, evidence-based treatment information can be very useful to the clinician. The information in this chapter not only serves to guide the clinician in treatment options, but also focuses the researcher on areas in need of further investigation.

Methodology

Electronic databases, including MEDLINE, Embase, the Cochrane Database of Systematic Reviews, the Cochrane Controlled Trials Registry, and the Cochrane Database of Abstracts of Reviews of Effects, were searched from 1990 to September 2008. A broad search strategy using a combination of subheadings and text words was employed, and included the following: exp Brain Neoplasms, Central Nervous System Neoplasms, exp Brain Neoplasms AND Central Nervous System Neoplasms (metasta$ or secondary).tw, exp Neoplasm Metastasis, (metasta$ or secondary).tw AND exp Neoplasm Metastasis, (metasta$ or secondary).tw AND exp Neoplasm Metastasis AND exp Brain Neoplasms

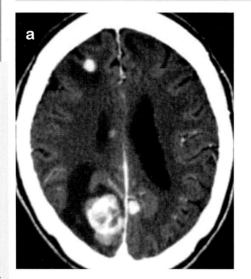

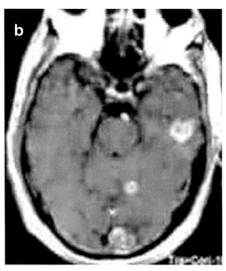

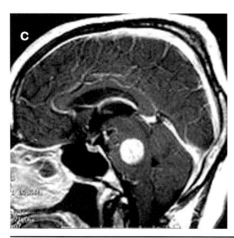

Figure 1. MRIs of brain metastases.

AND Central Nervous System Neoplasms, exp Brain Neoplasms/sc (Secondary), ([metasta$ or secondary] adj3 [brain or cereb$ or intercranial]).tw, exp Brain Neoplasms/sc (Secondary) AND ([metasta$ or secondary] adj3 [brain or cereb$ or intercranial]).tw, animals/not (animals/and humans/).

The search of the bibliographic databases yielded 16,966 articles, which were subsequently narrowed down by a series of reviews.

Radiation therapy

WBRT remains an important part of the standard treatment regimen for patients with metastatic brain lesions. This section reviews the evidence for WBRT and altered dose fractions along with the role of histopathology in outcomes. In addition, the role of WBRT and surgery is compared with WBRT alone in patients with newly diagnosed, single metastatic lesions that are surgically accessible.

Evidence from three randomized controlled trials (RCTs) [6-8] supports the use of surgical resection plus postoperative WBRT, as compared with WBRT alone, for the treatment of a newly diagnosed, surgically accessible single brain metastasis **(Ia/A)**. This level of evidence only applies to patients with limited extracranial disease who spend more than 50% of the day out of bed. In addition, the data do not apply to radiosensitive tumor histologies such as small-cell lung cancer (SCLC), leukemia, lymphoma, germ-cell tumors, and multiple myeloma.

The trial by Patchell *et al* consisted of 48 patients with known systemic cancer and a Karnofsky Performance Score (KPS) of at least 70 [6]. The patients were treated with WBRT and either biopsy or complete surgical resection. Patients with acute neurologic deterioration and radiosensitive tumors (SCLC, germ-cell tumors, lymphoma, leukemia, or multiple myeloma) were excluded. There was a statistically significant increase in the survival of the surgical group (40 weeks) compared with the non-surgical group (15 weeks) **(Ib/A)**. Furthermore, duration of functional independence, freedom from death due to neurologic compromise, and time to recurrence of a new brain metastasis were all significantly longer in the surgical group **(Ib/A)**.

Another multicenter randomized trial of 63 patients comparing surgical resection and WBRT with WBRT alone was performed by Vecht *et al* in the Netherlands [7]. The included patients spent no longer than 50% of their time in bed and did not require continuous nursing care. This trial showed significantly longer survival times in the surgical group (10 vs. 6 months). The benefit was only seen in patients younger than 60 years and without progressive systemic disease who were within 3 months of diagnosis **(Ib/A)**.

The final multicenter randomized trial, performed in Canada by Mintz *et al* with 84 patients, found no statistically significant difference in overall survival, causes of death, or quality of life in patients treated with WBRT plus surgery or WBRT alone [8] **(Ib/A)**. This trial included patients younger than 80 years with a KPS of at least 50. In contrast to the previous trials, these patients could spend more than 50% of their day in bed. Another further reason for the different results could be the lack of mandatory MRI scans in patients included in the study, giving rise to the possibility that additional lesions were present that were not seen on preoperative CT.

Three further level II studies have shown a survival benefit with surgical resection and WBRT compared with WBRT alone [9-11]. Taken together, there is level Ia/A evidence supporting the use of surgical resection with WBRT rather than WBRT alone.

Optimal WBRT dosing and fractionation schedule

Altering dosing or fractionation schedules of WBRT from a standard of 30Gy in 10 fractions (or a biologically effective dose of 39Gy10) does not significantly change the neurocognitive outcome, local control, or median survival in adults with a newly diagnosed brain metastasis **(Ia/A)**. This is based on 10 level I studies, including nine RCTs [12-20] and one randomized Phase I/II trial [21]. None of these trials demonstrated a significant survival benefit relative to the dose schedule.

Given the large number of primary neoplasms that can metastasize to the brain, WBRT outcomes based on tumor histopathology have also been analyzed. To date, there are insufficient data to make any evidence-based recommendations on this topic. Further work is needed in this area.

Surgical resection

Surgical resection plus WBRT versus surgical resection alone

These topics were reviewed in detail by Kalkanis *et al* in the 2010 evidence-based practice guidelines [22] for metastatic brain tumors adopted by the American Association of Neurological Surgeons (AANS), the Congress of Neurological Surgeons (CNS), and the Joint Section on Tumors. The outcomes of patients undergoing WBRT alone for brain metastasis are poor and in the range of 3-6 months [7, 8, 23]. In the previous section, we described how the combination of surgical resection and WBRT is superior to WBRT alone in terms of mortality in patients with a newly diagnosed brain metastasis. Over half a million people are diagnosed with new brain metastases every year in the USA [1, 2]. About one-third of these individuals will be candidates for surgical resection and WBRT. Given the known side effects of radiation therapy, surgical resection alone has been compared with the regimen of surgical resection followed by WBRT.

There is level Ib/A evidence for improved tumor control with surgical resection and WBRT compared with surgical resection alone, based on one RCT [3] and three retrospective cohort studies [24-26]. In the RCT, 95 patients with a KPS of more than 70 and complete surgical resection (based on MRI) were randomized to WBRT or no further treatment [3]. Tumor recurrence was 18% in the surgery plus WBRT group, compared with 70% in the surgery-alone group (p<0.001) **(Ib/A)**. This lower recurrence rate with WBRT was found to be true both for *de novo* lesions and recurrences at the original resection site. Although the study was not powered to look for overall survival, fewer people in the WBRT group died from neurologic causes (surgery

44% vs. surgery and WBRT 14%; p<0.003). The degree of functional independence did not differ significantly between the two groups.

Surgical resection plus WBRT versus SRS plus WBRT

One small RCT [27] and two retrospective cohort studies [28, 29] have compared surgical resection plus WBRT to SRS alone for the initial treatment of a newly diagnosed brain metastasis. The randomized trial was a multicenter study by Muacevic et al in Germany [27]. A total of 64 adult patients with a KPS of more than 70 and single small (<3cm) metastatic lesions were randomized to surgical resection and WBRT, or SRS alone. The only outcome that was statistically different between the groups was recurrence at distant brain sites, which was significantly higher in the SRS-alone group (p=0.04) **(Ib/A)**. Overall survival (the primary outcome) and duration of freedom from local recurrence did not significantly differ between the groups. This trial originally planned to enroll 242 patients but had to close prematurely due to poor patient accrual, which was one-quarter of the goal number.

Although no prospective studies have compared surgical resection and WBRT versus SRS and WBRT, four retrospective cohort studies have at least partially addressed this important comparison. In three of the studies, overall survival did not differ between the groups [30-32] **(III/B)**. In the other study, however, both overall survival and freedom from local recurrence were significantly longer in the group that received resection and WBRT [33] **(III/B)**. A flaw in this study was that the patients in the SRS arm were generally poorer resection candidates and thus in poorer condition overall. Furthermore, the three negative studies all showed greater freedom from local recurrence in the SRS and WBRT group [30-32]. None of the four studies showed a significant difference in the duration of freedom from recurrence at distant brain sites. Based on the above studies, there is level III/B evidence that surgical resection with WBRT, and SRS with WBRT, both represent effective treatment strategies resulting in equal survival.

Furthermore, based on these studies, there is level IIb/B evidence that lesions larger than 3cm or those causing a significant mass effect may have better outcomes with surgical resection. Radiosurgery is recommended for single surgically inaccessible lesions of less than 3cm in diameter.

Areas of future research

While surgical resection of multiple brain metastases is often performed when there are two lesions accessible through the same craniotomy, there is no robust comparative prospective evidence to offer any survival or outcomes comparisons relating to this practice. Further studies need to be conducted in this area – along with addressing the question of using postoperative SRS to the resection cavity, which is a treatment option currently being offered at many institutions throughout the USA. Given the relatively small differences in survival rates, further studies should also focus on overall functional status, neurocognitive outcomes, and quality-of-life measures.

Stereotactic radiosurgery

SRS has emerged as a treatment modality that is less invasive yet still able to treat neoplastic lesions while potentially sparing healthy brain (Figure 2). A detailed systematic review with evidence-based guidelines on this topic was published by Linskey et al in 2010 [34].

Two prospective RCTs have compared SRS and WBRT to WBRT alone in newly diagnosed patients with brain lesions. Only single-dose SRS was evaluated in each of these studies. The Radiation Therapy Oncology Group led a multicenter trial comparing these treatment modalities in patients with one to three solid brain metastases (diameter <4cm) and a KPS of more than 70 [5]. The primary endpoint was median survival, which was measured in 133 patients undergoing WBRT plus SRS and 139 patients undergoing WBRT alone. The results showed statistically significant improved survival (6.5 vs. 5.7 months), superior 1-year local control (progression in 71% vs. 82% of patients), and

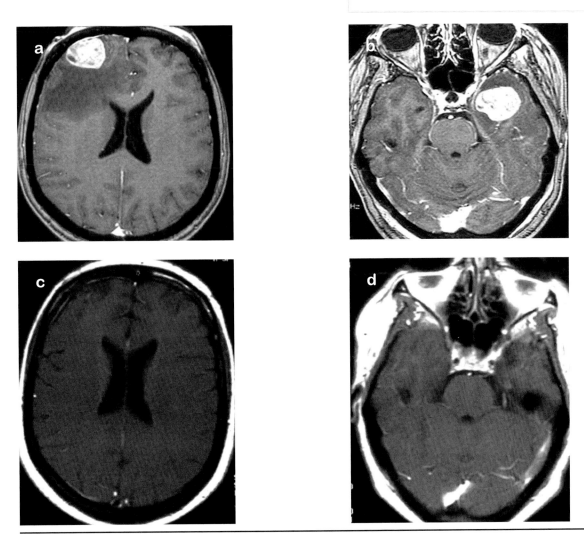

Figure 2. Two different MRI slice images from the same patient (a, b) before and (c, d) after being treated with stereotactic radiosurgery for brain metastases.

improved KPS in the WBRT plus SRS arm in patients with a single metastatic lesion **(Ib/A)**. Local control and improved KPS were secondary endpoints assessed with post hoc analysis. Kondziolka *et al* performed the second RCT in patients with two to four solid metastatic lesions (diameter <2.5cm) and a KPS of less than 70 [4]. There were 14 patients in the WBRT-alone arm and 13 in the WBRT plus SRS arm. The primary endpoint was image-defined local control. The study was stopped prematurely because of significant positive tumor control in the WBRT plus SRS arm during the interim analysis: the local failure rate was 8% in the WBRT plus SRS arm compared with 100% in the WBRT arm. Furthermore, median time to progression at the original site was

significantly longer in the WBRT plus SRS arm (36 vs. 6 months). The premature closure of the study did not give it enough power to measure differences in median survival.

Given the results from the above RCTs, and from three other retrospective studies [35-37], there is level Ia/A evidence supporting single-dose SRS along with WBRT leading to significantly longer patient survival than WBRT alone in patients with single metastatic brain tumors and a KPS of more than 70. There is level IIa/B evidence demonstrating that single-dose SRS plus WBRT is superior in terms of local tumor control and maintaining functional status when compared with WBRT alone for patients with fewer than four metastatic lesions with a KPS of more than 70. There is level III/B evidence that SRS plus WBRT leads to longer patient survival, compared with WBRT alone, in patients with two or three metastatic lesions.

Only one RCT has compared WBRT plus SRS with SRS alone: a multi-institutional trial by Aoyama et al in Japan [38, 39]. The inclusion criteria were one to four solid brain metastases (diameter <3cm) and a KPS of more than 70. Of note, the SRS dose in the combined SRS plus WBRT arm was reduced by 30%. The primary endpoint was median survival, which was not found to be statistically different between the groups (8 vs. 7.5 months) (Ib/A). There was also no difference in 1-year local control (73% vs. 89%) or neurologic cause of death. The secondary endpoint of distant brain site recurrence was significantly greater for the SRS-alone arm (74% vs. 47%), as was the chance of requiring salvage therapy in the form of WBRT or SRS (43% vs. 15%).

A three-arm prospective cohort study performed by Li et al also compared WBRT plus WBRT with SRS or WBRT alone [36]. This study was limited to patients with SCLC or non-small-cell lung cancer (NSCLC), a KPS greater than 60, and single brain metastases (diameter <4.5cm). The authors found no significant differences in median survival or local progression (IIa/B). A further nine retrospective cohort studies have also addressed this issue [40-48]. Together, these data provide level IIa/B evidence that single-dose SRS alone provides a similar survival advantage to the regimen of WBRT plus SRS. There is some level IIa/B evidence of improved distant brain site control with WBRT; it is therefore recommended that patients receiving only SRS undergo close imaging surveillance so that early salvage therapy can be initiated at recurrence.

No RCTs have compared SRS alone with WBRT alone. In the Li et al three-arm prospective cohort study, however, two of the arms investigated SRS alone and WBRT alone [36]. Patients in the SRS arm experienced significantly longer survival (9.3 vs. 5.7 months), median time to progression (6.9 vs. 4 months), and neuroimaging tumor response (87% vs. 38%). These data, together with data from four other retrospective [49-52] cohort studies, yield level III/B evidence supporting SRS alone as superior to WBRT

alone for survival in patients with up to three metastatic brain lesions.

Chemotherapy

The AANS/CNS evidence-based guidelines for the role of chemotherapy in brain metastases were published in 2010 [53]. The primary therapeutic modality for systemic metastases remains chemotherapy. However, the efficacy of chemotherapy in the brain has always been a concern because of the presence of the blood-brain barrier and its ability to exclude or greatly dilute agents delivered to the central nervous system. There is even some evidence that active transport via efflux pumps may play a role in the protective function of the blood-brain barrier [54]. It is also believed that brain metastases are preselected to be chemoresistant because only resistant cells are able to survive systemic chemotherapy and reach the brain. But even in previously untreated SCLC, the response rate of intracranial metastases remains lower than that of extracranial lesions [55].

Four RCTs have compared WBRT with WBRT plus chemotherapy. The first was a multi-institutional RCT that investigated WBRT and carboplatin in patients with metastatic NSCLC [56]. The patients had histologically proven NSCLC, with a WHO performance status of 0, 1, or 2, and at least one brain metastasis based on MRI or CT, and had either refused surgery or presented with lesions deemed inoperable. The primary endpoint was overall survival. Median survival was similar for the WBRT and WBRT plus carboplatin groups (4.4 vs. 3.7 months) (Ib/A). Unfortunately, the trial was halted because of failed accrual and was unable to show improved survival. Furthermore, the WHO performance status tended to be lower in the WBRT group.

Another RCT, performed by Ushio et al, included all lung cancer subtypes in patients with projected survival of at least 4 months [57]. Patients were excluded if they had received any prior chemotherapy. The study utilized three arms:

- WBRT.
- WBRT plus chloroethyl nitrosourea (CCNU).
- WBRT, CCNU, and tegafur.

The primary endpoint was tumor control, with survival tabulated as a secondary endpoint. The tumor response rates were 36%, 69%, and 74%, respectively. The only statistically significant difference was between WBRT and the combination of WBRT, CCNU, and tegafur for tumor control. There were no differences in survival **(Ib/A)**.

Another RCT of 48 patients did not show improved survival when temozolomide (TMZ) was added to WBRT (see later) [58]. It did, however, show improvements in tumor response rates and neurologic function in the TMZ group. Conversely, the final RCT did not find any difference in survival or tumor response rate with TMZ added to WBRT [59] **(Ib/A)**.

Given the above studies, there is level Ia/A evidence that adding chemotherapy to WBRT does not improve survival. However, most of the RCTs were conducted with patients with NSCLC and breast cancer and may not be applicable to other histologies. In addition, some of the RTCs did show improved response rates with chemotherapy and further trials in this area are warranted. These data do not apply to chemosensitive tumors such as germinomas metastatic to the brain.

Re-treatment

The median survival of patients with untreated brain metastases is 4 weeks, with death typically from neurologic causes [60]. There are few data and little consensus on managing recurrent metastases, given most studies have been performed with newly diagnosed patients. Detailed guidelines on this topic were published by Ammirati *et al* in 2010 [61].

Only three retrospective case series have looked at the effects of repeating WBRT in patients with brain recurrence following previous treatment. The average reirradiation dose ranged from 20 to 25Gy over multiple fractions. Post-WBRT survival was 4-5 months in all series [62-64] **(III/B)**.

Four case series have evaluated surgical resection for recurrent or progressive brain metastases [65-68]. Survival ranged from 8.9 to 11.5 months, and median time to recurrence at local and distant sites was 5.0-8.4 months **(III/B)**.

Only one prospective Phase I/II study has been performed to investigate SRS for recurrent/progressive brain metastases. This study included 12 patients who had been previously treated with WBRT and who had progressive metastatic lesions with at least 3 months' projected survival. The overall median survival was 6 months.

The role of chemotherapy for recurrent brain metastases has been evaluated by five prospective, single-arm Phase II studies [69-73]. Agents used in these studies included cisplatin, TMZ, thalidomide, vinorelbine, fotemustine, and cisplatin. Median survival was 3.5-6.6 months.

The target population for all of these studies was adults with progressive or recurrent brain metastases who had previously been treated with WBRT, surgical resection, or SRS.

There is only enough evidence to give a level III/B recommendation for individualization of care based on functional status, extent of systemic and intracranial disease, previous treatment type, primary cancer type, progression at original or distant site, and enrollment in clinical trials. Taking these factors into account, no further treatment, WBRT or SRS, or surgical excision can be recommended. There is far less evidence for recommending chemotherapy.

Prophylactic anticonvulsants

The role of prophylactic anticonvulsants in the setting of brain metastases remains unclear. It is thought that brain metastases are unlikely to be as epileptogenic as primary gliomas due to their less infiltrative nature. Evidence-based guidelines on this topic were published by Mikkelsen *et al* in 2010 [74].

One underpowered RCT, performed by Forsyth *et al*, analyzed anticonvulsant use for brain metastases [75]. The study included 100 patients with all types of brain tumor, stratified by primary or metastatic tumor. Patients were excluded if they had known seizures, a life expectancy of less than 4 weeks, allergies to antiepileptic drugs, a history of substance abuse or were pregnant. Most of the patients were treated with phenytoin, with the primary outcome of seizure occurrence at 3 months. The trial was terminated early because the anticipated seizure rate in the no-anticonvulsant arm was only 10%. This put the anticipated seizure rate outside the 95% confidence interval at 20%. In addition, the 3-month mortality rate was significantly higher than expected (30% vs. 15%). These factors greatly lowered the power of the study. The authors reported no difference in seizure incidence between those who received anticonvulsants and those who did not.

Given the above data, and taking into account the known side effects of anticonvulsants, there is level III/B evidence for not using routine anticonvulsant prophylaxis in patients with newly diagnosed brain metastases. There is still a need for future studies addressing this issue.

Steroids

It is well known that glucocorticoids can be used to help control cerebral edema, and dexamethasone is generally chosen because of its minimal mineralocorticoid activity. Steroids, however, are not without side effects, which include myopathy, insulin resistance, and gastrointestinal bleeding. The recommendations for steroid use are variable, despite a considerable body of literature on the subject. The role of steroids, including when and whether to use them and at what dose, is addressed in this section. Detailed evidence-based clinical guidelines on this topic were published by Ryken et al in 2010 [76].

Vecht et al published a randomized study of 4, 6, and 16mg/day dosing of dexamethasone [77]. Patients with a KPS of less than 80 with brain metastases were evaluated to find the minimal effective dose of oral dexamethasone, with KPS as the outcome measure. Although there was some improvement in all the groups, the authors found no advantage to the higher dosing in patients who were not thought to be in immediate danger of herniation. The authors concluded that doses of 4 and 8mg/day were equivalent in improving neurologic function, when compared with 16mg/day, in moderately symptomatic patients **(Ib/A)**.

Wolfson et al prospectively evaluated 12 patients with brain metastases to determine the indications for glucocorticoids [78]. Because of its small size and lack of statistical analysis, no conclusions can be drawn from this trial.

A level III/B recommendation can be made for the use of corticosteroids (4-8mg/day) to provide temporary relief of symptoms related to elevated intracranial pressure. A level III/B recommendation can also be made for using dexamethasone 16mg/day in patients experiencing severe symptoms of elevated intracranial pressure because of brain metastases causing brain edema. A level III/B recommendation for dexamethasone as the glucocorticoid of choice can also be made, along with the suggestion that the dose should be tapered over a period of 2 weeks or longer.

Emerging and investigational therapies

Clearly, uniformly successful control of brain metastasis has not been achieved. Even if relatively good control is achieved, the various treatment modalities are associated with significant toxicity. A number of new treatment modalities are emerging, including radiation sensitizers, local irradiation with balloon-based brachytherapy, stereotactic radiation sources, local chemotherapy with BCNU-impregnated polymers, and molecular targeting. This section discusses emerging modalities that have reached the point of assessment in clinical trials. Evidence-based guidelines for emerging metastatic brain tumor treatment modalities were published by Olson et al in 2010 [79].

Motexafin gadolinium

Motexafin gadolinium (MGd) is an MRI-detectable metallotexaphrin that accumulates in a significantly higher concentration within tumors than in normal tissue. Although its exact mechanism of action is unknown, it is thought to act as a radiation sensitizer and modifier. Two RCTs and one prospective single-arm study have evaluated this agent.

The single-arm study was published by Carde *et al* and established intravenous MGd 5mg/day as the best-tolerated dose when combined with 30Gy of WBRT given in 10 fractions [80]. This led to an RCT of 401 patients with brain metastases comparing WBRT with WBRT plus MGd [81]. The study did not show any difference in median survival or tumor response **(Ib/A)**. There was, however, a 0.5-month delay in neurologic progression in the MGd plus WBRT group, particularly in patients with lung cancer. A subsequent international Phase III study was conducted, which randomized 554 patients with NSCLC to WBRT or WBRT plus MGd, with neurologic progression as the primary endpoint. Overall, no statistically significant difference was found **(Ib/A)**. Interestingly, when patients outside North America were excluded, there was a significant increase in time to neurologic progression in the WBRT plus MGd group (from 8.8 to 24.2 months). This turned out to be a function of WBRT being initiated within 3 weeks of diagnosis, rather than geography.

Efaproxiral

Efaproxiral is a radiation sensitizer that is believed to cause a conformational change in hemoglobin. This is thought to lead to decreased oxygen-binding capacity, which ultimately results in more free oxygen in the tumor cells and increased radiation sensitization. Two Phase II studies have been performed with efaproxiral, but neither showed any improvement in survival or any other endpoint.

There is level IIa/B evidence that early use of efaproxiral with WBRT may prolong neurologic progression. There is also IIa/B evidence, however, suggesting that efaproxiral does not provide any survival benefit when combined with WBRT.

Interstitial modalities

Interstitial modalities consist of brachytherapy, defined as therapy placed inside or next to the area being treated. These modalities are appealing because of the potential to maximize therapy exposure to the metastatic pathology while sparing normal brain. No prospective studies have yet evaluated interstitial radiosurgery. However, one retrospective cohort study has been conducted by Ostertag and Kreth, which involved the implantation of ^{125}I seeds for spherical brain metastases of diameter 4cm or less, with 60Gy applied to the rim of the lesions [82]. The study compared WBRT and ^{125}I versus ^{125}I alone. No difference was found between these groups **(III/B)**. Two case series have also looked at [125]I [83, 84]. Both supported the feasibility of this modality, but did not offer any evidence for increased efficacy when added to WBRT.

Rogers *et al* evaluated the role of the GliaSite Radiation Therapy System in the post-resection surgical bed of patients with metastatic tumors in a Phase II study [85]. This system involves implantation of a balloon connected to a subcutaneous reservoir that can be injected with liquid [125]I. Median survival was 40 weeks at 1-year follow-up, and tumor progression was only involved in four of 35 deaths. These data were prospectively obtained with no comparator group.

Two single-arm studies have evaluated surgery and local chemotherapy with or without WBRT. Ewend *et al* prospectively evaluated 25 cases of newly diagnosed solitary metastatic lesions treated with surgical resection, Gliadel Wafer, and WBRT [86]. The primary outcome was toxicity, with a median follow-up of 36 weeks. Median survival was 33 weeks but there were no comparative data, thus relegating this to level III evidence. Nakagawa *et al* investigated the use of intracavitary 5-fluoro-2-deoxyuridine (FdUrd), which inhibits tumor DNA synthesis via its metabolite, in six patients with brain metastases [87]. An Ommaya reservoir was placed over the resection cavity with daily infusions of FdUrd. The authors did not note any adverse events; however, no comparative data were obtained **(III/B)**.

Two case series have investigated interstitial radiosurgery with the Photon Radiosurgery System [88, 89]. Both studies lacked comparative data, but showed median survival of 8 months and 1-year survival of 53% **(III/B)**.

Based on the current data, there is no evidence to support the use of new or existing interstitial radiation, chemotherapy, or other modalities outside of clinical trials.

Molecularly targeted therapy

Our understanding of the molecular mechanisms of tumor growth, proliferation, and spread is growing. While isolated treatment responses have been reported, there is currently no level I evidence for the use of molecularly targeted therapies in brain metastasis.

Gefitinib, which inhibits multiple receptor tyrosine kinases including epidermal growth factor receptor, is approved for use in advanced NSCLC. A few case reports and single-arm prospective studies have demonstrated tumor response or stabilization in most patients treated with gefitinib for NSCLC metastasizing to the brain [90-95].

Agents that target angiogenesis such as bevacizumab (a monoclonal antibody against vascular epidermal growth factor receptor) are also being evaluated for their role in brain metastases. Most of these studies are designed to evaluate safety rather than efficacy, and thus no evidence-based treatment recommendations can yet be made.

Clearly, given the promising theoretical advantage of molecularly targeted therapies, prospective studies focusing on survival, tumor control, and quality of life are warranted.

Temozolomide and fotemustine

A number of studies have evaluated the effectiveness of TMZ in the treatment of brain metastases. In most of these studies, melanoma was the primary tumor treated. Antonadou *et al* carried out a randomized Phase II study of TMZ in metastatic lung, breast, or unknown cancers [58]. A total of 48

patients were randomized to WBRT or WBRT and TMZ. The WBRT plus TMZ patients showed a tumor response rate of 96%, compared with 67% for the WBRT group (p<0.017). There was no difference in survival rates **(Ib/A)**. Verger *et al* also performed a Phase II study in which patients with any metastatic source were randomized to WBRT or WBRT plus TMZ [59]. This study demonstrated significantly increased progression-free survival in the WBRT plus TMZ group (72% vs. 54%) **(Ib/A)**. Two retrospective cohort studies have together not shown a survival advantage of adding TMZ to WBRT [96, 97]**(III/B)**.

Fotemustine has been studied in one RCT involving 76 cases of metastatic melanoma [98]. The study compared fotemustine and WBRT with WBRT alone. There were no significant differences in survival, response rate, or tumor control between the groups.

Taken together, these studies provide level III/B evidence for the use of WBRT and TMZ or fotemustine for the treatment of metastatic brain lesions, depending on the individual circumstances. There is level IIa/B evidence that TMZ and WBRT is a reasonable option for brain metastases.

Although these investigational therapies are very promising, they have not yet yielded level I evidence. More research into these and even newer modalities will undoubtedly result in improved patient care.

Conclusions

When properly understood and utilized, evidence-based recommendations can be an extremely useful tool in neuro-oncology. Such guidelines not only provide a scientifically secure base for clinical practice but also, through an exhaustive review of the available literature, highlight critical gaps in our current knowledge, which then can help direct future research. The systematic evidence-based guidelines for metastatic brain tumors that have been referenced throughout this chapter are summarized below.

Recommendations	Evidence level

- Surgical resection plus postoperative WBRT is recommended over WBRT alone in patients with limited extracranial disease and good functional status (<50% of day in bed). — Ia/A
- Surgical resection and WBRT result in superior local and distant brain control when compared with surgical resection alone. — Ia/A
- Altering the dose or fractionation schedule of WBRT does not result in differences in local control, neurocognitive outcomes, or median survival when compared with the standard dose/fractionation scheme (30Gy in 10 fractions or a biologically effective dose of 39Gy10). — Ia/A
- Surgical resection and WBRT result in equal survival rates when compared with SRS and WBRT. This is only applicable to lesions of less than 3cm in maximum diameter and those not causing significant mass effect (>1cm midline shift). — IIa/B
- SRS alone may result in similar functional and survival outcomes compared with surgical resection plus WBRT if patients have close follow-up for distant site failure so that salvage SRS is possible. — III/B
- Single-dose SRS with WBRT results in longer survival compared with WBRT alone in patients with a KPS of more than 70 and only a single metastasis. — Ia/A
- Single-dose SRS with WBRT results in improved local tumor control and functional status compared with WBRT alone for patients with one to four metastatic lesions and a KPS of more than 70. — Ia/A
- Single-dose SRS with WBRT may lead to longer survival times when compared with WBRT alone in patients with two or three metastatic lesions. — IIa/B
- Single-dose SRS may lead to improved survival compared with WBRT alone for patients with single or multiple metastases and a KPS of less than 70. — III/B
- Single-dose SRS alone may provide similar survival rates when compared with single-dose SRS plus WBRT only where there is very close surveillance for distant recurrence so that salvage therapy can be initiated early. — IIa/B
- Routine use of chemotherapy after WBRT has not been shown to increase survival. Since most of the studies evaluated mainly patients with NSCLC and breast cancer, effectiveness in other histologies cannot be ruled out. — Ia/A
- The use of radiation sensitizers (MGd or efaproxiral) is not recommended for treating brain metastases outside the setting of a clinical trial. — IIa/B
- Metastatic melanoma to the brain can be treated with WBRT and TMZ. — IIa/B

Chapter 17

References

1. Gavrilovic IT, Posner JB. Brain metastases: epidemiology and pathophysiology. *J Neurooncol* 2008; 75(1): 5-14.
2. American Cancer Society. Cancer Facts and Figures. 2008. Available from: www.cancer.org/docroot/stt/content/stt_1x_cancer_facts_and_figures_2008.asp. Accessed 10 November, 2010.
3. Patchell RA, Tibbs PA, Regine WF, *et al*. Postoperative radiotherapy in the treatment of single metastases to the brain: a randomized trial. *JAMA* 1998; 280(17): 1485-9.
4. Kondziolka D, Patel A, Lunsford LD, Kassam A, Flickinger JC. Stereotactic radiosurgery plus whole brain radiotherapy versus radiotherapy alone for patients with multiple brain metastases. *Int J Radiat Oncol Biol Phys* 1999; 45(2): 427-34.

Chapter 17

5. Andrews DW, Scott CB, Sperduto PW, *et al*. Whole brain radiation therapy with or without stereotactic radiosurgery boost for patients with one to three brain metastases: Phase III results of the RTOG 9508 randomised trial. *Lancet* 2004; 363(9422): 1665-72.

6. Patchell RA, Tibbs PA, Walsh JW, *et al*. A randomized trial of surgery in the treatment of single metastases to the brain. *N Engl J Med* 1990; 322(8): 494-500.

7. Vecht CJ, Haaxma-Reiche H, Noordijk EM, *et al*. Treatment of single brain metastasis: radiotherapy alone or combined with neuro-surgery? *Ann Neurol* 1993; 33(6): 583-90.

8. Mintz AH, Kestle J, Rathbone MP, *et al*. A randomized trial to assess the efficacy of surgery in addition to radiotherapy in patients with a single cerebral metastasis. *Cancer* 1996; 78(7): 1470-6.

9. Ampil FL, Nanda A, Willis BK, Nandy I, Meehan R. Metastatic disease in the cerebellum. The LSU experience. *Am J Clin Oncol* 1996; 19(5): 509-11.

10. Rades D, Kieckebusch S, Haatanen T, Lohynska R, Dunst J, Schild SE. Surgical resection followed by whole brain radiotherapy versus whole brain radiotherapy alone for single brain metastasis. *Int J Radiat Oncol Biol Phys* 2008; 70(5): 1319-24.

11. Sause WT, Crowley JJ, Morantz R, *et al*. Solitary brain metastasis: results of an RTOG/SWOG protocol evaluation surgery + RT versus RT alone. *Am J Clin Oncol* 1990; 13(5): 427-32.

12. Borgelt B, Gebler R, Larson M, Hendrickson F, Griffin T, Roth R. Ultra-rapid high-dose irradiation schedules for the palliation of brain metastases: final results of the first two studies by Radiation Therapy Oncology Group. *Int J Radiat Oncol Biol Phys* 1981; 7(12): 1633-8.

13. Chatani M, Matayoshi Y, Masaki N, Inoue T. Radiation therapy for brain metastases from lung carcinoma. Prospective randomized trial according to the level of lactate dehydrogenase. *Strahlenther Onkol* 1994; 170(3): 155-61.

14. Chatani M, Teshima T, Hata K, Inoue T, Suzuki T. Whole brain irradiation for metastases from lung carcinoma. A clinical investigation. *Acta Radiol Oncol* 1985; 24(4): 311-4.

15. Davey P, Hoegler D, Ennis M, Smith J. A Phase III study of accelerated versus conventional hypofractionated whole brain irradiation in patients of good performance status with brain metastases. *Radiother Oncol* 2008; 88(2): 173-6.

16. Haie-Meder C, Pellae-Cosset B, Laplanche A, *et al*. Results of a randomized clinical trial comparing two radiation schedules in the palliative treatment of brain metastases. *Radiother Oncol* 1993; 26(2): 111-6.

17. Komarnicky LT, Phillips TL, Martz K, Asbell S, Isaacson S, Urtasun R. A randomized Phase III protocol for the evaluation of misonidazole combined with radiation in the treatment of patients with brain metastases (RTOG-7916). *Int J Radiat Oncol Biol Phys* 1991; 20(1): 53-8.

18. Kurtz JM, Gleber R, Brady LW, Carella RJ Cooper JS. The palliation of brain metastases in a favorable patient population: a randomized clinical trial by the Radiation Therapy Oncology Group. *Int J Radiat Oncol Biol Phys* 1981; 7(7): 891-5.

19. Murray KJ, Scott C, Greenberg HM, *et al*. A randomized Phase III study of accelerated hyperfractionation versus standard in patients with unresected brain metastases: a report of the Radiation Therapy Oncology Group (RTOG) 9104. *Int J Radiat Oncol Biol Phys* 1997; 39(3): 571-4.

20. Priestman TJ, Dunn J, Brada M, Rampling R, Baker PG. Final results of the Royal College of Radiologists trial comparing two different radiotherapy schedules in the treatment of cerebral metastasis. *Clin Oncol* (R Coll Radiol) 1996; 8(5): 308-15.

21. Sause WT, Scott C, Krisch R, *et al*. Phase I/II trial of accelerated fractionation in brain metastases RTOG 85-28. *Int J Radiat Oncol Biol Phys* 1993; 26(4): 653-7.

22. Kalkanis SN, Kondziolka D, Gaspar LE, *et al*. The role of surgical resection in the management of newly diagnosed brain metastases: a systematic review and evidence-based clinical practice guideline. *J Neurooncol* 2010; 96(1): 33-43.

23. Kalkanis SN, Linskey ME. Evidence-based clinical practice parameter guidelines for the treatment of patients with metastatic brain tumors: introduction. *J Neurooncol* 2009; 96(1): 7-10.

24. Armstrong JG, Wronski M, Galicich J, Arbit E, Leibel SA, Burt M. Postoperative radiation for lung cancer metastatic to the brain. *J Clin Oncol* 1994; 12(11): 2340-4.

25. Hagen NA, Cirrincione C, Thaler HT, DeAngelis LM. The role of radiation therapy following resection of single brain metastasis from melanoma. *Neurology* 1990; 40(1): 158-60.

26. Skibber JM, Soong SF, Austin L, Balch CM, Sawaya RE. Cranial irradiation after surgical excision of brain metastases in melanoma patients. *Ann Surg Oncol* 1996; 3(2): 118-23.

27. Muacevic A, Wowra B, Siefert A, Tonn JC, Steiger HJ, Kreth FW. Microsurgery plus whole brain irradiation versus Gamma Knife surgery alone for treatment of single metastases to the brain: a randomized controlled multicentre Phase III trial. *J Neurooncol* 2008; 87(3): 299-307.

28. Muacevic A, Kreth FW, Horstmann GA, *et al*. Surgery and radiotherapy compared with Gamma Knife radiosurgery in the treatment of solitary cerebral metastases of small diameter. *J Neurosurg* 1999; 91(1): 35-43.

29. Rades D, Bohlen G, Pluemer A, *et al*. Stereotactic radiosurgery alone versus resection plus WBRT for 1 or 2 brain metastases in recursive portioning analysis class 1 and 2 patients. *Cancer* 2007; 109(12): 2515-21.

30. Garell PC, Hitchon PW, Wen BC, Mellenberg DE, Torner J. Stereotactic radiosurgery versus microsurgical resection for the initial treatment of metastatic cancer to the brain. *J Radiosurg* 1999; 2(1): 1-5.

31. Schöggl A, Kitz K, Reddy M, *et al*. Defining the role of stereotactic radiosurgery versus microsurgery in the treatment of single brain metastases. *Acta Neurochir* (Wien) 2000; 142(6): 621-6.

32. O'Neill BP, Iturria NJ, Link MJ, Pollock BE, Ballman KV, O'Fallon JR. A comparison of surgical resection and stereotactic radiosurgery in the treatment of solitary brain metastases. *Int J Radiat Oncol Biol Phys* 2003; 55(5): 1169-76.

33. Bindal AK, Bindal RK, Hess KR, *et al*. Surgery versus radiosurgery in the treatment of brain metastasis. *J Neurosurg* 1996; 84(5): 748-54.

34. Linskey ME, Andrews DW, Asher AL, et al. The role of stereotactic radiosurgery in the management of patients with newly diagnosed brain metastases: a systematic review and evidence-based clinical practice guideline. J Neurooncol 2010; 96(1): 45-68.

35. Sanghavi SN, Miranpuri SS, Chappell R, et al. Radiosurgery for patients with brain metastases: a multi-institutional analysis, stratified by the RTOG recursive partitioning analysis method. Int J Radiat Oncol Biol Phys 2001; 51(2): 426-34.

36. Li B, Yu J, Suntharalingam M, et al. Comparison of three treatment options for single brain metastasis for lung cancer. Int J Cancer 2000; 90(1): 37-45.

37. Want LG, Guo Y, Zhang X, et al. Brain metastasis: experience of the Xi-Jing Hospital. Stereotact Funct Neurosurg 2002; 78(2): 70-83.

38. Aoyama H, Shirato H, Tago M, et al. Stereotactic radiosurgery plus whole-brain radiation therapy vs. stereotactic radiosurgery alone for treatment of brain metastases: a randomized controlled trial. JAMA 2006; 295(21): 2483-91.

39. Aoyama H, Tago M, Kato N, et al. Neurocognitive function of patients with brain metastasis who received either whole brain radiotherapy plus stereotactic radiosurgery or radiosurgery alone. Int J Radiat Oncol Biol Phys 2007; 68(5): 1388-95.

40. Chidel MA, Suh JH, Reddy CA, Chao ST, Lundbeck MF, Barnett GH. Application of recursive partitioning analysis and evaluation of the use of whole brain radiation among patients treated with stereotactic radiosurgery for newly diagnosed brain metastases. Int J Radiat Oncol Biol Phys 2000; 47(4): 993-9.

41. Combs SE, Schulz-Ertner D, Thilmann C, Edler L, Debus J. Treatment of cerebral metastases from breast cancer with stereotactic radiosurgery. Strahlenther Onkol 2004; 180(9): 590-6.

42. Hoffman R, Sneed PK, McDermott MW, et al. Radiosurgery for brain metastases from primary lung carcinoma. Cancer J 2001; 7(2): 121-31.

43. Jawahar A, Willis BK, Smith DR, Ampil F, Datta R, Nanda A. Gamma Knife radiosurgery for brain metastases: do patients benefit from adjuvant external-beam radiotherapy? An 18-month comparative analysis. Stereotact Funct Neurosurg 2002; 79(3-4): 262-71.

44. Noel G, Medioni J, Valery CA, et al. Three irradiation treatment options including radiosurgery for brain metastases from primary lung cancer. Lung Cancer 2003; 41(3): 333-43.

45. Pirzkall A, Debus J, Lohr F, et al. Radiosurgery alone or in combination with whole-brain radiotherapy for brain metastases. J Clin Oncol 1998; 16(11): 3563-9.

46. Sneed PK, Lamborn KR, Forstner JM, et al. Radiosurgery for brain metastases: is whole brain radiotherapy necessary? Int J Radiat Oncol Biol Phys 1999; 43(3): 549-58.

47. Sneed PK, Suh JH, Goetsch SJ, et al. A multi-institutional review of radiosurgery alone vs. radiosurgery with whole brain radiotherapy as the initial management of brain metastases. Int J Radiat Oncol Biol Phys 2002; 53(3): 519-26.

48. Varlotto JM, Flickinger JC, Niranjan A, Bhatnagar A, Kondziolka D, Lunsford LD. The impact of whole-brain radiation therapy on the long-term control and morbidity of patients surviving more than one year after Gamma Knife radiosurgery for brain metastases. Int J Radiat Oncol Biol Phys 2005; 62(4): 1125-32.

49. Lee YK, Park NH, Kim JW, Song YS, Kang SB, Lee HP. Gamma-Knife radiosurgery as an optimal treatment modality for brain metastases from epithelial ovarian cancer. Gynecol Oncol 2008; 108(3): 505-9.

50. Rades D, Pluemer A, Veninga T, Hanssens P, Dunst J, Schild SE. Whole-brain radiotherapy versus stereotactic radiosurgery for patients in recursive partitioning analysis classes 1 and 2 with 1 to 3 brain metastases. Cancer 2007; 110(10): 2285-92.

51. Datta R, Jawahar A, Ampil FL, Shi R, Nanda A, D'Agostino H. Survival in relation to radiotherapeutic modality for brain metastasis: whole brain irradiation vs. Gamma Knife radiosurgery. Am J Clin Oncol 2004; 27(4): 420-4.

52. Kocher M, Maarouf M, Bendel M, Voges J, Muller RP, Sturm V. Linac radiosurgery versus whole brain radiotherapy for brain metastases. A survival comparison based on the RTOG recursive partitioning analysis. Strahlenther Onkol 2004; 180(5): 263-7.

53. Mehta MP, Paleologos NA, Mikkelsen T, et al. The role of chemotherapy in the management of newly diagnosed brain metastases: a systematic review and evidence-based clinical practice guideline. J Neurooncol 2010; 96(1): 71-83.

54. Gerstner ER, Fine RL. Increased permeability of the blood-brain barrier to chemotherapy in metastatic brain tumors: establishing a treatment paradigm. J Clin Oncol 2007; 25(16): 2306-12.

55. Seute T, Leffers P, Wilmink JT, ten Velde GP, Twijnstra A. Response of asymptomatic brain metastases from small-cell lung cancer to systemic first-line chemotherapy. J Clin Oncol 2006; 24(13): 2079-83.

56. Guerrieri M, Wong K, Ryan G, Millward M, Quong G, Ball DL. A randomised Phase III study of palliative radiation with concomitant carboplatin for brain metastases from non-small cell carcinoma of the lung. Lung Cancer 2004; 46(1): 107-11.

57. Ushio Y, Arita N, Hayakawa T, et al. Chemotherapy of brain metastases from lung carcinoma: a controlled randomized study. Neurosurgery 1991; 28(2): 201-5.

58. Antonadou D, Paraskevaidis M, Sarris G, et al. Phase II randomized trial of temozolomide and concurrent radiotherapy in patients with brain metastases. J Clin Oncol 2002; 20(17): 3644-50.

59. Verger E, Gil M, Yaya R, et al. Temozolomide and concomitant whole brain radiotherapy in patients with brain metastases: a Phase II randomized trial. Int J Radiat Oncol Biol Phys 2005; 61(1): 185-91.

60. Patchell RA. The management of brain metastases. Cancer Treat Rev 2003; 29(6): 533-40.

61. Ammirati M, Cobbs CS, Linskey ME, et al. The role of retreatment in the management of recurrent/progressive brain metastases: a systematic review and evidence-based clinical practice guideline. J Neurooncol 2010; 96(1): 85-96.

62. Cooper JS, Steinfeld AD, Lerch IA. Cerebral metastases: value of reirradiation in selected patients. Radiology 1990; 174(3: Pt 1): 883-5.

63. Sadikov E, Bezjak A, Yi QL, *et al.* Value of whole brain re-irradiation for brain metastases - single centre experience. *Clin Oncol* (R Coll Radiol) 2007; 19(7): 532-8.

64. Wong WW, Schild SE, Sawyer TE, Shaw EG. Analysis of outcome in patients reirradiated for brain metastases. *Int J Radiat Oncol Biol Phys* 1996; 34(3): 585-90.

65. Arbit E, Wroski M, Burt M, Galicich JH. The treatment of patients with recurrent brain metastases. A retrospective analysis of 109 patients with nonsmall cell lung cancer. *Cancer* 1995; 76(5): 765-73.

66. Bindal RK, Sawaya R, Leavens ME, Hess KR, Taylor SH. Reoperation for recurrent metastatic brain tumors. *J Neurosurg* 1995; 83(4): 600-4.

67. Truong MT, St Clair EG, Donahue BR, *et al.* Results of surgical resection for progression of brain metastases previously treated by Gamma Knife radiosurgery. *Neurosurgery* 2006; 59(1): 86-97.

68. Vecil GG, Suki D, Maldaun MV, Lang FF, Sawaya R. Resection of brain metastases previously treated with stereotactic radiosurgery. *J Neurosurg* 2005; 102(2): 209-15.

69. Abrey LE, Olson JD, Raizer JJ, *et al.* A Phase II trial of temozolomide for patients with recurrent or progressive brain metastases. *J Neurooncol* 2001; 53(3): 259-65.

70. Christodoulou C, Bafaloukos D, Linardou H, *et al.* Temozolomide (TMZ) combined with cisplatin (CDDP) in patients with brain metastases from solid tumors: a Hellenic Cooperative Oncology Group (HeCOG) Phase II study. *J Neurooncol* 2005; 71(1): 61-5.

71. Giorgio CG, Giuffrida D, Pappalardo A, *et al.* Oral temozolomide in heavily pre-treated brain metastases from non-small cell lung cancer: Phase II study. *Lung Cancer* 2005; 50(2): 247-54.

72. Hwu WJ, Lis E, Menell JH, *et al.* Temozolomide plus thalidomide in patients with brain metastases from melanoma: a Phase II study. *Cancer* 2005; 103(12): 2590-7.

73. Iwamoto FM, Omuro AM, Raizer JJ, *et al.* A Phase II trial of vinorelbine and intensive temozolomide for patients with recurrent or progressive brain metastases. *J Neurooncol* 2008; 87(1): 85-90.

74. Mikkelsen T, Paleologos NA, Robinson PD, *et al.* The role of prophylactic anticonvulsants in the management of brain metastases: a systematic review and evidence-based clinical practice guideline. *J Neurooncol* 2010; 96(1): 97-102.

75. Forsyth PA, Weaver S, Fulton D, *et al.* Prophylactic anticonvulsants in patients with brain tumour. *Can J Neurol Sci* 2003; 30(2): 106-12.

76. Ryken TC, McDermott M, Robinson PD, *et al.* The role of steroids in the management of brain metastases: a systematic review and evidence-based clinical practice guidelines. *J Neurooncol* 2010; 96(1): 103-14.

77. Vecht CJ, Hovestadt A, Verbiest HB, Vliet JJ, Putten WL. Dose-effect relationship of dexamethasone on Karnofsky performance in metastatic brain tumors: a randomized study of doses of 4, 8, and 16mg per day. *Neurology* 1994; 44(4): 675-80.

78. Wolfson AH, Snodgrass SM, Schwade JG, *et al.* The role of steroids in the management of metastatic carcinoma to the brain. A pilot prospective trial. *Am J Clin Oncol* 1994; 17(3): 234-8.

79. Olson JJ, Paleologos NA, Gaspar LE, *et al.* The role of emerging and investigational therapies for metastatic brain tumors: a systematic review and evidence-based clinical practice guideline of selected topics. *J Neurooncol* 2010; 96(1): 115-42.

80. Carde P, Timmerman R, Mehta MP, *et al.* Multicenter Phase Ib/II trial of the radiation enhancer motexafin gadolinium in patients with brain metastases. *J Clin Oncol* 2001; 19(7): 2074-83.

81. Mehta MP, Rodrigus P, Terhaard CH, *et al.* Survival and neurologic outcomes in a randomized trial of motexafin gadolinium and whole-brain radiation therapy in brain metastases. *J Clin Oncol* 2003; 21(13): 2529-36.

82. Ostertag CB, Kreth FW. Interstitial iodine-125 radiosurgery for cerebral metastases. *Br J Neurosurg* 1995; 9(5): 593-603.

83. Alesch F, Hawliczek R, Koos WT. Interstitial irradiation of brain metastases. *Acta Neurochir* 1995; 63(Suppl.): 29-34.

84. Bernstein M, Cabantog A, Laperriere N, Leung P, Thomason C. Brachytherapy for recurrent single brain metastasis. *Can J Neurol Sci* 1995; 22(1): 13-6.

85. Rogers LR, Rock JP, Sills AK, *et al.* Results of a Phase II trial of the GliaSite radiation therapy system for the treatment of newly diagnosed, resected single brain metastases. *J Neurosurg* 2006; 105(3): 375-84.

86. Ewend MG, Brem S, Gilbert M, *et al.* Treatment of single brain metastasis with resection, intracavity carmustine polymer wafers, and radiation therapy is safe and provides excellent local control. *Clin Cancer Res* 2007; 13(12): 3637-41.

87. Nakagawa H, Maeda N, Tsuzuki T, *et al.* Intracavitary chemotherapy with 5-fluoro-2'-deoxyuridine (FdUrd) in malignant brain tumors. *Jpn J Clin Oncol* 2001; 31(6): 251-8.

88. Curry WT Jr, Cosgrove GR, Hochberg FH, Loeffler J, Zervas NT. Stereotactic interstitial radiosurgery for cerebral metastases. *J Neurosurg* 2005; 103(4): 630-5.

89. Nakamura O, Matsutani M, Shitara N, *et al.* New treatment protocol by intra-operative radiation therapy for metastatic brain tumours. *Acta Neurochir* 1994; 131(1-2): 91-6.

90. Hotta K, Kiura K, Ueoka H, *et al.* Effect of gefitinib ('Iressa', ZD1839) on brain metastases in patients with advanced non-small-cell lung cancer. *Lung Cancer* 2004; 46(2): 255-61.

91. Namba Y, Kijima T, Yokota S, *et al.* Gefitinib in patients with brain metastases from non-small-cell lung cancer: review of 15 clinical cases. *Clin Lung Cancer* 2004; 6(2): 123-8.

92. Shimato S, Mitsudomi T, Kosaka T, *et al.* EGFR mutations in patients with brain metastases from lung cancer: association with the efficacy of gefitinib. *Neuro-Oncol* 2006; 8(2): 137-44.

93. Ceresoli GL, Cappuzzo F, Gregorc V, Bartolini S, Crino L, Villa E. Gefitinib in patients with brain metastases from non-small-cell lung cancer: a prospective trial. *Ann Oncol* 2004; 15(7): 1042-7.

94. Chiu CH, Tsai CM, Chen YM, Chiang SC, Liou JL, Perng RP. Gefitinib is active in patients with brain metastases from non-small cell lung cancer and response is related to skin toxicity. *Lung Cancer* 2005; 47(1): 129-38.

95. Wu C, Li YL, Wang ZM, Li Z, Zhang TX, Wei Z. Gefitinib as palliative therapy for lung adenocarcinoma metastatic to the brain. *Lung Cancer* 2007; 57(3): 359-64.

96. Conill C, Jorcano S, Domingo-Domenech J, *et al.* Whole brain irradiation and temozolomide-based chemotherapy in melanoma brain metastases. *Clin Transl Oncol* 2006; 8(4): 266-70.

97. Panagiotou IE, Brountzos EN, Kelekis DA, Papathanasiou MA, Bafaloukos DI. Cerebral metastases of malignant melanoma: contemporary treatment modalities and survival outcome. *Neoplasma* 2005; 52(2): 150-8.

98. Mornex F, Thomas L, Mohr P, *et al.* A prospective randomized multicentre Phase III trial of fotemustine plus whole brain irradiation versus fotemustine alone in cerebral metastases of malignant melanoma. *Melanoma Res* 2003; 13(1): 97-103.

Chapter 17

Brain metastases

Chapter 18

Pituitary tumors

Michael C Oh MD PhD
Resident Physician

Manish K Aghi MD PhD
Assistant Professor

DEPARTMENT OF NEUROLOGICAL SURGERY, UNIVERSITY OF CALIFORNIA, SAN FRANCISCO, CALIFORNIA, USA

Introduction

Pituitary tumors represent 10-15% of primary intracranial neoplasms [1]. More than 90% of pituitary tumors are pituitary adenomas [1, 2]. These are WHO grade I tumors [3], the only brain tumor grade considered benign due to the rarity of transformation to a higher grade. Pituitary adenomas are microadenomas when below 1cm in diameter, and macroadenomas when 1cm or larger (Figure 1). Pituitary adenomas can be endocrine active adenomas (EAAs), which secrete pituitary hormones, or non-functioning pituitary adenomas (NFPAs), which do not secrete hormones; both are equally common [4].

Pituitary adenomas can cause symptoms ranging from hormonal hypersecretion by EAAs to mass effect caused by large EAAs or NFPAs. Most EAAs release prolactin, adrenocorticotrophic hormone (ACTH), or growth hormone (GH), causing hyperprolactinemia, Cushing's disease, and acromegaly, respectively. Rarely, EAAs release gonadotropins (follicle-stimulating hormone, luteinizing hormone) or thyroid-stimulating hormones [5]. EAAs, symptomatic NFPAs, and asymptomatic NFPAs with mass effect warrant treatment. The role for surgery versus serial imaging of asymptomatic NFPAs remains undefined, but suggestions have emerged from natural progression studies of pituitary adenomas. Transsphenoidal resection is the primary treatment for most pituitary adenomas except prolactin-secreting adenomas (prolactinomas) or incompletely resectable GH-secreting adenomas, which are often treated medically.

Recent autopsy and radiographic studies suggest that pituitary tumors are far more prevalent than previously thought. As patients are imaged more frequently for other reasons, the prevalence of incidentally found pituitary adenomas, or 'incidentalomas,' has risen significantly. Therefore, the diagnosis and management of pituitary tumors will become more relevant not only to specialists, but also to primary care providers. In this chapter, we review the evidence published to date on pituitary tumors, with most recommendations based on III/B or IV/C levels of evidence.

Methodology

A National Library of Medicine computerized literature search was performed of publications from 1990 to 2010 using each of the following headings

Chapter 18

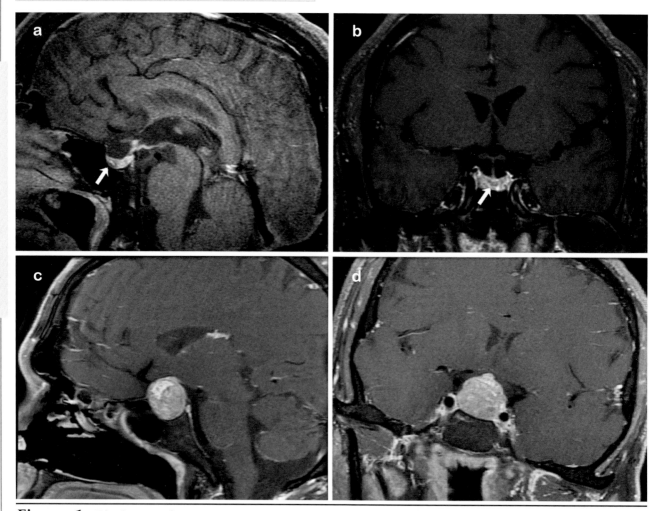

Figure 1. Pituitary adenomas are microadenomas (a, b) when below 1cm in diameter, and macroadenomas (c, d) when 1cm or larger. a, b) A 53-year-old man presented with symptoms consistent with acromegaly and was found to have a 3mm pituitary microadenoma associated with partially empty sella on T1-weighted MRI with gadolinium. His insulin-like growth factor-1 level returned to normal after resection. c, d) A 35-year-old man presented with headache and was found to have a 2.3cm pituitary macroadenoma. He had no visual deficits despite the lateral displacement of optic tracts (d). The patient underwent gross total resection with transient diabetes insipidus following the surgery. His pathology and pituitary hormone panel were consistent with a non-functioning pituitary macroadenoma.

separately to build a wide database of articles: 'pituitary adenoma,' 'prolactinoma,' 'acromegaly,' 'Cushing's disease,' 'transsphenoidal,' 'dopamine agonist,' and 'incidentaloma.' These articles were then reviewed to determine the level of evidence they presented. The bibliographies of these articles were also reviewed for other possible inclusions.

Management of pituitary incidentalomas

Because of their indolent nature and the fact that reporting benign tumors such as pituitary adenomas to cancer registries has only recently become mandatory and only for certain registries, the prevalence of pituitary tumors can only be estimated from small geographic studies. These estimate a prevalence of 94 per 100,000 [6, 7]. The incidence of pituitary tumors was recently reported by the Central Brain Tumor Registry of the United States (CBTRUS), which began mandating pituitary tumor reporting in 2004. In 2010, CBTRUS reported the 2004-2006 incidence of pituitary tumors to be 2.4 per 100,000 person-years adjusted to the 2000 US standard population [2].

Autopsy studies and studies of MRIs performed on healthy volunteers suggest that pituitary tumors are 700 times more prevalent than registry studies suggest. These autopsy and radiographic studies indicate that the prevalence of pituitary tumors, which are mostly asymptomatic, is 16.7% (14.4% from autopsy studies and 22.5% from healthy volunteer radiographic studies), which represents one in six people [8, 9]. Furthermore, immunohistochemistry has revealed that 22-66% of pituitary tumors found at autopsy stain for prolactin [10-12]. One study evaluating 3,048 autopsies found 334 pituitary tumors, of which only two were macroadenomas. The median tumor size was 1.6mm, suggesting that most of these tumors were clinically insignificant during life.

The growing use of cranial imaging for reasons such as trauma, headache, or vertigo is bringing some people with pituitary tumors to diagnosis during life, increasing the prevalence of incidentally found pituitary tumors (called 'incidentalomas'; Figure 2). Thus, one must understand the natural progression of these tumors in order to choose between surgery versus observation through serial imaging.

Observation versus surgery

A meta-analysis of 11 studies has provided insight into the progression of pituitary adenomas observed with serial imaging rather than surgery (Table 1) [10]. These studies included 513 NFPAs (51% macroadenomas, 49% microadenomas) observed for 2.3-8 years. Only 11% of microadenomas grew, while 29% of macroadenomas grew. Some tumors (6% of microadenomas, 13% of macroadenomas) spontaneously decreased in size. In a series of 37 macroadenomas observed for an average of 5 years, 11% developed apoplexy or intratumoral hemorrhage with devastating symptoms such as irreversible vision loss [13]. Because of their propensity to grow and cause mass effect and sometimes apoplexy, surgery is recommended for incidentally found macroadenomas [10, 14, 15] **(III/B)**.

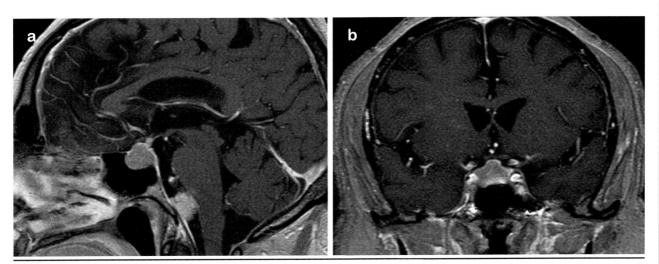

Figure 2. Incidentaloma found during work-up for syncope. A 78-year-old man underwent T1-weighted MRI with gadolinium for a syncope work-up, which revealed a 1.6cm pituitary mass. His pituitary hormone panel showed mild hypopituitarism with a slightly elevated prolactin level, probably secondary to the mass effect on the stalk as pathology was consistent with a non-functioning pituitary adenoma. Following surgery, all hormone levels returned to normal except for a mild growth hormone deficiency.

Table 1. Results of 11 series from 1990 to 2007 in which pituitary incidentalomas were followed with serial imaging.

Reference	Growth rate, n (%)			Mean follow-up (years)	Comments
	Microadenoma	Macroadenoma	Overall		
Reincke et al, 1990 [84]	1/7 (14)	2/7 (29)	3/14 (21)	8	-
Donovan and Corenblum, 1995 [16]	0/15 (0)	4/16 (25)	4/31 (13)	6.4	Apoplexy in 1/31 (macroadenoma) during follow-up
Nishizawa et al, 1998 [85]	Not stated	2/28 (7)	2/28 (7)	5.6	Apoplexy in 1/28 (macroadenoma) during follow-up
Feldkamp et al, 1999 [86]	1/31 (3)	5/19 (26)	6/50 (12)	2.7	-
Igarashi et al, 1999 [87]	0/1 (0)	6/22 (27)	6/23 (26)	5.1	-
Sanno et al, 2003 [88]	20/165 (12)	10/74 (14)	30/239 (13)	2.3	-
Fainstein Day et al, 2004 [19]	1/11 (9)	1/7 (14)	2/18 (11)	3.2	-
Oyama et al, 2005 [89]	Not stated	Not stated	28/126 (22)	2.3	Apoplexy in 1/126 (1%) during follow-up
Arita et al, 2006 [13]	2/5 (40)	19/37 (51)	21/42 (50)	5.2	10/37 macroadenomas became symptomatic during follow-up, 4/37 macroadenomas developed apoplexy during follow-up
Dekkers et al, 2007 [90]	No cases	14/28 (50)	14/28 (50)	7.1	-
Karavitaki et al, 2007 [91]	2/16 (13)	12/24 (50)	14/40 (35)	3.6	-
Total	**27/251 (11)**	**75/262 (29)**	**130/639 (20)**	**4.2**	**Apoplexy reported in 7/221 (3%) adenomas during follow-up; apoplexy in 6/93 macroadenomas (6%)**

Incidentally found microadenomas can be followed with repeat imaging as tumor growth is infrequent, with surgery offered if there is growth [15-17] **(III/B)**. Currently, no randomized trials have been performed to confirm these recommendations.

Because pituitary incidentalomas can be EAAs and because incidentalomas can cause asymptomatic hypopituitarism from gland or stalk compression that might warrant medical treatment or influence decision-making regarding whether to offer surgery, screening for hormonal over- or undersecretion by a full pituitary laboratory panel is recommended regardless of tumor size **(IV/C)**. While there are cost-effectiveness arguments against a full endocrine screening panel [18], other studies have indicated that incidentally found EAAs are frequent enough to warrant a full laboratory work-up. For example, one group found that among 46 incidental macroadenomas, 15% were prolactinomas based on laboratory evaluation [19]. Moreover, among 17 patients who underwent surgery, immunohistochemistry showed that 70% of tumors stained for hormones. Other studies have found that subclinical pituitary hormone elevation can increase health risks [20].

Another debate is whether pituitary tumors found in patients with headaches who undergo cranial imaging followed by normal laboratory evaluation should be considered incidentalomas or symptomatic NFPAs. Headache is present in 33-72% of pituitary tumor patients [21-23] and 48% of primary and metastatic brain tumor patients [24], similar to the 47% prevalence of headache in the general population [25]. A retrospective study published in 2009 reviewed 41 patients with pituitary microadenomas to see if headaches improved following transsphenoidal surgery [26]. This study showed that 85% of patients had headache improvement, while 58% had complete resolution. EAA patients exhibited similar improvements in headaches. Although these results need confirmation, the study suggests that microadenomas in patients with headaches may not be incidentalomas, but may instead cause the headaches. Given the relatively low morbidity of transsphenoidal surgery and the potential to improve headaches, surgery may be appropriate for microadenoma patients with intractable headaches.

Surgical resection of pituitary tumors

The goals of surgical resection of pituitary tumors are to completely remove the tumor to reduce or normalize elevated pituitary hormones produced by EAAs, and prevent further decline or reverse symptoms of mass effect caused by either NFPAs or EAAs, which may include visual field defect, hypopituitarism, and headache.

For the past few decades, surgery for pituitary tumors has involved using a microscope with an endonasal speculum via a transseptal transsphenoidal approach, with fluoroscopy or neuronavigation for intraoperative localization. Transcranial approaches are needed in 10% of cases for large pituitary tumors with significant extrasellar components [27]. Over the last decade, endoscopic pituitary surgery has gained in popularity. Advantages over microscope-based surgery included angled scopes, which improve visualization and resection of tumor in the suprasellar, infrasellar, and parasellar (lateral to the sellar) spaces [28]. For example, a 36-patient series reported a 72% gross total resection rate of pituitary tumors invading the cavernous sinus [28].

The endoscopic approach has also been reported to offer better sinonasal function preservation, reduced length of hospitalization, decreased pain postoperatively, less blood loss, and less lumbar drain usage [29]. The microscope, however, allows a three-dimensional view of the surgical field, while an endoscope with a monitor may provide inferior resolution. Furthermore, postoperative pain, complications, blood loss, and length of hospital stay are already quite low with microscopic-based surgery [29].

Arguments for or against the endoscopic versus microscope-based approaches have not been tested by randomized studies. A meta-analysis of nine studies showed that pituitary tumors can be removed endoscopically with good short-term outcomes and low complication rates [30]. Complete tumor removal was achieved in 78% of patients, with 81-84% remission rates for EAAs. Visual field deficits improved in 62-100% of patients with deficits. A retrospective cohort study found that endoscopic and microscopic pituitary tumor resection produced similar operative results and complication rates [29] **(III/B)**.

Thus, endoscopy may allow an experienced neurosurgeon to completely resect tumors invading the cavernous sinus that were previously incompletely resectable. For non-invasive adenomas, however, the choice between endoscopic versus microscope-based surgery is made according to surgeon preference, previous surgical experience, and available resources. Hopefully, future long-term studies with a large sample size will compare endoscopic versus microscope-based pituitary surgery and allow an informed choice between the methods, accounting for patient- and tumor-specific factors.

Symptomatic non-functioning pituitary adenomas

Clinically, NFPAs are characterized by a lack of symptoms of pituitary hormone over-production. However, many NFPAs release subclinical levels of pituitary hormones [14, 15]; up to 90% of NFPAs produce gonadotropins when analyzed by immunohistochemistry [31, 32]. The significance of staining for hormones in NFPAs remains undefined, but small series with ACTH-positive NFPAs suggest more aggressive behavior compared with ACTH-negative NFPAs [23]. NFPAs comprise 25% of pituitary adenomas [32] and half of surgical pituitary tumors [4].

NFPAs cause symptoms from mass effect, through compressing intrasellar structures (headache or hypopituitarism), parasellar structures (palsies of cranial nerves in the cavernous sinuses lateral to the sella), or suprasellar structures (optic neuropathy). Headache is the most common presenting symptom of mass effect. It is more common in macroadenomas but also present in microadenomas [26], likely from increased intrasellar pressure or dural stretch. Compression of portal vessels and the pituitary stalk can also cause hypopituitarism, most commonly hypogonadism (43%) [22]. Because NFPAs can cause hypopituitarism that is medically correctable once identified and because the diagnosis of NFPA is made by excluding pituitary hormone over-production, which

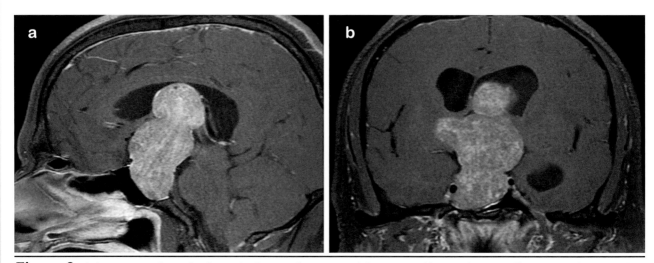

Figure 3. A large non-functioning pituitary adenoma with suprasellar and parasellar extensions. A 31-year-old man presented with a history of visual loss in the left eye 2 years previously, with progressively worsening headaches, somnolence, nausea, and vomiting. T1-weighted MRI with gadolinium showed suprasellar extension of the tumor into the third and left lateral ventricle on both a) sagittal and b) coronal images. Parasellar invasion into the bilateral cavernous sinus is visible on the coronal image (b). The patient presented with hypopituitarism and obstructive hydrocephalus, requiring an external ventricular drain. He underwent transsphenoidal resection, followed by an interhemispheric approach to resect the tumor in the third and left lateral ventricle, and ventriculoperitoneal shunt placement.

will influence the management strategy, a complete endocrine laboratory panel should be checked in patients with pituitary adenomas [14, 15, 22] (III/B).

Large NFPAs can grow with suprasellar or parasellar extension (Figure 3) and cause mass effect by compressing structures. Suprasellar extension can compress the optic chiasm and cause bitemporal hemianopsia. Although early decompression can reverse visual field defects, prolonged compression causes optic nerve atrophy and decreased visual acuity. Lateral extension into the cavernous sinuses can cause cranial neuropathies, leading to ptosis, ophthalmoplegia, and diplopia (cranial nerves III, VI, and IV in the order of frequency). These symptoms may be reversible with decompression following early tumor resection [33] (III/B).

Tumor resection and radiation therapy

Tumor resection via a transsphenoidal approach is the main treatment for symptomatic NFPAs [31] (III/B). Patients with macroadenomas causing symptomatic mass effect with visual field defects [10, 14] or hypopituitarism [34] should undergo surgery; early resection decompresses structures subject to mass effect and can reverse these symptoms (III/B).

Management strategies for residual NFPA after transsphenoidal surgery include observation with serial imaging versus radiation [35, 36]. Although there are no randomized clinical trials, controlled prospective studies show that stereotactic Gamma Knife radiosurgery halts NFPA growth, often decreasing tumor size. In one study, a group not receiving Gamma Knife treatment following transsphenoidal NFPA resection was 51.1% recurrence-free at 5 years, while a group receiving a mean margin dose of 16.5Gr was 89.8% recurrence-free [37] (IIa/B). Another study showed that the tumor reduction was radiation-dose-dependent: patients receiving below 17Gr had a 20% reduction in tumor size, while those receiving 21-23Gr had a 40% reduction at 3 years [38] (III/B).

The most significant long-term toxicity, hypopituitarism, occurs in slightly more than 10% of patients [39, 40]. Other side effects, including optic apparatus damage, strokes, and new cranial nerve deficits, occur in well below 1% of patients [41]. Because of the risk of hypopituitarism and the possibility that residual adenoma may remain stable over many years, radiosurgery is often utilized only for residual adenomas that grow on serial imaging or for recurrence after a gross total resection (III/B).

Medical therapies

Studies are underway to investigate medical therapies for residual NFPAs. NFPA cells express dopamine and somatostatin receptors, and studies indicate that dopamine agonists or somatostatin analogs can cause tumor reduction in some patients [42-44]. However, there are currently no long-term, placebo-controlled clinical trials to confirm the efficacy of these agents in treating residual NFPAs.

Prolactinomas

Prolactinomas are the most common EAA, comprising 40% of pituitary tumors [45, 46]. Patients usually present with decreased libido, nipple discharge, amenorrhea in women, and infertility. Because amenorrhea is readily detected in women while decreased libido is often not reported by men, women often present with microprolactinomas and men with macroprolactinomas. Asymptomatic microprolactinomas grow slowly and therefore may not warrant treatment; only nine of 139 women (7%) with microprolactinomas in six studies had tumor growth during untreated follow-up averaging 8 years [46].

Medical therapy

Over the last 25 years, dopamine agonists have become the main treatment for prolactinomas, including symptomatic microprolactinomas and macroprolactinomas causing mass effect symptoms such as gradual visual loss. Dopamine agonists bind the D2 receptor on prolactinomas, causing cell death. In a 1985 prospective multicenter trial, the dopamine agonist bromocriptine normalized prolactin levels in 18 of 27 patients, with tumors decreasing in size as early as 6 weeks after administration. Tumor size

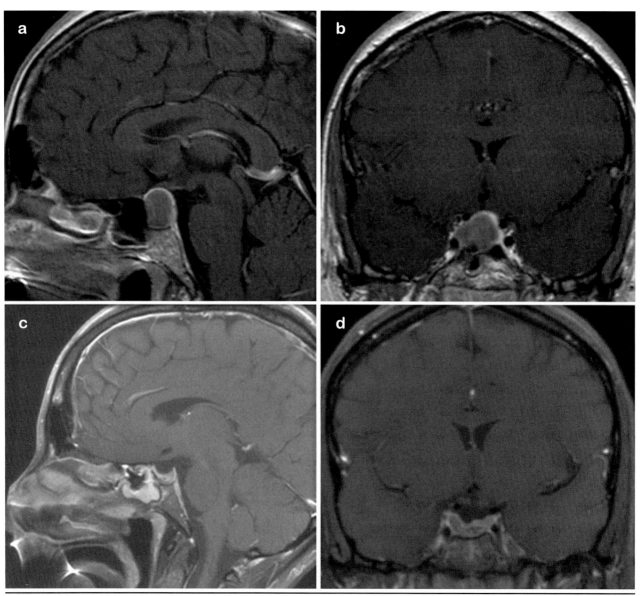

Figure 4. Cystic component of a prolactinoma requiring surgical treatment. A 38-year-old woman with a cystic pituitary tumor seen on a) sagittal and b) coronal T1-weighted gadolinium-enhanced pituitary MRI. The patient had amenorrhea for 2 years after childbirth and was found to have a serum prolactin level of 85ng/mL. The prolactin normalized with dopamine agonist therapy but the MRI did not change, and the patient continued to have a large cystic mass causing mass effect on the overlying optic chiasm. While there were no visual symptoms, the presence of mass effect on the optic chiasm and the lack of a radiographic response with medical management led to a transsphenoidal resection with cyst drainage. This decompressed the optic chiasm and led to a postoperative MRI with no residual pituitary tumor seen on c) sagittal and d) coronal T1-weighted gadolinium-enhanced fat-saturated pituitary MRI.

decreased by more than 50% in 13 patients (46%), by approximately 50% in five patients (18%), and by 10-25% in nine patients (36%) [47] **(III/B)**. Visual fields improved in nine of 10 patients who had deficits, confirming that medical treatment could treat tumor mass effect. These results with medical therapy of prolactinomas resemble those achieved with surgery. A meta-analysis of 34 series showed that 74% of microadenomas and 32% of macroadenomas had normal prolactin levels 1-12 weeks following surgery [48]. Thus, dopamine agonist therapy has become the standard treatment for prolactinomas, although a randomized trial comparing medical with surgical treatment has yet to be performed.

Surgery

Transsphenoidal surgery is recommended for prolactinomas only in the following circumstances **(IV/C)**:

- The tumor is cystic, as cysts will not shrink with dopamine agonist therapy (Figure 4).
- Inadequate prolactin reduction or tumor growth occurs despite high dopamine agonist doses.
- A female patient desires fertility, which may not occur with dopamine agonists.
- There is intratumoral hemorrhage with mass effect or apoplexy [41], which will not resolve with dopamine agonist therapy.
- The patient presents with rapid visual loss or rapid visual loss occurs while on dopamine agonist therapy.

Cabergoline

A dopamine agonist that has recently supplanted bromocriptine is cabergoline, which is a longer-acting dopamine D2 receptor agonist than bromocriptine. Direct comparison of cabergoline with bromocriptine in a randomized multicenter trial involving 459 women showed that cabergoline is more effective and better tolerated. Normal prolactin levels were achieved in 59% of women treated with bromocriptine, while cabergoline restored normal prolactin levels in 83% [49]. Amenorrhea persisted in

7% of women taking cabergoline versus 16% for bromocriptine, and 3% stopped cabergoline due to drug intolerance versus 12% for bromocriptine [49]. These findings were confirmed by another multicenter randomized double-blind study involving 120 women, in which prolactin normalization occurred in 93% of patients taking cabergoline and 48% of patients taking bromocriptine [50]. Because of these two randomized trials, cabergoline has replaced bromocriptine as the dopamine agonist of choice for prolactinomas **(Ib/A)**. Surgery is reserved for the indications above, and radiation is rarely used given the efficacy of medical therapy.

Furthermore, a prospective study from 2008 showed that higher cabergoline doses can restore prolactin levels to normal irrespective of the treatment history [51] **(IIa/B)**. Even patients previously resistant to other dopamine agonists responded to cabergoline, with 35% of patients in remission within a year [51]. Cabergoline is also more effective than bromocriptine in terms of the ability to withdraw medication without prolactin elevation after prolactin has normalized – the ultimate goal with medically managed prolactinomas. Although no randomized comparison has been performed, numerous series have reported 0-44% rates of maintaining normal prolactin 2-48 months after bromocriptine withdrawal, compared with 10-69% rates 3-60 months after cabergoline withdrawal [43] **(III/B)**.

Cushing's disease

Cushing's disease comprises 60-80% of Cushing's syndrome cases [52, 53]. In Cushing's disease, ACTH is oversecreted by a pituitary tumor, causing bilateral adrenal gland hyperplasia and oversecretion of cortisol, adrenal androgens, and 11-deoxycorticosterone. Clinical features of Cushing's disease include central weight gain and redistribution of fat (moon face, supraclavicular and dorsocervical fat pads), severe fatigue, muscle atrophy, hypertension, skin thinning with striae, osteoporosis, immunosuppression, hirsutism, and psychiatric problems (depression, cognitive impairment) [54].

Transsphenoidal surgery

Unlike prolactinomas, no drugs directed at ACTH-releasing pituitary tumors achieve remission and tumor reduction in a timely fashion with acceptable morbidity. Achieving timely remission is important; reports of 20% mortality 15 years after curative transsphenoidal surgery in Cushing disease patients, compared with 10% in patients undergoing surgery for NFPAs, suggest long-term effects on survival of transient hypercortisolemia that correlate with hypercortisolemia duration and do not disappear with cortisol normalization [55, 56]. Thus, timely transsphenoidal surgery is the first-line therapy for Cushing's disease, with a 65-90% remission rate [53, 57] **(III/B)**. The recurrence rate of Cushing's disease, reported to be 5-13% at 5 years and 10-20% at 10 years [53, 57], depends on the surgeon's experience and the degree of tumor extension into surrounding structures. In Cushing's disease, the causative tumors are typically small, with one series reporting 9% macroadenomas, 57% microadenomas, and 34% normal MRIs [57]. High remission and low recurrence occur in patients with microadenomas [57], no cavernous sinus invasion, and subnormal immediate postoperative cortisol levels.

In one series in which patients with microadenomas and no tumors on preoperative MRIs underwent repeat surgery within 6 weeks of unsuccessful transsphenoidal surgery, remission rates increased from 79% to 90% for patients with normal MRIs and from 90% to 97% for patients with microadenoma [57]. Repeat transsphenoidal surgery for recurrent Cushing's disease has been reported to have a remission rate of 50-77% [57-60]. Thus, patients with Cushing's disease who do not achieve remission or who experience disease recurrence after initial transsphenoidal surgery are offered repeat transsphenoidal surgery, unless the residual or recurrent tumor is in the cavernous sinus **(III/B)**. Again, the remission rate depends on the surgeon's experience and whether tumors can be identified on imaging studies [57].

Radiotherapy

Conventional fractionated external-beam radiation and stereotactic radiosurgery have also been employed to treat recurrent Cushing's disease, with similar remission rates of 40-70% [61-63] **(III/B)**. There are some reports that the effects of Gamma Knife radiosurgery may be more rapid in onset than those of conventional radiotherapy, but this remains to be confirmed. The most common complication following radiotherapy is hypopituitarism (16-55%) [64, 65]. Other complications, such as cranial neuropathy, occur in less than 1% of patients, but are more frequent if radiation is delivered a second time [65].

Medical therapy

Three classes of drugs are used to treat Cushing's disease in patients who do not achieve remission with surgery or radiation. All require lifelong administration and cortisol monitoring for periodic dose adjustment.

The first category is drugs that inhibit steroidogenesis. An example is ketoconazole, the current drug of choice for Cushing's disease, which normalizes cortisol in 45% of patients but causes hepatic dysfunction in 12% [66]. Drugs such as ketoconazole treat the hypercortisolemia but not the ACTH-secreting tumor, which can grow during inhibited cortisol production [66, 67].

The second category of drugs is cortisol-receptor antagonists such as mifepristone. These remain under investigation and are not in widespread use. The third category is drugs modulating ACTH release. This approach is appealing because it targets the adenoma itself, eliminating side effects such as hyperpigmentation associated with ACTH hypersecretion and reducing adenoma size.

Corticotrophic pituitary adenoma cells express somatostatin receptor subtypes sst1, sst2, and sst5 [68] and 75% express dopamine D2 receptors [69]. Studies are currently underway to determine whether somatostatin analogs and dopamine agonists are effective in treating Cushing's disease. Unlike the commonly used somatostatin analog, octreotide, which only activates sst2, pasireotide (SOM230) has high affinity for sst1-3 and sst5, which makes it attractive because it targets all somatostatin receptors on corticotrophic adenomas. A Phase I/II clinical trial of pasireotide showed reduced urine cortisol in 76% and normal urine cortisol in 17% of patients during a 15-day treatment period [70]. Positive results have also been seen with the dopamine agonist cabergoline. In 20 patients with recurrent Cushing's disease treated with cabergoline, 40% of patients had controlled urine cortisol levels after 2 years, with tumor reduction in 20% [71]. Larger clinical trials are needed to confirm these findings.

Recurrent disease

Hypophysectomy is another surgical option for recurrence, but the risk of pituitary insufficiency is higher than with selective adenomectomy (50% vs. 5%) [59], making it less appealing than radiation. Bilateral adrenalectomy is a definitive treatment for recurrent Cushing's disease, although permanent hypoadrenalism means patients require lifelong replacement therapy. Bilateral adrenalectomy carries high morbidity [72], and repeat transsphenoidal surgery is therefore the recommended initial therapy for recurrent Cushing's disease, followed in order by radiation, ketoconazole, hypophysectomy, and bilateral adrenalectomy [53, 54] **(IV/C)**.

Acromegaly

GH-secreting adenomas cause acromegaly, characterized by dysmorphic features including widening of the nose, cheekbones, and fingers; frontal bossing; thickened lips and tongue; increased hand and foot size; and medical comorbidities such as hypertension, congestive heart failure, chronic obstructive pulmonary disease, diabetes, osteoarthropathies, and sleep apnea [73]. A meta-analysis of 16 studies suggests that mortality is increased by 72% in patients with acromegaly because of these medical comorbidities, with a 10-year decrease in life expectancy compared with the general population [74]. Morbidity and mortality rates

correlate with the degree to which GH levels are elevated [74, 75]. Thus, the goals of therapy are to reverse acromegaly symptoms by reducing GH and insulin-like growth factor (IGF)-1 levels and decrease tumor size [76, 77]. Whether morbidity and mortality rates can be normalized to those of the general population is unclear. Some studies have observed that, as in Cushing's disease, mortality remains elevated in patients with acromegaly even after IGF-1 normalization [74], possibly due to irreversible physiological effects of elevated GH.

Transsphenoidal surgery

As in Cushing's disease, transsphenoidal surgery is the accepted first-line treatment for acromegaly except when complete resection is unlikely, in which case medical therapy may be considered [77] **(III/B)**. Outcomes depend on the surgeon's experience, tumor size, and presurgical GH level. IGF-1 levels are normalized in 75-95% of microadenomas and 40-68% of macroadenomas following transsphenoidal surgery [77-79] **(III/B)**.

Medical therapy

Currently, three classes of drugs are available for acromegaly: somatostatin analogs, which inhibit GH release and cause tumor shrinkage (e.g., octreotide LAR, lanreotide Autogel); the dopamine agonist cabergoline; and the GH receptor antagonist pegvisomant. A recent trial randomized newly diagnosed patients with acromegaly to octreotide versus transsphenoidal surgery. Although the surgery group had a higher 48-week remission rate (39% vs. 28%), the difference was not statistically significant [80] **(Ib/A)**. Tumor size also decreased in both groups, with slightly more patients experiencing significant shrinkage (>20%) in the surgery group (95% vs. 73%).

The GH receptor antagonist, pegvisomant, normalizes IGF-1 in 56% of patients with acromegaly [81]. However, blocking the GH receptor can upregulate tumor GH production and cause tumor growth, with 5% of acromegaly patients on pegvisomant experiencing more than 25% volumetric tumor growth [82]. Thus, pegvisomant is a second choice for the medical management of acromegaly after somatostatin analogs **(IV/C)** [77]. Among the dopamine agonists, only cabergoline has efficacy in acromegaly. Cabergoline is most useful when combined with somatostatin analogs in patients who fail to achieve remission with monotherapy [43, 44, 77].

Radiotherapy

Further study of radiation is required, including randomized trials, to better define its role in treating acromegaly. While reported radiosurgery remission rates in acromegaly range from 17% to 60% [73, 77], because the mean time to remission ranges from 1 to 5 years, radiation is generally utilized after failure of surgery and somatostatin analogs.

Recommendations

Unlike with Cushing's disease and prolactinomas, all three approaches (surgery, medication, and radiation) can be similarly successful in acromegaly and can play a role in management. Thus, an expert panel, the Acromegaly Consensus Group, formed in 2000, publishes guidelines for acromegaly management, most recently in 2009. The recommendations are that tumors deemed completely resectable undergo surgery, with somatostatin analogs used for patients who fail to achieve remission after surgery. Tumors that are deemed incompletely resectable are treated with somatostatin analogs. Patients who fail to achieve remission on somatostatin analogs are treated with pegvisomant if there is no mass effect on MRI, because the tumor growth that can occur with pegvisomant would be

tolerated, or with radiation if there is mass effect on MRI [77] **(IV/C)**.

Partial surgical debulking prior to medical therapy may improve the response to somatostatin analogs such as octreotide, but more studies are needed to confirm this. Some studies have also suggested the converse: that preoperative octreotide increases postoperative cure rates. In one study, newly diagnosed patients with acromegaly were randomized to immediate surgery versus octreotide pretreatment for 6 months before surgery. Pretreated patients had a higher remission rate than non-pretreated patients, as defined by IGF-1 normalization (45% vs. 23%) [83] **(Ib/A)**. However, other studies have found no benefits with somatostatin analog pretreatment, and more studies are therefore needed to confirm these findings [77].

Conclusions

Pituitary tumors pose numerous challenges that are best addressed through the combined efforts of endocrinologists, neurosurgeons, and radiation oncologists. A complete endocrine laboratory panel is a critical first step because it defines the adenoma type (EAA vs. NFPA), which influences treatment choice, and because it assesses for hypopituitarism that can occur with EAAs or NFPAs and can be medically corrected. Surgery remains the main treatment for many pituitary tumors, but medical therapy has replaced surgery for certain tumors such as prolactinomas and incompletely resectable GH-secreting tumors. Ongoing work to identify new drugs and enhance surgical techniques will continue the improvements that have already been made in remission rates and quality of life for patients with pituitary tumors.

Recommendations	Evidence level

- Incidentally found pituitary macroadenomas have a propensity to grow and should be resected by surgery to prevent mass effect, while incidentally found non-functioning microadenomas can be observed with serial imaging. **III/B**
- Symptomatic non-functioning pituitary macroadenomas causing mass effect (visual field cut, panhypopituitarism, headaches) should be surgically resected, as early decompression may reverse symptoms of mass effect. **III/B**
- Headache can be a symptom of a pituitary microadenoma that may respond to surgical resection. **IV/C**
- Residual NFPA that grows during serial imaging or recurrent NFPA lateral to the sella can be treated with Gamma Knife radiosurgery. **III/B**
- The dopamine agonist cabergoline is first-line therapy for prolactinomas (both macroadenomas and microadenomas), with surgery indicated for patients who fail medical management or present with rapid visual loss, tumors with cystic or hemorrhagic components, or tumors in women who desire pregnancy. **III/B**
- Transsphenoidal surgery is the first-line therapy for Cushing's disease; repeat surgery is used for patients who fail to achieve remission after initial surgery or where disease recurs. **III/B**
- Transsphenoidal surgery is the first-line therapy for acromegaly in completely resectable cases, with medical therapy used for incompletely resectable tumors. **III/B**

Chapter 18

References

1. Monson JP. The epidemiology of endocrine tumours. *Endocr Relat Cancer* 2000; 7: 29-36.
2. Central Brain Tumor Registry of the United States. 2009-2010 CBTRUS Statistical Report: Primary Brain and Central Nervous System Tumors Diagnosed in the United States in 2004-2006. 2010. Available from www.cbtrus.org. Accessed April 4, 2010.
3. Louis DN, Ohgaki H, Wiestler OD, *et al*. The 2007 WHO classification of tumours of the central nervous system. *Acta Neuropathol* 2007; 114: 97-109.
4. Saeger W, Ludecke DK, Buchfelder M, Fahlbusch R, Quabbe HJ, Petersenn S. Pathohistological classification of pituitary tumors: 10 years of experience with the German Pituitary Tumor Registry. *Eur J Endocrinol* 2007; 156: 203-16.
5. Beck-Peccoz P, Persani L, Mannavola D, Campi I. Pituitary tumours: TSH-secreting adenomas. *Best Pract Res Clin Endocrinol Metab* 2009; 23: 597-606.
6. Daly AF, Rixhon M, Adam C, Dempegioti A, Tichomirowa MA, Beckers A. High prevalence of pituitary adenomas: a cross-sectional study in the province of Liege, Belgium. *J Clin Endocrinol Metab* 2006; 91: 4769-75.
7. Davis JR, Farrell WE, Clayton RN. Pituitary tumours. *Reproduction* 2001; 121: 363-71.
8. Ezzat S, Asa SL, Couldwell WT, *et al*. The prevalence of pituitary adenomas: a systematic review. *Cancer* 2004; 101: 613-9.
9. Daly AF, Burlacu MC, Livadariu E, Beckers A. The epidemiology and management of pituitary incidentalomas. *Horm Res* 2007; 68(Suppl. 5): 195-8.
10. Molitch ME. Pituitary tumours: pituitary incidentalomas. *Best Pract Res Clin Endocrinol Metab* 2009; 23: 667-75.
11. Molitch ME. Nonfunctioning pituitary tumors and pituitary incidentalomas. *Endocrinol Metab Clin North Am* 2008; 37: 151-71, xi.
12. Buurman H, Saeger W. Subclinical adenomas in postmortem pituitaries: classification and correlations to clinical data. *Eur J Endocrinol* 2006; 154: 753-8.
13. Arita K, Tominaga A, Sugiyama K, *et al*. Natural course of incidentally found nonfunctioning pituitary adenoma, with special reference to pituitary apoplexy during follow-up examination. *J Neurosurg* 2006; 104: 884-91.
14. Dekkers OM, Pereira AM, Romijn JA. Treatment and follow-up of clinically nonfunctioning pituitary macroadenomas. *J Clin Endocrinol Metab* 2008; 93: 3717-26.
15. Greenman Y, Stern N. Non-functioning pituitary adenomas. *Best Pract Res Clin Endocrinol Metab* 2009; 23: 625-38.
16. Donovan LE, Corenblum B. The natural history of the pituitary incidentaloma. *Arch Intern Med* 1995; 155: 181-3.

17. Suzuki M, Minematsu T, Oyama K, *et al*. Expression of proliferation markers in human pituitary incidentalomas. *Endocr Pathol* 2006; 17: 263-75.

18. King JT Jr, Justice AC, Aron DC. Management of incidental pituitary microadenomas: a cost-effectiveness analysis. *J Clin Endocrinol Metab* 1997; 82: 3625-32.

19. Fainstein Day P, Guitelman M, Artese R, *et al*. Retrospective multicentric study of pituitary incidentalomas. *Pituitary* 2004; 7: 145-8.

20. Angeli A, Terzolo M. Adrenal incidentaloma - a modern disease with old complications. *J Clin Endocrinol Metab* 2002; 87: 4869-71.

21. Abe T, Matsumoto K, Kuwazawa J, Toyoda I, Sasaki K. Headache associated with pituitary adenomas. *Headache* 1998; 38: 782-6.

22. Ferrante E, Ferraroni M, Castrignano T, *et al*. Non-functioning pituitary adenoma database: a useful resource to improve the clinical management of pituitary tumors. *Eur J Endocrinol* 2006; 155: 823-9.

23. Scheithauer BW, Jaap AJ, Horvath E, *et al*. Clinically silent corticotroph tumors of the pituitary gland. *Neurosurgery* 2000; 47: 723-9; discussion 729-30.

24. Forsyth PA, Posner JB. Headaches in patients with brain tumors: a study of 111 patients. *Neurology* 1993; 43: 1678-83.

25. Jensen R, Stovner LJ. Epidemiology and comorbidity of headache. *Lancet Neurol* 2008; 7: 354-61.

26. Fleseriu M, Yedinak C, Campbell C, Delashaw JB. Significant headache improvement after transsphenoidal surgery in patients with small sellar lesions. *J Neurosurg* 2009; 110: 354-8.

27. Buchfelder M, Schlaffer S. Surgical treatment of pituitary tumours. *Best Pract Res Clin Endocrinol Metab* 2009; 23: 677-92.

28. Kitano M, Taneda M, Shimono T, Nakao Y. Extended transsphenoidal approach for surgical management of pituitary adenomas invading the cavernous sinus. *J Neurosurg* 2008; 108: 26-36.

29. Higgins TS, Courtemanche C, Karakla D, *et al*. Analysis of transnasal endoscopic versus transseptal microscopic approach for excision of pituitary tumors. *Am J Rhinol* 2008; 22: 649-52.

30. Tabaee A, Anand VK, Barron Y, *et al*. Endoscopic pituitary surgery: a systematic review and meta-analysis. *J Neurosurg* 2009; 111: 545-54.

31. Jaffe CA. Clinically non-functioning pituitary adenoma. *Pituitary* 2006; 9: 317-21.

32. Katznelson L, Alexander JM, Klibanski A. Clinical review 45: clinically nonfunctioning pituitary adenomas. *J Clin Endocrinol Metab* 1993; 76: 1089-94.

33. Kim SH, Lee KC. Cranial nerve palsies accompanying pituitary tumour. *J Clin Neurosci* 2007; 14: 1158-62.

34. Arafah BM. Reversible hypopituitarism in patients with large nonfunctioning pituitary adenomas. *J Clin Endocrinol Metab* 1986; 62: 1173-9.

35. Brada M, Jankowska P. Radiotherapy for pituitary adenomas. *Endocrinol Metab Clin North Am* 2008; 37: 263-75, xi.

36. Kanner AA, Corn BW, Greenman Y. Radiotherapy of nonfunctioning and gonadotroph adenomas. *Pituitary* 2009; 12: 15-22.

37. Picozzi P, Losa M, Mortini P, *et al*. Radiosurgery and the prevention of regrowth of incompletely removed nonfunctioning pituitary adenomas. *J Neurosurg* 2005; 102(Suppl.): 71-4.

38. Pamir MN, Kilic T, Belirgen M, Abacioglu U, Karabekiroglu N. Pituitary adenomas treated with Gamma Knife radiosurgery: volumetric analysis of 100 cases with minimum 3-year follow-up. *Neurosurgery* 2007; 61: 270-80.

39. Losa M, Valle M, Mortini P, *et al*. Gamma Knife surgery for treatment of residual nonfunctioning pituitary adenomas after surgical debulking. *J Neurosurg* 2004; 100: 438-44.

40. Kong DS, Lee JI, Lim do H, *et al*. The efficacy of fractionated radiotherapy and stereotactic radiosurgery for pituitary adenomas: long-term results of 125 consecutive patients treated in a single institution. *Cancer* 2007; 110: 854-60.

41. Castinetti F, Regis J, Dufour H, Brue T. Role of stereotactic radiosurgery in the management of pituitary adenomas. *Nat Rev Endocrinol* 2010; 6: 214-23.

42. Colao A, Di Somma C, Pivonello R, Faggiano A, Lombardi G, Savastano S. Medical therapy for clinically non-functioning pituitary adenomas. *Endocr Relat Cancer* 2008; 15: 905-15.

43. Colao A, Pivonello R, Di Somma C, Savastano S, Grasso LF, Lombardi G. Medical therapy of pituitary adenomas: effects on tumor shrinkage. *Rev Endocr Metab Disord* 2009; 10: 111-23.

44. Colao A, Filippella M, Pivonello R, Di Somma C, Faggiano A, Lombardi G. Combined therapy of somatostatin analogues and dopamine agonists in the treatment of pituitary tumours. *Eur J Endocrinol* 2007; 156(Suppl. 1): S57-63.

45. Gillam MP, Molitch ME, Lombardi G, Colao A. Advances in the treatment of prolactinomas. *Endocr Rev* 2006; 27: 485-534.

46. Colao A. Pituitary tumours: the prolactinoma. *Best Pract Res Clin Endocrinol Metab* 2009; 23: 575-96.

47. Molitch ME, Elton RL, Blackwell RE, *et al*. Bromocriptine as primary therapy for prolactin-secreting macroadenomas: results of a prospective multicenter study. *J Clin Endocrinol Metab* 1985; 60: 698-705.

48. Molitch ME. Medical management of prolactin-secreting pituitary adenomas. *Pituitary* 2002; 5: 55-65.

49. Webster J, Piscitelli G, Polli A, Ferrari CI, Ismail I, Scanlon MF. A comparison of cabergoline and bromocriptine in the treatment of hyperprolactinemic amenorrhea. Cabergoline Comparative Study Group. *N Engl J Med* 1994; 331: 904-9.

50. Pascal-Vigneron V, Weryha G, Bosc M, Leclere J. [Hyperprolactinemic amenorrhea: treatment with cabergoline versus bromocriptine. Results of a national multicenter randomized double-blind study.] *Presse Med* 1995; 24: 753-7.

51. Ono M, Miki N, Kawamata T, *et al*. Prospective study of high-dose cabergoline treatment of prolactinomas in 150 patients. *J Clin Endocrinol Metab* 2008; 93: 4721-7.

52. Bertagna X, Guignat L, Groussin L, Bertherat J. Cushing's disease. *Best Pract Res Clin Endocrinol Metab* 2009; 23: 607-23.

53. Biller BM, Grossman AB, Stewart PM, *et al*. Treatment of adrenocorticotropin-dependent Cushing's syndrome: a consensus statement. *J Clin Endocrinol Metab* 2008; 93: 2454-62.

54. Aghi MK. Management of recurrent and refractory Cushing disease. *Nat Clin Pract Endocrinol Metab* 2008; 4: 560-8.

55. Dekkers OM, Biermasz NR, Pereira AM, *et al*. Mortality in patients treated for Cushing's disease is increased, compared with patients treated for nonfunctioning pituitary macroadenoma. *J Clin Endocrinol Metab* 2007; 92: 976-81.

56. Lindholm J, Juul S, Jorgensen JO, *et al*. Incidence and late prognosis of Cushing's syndrome: a population-based study. *J Clin Endocrinol Metab* 2001; 86: 117-23.

57. Aghi MK, Petit J, Chapman P, *et al*. Management of recurrent and refractory Cushing's disease with reoperation and/or proton beam radiosurgery. *Clin Neurosurg* 2008; 55: 141-4.

58. Benveniste RJ, King WA, Walsh J, Lee JS, Delman BN, Post KD. Repeated transsphenoidal surgery to treat recurrent or residual pituitary adenoma. *J Neurosurg* 2005; 102: 1004-12.

59. Friedman RB, Oldfield EH, Nieman LK, *et al*. Repeat transsphenoidal surgery for Cushing's disease. *J Neurosurg* 1989; 71: 520-7.

60. Hofmann BM, Hlavac M, Kreutzer J, Grabenbauer G, Fahlbusch R. Surgical treatment of recurrent Cushing's disease. *Neurosurgery* 2006; 58: 1108-18.

61. Castinetti F, Nagai M, Dufour H, *et al*. Gamma Knife radiosurgery is a successful adjunctive treatment in Cushing's disease. *Eur J Endocrinol* 2007; 156: 91-8.

62. Devin JK, Allen GS, Cmelak AJ, Duggan DM, Blevins LS. The efficacy of linear accelerator radiosurgery in the management of patients with Cushing's disease. *Stereotact Funct Neurosurg* 2004; 82: 254-62.

63. Estrada J, Boronat M, Mielgo M, *et al*. The long-term outcome of pituitary irradiation after unsuccessful transsphenoidal surgery in Cushing's disease. *N Engl J Med* 1997; 336: 172-7.

64. Oyesiku NM. Stereotactic radiosurgery for Cushing disease: a review. *Neurosurg Focus* 2007; 23: E14.

65. Jagannathan J, Sheehan JP, Pouratian N, Laws ER, Steiner L, Vance ML. Gamma Knife surgery for Cushing's disease. *J Neurosurg* 2007; 106: 980-7.

66. Castinetti F, Morange I, Jaquet P, Conte-Devolx B, Brue T. Ketoconazole revisited: a preoperative or postoperative treatment in Cushing's disease. *Eur J Endocrinol* 2008; 158: 91-9.

67. Engelhardt D, Weber MM. Therapy of Cushing's syndrome with steroid biosynthesis inhibitors. *J Steroid Biochem Mol Biol* 1994; 49: 261-7.

68. Hofland LJ, van der Hoek J, Feelders R, *et al*. The multi-ligand somatostatin analogue SOM230 inhibits ACTH secretion by cultured human corticotroph adenomas via somatostatin receptor type 5. *Eur J Endocrinol* 2005; 152: 645-54.

69. Pivonello R, Ferone D, de Herder WW, *et al*. Dopamine receptor expression and function in corticotroph pituitary tumors. *J Clin Endocrinol Metab* 2004; 89: 2452-62.

70. Boscaro M, Ludlam WH, Atkinson B, *et al*. Treatment of pituitary-dependent Cushing's disease with the multireceptor

ligand somatostatin analog pasireotide (SOM230): a multicenter, Phase II trial. *J Clin Endocrinol Metab* 2009; 94: 115-22.

71. Pivonello R, De Martino MC, Cappabianca P, *et al*. The medical treatment of Cushing's disease: effectiveness of chronic treatment with the dopamine agonist cabergoline in patients unsuccessfully treated by surgery. *J Clin Endocrinol Metab* 2009; 94: 223-30.

72. O'Riordain DS, Farley DR, Young WF Jr, Grant CS, van Heerden JA. Long-term outcome of bilateral adrenalectomy in patients with Cushing's syndrome. *Surgery* 1994; 116: 1088-93.

73. Aghi M, Blevins LS Jr. Recent advances in the treatment of acromegaly. *Curr Opin Endocrinol Diabetes Obes* 2009; 16: 304-7.

74. Dekkers OM, Biermasz NR, Pereira AM, Romijn JA, Vandenbroucke JP. Mortality in acromegaly: a meta-analysis. *J Clin Endocrinol Metab* 2008; 93: 61-7.

75. Orme SM, McNally RJ, Cartwright RA, Belchetz PE. Mortality and cancer incidence in acromegaly: a retrospective cohort study. United Kingdom Acromegaly Study Group. *J Clin Endocrinol Metab* 1998; 83: 2730-4.

76. Chanson P, Salenave S, Kamenicky P, Cazabat L, Young J. Pituitary tumours: acromegaly. *Best Pract Res Clin Endocrinol Metab* 2009; 23: 555-74.

77. Melmed S, Colao A, Barkan A, *et al*. Guidelines for acromegaly management: an update. *J Clin Endocrinol Metab* 2009; 94: 1509-17.

78. Freda PU. How effective are current therapies for acromegaly? *Growth Horm IGF Res* 2003; 13(Suppl. A): S144-51.

79. Nomikos P, Buchfelder M, Fahlbusch R. The outcome of surgery in 668 patients with acromegaly using current criteria of biochemical 'cure'. *Eur J Endocrinol* 2005; 152: 379-87.

80. Colao A, Cappabianca P, Caron P, *et al*. Octreotide LAR vs. surgery in newly diagnosed patients with acromegaly: a randomized, open-label, multicentre study. *Clin Endocrinol (Oxf)* 2009; 70: 757-68.

81. Trainer PJ, Ezzat S, D'Souza GA, Layton G, Strasburger CJ. A randomized, controlled, multicentre trial comparing pegvisomant alone with combination therapy of pegvisomant and long-acting octreotide in patients with acromegaly. *Clin Endocrinol (Oxf)* 2009; 71: 549-57.

82. Buhk JH, Jung S, Psychogios MN, *et al*. Tumor volume of growth hormone-secreting pituitary adenomas during treatment with pegvisomant: a prospective multicenter study. *J Clin Endocrinol Metab* 2010; 95: 552-8.

83. Carlsen SM, Lund-Johansen M, Schreiner T, *et al*. Preoperative octreotide treatment in newly diagnosed acromegalic patients with macroadenomas increases cure short-term postoperative rates: a prospective, randomized trial. *J Clin Endocrinol Metab* 2008; 93: 2984-90.

84. Reincke M, Allolio B, Saeger W, Menzel J, Winkelmann W. The 'incidentaloma' of the pituitary gland. Is neurosurgery required? *JAMA* 1990; 263: 2772-6.

85. Nishizawa S, Ohta S, Yokoyama T, Uemura K. Therapeutic strategy for incidentally found pituitary tumors ('pituitary

incidentalomas'). *Neurosurgery* 1998; 43: 1344-8; discussion 1348-50.

86. Feldkamp J, Santen R, Harms E, Aulich A, Modder U, Scherbaum WA. Incidentally discovered pituitary lesions: high frequency of macroadenomas and hormone-secreting adenomas - results of a prospective study. *Clin Endocrinol (Oxf)* 1999; 51: 109-13.

87. Igarashi T, Saeki N, Yamaura A. Long-term magnetic resonance imaging follow-up of asymptomatic sellar tumors - their natural history and surgical indications. *Neurol Med Chir (Tokyo)* 1999; 39: 592-8; discussion 598-9.

88. Sanno N, Oyama K, Tahara S, Teramoto A, Kato Y. A survey of pituitary incidentaloma in Japan. *Eur J Endocrinol* 2003; 149: 123-7.

89. Oyama K, Sanno N, Tahara S, Teramoto A. Management of pituitary incidentalomas: according to a survey of pituitary incidentalomas in Japan. *Semin Ultrasound CT MR* 2005; 26: 47-50.

90. Dekkers OM, Hammer S, de Keizer RJ, *et al.* The natural course of non-functioning pituitary macroadenomas. *Eur J Endocrinol* 2007; 156: 217-24.

91. Karavitaki N, Collison K, Halliday J, *et al.* What is the natural history of nonoperated nonfunctioning pituitary adenomas? *Clin Endocrinol (Oxf)* 2007; 67: 938-43.

Chapter 18

Chapter 19

Surgery for glioblastoma

Nader Sanai MD

Director, Neurosurgical Oncology;

Director, Barrow Brain Tumor Research Center

DIVISION OF NEUROSURGICAL ONCOLOGY AND BARROW BRAIN TUMOR RESEARCH CENTER, BARROW NEUROLOGICAL INSTITUTE, PHOENIX, ARIZONA, USA

Introduction

Standard treatment for glioblastoma multiforme (GBM), the most common primary malignant brain tumor, includes microsurgical resection followed by concomitant chemotherapy and radiation therapy [1]. Unfortunately, despite decades of refinement, this multimodal approach still leads to a median survival of just 12-14 months, with the exception of a select group of patients who have MGMT promoter methylation and are treated with temozolomide (46% 2-year overall survival) [1, 2]. Thus, beyond establishing the histologic diagnosis and decompressing tumor mass effect, the value of microsurgical resection of GBMs remains controversial. In the last decade, however, mounting evidence has suggested that more extensive surgical resection is associated with better survival in patients with GBM [3]. While these data have helped establish a precarious and frequently debated consensus that more extensive GBM resection improves patient outcomes, the impracticality of conducting a randomized clinical trial limits our ability to quantify the value of greater tumor resection. Simply put, how much tumor resection is enough to make a difference?

Methodology

A National Library of Medicine computerized literature search was performed of publications from 1966 to 2012 using each of the following headings separately to build a wide database of articles: 'glioma,' 'glioblastoma,' 'intraoperative mapping,' and 'extent of resection.' These headings were then combined with the heading 'evidence-based' to select articles of that nature. The bibliographies of these articles were reviewed for other possible inclusions.

Glioblastoma pathology and pathogenesis

Even within the conventional GBM category of the WHO, the cellular composition of GBM is heterogeneous and may include fibrillary, gemistocytic, and occasional giant cells. Neoplastic fibrillary astrocytes contain enlarged, elongated to irregularly shaped, hyperchromatic nuclei, scant cytoplasm, and variable glial fibrillary acidic protein-immunoreactive processes that form a loose, fibrillary matrix. Diagnosis is based upon morphologic criteria and depends upon the presence of microvascular proliferation or tumor necrosis.

GBM may arise through two distinct pathways of neoplastic progression. Tumors that progress from lower-grade (WHO grades II or III) astrocytic tumors, termed secondary GBM, typically display both well-differentiated and poorly differentiated foci. Secondary GBMs develop in younger patients (fifth to sixth decade), with time to progression from lower-grade lesions ranging from months to decades. In contrast, primary GBMs develop in older individuals (sixth to seventh decade), have short clinical histories (<3 months), and arise *de novo* without any evidence of a lower-grade precursor. Primary and secondary

GBMs also harbor distinct molecular genetic abnormalities [4]:

* Primary GBMs are characterized by relatively high frequencies of *EGFR* amplification, *PTEN* deletion, and *CDKN2A* (p16) loss.
* Secondary GBMs often contain *TP53* mutations, especially those involving codons 248 and 273 or G:C→A:T mutations at CpG sites.

The value of extent of resection

In 2009, the Central Brain Tumor Registry of the United States reported 12% survival at 2 years, 5% at

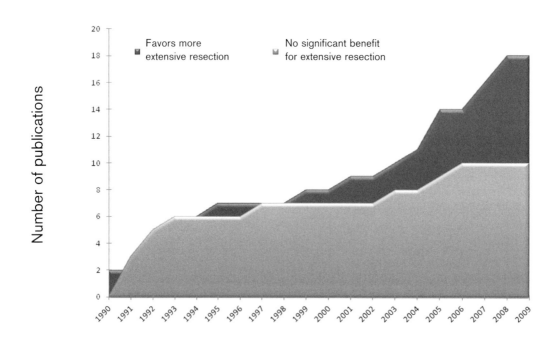

Figure 1. Cumulative literature examining extent of resection for high-grade gliomas. In terms of either overall survival or progression-free survival, mounting evidence demonstrates a value for greater extent of resection when treating WHO grade III or IV gliomas.

5 years, and 3% at 10 years for GBM. The current standard of care for patients at most large brain tumor centers involves gross total resection, followed by temozolomide chemotherapy and fractionated radiotherapy **(Ib/A)**. While microsurgical resection remains a critical therapeutic modality for GBMs, particularly to establish a histologic diagnosis and decompress tumor mass effect, there remains no general consensus in the literature regarding the efficacy of extent of resection (EOR) in improving patient outcomes. With the exception of WHO grade I tumors, gliomas are generally difficult to cure with surgery alone, and most patients will experience some form of tumor recurrence.

For all GBMs, the identification of universally applicable prognostic factors and treatment options remains a great challenge. Among the many tumor- and treatment-related parameters, only patient age and tumor histology have been identified as reliable predictors of patient prognosis, although functional status can also be statistically significant. While the importance of glioma resection in obtaining tissue diagnosis and to alleviate symptoms is clear, a lack of level I evidence prevents similar certainty in assessing the influence of EOR. In fact, despite significant advances in brain tumor imaging and intraoperative technology during the last 15 years, the effect of glioma resection in extending tumor-free progression and patient survival remains unknown.

In the last decade, however, mounting evidence has suggested that greater microsurgical EOR is associated with better survival in patients with GBM (Figure 1). While most of these studies provide level III evidence, the impracticality of conducting a randomized clinical trial limits our ability to more accurately quantify the value of greater tumor resection.

Current studies of extent of resection

In the last decade, seven studies focusing solely on GBMs have examined the impact of EOR (Table 1) [5-11]. With one exception, each of these studies demonstrated through multivariate analysis a statistically significant overall or progression-free survival benefit with greater EOR.

To date, the most rigorous study to quantify the exact survival benefit of EOR for GBM patients was performed by Lacroix *et al* in 2001 [6]. This retrospective analysis combined 416 newly diagnosed and recurrent GBM patients, and concluded that an EOR of 98% or greater is necessary to significantly improve survival **(III/B)**. In the modern era, this report serves as a critical study of reference for the neurosurgical community, justifying the 'all-or-none' approach that is commonly practiced in the surgical management of GBM [12]. However, while a mixture of newly diagnosed and recurrent GBMs amplified the overall sample size in this study, considerable differences in demographics, biology, and outcomes are known to distinguish these two populations. Furthermore, an infolded subgroup analysis of 233 newly diagnosed GBM patients was insufficiently powered, given that nearly half (46%) of the patients had 98% or greater tumor resection.

Weakness in statistical methodologies plagued both approaches, as the value of EOR was assessed using a 'minimum p-value method' [13]. This putative strategy attempts to define a statistical cut-off by arbitrarily categorizing the dataset into two groups on the basis of a single variable (e.g., EOR). Unfortunately, previous oncology studies have demonstrated that this statistical tactic can be misleading and associated with a 10-fold increase in the false-positive rate [13]. Furthermore, inclusion of such a determined cut-off as a binary variable in a Cox multiple regression analysis can lead to an inflated effect at the expense of other variables that may be more important. Taken together, these study design deficiencies severely hampered a valuable opportunity to detect the 'threshold value' beyond which GBM EOR improves outcomes. Nevertheless, in the absence of a more comprehensive analysis, the Lacroix EOR study has endured for a decade as a mainstay in our current GBM management paradigm.

Class I evidence

Since then, other attempts to further refine our understanding of EOR impact on GBMs have emerged, although none as meticulous. In 2003, the first prospective randomized clinical trial examining

Table 1. Overview of recent publications examining extent of resection for glioblastoma.

Reference	n	Extent of resection (no. patients)	Overall survival, p-value	Progression-free survival, p-value	Patients with radiotherapy (%)	Patients with chemotherapy (%)	Level of evidence
Lacroix *et al*, 2001 [6]	416	<98% ≥98%	<0.0001	NA	100	NA	III/B
Vuorinen *et al*, 2003 [11]	30	GTR (15) Biopsy (15)	0.035	NS	100	0	Ib/A
Lamborn *et al*, 2004 [7]	832	GTR (101) STR (469) Biopsy (86)	<0.001	NA	100	100	III/B
Ushio *et al*, 2005 [8]	105	GTR (35) PR (57) Biopsy (13)	0.018	0.0042	100	100	III/B
Stark *et al*, 2005 [9]	267	GTR (167) STR (80) PR (14)	0.014	NA	83.1	21.3	III/B
Pope *et al*, 2005 [5]	110	<20% 20-89% 90-99% 100%	NS	NA	100	NA	III/B
Stummer *et al*, 2008 [10]	243	GTR (122) STR (121)	<0.0001	NA	100	0	Ib/A
Sanai *et al*, 2010 [16]	500	<78% ≥78%	<0.0001	NA	100	100	III/B

GTR = gross total resection; NA = not assessed; NS = not significant; PR = partial resection; STR = subtotal resection

biopsy versus resection for GBM patients was reported. This study, by Vuorinen *et al*, recruited 30 elderly patients (>65 years) with WHO grade III and IV gliomas, randomizing them to tumor resection or stereotactic biopsy [11]. The impact on each arm was assessed in terms of overall survival. For patients who underwent resection, the median overall survival was 171 days, as compared with 85 days for stereotactic biopsy **(Ib/A)**.

In 2004, Lamborn *et al* pooled the combined experiences of 832 patients with WHO grade IV gliomas who had received subsequent radiation and chemotherapy into three categories: gross total resection (n=101), subtotal resection (n=469), and biopsy (n=86) [7]. Recursive partitioning analysis was used to analyze overall survival, revealing a statistically significant association with EOR (p<0.001) **(III/B)**. Similarly, a 2005 retrospective review by Ushio *et al*

Chapter 19

examined 105 patients with WHO grade IV gliomas who were similarly grouped into the same EOR categories as above (n=35, 57, and 13, respectively) [8]. Using both progression-free survival and overall survival as outcome measures, greater EOR was a significant predictor for each (p=0.0042 and p=0.018, respectively) **(III/B)**. That same year, Stark *et al* described a series of 267 patients subdivided into gross total (n=167), subtotal (n=80), and partial (n=14) resections [9]. In this study, univariate analysis again demonstrated an association between EOR and overall survival (p=0.014).

In contrast, and also published in 2005, Pope *et al* reported an experience with 110 patients whose EORs were volumetrically analyzed and categorized into four groups: <20%, 20-89%, 90-99%, and 100% [5]. Unlike the Lacroix study, however, this volumetric analysis demonstrated no significant association between EOR and overall survival, although with considerably fewer patients enrolled **(III/B)**. In 2008, the 5-ALA Glioma Study Group reported their results with 243 GBM patients who had previously been randomized to conventional white light versus 5-aminolevulinic acid (5-ALA) tumor fluorescence during microsurgical resection, a study that was ended after early results demonstrated a nearly two-fold improvement in EOR with 5-ALA. Interestingly, restratification of the original randomized trial results enabled an analysis controlling for 16 pre- and postoperative variables to adjust for potential bias. The gross total resection subgroup (n=122) had a median overall survival of 16.7 months, as compared with 11.8 months for the subtotal resection subgroup (n=121) [10]. Multivariate analysis demonstrated this relationship to be highly significant (p<0.0001) **(Ib/A)**. Of note, this study's design included strict inclusion criteria, allowed only GBM histology, and featured randomized groups that were then actively balanced on the basis of EOR. It remains one of the most rigorous analyses of EOR and survival with GBM.

An extent of resection threshold

Despite these multiple studies emphasizing the importance of greater EOR, the value of subtotal resection for GBM remains unknown. While the body of modern literature described above indicates that gross total resection can improve overall survival, it remains unclear how much of this benefit carries over to subtotal resection.

To address this issue and calculate a threshold for GBM EOR, we recently completed a study of 500 newly diagnosed GBM patients that strongly suggests that EOR is of paramount importance, even when gross total resection is not possible [14]. We identified 500 consecutive, newly diagnosed supratentorial GBM patients treated at the University of California, San Francisco from 1997 to 2009. Clinical, radiographic, and outcome parameters were measured for each patient, including MRI-based volumetric tumor analysis. Patients had a median age of 60.0 years and presented with a median Karnofsky Performance Score of 80. Mean clinical follow-up was 15.3 months and no patient was unaccounted for. All patients underwent resection followed by chemo- and radiation therapy. The median postoperative tumor volume was $2.3cm^3$, equating to a 96% EOR.

The median overall survival was 12.2 months. Using Cox proportional hazards analysis, younger age, lower Karnofsky Performance Score, and greater EOR were predictive of survival (p<0.0001). Importantly, a significant survival advantage was seen with as little as 78% EOR and stepwise improvement in survival was evident even in the 95-100% range (Figure 2). A recursive partitioning analysis validated these findings and provided additional risk stratification parameters related to age, EOR, and tumor burden. This study supports a paradigm shift for glioma surgery, justifying microsurgical resection for newly diagnosed GBMs when at least 78% of the tumor volume can be safely resected **(III/B)**. The analysis also underscores the value of reducing tumor burden to shape outcome, particularly since tumor responses to radiation and chemotherapy are likely non-linear and subject to change by the quantity and distribution of remaining tumor cells. Nevertheless, in cases where a 78% EOR does not seem possible, tumor debulking remains a reasonable option to alleviate symptoms due to mass effect and establish a diagnosis.

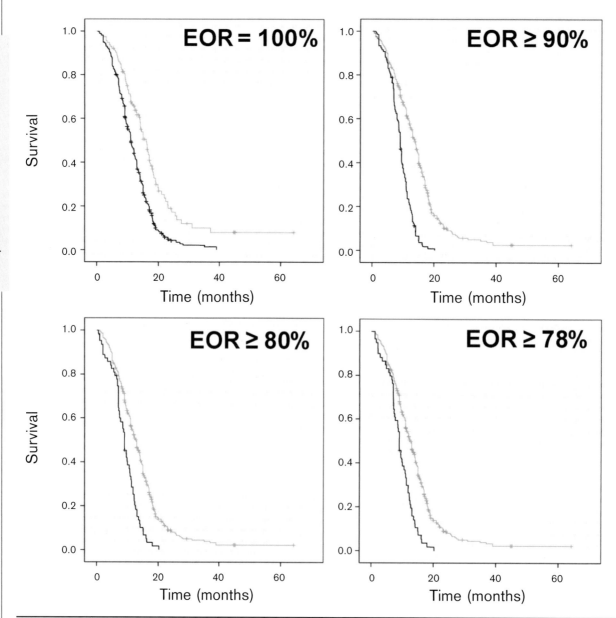

Figure 2. Select Kaplan-Meier survival curves for 100%, 90%, 80%, and 78% extent of resection thresholds (grey). Corresponding median overall survival (black) times beyond each threshold value were 16, 13.8, 12.8, and 12.5 months, respectively.

Persistent challenges in examining extent of resection

Despite these recent data, many critical questions remain unanswered in the literature regarding the value of EOR for GBMs. Specifically, it is unclear whether the emerging correlation between aggressive glioma resection and overall survival holds true for both first-time and recurrent operations. The effect of EOR for different ages and histologic subtypes must also be studied further. In addition, the question of the impact of surgical resection on patient survival must be asked in the context of current prognostic factors (e.g., 1p/19q and MGMT methylation status), as well as with respect to specific adjuvant therapy regimens. Future studies linking EOR and outcomes should use these markers as stratification factors in the analysis.

Additional challenges relate to study design sensitivity and certain statistical methodologies, which can limit the ability to detect small, yet meaningful, improvements in patient outcomes following microsurgical resection. This masking effect is likely worsened by both the short life expectancy of these patients and the highly aggressive nature of the disease. These formidable limitations, however, can be overcome with a statistically robust analysis of a large, homogenous population of GBM patients, emphasizing the need for large-scale data collection within each major brain tumor center and across multicenter consortia.

Assessing the evidence for glioblastoma extent of resection: progress to date

The value of EOR for gliomas remains a longstanding topic of debate. Interestingly, the most compelling evidence exists for low-grade gliomas [3], where volumetric analyses have shown, both in hemispheric [15] and insular [16] low-grade gliomas, that greater EOR portends better overall, progression-free, and malignant progression-free survival. For high-grade gliomas, however, the evidence is less consistent and robust: level I evidence is scarce, owing at least in part to the ethical and logistical challenges related to randomizing for subtotal resection.

As described above, one prospective randomized study does exist, comparing biopsy versus debulking for elderly patients with GBM [12]. Although the study demonstrated a survival benefit (5.7 vs. 2.8 months) with greater EOR, it was unblinded, underpowered, and without adjuvant chemotherapy. More recently, the 5-ALA Glioma Study Group evaluated EOR in 260 patients enrolled in a prospective, randomized, multicenter trial examining intraoperative 5-ALA-mediated tumor fluorescence versus conventional white light for high-grade glioma resection [17]. Although the difference in observed rates of complete resection (65% for 5-ALA vs. 36% for white light) presented an unprecedented opportunity to study the impact of EOR, this study was limited by several factors, including investigator bias (surgeons were unblinded), absence of intraoperative neuronavigation, minimal (<10%) adjuvant chemotherapy, and use of 6-month progression-free survival as the sole outcome measure. In the follow-up study described above, however, a more stringent analysis of the original dataset was performed, focusing on the 243 randomized patients with WHO grade IV gliomas and restratifying them on the basis of complete versus incomplete resection [10]. Sixteen pre- and postoperative variables were then controlled for across both groups, producing one of the most controlled EOR analyses to date. However, although a 4.9-month survival benefit (16.7 vs. 11.8 months for complete and incomplete resections, respectively) was reported, the value of a subtotal resection was not assessed beyond these two categories.

Thus, the most comprehensive work published to date on the value of EOR suggests that an EOR of 98% or more is necessary to impact GBM patient survival [6]. While these data are valuable, they nonetheless offer little hope for patients without a complete radiographic resection. Nevertheless, the 'all-or-none' conceptualization of glioma management has filtered into the mainstream of medical literature. One recent high-grade glioma case analysis published in *JAMA* concluded that "Data presented so far show no continuous correlation between the EOR and survival; only maximal or gross total resections affect survival" [13]. However, as detailed above, findings from our recently completed volumetric study on EOR of newly diagnosed GBM challenge this doctrine by demonstrating that an EOR of 78% or more can impact patient survival. Interestingly, this trend continues even as EOR climbs up to the highest levels of resection.

Conclusions

While the value of EOR for GBMs remains a topic of debate, particularly for incomplete resections, the summations of these works overwhelmingly substantiate the value of EOR for the vast majority of patients with GBM. In the modern neurosurgical era, attaining an EOR beyond the 78% threshold should be of critical concern to the neurosurgeon treating any GBM patient.

Recommendations	Evidence level
◆ The current standard of care for patients at most large brain tumor centers involves gross total resection, followed by temozolomide chemotherapy and fractionated radiotherapy.	Ib/A
◆ For GBM, microsurgical resection generates a survival benefit as compared with stereotactic biopsy.	Ib/A
◆ Greater EOR during microsurgical resection of GBM provides a survival benefit.	Ib/A
◆ The minimum level of GBM EOR providing a survival benefit is 78%.	III/B

References

1. Stupp R, Mason WP, van den Bent MJ, et al. Radiotherapy plus concomitant and adjuvant temozolomide for glioblastoma. N Engl J Med 2005; 352(10): 987-96.

2. Hegi ME, Diserens AC, Gorlia T, et al. MGMT gene silencing and benefit from temozolomide in glioblastoma. N Engl J Med 2005; 352(10): 997-1003.

3. Sanai N, Berger MS. Glioma extent of resection and its impact on patient outcome. Neurosurgery 2008; 62(4): 753-64; discussion 264-6.

4. Ohgaki H, Kleihues P. Genetic pathways to primary and secondary glioblastoma. Am J Pathol 2007; 170(5): 1445-53.

5. Pope WB, Sayre J, Perlina A, Villablanca JP, Mischel PS, Cloughesy TF. MR imaging correlates of survival in patients with high-grade gliomas. AJNR Am J Neuroradiol 2005; 26(10): 2466-74.

6. Lacroix M, Abi-Said D, Fourney DR, et al. A multivariate analysis of 416 patients with glioblastoma multiforme: prognosis, extent of resection, and survival. J Neurosurg 2001; 95(2): 190-8.

7. Lamborn KR, Chang SM, Prados MD. Prognostic factors for survival of patients with glioblastoma: recursive partitioning analysis. Neuro Oncol 2004; 6(3): 227-35.

8. Ushio Y, Kochi M, Hamada J, Kai Y, Nakamura H. Effect of surgical removal on survival and quality of life in patients with supratentorial glioblastoma. Neurol Med Chir (Tokyo) 2005; 45(9): 454-60; discussion 60-1.

9. Stark AM, Nabavi A, Mehdorn HM, Blomer U. Glioblastoma multiforme - report of 267 cases treated at a single institution. Surg Neurol 2005; 63(2): 162-9.

10. Stummer W, Reulen HJ, Meinel T, et al. Extent of resection and survival in glioblastoma multiforme: identification of and adjustment for bias. Neurosurgery 2008; 62(3): 564-76.

11. Vuorinen V, Hinkka S, Farkkila M, Jaaskelainen J. Debulking or biopsy of malignant glioma in elderly people - a randomised study. Acta Neurochir (Wien) 2003; 145(1): 5-10.

12. Warnke PC. A 31-year-old woman with a transformed low-grade glioma. JAMA 2010; 303(10): 967-76.

13. Altman DG, Lausen B, Sauerbrei W, Schumacher M. Dangers of using 'optimal' cutpoints in the evaluation of prognostic factors. J Natl Cancer Inst 1994; 86(11): 829-35.

14. Sanai N, Polley MY, McDermott MW, Parsa AT, Berger MS. An extent of resection threshold for newly diagnosed glioblastomas. J Neurosurg 2011; 115(1): 3-8.

15. Smith JS, Chang EF, Lamborn KR, et al. Role of extent of resection in the long-term outcome of low-grade hemispheric gliomas. J Clin Oncol 2008; 26(8): 1338-45.

16. Sanai N, Polley MY, Berger MS. Insular glioma resection: assessment of patient morbidity, survival, and tumor progression. J Neurosurg 2010; 112(1): 1-9.

17. Stummer W, Pichlmeier U, Meinel T, Wiestler OD, Zanella F, Reulen HJ. Fluorescence-guided surgery with 5-aminolevulinic acid for resection of malignant glioma: a randomised controlled multicentre Phase III trial. Lancet Oncol 2006; 7(5): 392-401.

Chapter 20

Stereotactic radiosurgery versus microsurgical resection for patients with vestibular schwannomas

Brian D Milligan MD, Neurosurgical Resident

Michael J Link MD, Professor of Neurosurgery

Bruce E Pollock MD, Professor of Neurosurgery

and Radiation Oncology

MAYO CLINIC COLLEGE OF MEDICINE, ROCHESTER, MINNESOTA, USA

Introduction

Evidence-based medicine involves identifying and interpreting the highest-quality scientific evidence for the purpose of making the best medical decisions in the care of individual patients [1]. In the late 1970s, Fletcher and Sackett defined a recommendation grading system based upon the available scientific 'levels of evidence' to rank the validity of evidence of preventive health care measures [2]. Grade A recommendations are made for a particular therapy when it has been studied with at least one randomized controlled trial (RCT) (level Ia/Ib evidence) with little variation in the direction or magnitude of the results. Grade B recommendations can be made with consistent level IIa (prospective cohort studies), IIb (prospective case-control series), or III studies (retrospective case-control or case series). Grade C recommendations can be made from level IV studies (expert opinions) or inconsistent or inconclusive studies of any level. By incorporating the best available evidence together with clinical experience and consideration of an individual's life situation and preferences, a physician is able to employ an evidence-based medicine practice.

A variety of reasons can limit the practicality of performing RCTs for a given therapy. First, the condition of interest may be rare and even when the efficacy difference between treatments is large, a sufficient number of patients must be enrolled to show this difference in a statistically meaningful way. Second, for benign tumors such as vestibular schwannomas (VSs) (Figure 1), the success of an operation in preventing tumor recurrence or progression may not be evident for 10 years or more after surgery. Thus, retrospective case series (level III evidence) may provide the best available data upon which to base clinical decisions for patients with benign tumors and extended life expectancies. Third, and particularly relevant to stereotactic radiosurgery (SRS), is the fact that few patients are willing to undergo randomization between open surgery and SRS. So although an RCT comparing outcomes after surgical resection and SRS for VS would likely yield valuable information, the 'trial-ability' of such proposed studies is low. For these and many other reasons, clinicians often have to base their decision-making on rather poor-quality evidence.

This chapter compares recent studies on VS resection and SRS according to evidence-based

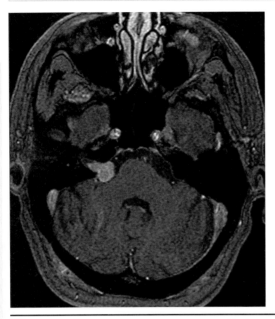

Figure 1. An axial post-gadolinium MRI showing a patient with a right-sided vestibular schwannoma.

medicine guidelines. Specifically, the SRS studies used in this chapter refer to single-session procedures as opposed to either multisession SRS (two to five fractions) or stereotactic radiation therapy (more than five fractions) [3].

Methodology

A limited review of recently published, commonly referred to studies on VS resection and SRS was performed. The studies were grouped according to the quality of the information provided (level I-IV; Table 1), and the conclusions summarized.

Results

Level Ia/Ib evidence

In 2002, Nikolopoulos and O'Donoghue reviewed the English-language literature published over the preceding 23 years (111 papers) and found no level I or IIa evidence to support either surgical resection or SRS as the preferred management for VS patients [4]. They concluded that the quality of evidence on this

topic was poor, and emphasized the need for better studies in the future. Ideally, an RCT would be performed to compare outcomes for VS patients having surgical resection or SRS. However, such a study would be difficult to perform because patients may be reluctant to undergo randomization between open brain surgery and an outpatient-based procedure performed under local anesthesia. In addition, many physicians who regularly manage VS patients are polarized in their thinking on this topic and would be unwilling to participate in an RCT.

Table 1. Comparison of surgical resection and radiosurgery by evidence-based medicine standards.

Level of evidence	Preferred treatment
Ia/Ib	No studies available
IIa	Radiosurgery [5, 13, 17]
III	Radiosurgery [7-9, 12, 18]
	Conflicting conclusions
IV	Conflicting opinions

Level IIa evidence

Recognizing the limitations outlined above, three groups have now published prospective cohort studies **(IIa/B)** comparing SRS and open surgery, each with notable strengths and/or weaknesses.

In 2006, we reported on a prospective cohort of 82 adult patients with unilateral, unoperated VS of less than 3cm in average diameter who underwent either surgical resection (n=36) or SRS (n=46) [5]. Patients undergoing resection were younger (48 vs. 54 years; p=0.03), but the groups were otherwise similar with regard to hearing loss, associated symptoms, and tumor size. The mean follow-up was 42 months (range 12-62 months). Importantly, blinded observers determined tumor size, facial weakness, and hearing

Chapter 20

Table 2. Prospective cohort series (level IIa evidence) comparing surgical resection and radiosurgery for patients with vestibular schwannomas.

| Study | Normal facial function (last follow-up) | | Functional hearing preserved (last follow-up) | | Quality of life (change in SF-36 scores vs. baseline) | | | |
| | | | | | Early (≤1 year) | | Late (>1 year) | |
	SRS	Surgery	SRS	Surgery	SRS	Surgery	SRS	Surgery
Pollock et al, 2006 [5]	96%[a,**]	75%[a,**]	63%[a,***]	5%[a,***]	No change	Decline in subscores of: Physical function* Bodily pain* Role-physical*** Energy-fatigue*	No change	Decline in bodily pain subscore*
Myrseth et al, 2009 [13]	98%[b,***]	54%[b,***]	68%[b,***]	0%[b,***]	No change	No change	No change	No change
Di Maio and Akagami 2009 [17]	73%[c]	76%[c]	8%[c]	16%[c]	No change	No change	No change	Total score improved***

a = blinded/objective; b = assessed by operating surgeon; c = patient reported/no objective assessment

* = p<0.05; ** = p<0.01; *** = p<0.001

SF-36 = Short Form-36

preservation. Facial nerve outcomes, preservation of serviceable hearing, and subscale scores of the Health Status Questionnaire (HSQ) measuring the patients' quality of life favored SRS at both early (≤1 year) and late (>1 year) time points (Table 2). The SRS group had lower mean Dizziness Handicap Inventory scores at last follow-up (16.5 vs. 8.4; p=0.02). There was no difference in radiographic tumor control (100% vs. 96%; p=0.50), although two SRS patients required shunting for hydrocephalus **(IIa/B)**.

In contrast to other groups' prospective studies, blinded, independent observers graded facial nerve outcomes, determined hearing preservation, and measured the tumors. So although this study was not an RCT, it does provide rigorous level IIa evidence comparing cranial nerve outcomes for VS patients undergoing either surgical resection or SRS. At every time point examined, patients who underwent SRS more often had normal facial movement and retained serviceable hearing compared with the microsurgical group. Despite the importance typically placed on cranial nerve function after VS management, the effect of treatment on patients' quality of life (QoL) is a more meaningful measure. Retrospective studies of patients following open VS resection have shown the following:

* More than half of patients felt their QoL was worse after surgery [6].
* Only one-third of patients resumed their normal activities of daily living within 1 month of their operation [7, 8].
* Patients experienced a significant decline in the physical functioning, role-physical, and social functioning components of the HSQ after VS resection when compared with published results for age-adjusted population-based controls [9-11].

The effect of SRS on QoL for VS patients in retrospective studies has been less significant than that of surgical resection [7-9, 12]. In our prospective study, the surgical resection group suffered a significant decline in several components of the HSQ at 3 months, 1 year, and at last follow-up compared with their preoperative level of functioning. The radiosurgical group, however, showed no decline in any subset of the HSQ at any point during the follow-up interval **(IIa/B)**.

Myrseth *et al* prospectively followed a cohort of patients with non-syndromic, unilateral VS of less than 2.5cm in posterior fossa diameter treated with SRS (n=60) or open surgery (n=28) [13]. SRS dosing was 12Gy to the 40% isodose line. The operating surgeons recorded cranial nerve status at baseline and 1- and 2-year follow-up. The SRS group more frequently had normal facial nerve function (98% vs. 54%, p<0.001) and serviceable hearing (68% vs. 0%, p<0.001). Although HSQ subscores were not significantly different, the radiosurgical group had better QoL at 2 years based on the Glasgow Benefit Inventory. The 2-year follow-up was too short for a valid comparison of tumor control between the groups [14, 15] **(IIa/B)**.

Although more favorable QoL outcomes were seen following SRS than resection for small- to medium-sized VS, the HSQ subscores did not differ significantly [13], making direct comparison with other prospective studies difficult. Cranial nerve outcomes after SRS were similar to those published by other groups [5, 7, 9, 12] using a margin dose of 12Gy. In the surgical group, which comprised less than one-third of the study population, cranial nerve outcomes were much poorer than those reported in large surgical series (normal facial function 81%, preserved functional hearing 51%) [16]. Surgical patients also had high rates of meningitis (7%), hemorrhage (5%), and cerebrospinal fluid leakage requiring re-operation (17%) **(IIa/B)**. This makes the results difficult to generalize to other groups and introduces a negative bias toward the surgical group.

The third prospective cohort study compared QoL (HSQ) among patients allocated to observation (n=47), radiation (SRS n=25; stereotactic radiation therapy n=23) and surgical resection (n=134) [17]. Baseline HSQ subscores were not different among the three groups. During the mean follow-up of 32 months, HSQ scores did not significantly change from baseline. In subgroup analysis, patients allocated to surgery for a tumor of more than 3cm in diameter had depressed QoL at baseline and were the only group to show improved QoL during follow-up. Cranial nerve outcomes were based upon patient self-reporting via questionnaire (Table 2). Interestingly, patients reported that hearing, tinnitus, and dizziness were the symptoms most commonly affecting QoL and not facial nerve function. Actuarial tumor control rates were not reported **(IIa/B)**.

In this study, it may be that the combination of a low rate of hearing preservation after both surgery and SRS (16% vs. 8%) and the significant patient-perceived impact of hearing loss, tinnitus, and dizziness on QoL resulted in similar QoL outcomes for the two treated groups. Facial function and hearing preservation rates were self-reported via questionnaire, introducing significant bias.

Level III evidence

Five retrospective case-control series have been performed comparing surgical resection with SRS [7-9, 12, 18]. These studies found that SRS had improved facial nerve outcomes and hearing preservation rates. Patients returned to work faster after SRS, and the costs associated with radiosurgical management were less than those of open surgery **(III/B)**. Table 3 outlines the major findings of these studies.

Large case series are available for surgical resection from the retrosigmoid [19, 20], translabyrinthine [21], and middle fossa approaches [22]. Likewise, large case series are available after radiosurgery performed with the Gamma Knife [14, 23-25] and modified linear accelerators [26]. Similar to expert opinions on this topic, advocates of surgical resection and SRS typically argue that the published results favor their particular method of treatment **(III/B)**.

Table 3. Retrospective case-control series (level III evidence) comparing surgical resection and radiosurgery for patients with vestibular schwannomas.

Treatment with better outcome

Study	Trigeminal nerve	Facial nerves	Hearing	Activities of daily living	Cost/charges
Pollock et al, 1995 [7]	No difference	Radiosurgery	Radiosurgery	Not tested	Radiosurgery
Van Roijen et al, 1997 [8]	No difference	No difference	Not tested	Radiosurgery	Radiosurgery
Karpinos et al, 2002 [18]	Radiosurgery	Radiosurgery	Radiosurgery	No difference	Not tested
Regis et al, 2002 [12]	Radiosurgery	Radiosurgery	Radiosurgery	Radiosurgery	Not tested
Myrseth et al, 2005 [9]	Not tested	Radiosurgery	Radiosurgery	Radiosurgery	Not tested

Chapter 20

Level IV evidence

Literature reviews have been published that promote both surgical resection [27, 28] and SRS [29] as the best treatment for VS patients **(IV/C)**. Ironically, the diametrically opposed opinions expressed in these different papers were derived from the same body of information (papers on VS resection and radiosurgery from the 1980s until the late 1990s).

Tumor control

As a consequence of low patient numbers and relatively short follow-ups, comparison studies to date have provided no meaningful information regarding tumor control rates after surgical resection or SRS of VS. It is generally accepted that VS recurrence after total excision is approximately 3%. Numerous series have published a similar failure rate after VS radiosurgery, although these patients were treated with higher radiation doses than are commonly used today [15]. Hasegawa et al has reported outcomes for 317 VS patients undergoing SRS between 1991 and

1998 [14]. The average tumor margin dose was 13.2Gy. At a mean follow-up of 7.8 years, the 10-year progression-free survival for patients with tumors less than 15cm^3 was 97%.

In 2009, we reported tumor control rates in 293 VS patients treated with SRS between 1990 and 2004 (Figure 2) [30]. Actuarial tumor control rates at 3 and 7 years were both 98% in the 16Gy group (n=88, treated before April 1997), but decreased to 96% and 90% (p=0.04), respectively, for those receiving 12Gy to the margin (n=205, treated after April 1997). Patients receiving the lower dose were treated with more isocenters (5.3 vs. 7.9; p<0.001) and a lower prescription isodose volume (volume per isocenter, 680 vs. 182mm^3). On multivariate analysis, only the number of isocenters was significantly associated with failure of tumor control (hazard ratio 1.1; 95% confidence interval 1.02-1.32).

It may be that prescription dose reduction and increased dose-plan conformality coupled with targeting errors related to image distortion inherent to MRI at the bone-tumor interface has led to under-

Chapter 20

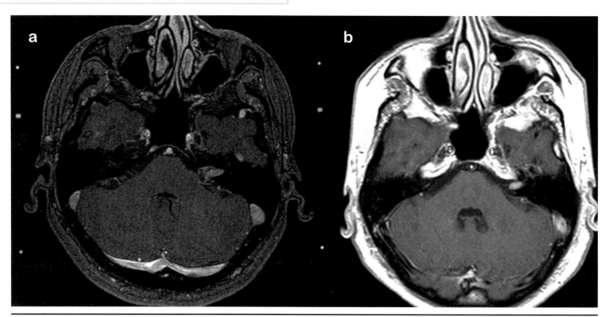

Figure 2. Axial post-gadolinium MRIs of a patient with a left-sided vestibular schwannoma. a)
At the time of and b) 135 months after stereotactic radiosurgery, showing the tumor to be decreased
in size.

dosing of the tumor border and subsequent failure of
tumor control. More data are needed to fully assess
long-term tumor control using the lower-dose
technique. If other investigators confirm an increased
failure rate for current lower-dose SRS, the published
results suggest that subsequent tumor removal in
these patients is more difficult, that patient outcomes
are poor compared with those of patients never
undergoing SRS, and that the cost savings
associated with SRS may be lost [31-33].

Other factors

A number of other factors need to be remembered
when comparing the different treatments for VS
patients. First, not every VS patient is suitable for
radiosurgery. Observation with serial imaging can be
used to effectively manage many elderly patients with
small or minimally symptomatic VSs [34]. In addition,
patients with large tumors and significant brainstem
compression and/or obstructive hydrocephalus are

poor candidates for radiosurgery. Finally, it is now recognized that
patients undergoing radiosurgery are at some risk for
developing radiation-induced neoplasms [35]. The best
estimate of this complication at this time is
approximately 0.01-0.1%, although this number may
increase as more patients are followed for longer
intervals after radiosurgery. By comparison, a series
of 707 patients operated on between 1987 and
2001 found the risk of death after VS resection to be
0.1% [21] **(III/B)**.

Conclusions

The best quality of evidence shows superior
outcomes for VS patients undergoing SRS
compared with surgical resection **(IIa/B or III/B)**.
Additional follow-up information on tumor control for
patients being treated with low-dose (12-13Gy)
techniques is needed to confirm that SRS is the best
strategy for the majority of VS patients **(III/B)**.

Recommendations

Evidence level

◆ SRS for small- to medium-sized VS is associated with better short- and long-term QoL, and with better facial nerve and hearing outcomes.

IIa/B

◆ SRS and microsurgery achieve similar tumor control rates in the treatment of small- to medium-sized VS.

III/B

◆ SRS is associated with lower direct costs than microsurgery for the treatment of small- to medium-sized VS.

III/B

References

1. Sackett DL, Rosenberg WM, Gray JA, Haynes RB, Richardson WS. Evidence-based medicine: what it is and what it isn't. *BMJ* 1996; 312: 71-2.

2. Canadian Task Force on the Periodic Health Examination. The periodic health examination. *CMAJ* 1979; 121: 1193-254.

3. Pollock BE, Lunsford LD. A call to define stereotactic radiosurgery. *Neurosurgery* 2004; 55: 1371-3.

4. Nikolopoulos TP, O'Donoghue GM. Acoustic neuroma management: an evidence-based medicine approach. *Otol Neurotol* 2002; 23: 534-41.

5. Pollock BE, Driscoll CL, Foote RL, *et al*. Patient outcomes after vestibular schwannoma management: a prospective comparison of microsurgical resection and stereotactic radiosurgery. *Neurosurgery* 2006; 58: 77-85.

6. Da Cruz MJ, Moffat DA, Hardy DG. Postoperative quality of life in vestibular schwannoma patients measured by the SF-36 Health Questionnaire. *Laryngoscope* 2000; 110: 151-5.

7. Pollock BE, Lunsford LD, Kondziolka D, *et al*. Outcome analysis of acoustic neuroma management: a comparison of microsurgery and stereotactic radiosurgery. *Neurosurgery* 1995; 36: 215-23.

8. Van Roijen L, Nijs HG, Avezaat CJ, *et al*. Costs and effects of microsurgery versus radiosurgery in treating acoustic neuromas. *Acta Neurochir* (Wein) 1997; 139: 942-8.

9. Myrseth E, Moller P, Pedersen P, Vassbotn FS, Wentzel-Larsen T, Lund-Johansen M. Vestibular schwannomas: clinical results and quality of life after microsurgery or Gamma Knife radiosurgery. *Neurosurgery* 2005; 56: 927-35.

10. Betchan SA, Walsh J, Post KD. Self-assessed quality of life after acoustic neuroma surgery. *J Neurosurg* 2003; 99: 818-23.

11. Martin HC, Sethi J, Lang DL, Neil-Dwyer G, Lutman ME, Yardley L. Patient-assessed outcomes after excision of acoustic neuroma: postoperative symptoms and quality of life. *J Neurosurg* 2001; 94: 211-6.

12. Regis J, Pellet W, Delsanti C, *et al*. Functional outcome after Gamma Knife surgery or microsurgery for vestibular schwannomas. *J Neurosurg* 2002; 97: 1091-100.

13. Myrseth E, Moller P, Pedersen PH, Lund-Johansen M. Vestibular schwannoma: surgery or Gamma Knife radiosurgery? A prospective, nonrandomized study. *Neurosurgery* 2009; 64: 654-63.

14. Hasegawa T, Fujitani S, Katsumata S, Kida Y, Yoshimoto M, Koike J. Stereotactic radiosurgery for vestibular schwannomas: analysis of 317 patients followed more than 5 years. *Neurosurgery* 2005; 57: 257-64.

15. Kondziolka D, Lunsford LD, McLaughlin MR, Flickinger JC. Long-term outcomes after radiosurgery for acoustic neuromas. *N Engl J Med* 1998; 339: 1426-33.

16. Samii M, Gerganov V, Samii A. Improved preservation of hearing and facial nerve function in vestibular schwannoma surgery via the retrosigmoid approach in a series of 200 patients. *J Neurosurg* 2006; 105: 527-35.

17. Di Maio S, Akagami R. Prospective comparison of quality of life before and after observation, radiation, or surgery for vestibular schwannomas. *J Neurosurg* 2009; 111: 855-62.

18. Karpinos M, The BS, Zeck O, *et al*. Treatment of acoustic neuroma: stereotactic radiosurgery vs. microsurgery. *Int J Radiat Oncol Biol Phys* 2002; 54: 1410-21.

19. Samii M, Matthies C. Management of 1000 vestibular schwannomas (acoustic neuromas): hearing function in 1000 tumor resections. *Neurosurgery* 1997; 40: 248-60.

20. Sampath P, Holliday MJ, Brem H, Niparko JK, Long DM. Facial nerve injury in acoustic neuroma (vestibular schwannoma) surgery: etiology and prevention. *Neurosurgery* 1997; 87: 60-6.

21. Sanna M, Taibah A, Russo A, Falcioni M, Agarwal M. Perioperative complications in acoustic neuroma (vestibular schwannoma) surgery. *Otol Neurotol* 2004; 25: 379-86.

22. Brackmann DE, Owens RM, Friedman RA, *et al*. Prognostic factors for hearing preservation in vestibular schwannoma surgery. *Am J Otol* 2000; 21: 417-24.

23. Flickinger JC, Kondziolka D, Niranjan A, Maitz A, Voynov G, Lunsford LD. Acoustic neuroma radiosurgery with marginal tumor doses of 12 to 13 Gy. *Int J Radiat Oncol Biol Phys* 2004; 60: 225-30.

24. Iwai Y, Yamanaka K, Shiotani M, Uyama T. Radiosurgery for acoustic neuromas: results of low-dose treatment. *Neurosurgery* 2003; 53: 282-7.

25. Petit JH, Hudes RS, Chen TT, Eisenberg HM, Simard JM, Chin LS. Reduced-dose radiosurgery for vestibular schwannomas. *Neurosurgery* 2001; 49: 1299-306.

26. Foote KD, Freidman WA, Buatti JM, Meeks SL, Bova FJ, Kubilis PS. Analysis of risk factors associated with radiosurgery for vestibular schwannoma. *J Neurosurg* 2001; 95: 440-9.

Chapter 20

27. Kaylie DM, McMenomey SO. Microsurgery vs. Gamma Knife radiosurgery for the treatment of vestibular schwannomas. *Arch Otolaryngol Head Neck Surg* 2003; 129: 903-6.

28. Sekhar LN, Gormley WB, Wright DC. The best treatment for vestibular schwannoma (acoustic neuroma): microsurgery or radiosurgery? *Am J Otol* 1996; 17: 676-82.

29. Pollock BE, Lunsford LD, Noren G. Vestibular schwannoma management in the next century: a radiosurgical perspective. *Neurosurgery* 1998; 43: 475-83.

30. Pollock BE, Link MJ, Foote RL. Failure rate of contemporary low-dose radiosurgical technique for vestibular schwannoma. *J Neurosurg* 2009; 111: 840-4.

31. Friedman RA, Brackmann DE, Hitselberger WE, Schwartz MS, Iqbal Z, Berliner KI. Surgical salvage after failed irradiation for vestibular schwannoma. *Laryngoscope* 2005; 115: 1827-32.

32. Lee DJ, Westra WH, Staecker H, Long D, Niparko JK. Clinical and histopathologic features of recurrent vestibular schwannomas (acoustic neuroma) after stereotactic radiosurgery. *Otol Neurotol* 2003; 24: 650-60.

33. Banerjee R, Moriarty JP, Foote RL, Pollock BE. Comparison of surgical and follow-up costs associated with microsurgical resection and stereotactic radiosurgery for vestibular schwannoma. *J Neurosurg* 2009; 108: 1220-4.

34. Raut VV, Walsh RM, Bath AP, *et al*. Conservative management of vestibular schwannomas-second review of a prospective longitudinal study. *Clin Otolaryngol* 2004; 29: 505-14.

35. Loeffler JS, Niemierko A, Chapman PH. Second tumors after radiosurgery: tip of the iceberg or a bump in the road? *Neurosurgery* 2003; 52: 1436-42.

Chapter 20

Chapter 21

Surgical resection of low-grade gliomas

Jason Beiko MD PhD

Assistant Professor 1

Daniel P Cahill MD PhD

Assistant Professor; Attending Neurosurgeon 2

1 SECTION OF NEUROSURGERY, UNIVERSITY OF MANITOBA, WINNIPEG, CANADA
2 DEPARTMENT OF NEUROSURGERY, MASSACHUSETTS GENERAL HOSPITAL,
HARVARD MEDICAL SCHOOL, BOSTON, MASSACHUSETTS, USA

Introduction

Gliomas are the most common intrinsic brain tumors [1]. Historically, there has been controversy about the timing of surgery and the impact of aggressive surgical resection on patient outcomes. For low-grade gliomas there are no randomized studies to guide the decision for early versus delayed surgery, or biopsy versus aggressive surgical resection. As such, the following questions remain topics of intense debate:

- Should surgical debulking be rendered at the time of diagnosis or after confirmation of radiographic progression?
- Does the extent of surgical resection (EOR) confer a survival benefit over and above other known prognostic factors and treatments?

In this chapter, we describe the evidence base examining the role of surgery in the management of these neoplasms.

Methodology

A US National Library of Medicine search was conducted using the search words 'low-grade glioma,' 'surgery,' 'extent of surgical resection,' and 'outcome.' The titles of the abstracts were carefully reviewed for relevance and pertinent articles identified and subsequently reviewed. The articles selected for review contained original research or were subset analyses of large multicenter randomized controlled trials that examined the role of surgical resection in patients with low-grade gliomas. In addition, the reference list of the selected articles was reviewed and further articles identified based on the criteria above.

Low-grade gliomas

According to the WHO histopathologic grading, gliomas are classified as pilocytic (grade I), low grade (grade II), and high grade or malignant, encompassing anaplastic gliomas (grade III) and glioblastomas (grade IV) [2]. WHO grade IV gliomas demonstrate microvascular proliferation and/or necrosis and, despite recent advances in treatment, patients have a median survival of less than 2 years [3]. Low-grade gliomas can further be subclassified by astrocytic, oligodendroglial, or mixed histology, reflecting the cell lineages of normal neural differentiation. This histologic differentiation has prognostic relevance, as evidenced by 5-year survival rates of 56% and 74%, respectively, for predominantly astrocytic versus predominantly oligodendroglial grade II gliomas [4]. Low-grade tumors are characteristically non-enhancing on MRI scans (Figure 1); indeed, the identification of contrast enhancement often raises the possibility of anaplastic transformation or malignant degeneration.

According to the Central Brain Tumor Registry of the United States (CBTRUS) 2010 statistical report on primary brain and central nervous system tumors, approximately 7,200 low-grade non-pilocytic astrocytomas, oligodendrogliomas, and mixed gliomas were diagnosed between 2004 and 2006, compared with approximately 27,000 glioblastomas [1]. As would be expected, low-grade gliomas are associated with a better prognosis than their high-grade counterparts. Nonetheless, these tumors are ultimately fatal in most patients, through an invasive growth pattern that impacts neurologic function, and malignant degeneration to a higher-grade lesion.

For high-grade malignant gliomas, carefully controlled cohort studies have demonstrated an independent contribution of maximal surgical resection to overall survival (OS) [5, 6]. However, molecular genetic studies of the alterations driving low-grade gliomas raise an important cautionary note when attempting to generalize these data from higher-grade tumor cohorts. Grade II gliomas are near-uniformly characterized by heterozygous mutation of the *IDH1* or *IDH2* genes [7-9]. *IDH* gene mutations are rarely seen in *de novo* high-grade gliomas, suggesting that grade II tumors do not 'progress' to become the lesions typically found in the higher grades [10]. The genetic alterations associated with progression of *IDH*-mutant tumors to a higher grade remain unknown.

Of course, this molecular observation only underscores what has been a longstanding clinical observation: a grade IV glioma arising from a

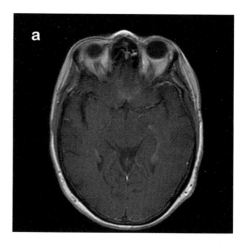

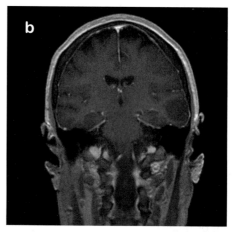

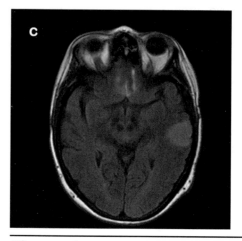

Figure 1. Figure 1. Preoperative contrast-enhanced a) axial and b) coronal T1-weighted images, and c) axial FLAIR images, demonstrating a non-enhancing tumor in the left temporal lobe of a 66-year-old woman, which was incidentally discovered during work-up for symptoms of positional vertigo. A gross total resection of the tumor was performed, with a pathologic diagnosis of grade II astrocytoma.

previously low-grade lesion – termed a 'secondary glioblastoma' – has a different natural history, and likely a different outcome when treated with surgery, radiation, or chemotherapy, compared with an *IDH*-wild-type primary glioblastoma. These molecular classifiers argue against routine clinical practice extending the results from randomized trials of glioblastomas (which are typically >95% primary glioblastomas, and thus *IDH*-wild type) to lower-grade tumors. For instance, the Phase III trial data supporting the use of combined radiation and temozolomide for glioblastomas might be favored as a rationale to treat lower-grade lesions with temozolomide [11]. However, given the different molecular genetic alterations within these tumors, this extension of clinical practice would not be evidence-based.

Six reasons are generally advanced in favor of more extensive surgery for low-grade gliomas:

- To decrease mass effect and improve neurologic function.
- To improve histologic sampling and increase diagnostic accuracy.
- To prevent or alleviate seizures.
- To prevent or delay malignant transformation.
- To improve progression-free survival (PFS) (and thus avoid further treatment with radiation or chemotherapy and their associated side effects).
- To improve OS.

However, more extensive surgery carries greater short-term risk, and thus the above considerations must be balanced against the following:

- Surgery may damage tumor-infiltrated normal neurologic pathways. These iatrogenic neurologic deficits can negatively impact outcome.
- The effects of surgery must be compared against less invasive treatment options, such as radiotherapy or chemotherapy.

The natural history of low-grade gliomas in the absence of surgery is not definitively known, especially in the modern era, when many lesions are

discovered incidentally in the absence of neurologic symptoms. Thus, there is no appropriate control cohort for comparison to determine the true impact of surgical intervention on the course of this malignancy.

It is nearly impossible to design a randomized trial of surgical resection for low-grade glioma due to the highly individualized nature of treatment. Thus, the best available evidence supporting extensive surgical resection comes from the examination of prognostic factors in prospective radiation treatment trials of low-grade gliomas, and through careful retrospective analyses of surgical case series, as described below.

Prospective data

There have been four large, prospective, multicenter trials of different radiation treatment regimens in low-grade gliomas (Table 1) [4, 12-14, 15, 16]. Although none of these trials was specifically designed to independently assess the contribution of surgical resection to patient outcomes, these studies nonetheless offer information collected in a prospective fashion on closely followed and uniformly treated patients.

Before reviewing these studies, it is important to clarify their limitations in assessing the impact of surgical resection on patient survival. One significant limitation is that each study used intraoperative surgeon impression to assess EOR, which does not have good correlation with postoperative MRI evaluations [14, 17]. EOR has been classically estimated as a percentage of removal, for example, less than 50% or 90-100%. With high-resolution MRI, EOR can now be more accurately calculated as the percentage of preoperative tumor volumetrically removed versus the postoperative scan.

More importantly, because there was no randomization, surgical resection in these studies could not be assessed as an isolated variable due to the close association with preoperative patient and tumor characteristics. The decision of whether to recommend surgery and the EOR is, by necessity, closely associated with patient factors such as age and performance status, and preoperative tumor

Table 1. Summary of prospective trials in low-grade glioma.

Reference	Description	n	Extent of resection	Main finding	Comment	Evidence level/ recommendation
Karim *et al*, 1996 [12]	An RCT comparing radiotherapy dosage in patients with supratentorial LGG (EORTC 22844)	343	Non-volumetric (estimated at the time of surgery)	EOR was predictive of outcome in both PFS and OS in both univariate and multivariate analyses	EOR coded as minimal/biopsy (<50%), bulk removal (50-89%), or total (90-100%)	III/B
Shaw *et al*, 2002 [4]	Analyzed data from NCCTG, RTOG, and ECOG	203	Method of determination not specified	GTR was associated with prolonged PFS in univariate and multivariate analyses	EOR coded as total, subtotal, or biopsy	III/B
Pignatti *et al*, 2002 [16]	Analyzed data from EORTC 22844 to determine prognostic variables in patients with supratentorial LGGs and validated the results with data from EORTC 22845	Statistical model constructed from EORTC 22844 (n=322) Model validated on EORTC 22845 (n=288)	Non-volumetric (estimated at the time of surgery)	Extensive (90-100%) EOR was positively associated with outcome in univariate but not multivariate analyses	These are the same data as from Karim *et al*, 1996 [12] (see above), but validated on EORTC 22845 EOR binarily coded as: extensive (90-100%) or non-extensive (<90%)	III/B
Shaw *et al*, 2008 [14]	Prospectively followed young patients (age <40 years) from RTOG protocol 9802 with neurosurgeon-determined GTR of LGG	111	MRI (pre- and postoperative images) to assess maximum residual tumor width	Residual tumor on postoperative MRI scan was negatively associated with PFS	Residual tumor coded as <1, 1-2, and >2cm	III/B

ECOG = European Cooperative Oncology Group; EOR = extent of resection; EORTC = European Organization for Research and Treatment of Cancer; GTR = gross total resection; LGG = low-grade glioma; NCCTG = North Central Cancer Treatment Group; OS = overall survival; PFS = progression-free survival; RCT = randomized control trial; RTOG = Radiation Therapy Oncology Group

features such as size and location relative to critical neurologic functional areas. For example, some neurosurgeons may limit the EOR in older patients with large tumors in eloquent regions of the brain to minimize the risk of postoperative neurologic deficit. Thus, although these studies provide some evidence supporting the impact of EOR on patient survival, their design precludes drawing causal relationships.

EORTC 22844/22845

The first two studies of note are the European Organisation for Research and Treatment of Cancer (EORTC) trials 22844 and 22845. These studies recruited 690 patients with low-grade cerebral astrocytoma, oligodendroglioma, or mixed oligoastrocytoma from 1985 to 1997. EORTC 22844 was a prospective, randomized, multicenter controlled trial primarily designed to compare the effects of low- and high-dose postoperative radiation in patients with low-grade glioma [12]. EORTC 22845 was a paired prospective, randomized, multicenter controlled trial designed to compare the outcomes between early versus delayed postoperative radiation in patients with low-grade glioma [13, 15, 16].

An initial report from EORTC 22844 at a minimum follow-up of 4.6 years analyzed 343 patients [12] **(III/B)**. Standard preoperative variables including age, performance status, tumor size, and histology, were assessed, along with neurosurgeon-determined EOR. The EOR was grouped as follows:

- Gross total resection (GTR) (90-100%).
- Subtotal resection (50-89%).
- Biopsy only (<50%).

When analyzed in both univariate and multivariate models, EOR was positively associated with both PFS and OS. In other words, patients with more tumor removed at surgery had longer PFS and OS. However, as previously mentioned, the EOR was not independently controlled in this study; therefore, its causal role in prolonging survival cannot be determined. Other factors that were prognostic in multivariate analyses were age, tumor size, histology, and neurologic status.

Illustrating this point in a further analysis, using a subset of 322 patients from the EORTC 22844 study, Pignatti *et al* assessed a wider array of clinical variables for their correspondence with outcome [16] **(III/B)**. In this case, however, EOR was grouped as a binary variable: biopsy to 89% resection versus 90-100% resection. Greater EOR was a significant predictor of OS in univariate analyses but was not significant in the final multivariate model, in accord with its close association with various preoperative factors. The final factors included in a prognostic scaling metric were age (>40 years), tumor diameter (>6cm), tumor crossing the midline, histology (astrocytic vs. oligodendroglial), and neurologic deficit. This model was then validated using OS data from 288 patients from EORTC 22845.

While EOR was not explicitly included in the final model, it was clearly related to three of the preoperative tumor and patient-specific features (i.e., tumor diameter, tumor crossing the midline, and neurologic deficit), all of which contributed to the final model. In particular, the investigators noted that both tumor crossing the midline (p=0.014) and tumor largest diameter (p=0.018) were closely associated with the EOR on multiple logistic regression. This observation further demonstrates the concept that EOR is not a truly independent variable, and thus its positive association with survival must be evaluated in this context.

NCCTG/RTOG/ECOG Intergroup

The North Central Cancer Treatment Group (NCCTG)/Radiation Therapy Oncology Group (RTOG)/Eastern Cooperative Oncology Group (ECOG) intergroup trial examined 203 patients with astrocytomas, oligodendrogliomas, or mixed oligoastrocytomas from 1986 to 1994, who were randomized to low-dose versus high-dose radiation [4] **(III/B)**. Although not part of the primary study design, EOR was used in both univariate and multivariate analyses to determine predictors of the various measures of outcome. In this study, the method used to determine EOR was not explicitly detailed, but EOR was ultimately classified as biopsy, subtotal resection, or GTR. The results showed that GTR was positively associated with PFS and OS in univariate analysis, and to PFS in exploratory multivariate models. These results are in accord with those from the EORTC analyses, but suffer from the same study limitations from confounding preoperative variables.

RTOG 9802

In a more recent prospective study, the RTOG protocol 9802 enrolled patients with low-grade gliomas from 1998 to 2002. Based on age and neurosurgeon-estimated EOR, patients in RTOG 9802 were dichotomized into low-risk and high-risk groups. Low-risk patients were younger than 40 years and had neurosurgeon-determined GTR. Patients in the low-risk group were then followed expectantly, while those in the high-risk group were treated with radiation alone or radiation in combination with chemotherapy. The findings in the low-risk portion of the study were the subject of a report by Shaw *et al* in 2008 [14]. One unique aspect of this study, which included the usual preoperative variables such as age, performance status, and tumor histology, was the assessment of pre- and postoperative MRI images. This allowed for a more objective assessment of postoperative residual tumor beyond the neurosurgeon-determined EOR. In this study, only 59% of postoperative MRI images were deemed to contain less than 1cm of residual tumor, suggesting that neurosurgeon estimates of EOR are not very accurate. The implication is that surgeon estimates of EOR from the previous studies may also be inaccurate, which could result in obscuring a true association of EOR with survival.

A potential benefit of this study is that by restricting enrollment to patients who only underwent surgeon-determined GTR, preoperative patient and tumor factors were less likely to influence EOR. Thus we can entertain a presumption of minimal bias, and an assessment of the impact of resection as an isolated factor can be attempted **(III/B)**. A similar logic was employed for higher-grade tumors, with a restratification analysis of the fluorescence-guided surgical trial data [6].

A total of 98 patients were prospectively followed in the low-risk group for a median period of 4.4 years. The usual prognostic factors such as age, performance status, and tumor histology, in addition to postoperative MRI-determined residual tumor, were assessed for their association with PFS and OS. The results showed that, in both univariate and multivariate analyses, patients with less than 1cm of postoperative residual tumor had significantly improved PFS. Because of the high OS in the low-risk group (99% at 2 years and 93% at 5 years), no prognostic factors reached statistical significance. This trial was the first prospective study to correlate MRI-determined residual tumor measurements with clinical outcome measures. By restricting patients in the study to those deemed by the neurosurgeon to have GTR, the positive association between surgery and PFS was less likely confounded by preoperative patient and tumor characteristics.

Summary of prospective data

Taken together, these studies demonstrate that reducing tumor volume at surgery, when pursued within the usual care of low-grade glioma patients, is associated with improved PFS and OS **(III/B)**. The positive association between tumor debulking and measures of survival should not be causally assumed, since the aforementioned study designs do not permit this type of assessment.

Retrospective studies

Because of the relative rarity of low-grade gliomas, an analysis of predictive factors from prospective trials suffers from the criticism of outdated practice by the time a study has accumulated enough cases for statistical significance. These criticisms stem from the following issues:

* Low-grade gliomas are increasingly discovered incidentally due to the broader utilization of MRI. Thus, these lesions are discovered earlier in their natural history than lesions studied in the past.
* In the last two decades, the risks of aggressive surgery have been substantially lowered by progressive improvements in intraoperative stereotactic navigation, functional cortical and subcortical mapping techniques [18-21], and intraoperative imaging techniques such as ultrasound [22] and MRI [23-25].
* Management of progressive disease with more effective chemotherapeutics, such as temozolomide and bevacizumab, has likely improved OS compared with earlier eras, potentially altering the impact of surgical resection on overall outcome.
* Incorporation of molecular typing information into pathologic classification has further sharpened the diagnostic categorization of these tumors, holding the potential to individualize treatment to subsets of patients who would maximally benefit from surgical resection compared with other treatment options such as radiotherapy or chemotherapy.

Table 2. Summary of retrospective trials in low-grade glioma.

Reference	Description	n	Extent of resection	Main finding	Comment	Evidence level/recommendation
Berger et al, 1994 [26]	Retrospective review of survival outcomes in patients with supratentorial LGG	53	Volumetric (CT and MRI)	EOR was negatively correlated with tumor progression Patients with 100% EOR had zero tumor recurrence during the study period (54 months)	Extent of resection volumetrically determined	III/B
Leighton et al, 1997 [27]	Retrospective review of survival outcomes in patients with supratentorial LGG	167	Non-volumetric (based on postoperative MRI and CT)	EOR was positively associated with OS in univariate and multivariate analyses	EOR coded as >90% or <90%	III/B
Smith et al, 2008 [28]	Retrospective review of survival outcomes in patients with supratentorial LGG	216	Volumetric (MRI)	Extent of resection was positively associated with PFS and OS		III/B
Chaichana et al, 2010 [29]	Retrospective review of survival outcomes in patients with supratentorial LGG	191	Non-volumetric (estimates of EOR based on MRI FLAIR signal)	GTR was negatively associated with malignant degeneration in both univariate and multivariate analyses GTR was negatively associated with tumor progression in univariate analyses	GTR was defined as zero post-operative MRI FLAIR signal; STR was defined as positive residual MRI FLAIR signal	III/B

EOR = extent of resection; GTR = gross total resection; LGG = low-grade glioma; OS = overall survival; PFS = progression-free survival; STR = subtotal resection

Well-designed retrospective studies can alleviate many of these concerns by reporting the outcomes of large patient groups cared for in single institutions over a relatively short period of time. This clinical practice setting enforces a strong standardization of care, as surgery is often performed by a single surgeon or small group of surgeons, and subsequent neuro-oncologic care adheres to a consistent practice pattern. Retrospective studies in low-grade gliomas are summarized in Table 2.

Berger *et al* were the first to demonstrate that imaging-determined volumetric EOR was associated with improved outcomes [26]. These investigators examined 53 patients from 1977 to 1990 in Seattle who had a minimum follow-up of 2 years after surgery and a histopathologic diagnosis of astrocytoma, oligodendroglioma, or oligoastrocytoma. Recurrence was seen in 10 of the 53 patients, with seven of these patients experiencing recurrence as a higher-grade

lesion. Patient subgroups were determined for preoperative (<10, 10-30, and >30cm^3) and residual (0, <10, and >10cm^3) tumor volumes and EOR (<50%, 50-89%, 90-99%, and 100%). In univariate analyses, smaller tumors, smaller residual volumes, and increased EOR were all associated with statistically significant increases in PFS. Interestingly, unlike the prospective trials noted above, age, histology, and postoperative treatment with radiotherapy did not demonstrate associations with PFS, perhaps due to the highly selected nature of the sample set [26] **(III/B)**.

Leighton *et al* examined 167 patients with low-grade glioma treated in Canada between 1979 and 1995 [27]. Though spanning a treatment era prior to the routine use of MRI, this retrospective study was well designed. Importantly, the authors restricted their analyses to just astrocytomas, oligodendrogliomas, and mixed tumors, explicitly excluding pilocytic astrocytomas or gemistocytic astrocytomas. Furthermore, the EOR was estimated by postoperative imaging, not surgeon-determined, and classified into two groups (minimal residual with >90% resected and bulky residual with <90% resected). Multivariate analyses identified age, histopathology, residual tumor, seizures, and performance status as factors predictive of OS [27] **(III/B)**.

Continuing the work from Berger *et al*, Smith *et al* examined 216 patients with low-grade glioma who underwent surgical resection in California between 1989 and 2005 [28]. Patients who only underwent biopsy were excluded from the analysis. Again, volumetric MRI imaging techniques were used to determine the residual tumor volume and EOR. Recognizing the potential for close association between tumor size and EOR, separate multivariate Cox proportional hazard models were generated for OS, PFS, and malignant PFS (MPFS). EOR was predictive of OS, and log preoperative tumor volume was predictive of PFS and MPFS in these multivariate analyses [28] **(III/B)**.

Examining 191 consecutive patients treated from 1996 to 2006 in Baltimore, Chaichana *et al* assessed predictors of PFS and MPFS in patients with grade II oligodendrogliomas, astrocytomas, and mixed tumors [29]. Biopsy patients were excluded because of the likelihood that histologic diagnostic sampling would prove inadequate. EOR was determined by comparison of preoperative MRI with postoperative imaging. GTR was defined as no residual MRI signal. In univariate analysis, GTR was positively associated with PFS. In univariate and multivariate analyses, GTR was positively associated with MPFS. Similar to other authors, these investigators reported a tight association between tumor size and GTR [29]. McGirt *et al* examined a subset of these patients, classifying EOR in 170

patients as GTR (38%), near total resection (<3mm rim of FLAIR residual, 23%), and subtotal resection (39%). Comparing the two extremes of GTR versus subtotal resection in a multivariate model, GTR was associated with longer OS and PFS [30] **(III/B)**.

Summary of retrospective data

Results from retrospective single-institution studies from the modern era are consistent with earlier prospective data. These newer retrospective studies were performed in the era of increased use of MRI imaging and utilized newer chemotherapeutic agents. The consensus from the retrospective studies presented is that surgical EOR is positively associated with improved PFS and OS in low-grade glioma patients **(III/B)**. However, as mentioned previously, the positive association between tumor debulking and measures of survival should not be causally assumed, since the study designs do not permit this type of assessment.

Conclusions

No randomized controlled trials have independently isolated EOR as a tested variable in patients with low-grade gliomas. As such, inferences about EOR in prolonging survival must be indirectly made from its correlation with various measures of survival. With this in mind, many high-quality prospective and retrospective studies have demonstrated a positive association between EOR and survival. Given that a randomized controlled trial is unlikely to occur, assessments of the role of EOR on survival must be based on the findings from prospective and retrospective studies. Therefore, insofar as it can be safely performed, the initial management of a low-grade glioma should include maximal surgical resection **(III/B)**.

Recommendations	Evidence level
◆ No randomized controlled trials have independently assessed EOR in patients with low-grade gliomas.	-
◆ Several major well-designed prospective and retrospective studies have shown that a greater EOR is positively associated with survival.	III/B

References

1. Central Brain Tumor Registry of the United States. 2009-2010 CBTRUS Statistical Report: Primary Brain and Central Nervous System Tumors Diagnosed in the United States in 2004-2006. 2010. Available from www.cbtrus.org.
2. Louis DN, Ohgaki H, Wiestler OD, *et al*. The 2007 WHO classification of tumours of the central nervous system. *Acta Neuropathol* 2007; 114(2): 97-109.
3. Stupp R, Hegi ME, Mason WP, *et al*. Effects of radiotherapy with concomitant and adjuvant temozolomide versus radiotherapy alone on survival in glioblastoma in a randomised Phase III study: 5-year analysis of the EORTC-NCIC trial. *Lancet Oncol* 2009; 10(5): 459-66.
4. Shaw E, Arusell R, Scheithauer B, *et al*. Prospective randomized trial of low- versus high-dose radiation therapy in adults with supratentorial low-grade glioma: initial report of a North Central Cancer Treatment Group/Radiation Therapy Oncology Group/Eastern Cooperative Oncology Group study. *J Clin Oncol* 2002 1; 20(9): 2267-76.
5. Vuorinen V, Hinkka S, Farkkila M, Jaaskelainen J. Debulking or biopsy of malignant glioma in elderly people - a randomised study. *Acta Neurochir* (Wien) 2003; 145(1): 5-10.
6. Stummer W, Reulen HJ, Meinel T, *et al*. Extent of resection and survival in glioblastoma multiforme: identification of and adjustment for bias. *Neurosurgery* 2008; 62(3): 564-76.
7. Parsons DW, Jones S, Zhang X, *et al*. An integrated genomic analysis of human glioblastoma multiforme. *Science* 2008; 321(5897): 1807-12.
8. Balss J, Meyer J, Mueller W, Korshunov A, Hartmann C, von Deimling A. Analysis of the *IDH1* codon 132 mutation in brain tumors. *Acta Neuropathol* 2008; 116(6): 597-602.
9. Yan H, Parsons DW, Jin G, *et al*. *IDH1* and *IDH2* mutations in gliomas. *N Engl J Med* 2009; 360(8): 765-73.
10. Nobusawa S, Watanabe T, Kleihues P, Ohgaki H. *IDH1* mutations as molecular signature and predictive factor of secondary glioblastomas. *Clin Cancer Res* 2009; 15(19): 6002-7.
11. Stupp R, Mason WP, van den Bent MJ, *et al*. Radiotherapy plus concomitant and adjuvant temozolomide for glioblastoma. *N Engl J Med* 2005; 352(10): 987-96.
12. Karim AB, Maat B, Hatlevoll R, *et al*. A randomized trial on dose-response in radiation therapy of low-grade cerebral glioma: European Organization for Research and Treatment of Cancer (EORTC) Study 22844. *Int J Radiat Oncol Biol Phys* 1996; 36(3): 549-56.
13. van den Bent MJ, Afra D, de Witte O, *et al*. Long-term efficacy of early versus delayed radiotherapy for low-grade astrocytoma and oligodendroglioma in adults: the EORTC 22845 randomised trial. *Lancet* 2005; 366(9490): 985-90.
14. Shaw EG, Berkey B, Coons SW, *et al*. Recurrence following neurosurgeon-determined gross-total resection of adult supratentorial low-grade glioma: results of a prospective clinical trial. *J Neurosurg* 2008; 109(5): 835-41.
15. Karim AB, Afra D, Cornu P, *et al*. Randomized trial on the efficacy of radiotherapy for cerebral low-grade glioma in the adult: European Organization for Research and Treatment of Cancer Study 22845 with the Medical Research Council study BRO4: an interim analysis. *Int J Radiat Oncol Biol Phys* 2002; 52(2): 316-24.
16. Pignatti F, van den Bent M, Curran D, *et al*. Prognostic factors for survival in adult patients with cerebral low-grade glioma. *J Clin Oncol* 2002; 20(8): 2076-84.
17. Nazzaro JM, Neuwelt EA. The role of surgery in the management of supratentorial intermediate and high-grade astrocytomas in adults. *J Neurosurg* 1990; 73(3): 331-44.
18. Duffau H, Capelle L, Denvil D, *et al*. Usefulness of intraoperative electrical subcortical mapping during surgery for low-grade gliomas located within eloquent brain regions: functional results in a consecutive series of 103 patients. *J Neurosurg* 2003; 98(4): 764-78.
19. Duffau H, Peggy Gatignol ST, Mandonnet E, Capelle L, Taillandier L. Intraoperative subcortical stimulation mapping of language pathways in a consecutive series of 115 patients with Grade II glioma in the left dominant hemisphere. *J Neurosurg* 2008; 109(3): 461-71.
20. Sanai N, Mirzadeh Z, Berger MS. Functional outcome after language mapping for glioma resection. *N Engl J Med* 2008; 358(1): 18-27.
21. Kim SS, McCutcheon IE, Suki D, *et al*. Awake craniotomy for brain tumors near eloquent cortex: correlation of intraoperative cortical mapping with neurological outcomes in 309 consecutive patients. *Neurosurgery* 2009; 64(5): 836-45; discussion 345-6.
22. Le Roux PD, Berger MS, Wang K, Mack LA, Ojemann GA. Low grade gliomas: comparison of intraoperative ultrasound characteristics with preoperative imaging studies. *J Neurooncol* 1992; 13(2): 189-98.
23. Claus EB, Horlacher A, Hsu L, *et al*. Survival rates in patients with low-grade glioma after intraoperative magnetic resonance image guidance. *Cancer* 2005; 103(6): 1227-33.

Chapter 21

Chapter 21

24. Hatiboglu MA, Weinberg JS, Suki D, *et al*. Impact of intraoperative high-field magnetic resonance imaging guidance on glioma surgery: a prospective volumetric analysis. *Neurosurgery* 2009; 64(6): 1073-81.

25. Gasco J, Tummala S, Mahajan NM, Weinberg JS, Prabhu SS. Simultaneous use of functional tractography, neuronavigation-integrated subcortical white matter stimulation and intraoperative magnetic resonance imaging in glioma surgery: technical note. *Stereotact Funct Neurosurg* 2009; 87(6): 395-8.

26. Berger MS, Deliganis AV, Dobbins J, Keles GE. The effect of extent of resection on recurrence in patients with low grade cerebral hemisphere gliomas. *Cancer* 1994; 74(6): 1784-91.

27. Leighton C, Fisher B, Bauman G, *et al*. Supratentorial low-grade glioma in adults: an analysis of prognostic factors and timing of radiation. *J Clin Oncol* 1997; 15(4): 1294-301.

28. Smith JS, Chang EF, Lamborn KR, *et al*. Role of extent of resection in the long-term outcome of low-grade hemispheric gliomas. *J Clin Oncol* 2008; 26(8): 1338-45.

29. Chaichana KL, McGirt MJ, Laterra J, Olivi A, Quinones-Hinojosa A. Recurrence and malignant degeneration after resection of adult hemispheric low-grade gliomas. *J Neurosurg* 2010; 112(1): 10-7.

30. McGirt MJ, Chaichana KL, Attenello FJ, *et al*. Extent of surgical resection is independently associated with survival in patients with hemispheric infiltrating low-grade gliomas. *Neurosurgery* 2008; 63(4): 700-7.

Introduction

Pediatric neurosurgery

Edward R Smith MD

Director, Pediatric Cerebrovascular Surgery 1;

Associate Professor of Surgery 2

1 DEPARTMENT OF NEUROSURGERY, CHILDREN'S HOSPITAL BOSTON, MASSACHUSETTS, USA
2 HARVARD MEDICAL SCHOOL, BOSTON, MASSACHUSETTS, USA

As surgeons, we are obliged to obtain informed consent before performing a procedure. We share our knowledge about the goals of the surgery, potential risks, and alternative approaches with our patients so that they know what to expect from the operation. While important, these discussions often occur after a decision has been made to embark upon a specific course of treatment. What is lacking – both for patients and physicians – is a clear understanding of the evidence that leads to choosing the treatment in the first place.

This book is designed to better our understanding of what currently exists – and to identify what gaps remain – in the evidence that guides our clinical decision-making in neurosurgery. Challenges to evidence-guided practice in neurosurgery are numerous, and the subspecialty of pediatric neurosurgery shares many of the problems well known to other fields, while also facing issues unique to the care of children with neurosurgical disease. Similar to our colleagues treating adult patients, we have small numbers of patients relative to other disciplines of medicine. We frequently rely on surrogate measures of outcome (e.g., angiographic obliteration of arteriovenous malformations as a measure of rebleeding risk, reduction in ventricle size as a measure of intracranial pressure, improved urodynamic parameters as a measure of spinal cord tethering) and there is a paucity of randomized controlled trials that address questions in need of answers.

Compounding these shared issues are the difficulties unique to treating a pediatric population. Attempts to measure outcomes are challenging enough when the goal is a return to baseline prior to the onset of illness. The ability to compare outcomes between different treatments is substantially more complicated when the baseline is dynamically changing in the setting of a developing child – in essence, moving the finish line while running the race. The inability of young children to adequately articulate the effects of illness or the changes resulting from interventions adds a remarkable level of complexity to the already difficult task of assessing the burden of disease or the efficacy of treatment. Paradoxically, the remarkable plasticity of the childhood nervous system may obscure treatment effect. It may be unclear if recovery is primarily the result of a specific intervention (or lack thereof) or due to the inherent regenerative capacity of a child's brain. Long-term follow-up to adequately assess delayed effects on development, late-term recurrences, and unforeseen complications is of paramount importance in the pediatric population. Lastly, clinical studies are often logistically more demanding with minors, frequently requiring additional stipulations, protections, and consents, which can serve as obstacles to recruiting and completing trials.

Yet, despite these challenges, some laudable efforts have been made. The most common problem faced by pediatric neurosurgeons – hydrocephalus – has recently been the subject of a series of well-designed clinical trials. Endoscopic shunt placement and shunt design trials stand as examples of attempts to better administer treatments for this remarkably frustrating condition [1-3]. The ongoing Management of Myelomeningocele Study stands as another effort of pediatric neurosurgeons to develop evidence-based practice patterns by using a multicenter approach to tackle a distinct childhood problem [4]. Some of the greatest successes in evidence-based neurosurgery have come from the study of pediatric brain tumors, such as medulloblastoma; while other pediatric conditions – such as Chiari malformations – remain among the most controversial in all of neurosurgery.

This section on pediatric neurosurgery seeks to review these four conditions: hydrocephalus, Chiari malformations, myelomeningocele, and medulloblastoma. They are among the most common entities faced by practitioners in this field and are thus important in their own right. They also serve to highlight some of the successes – and failures – of efforts to develop evidence-based guidelines for treatment. The authors of these chapters are experts in their fields and bring a wealth of experience to bear on this spectrum of disease. It is hoped that these authoritative reviews will serve to clarify the best knowledge that currently exists in these critical areas, illuminating the path toward more informed – and effective – treatments for children afflicted with these conditions.

References

1. Drake JM, Kestle JR, Milner R, *et al*. Randomized trial of cerebrospinal fluid shunt valve design in pediatric hydrocephalus. *Neurosurgery* 1998; 43: 294-303; discussion 303-5.
2. Kestle JR, Drake JM, Cochrane DD, *et al*. Lack of benefit of endoscopic ventriculoperitoneal shunt insertion: a multicenter randomized trial. *J Neurosurg* 2003; 98: 284-90.
3. Kestle J, Drake J, Milner R, *et al*. Long-term follow-up data from the Shunt Design Trial. *Pediatr Neurosurg* 2000; 33: 230-6.
4. Sutton LN. Fetal surgery for neural tube defects. *Best Pract Res Clin Obstet Gynaecol* 2008; 22: 175-88.

Introduction

Chapter 22

Chiari I malformation in children

Todd C Hankinson MD MBA, Assistant Professor of Neurosurgery 1
R Shane Tubbs PhD PA-C, Researcher 2
John C Wellons III MD, Associate Professor 3

1 CHILDREN'S HOSPITAL COLORADO, UNIVERSITY OF COLORADO DENVER, AURORA, COLORADO, USA
2 CHILDREN'S OF ALABAMA, BIRMINGHAM, ALABAMA, USA
3 DIVISION OF NEUROSURGERY; DIVISION OF PEDIATRIC NEUROSURGERY, CHILDREN'S OF ALABAMA, UNIVERSITY OF ALABAMA BIRMINGHAM, BIRMINGHAM, ALABAMA, USA

Introduction

Chiari malformation type I (CM1) is characterized by a varying degree of herniation of the cerebellar tonsils through the foramen magnum, generally greater than 5mm (Figure 1). This condition may be found incidentally or present through myriad symptom complexes. Headache is the most common presenting symptom, while hydrocephalus is encountered in less than 10% of patients. One common presentation is scoliosis, which is found in 10-20% of these patients. Syringomyelia, which may or may not be the underlying etiology of the scoliosis, is present in 12-85% of patients [1-3] (Figure 2). Barring a reversible underlying cause in acquired cases (e.g., those secondary to hydrocephalus), surgery is the only effective treatment for symptomatic patients.

If hydrocephalus is present, cerebrospinal fluid (CSF) diversion through ventriculoperitoneal shunt or endoscopic third ventriculostomy [4] should be completed prior to any other surgical intervention. In the absence of hydrocephalus, the first-line surgical management for CM1 is posterior fossa

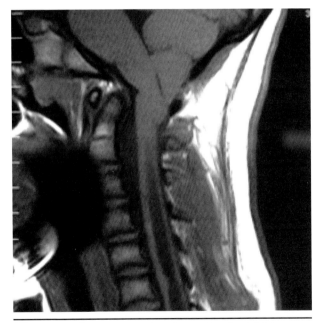

Figure 1. T1-weighted sagittal MRI scan demonstrating a Chiari malformation type I with morphologic changes of the cerebellar tonsils and cervical syringomyelia.

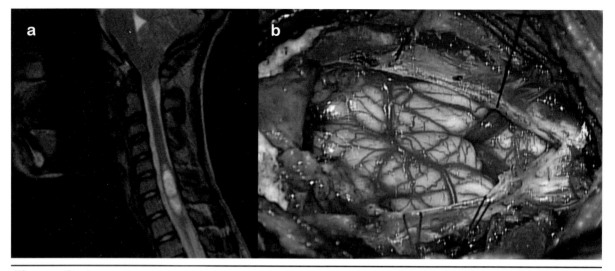

Figure 2. a) T2-weighted sagittal MRI scan demonstrating a Chiari malformation type I with cervical syringomyelia. b) Intraoperative photograph demonstrating the appearance of the cerebellar tonsils and dorsal craniocervical junction after dural opening.

decompression through a midline suboccipital craniectomy and removal of the dorsal arch of the atlas with or without dural opening. This chapter discusses the current literature regarding the role of opening the dura as a component of posterior fossa decompression, an area of debate in pediatric neurosurgery. When dural opening with duraplasty is chosen, the surgeon may elect to perform further maneuvers, such as cerebellar tonsillar reduction or resection. The surgeon may also select not to close the dura. Despite the fact that all of these techniques have been individually reported with favorable outcomes [5-8], few studies have directly compared dural opening with and without additional intradural maneuvers [6, 8]. This chapter, therefore, does not specifically address decision-making with regard to the completion of further intradural maneuvers after dural opening. It instead focuses on the current literature examining outcomes following posterior fossa decompression without dural opening (PFD) compared with posterior fossa decompression with duraplasty (PFDD).

Brief overview of surgical technique

For PFD or PFDD, the patient is positioned prone with the head in a neutral position and the neck flexed. For PFDD, the incision generally extends from a point just below the inion to the spinous process of C2. For PFD, a shorter incision (approximately 5cm) centered on the occipitocervical junction may be employed. For both procedures, the avascular plane (nuchal ligament) between the paraspinous muscles is followed down to the bone and a subperiosteal dissection is then performed. A moderate suboccipital craniectomy, often the width of the foramen magnum, is completed along with removal of the dorsal arch of the atlas. If dural opening is not performed (PFD), some surgeons will close at this point; others will open or split the outer layer of the dura to promote some degree of dural relaxation. Ultrasound may be used to assess tonsillar mobility if the dura is not opened. When dural opening is performed (PFDD), all layers of the dura are opened.

In our institution, the opened arachnoid is clipped to the dural edge. Arachnoid adhesions or veils potentially obstructing the outflow of CSF from the foramen of Magendie [9] are removed and the floor of the fourth ventricle is examined. A portion of the occipital pericranium is harvested through a separate incision and duraplasty is completed. The wound is closed in anatomic layers.

Methodology

A Medline-Ovid search was completed using each of the terms 'Chiari malformation,' 'syringomyelia,' 'syrinx,' and 'syringohydromyelia' in combination with 'child' or 'pediatric.' Relevant papers were identified and their reference lists were manually reviewed. Publications were considered relevant if they reported the results of PFD or PFDD for the surgical treatment of CM1 in a population of patients younger than 18 years. Studies in which a large majority of patients were treated using methods other than PFD or PFDD were excluded unless the results of the subset of patients treated with PFD or PFDD could be readily extracted.

The included studies were divided into three categories based upon the surgical techniques studied. The first group of papers included works that directly compared PFD with PFDD. The second group included studies in which all patients were treated with PFD. The third group included studies in which all patients were treated with PFDD. Three outcome parameters were assessed:

- Improvement of clinical signs/symptoms.
- Syrinx resolution.
- Scoliosis progression.

Studies comparing dural opening with non-dural opening

At this time, there is no level I or IIa evidence comparing PFD with PFDD. Among the studies that have directly compared the two surgical techniques, there are two published surveys [10, 11] **(IV/C)** and a meta-analysis [12] that is composed of five retrospective cohort studies [6, 8, 13-15] and two prospective cohort studies [16, 17] **(IIb/B)** (Table 1).

Table 1. Rates of symptom and syrinx improvement and reoperation in studies including both PFD and PFDD.

Reference	n	Dural opening	Clinical improvement, n (%)	Syrinx improvement, n (%)	Scoliosis stable/improvement, n (%)
Munshi et al, 2000 [14]	11	N	8 (72.7)	3 (50.0, n=6)	NR
	21[a]	Y	18 (85.7)	7 (63.6, n=11)	NR
Ventureyra et al, 2003 [15]	6	N	4 (66.7)	0 (0, n=2)	NR
	10	Y	10 (100)	5 (100, n=5)	NR
Navarro et al, 2004 [8]	56[b]	N	40[b] (72.2)	NR	NR
	24[b]	Y	16[b] (68.4)	NR	NR
	29[b]	Y[c]	17[b] (60.8)	NR	NR
Limonadi et al, 2004 [16]	12	N	1.67[d]	NR	NR
	12	Y	1.53[d]	7 (70, n=10)	NR
Yeh et al, 2006 [17]	40	N	36 (90.0)	4 (66.7)	1 (100)
	85	Y	83 (97.6)	17 (85)	9 (100)
Galarza et al, 2007 [6]	20	N	4 (33.3, n=12)	2 (40, n=5)	NR
	21	Y	11 (73.3, n=15)	0 (0, n=2)	NR
	19	Y[c]	8 (88.9, n=9)	7 (100, n=7)	NR

[a] = dural opening as initial procedure; [b] = extrapolated from percentages; [c] = with intradural maneuvers; [d] = aggregate scoring system with range from -1 to 2, with 2 = all preoperative symptoms resolved (p=not significant); NR = not reported

Durham and Fjeld-Olenec concluded there was no statistically significant difference in clinical outcomes between the PFD and PFDD populations, specifically with regard to symptom improvement and syringomyelia [12]. In summary, rates of clinical improvement were 65% in the PFD patients and 79% in the PFDD patients. Rates of radiologic syrinx improvement were influenced by small numbers in some studies, but were 56% in the PFD patients and 87% in those undergoing PFDD. The authors were able to conclude that patients who undergo duraplasty are less likely to require reoperation (2.1% vs. 12.6%) for persistent or recurrent symptoms, but are more likely to suffer CSF-related complications (18.5% vs. 1.8%). The authors also acknowledged their conclusions were limited by the patient selection methods of the studies they examined. Specifically, five papers used intraoperative ultrasound to help determine whether to perform a dural opening [8, 13, 15-17]. The inherent subjectivity of this technique limits the degree to which the findings of each work may be generalized. In addition, no study included a randomization or blinding process.

Reporting expert opinion through a survey of attendees at the 1998 annual meeting of the pediatric section of the American Association of Neurological Surgeons **(IV/C)**, Haroun et al reported that 25% of respondents would perform PFD for children with symptomatic CM1, while 32% recommended PFDD and 55% recommended PFDD with further intradural manipulations, such as tonsillar manipulation (some respondents chose more than one intervention) [10]. International survey data published by Schijman and Steinbok demonstrated that 76% of pediatric neurosurgeons always open the dura mater when treating CM1 [11] **(IV/C)**.

Studies of PFD without dural opening

There is significant literature retrospectively examining the results of PFD and PFDD. As previously stated, outcomes may be assessed through three general categories: clinical improvement, syrinx resolution, and scoliosis progression.

As mentioned previously, multiple groups have employed intraoperative ultrasound as a tool to help guide their decision-making with regard to dural opening in children with CM1 [8, 17-20]. Three studies have provided electrophysiologic evidence that neurologic improvement can be achieved without a dural opening [20-22] **(III/B)**. These authors found that improved conduction of nerve impulses through the brain stem occurs following bony decompression rather than after dural opening. Yeh et al reported that factors associated with adequate decompression without duraplasty included age younger than 1 year [17]. Factors that were more likely to be associated with the need for duraplasty included spinal symptoms (motor, sensory, or scoliosis) and a greater magnitude of tonsillar descent at presentation.

Clinical outcome

Most studies that have reported rates of clinical and radiologic improvement following PFD also included patients who were treated with PFDD and are therefore referenced in the preceding section. Two Italian reports demonstrated excellent results in retrospective series of patients who underwent PFD alone [23, 24] **(III/B)**. Genitori et al performed PFD in 26 patients [24]. A total of 16 patients (61.5%) did not have syringomyelia. Thirteen of these (81.3%) experienced complete symptom resolution and the remaining three (18.8%) experienced partial resolution following PFD. Among the 10 patients with syringomyelia (38.5%), symptoms improved or resolved in all cases with the exception of one of three cases of scoliosis (33.3%) and one of five cases of sensory loss (20%). Rates of complete symptom resolution ranged from 25% (sensory loss) to 100% (vertigo). Two patients (7.7%) required reoperation. In a retrospective review of their experience using PFD to treat 30 children with CM1, Caldarelli et al reported that 28 patients (93.3%) demonstrated a significant improvement in their clinical condition after 4.7 years of follow-up [23].

Syrinx resolution

As previously mentioned, in the series of Genitori et al, 10 of 26 patients (38.5%) presented with syringomyelia [24]. Following PFD, complete syrinx resolution occurred in eight patients (80%). The remaining two children (20%) had an initial clinical improvement but suffered persistent syringomyelia and underwent PFDD. Caldarelli *et al* reported that 12 of 30 patients (40%) presented with syringomyelia [23]. Postoperatively, six of these patients (50%) experienced a decrease in the size of the syrinx. Two patients (16.7%) demonstrated recurrent symptoms and postoperative syrinx growth (one *de novo* and another who had a syrinx preoperatively) and required reoperation. The authors argued that radiologic change (either in syrinx size or posterior fossa subarachnoid volume) was not mandatory for a successful result if the presenting signs and symptoms are significantly improved. Wetjen *et al* also argued that the absence of syrinx distention is more important than complete collapse [25].

In the PFD groups of the studies included in their meta-analysis, Durham and Fjeld-Olenec reported an aggregate 56.3% rate of syrinx reduction (nine of 16 patients), which was not statistically different from the 87% rate (40 of 46 patients) calculated for the PFDD group in their analysis [12] **(IIb/B)**.

Scoliosis improvement

Very few patients with scoliosis who have undergone PFD have been reported. In the previously discussed Italian studies, Genitori *et al* reported improvement in two of three patients [24] and Caldarelli *et al* reported mild improvement in two of two patients [23]. In their series of 21 patients with CM1, syringomyelia and scoliosis, Attenello *et al* described a single patient who underwent PFD [26]. This patient had progression of scoliosis and underwent reoperation with duraplasty.

Studies of PFD with dural opening

As previously mentioned, there is significant literature describing the application of PFDD for the treatment of CM1. Most of the data are retrospective and from single institutions **(III/B)**.

Clinical outcome

Tubbs *et al* reported relief of preoperative symptoms in 83% of 130 patients treated with PFDD [3]. Headache persisted to some extent in 12% and perioperative complications occurred in 2.3%. In smaller series using PFDD (with or without further intradural manipulation), clinical improvement ranges from 92% to 100% with reported complication rates of 0-16.7% [7, 21, 22, 27-32]. In a retrospective study comparing duraplasty materials (autograft vs. synthetic allograft), Attenello *et al* reported mild to moderate symptom recurrence at 16 months' follow-up in 14 out of 67 patients (20.9%), with four of these patients (6%) requiring revision decompression. Pseudomeningocele was identified radiographically in 10 patients (17%), but only one became symptomatic. A total of five patients (7%) suffered CSF-related complications: two (3%) with CSF leak and two (3%) with aseptic meningitis [33].

Syrinx resolution

There is a wide range of reported improvement rates (55-100%) with regard to syringomyelia following PFDD for CM1 [7, 18, 21, 22, 27, 29, 31-33]. This variability is likely multifactorial, but small sample sizes and the lack of a standard definition of 'syrinx improvement' are certainly significant contributing factors. As previously mentioned, Durham and Fjeld-Olenec [12] calculated an overall rate of 87% syrinx reduction in the PFDD arms of studies that directly compared PFD with PFDD.

In the report from Tubbs *et al*, only eight of 75 syringes (10.7%) failed to improve following PFDD [3]. Seven of these (87.5%) improved with repeat PFDD [34] **(III/B)**. No radiographic parameters predicted failure of syrinx response. In a retrospective review of 49 consecutive cases (46 PFDD, three PFD), Attenello *et al* reported a 55% syrinx improvement rate 14 months postoperatively [18]. A total of 26 patients (56.5%) in the PFDD group had syrinx improvement, while one of three who underwent PFD improved. Overall, five patients (10.2%) required repeat decompression; one (2%) due to syrinx expansion at 5 months after PFDD. Complications included aseptic meningitis and wound

Table 2. Postoperative outcome of scoliosis in children with CM1.

Reference	n	Age	Surgical procedure	Curve stabilization, n (%)	Curve improvement, n (%)	Curve progression, n (%)	Spinal fusion, n (%)
Muhonen et al, 1992 [46]	11	10.1	PFDD + TOD	1 (9)	8 (73)	2 (18)	1 (9)
Isu et al, 1992 [38]	6	NR	NR	2 (33)	4 (67)	0	0
Ghanem et al, 1997 [44]	7	10.3	PFDD	1 (14)	1 (14)	5 (72)	5 (72)
Hida et al, 1999 [45]	13	10.2	PFDD + SSS	5 (38)	5 (38)	3 (23)	3 (23)
Sengupta et al, 2000 [48]	16	11	PFDD	1 (6)	5 (31)	10 (63)	8 (50)
Eule et al, 2002 [41]	8	NR	PFDD	1 (13)	4 (50)	3 (37)	0
Farley et al, 2002 [42]	9	8	PFDD + SSS	3 (33)	0	6 (67)	5 (56)
Özerdemoglu et al, 2003 [47]	18	16.9	PFD/PFDD + SSS	3 (17)	7 (39)	8 (44)	3 (17)
Brockmeyer et al, 2003 [40]	21	8.7	PFDD	4 (19)	9 (43)	8 (38)	4 (19)
Flynn et al, 2004 [43]	15	9.0	PFD/PFDD + SSS	4 (27)	2 (13)	9 (60)	7 (47)

CM1 = Chiari malformation type I; NR = not reported; PFD = posterior fossa decompression; SSS = syringosubarachnoid shunt; TOD = transoral decompression

breakdown in two patients (4%) each and pseudomeningocele in one patient (2%). None of these complications required reoperation.

An area that merits additional investigation is the expected interval and magnitude of syrinx collapse following PFD or PFDD. Although a subjectively significant decrease in syrinx size on the first postoperative imaging examination is reassuring to the surgeon, complete resolution of the fluid collection is likely unnecessary [23, 25] and syringes may dissipate after a prolonged interval [35].

Scoliosis progression

Scoliosis in the context of CM1 is usually associated with syringomyelia [36]. The causal relationship between syringomyelia and scoliosis is incompletely understood, but it has been postulated that lower motor neuron injury secondary to compression from syrinx expansion imbalances innervation to the trunk musculature, predisposing the patient to scoliosis [37-39]. Consistent with this theory, multiple authors have reported scoliosis improvement or stabilization following PFDD in children with CM1 (Table 2). In retrospective studies of patients treated primarily with PFDD, rates of scoliosis improvement are 0-73% and rates of progression are 18-72% [3, 40-48]. This demonstrates that CM1 treatment may slow or halt scoliosis progression in some cases, although there remains a considerable risk of progression (III/B).

In some series, children younger than 8-10 years have been less likely to suffer from scoliosis progression [40, 41, 46-48]. While a smaller presenting Cobb angle has been associated with superior outcomes, Brockmeyer et al reported that a decrease in syrinx size did not necessarily correlate with scoliosis improvement [40]. In 20 pediatric patients with CM1-associated scoliosis treated by PFDD, Attenello et al reported similar proportions, 40% and 45%, respectively, improved and progressed [26]. The authors reported that an increased magnitude of scoliosis curve at presentation was predictive of scoliosis progression, as were thoracolumbar junction scoliosis and a lack of postoperative radiologic syrinx response.

Conclusions

Surgical decision-making for children with CM1 may be considered in two steps:

- When to operate.
- What operation to perform.

With increasing availability of MRI, neurosurgeons are asked to evaluate many asymptomatic and minimally symptomatic children with tonsillar herniation. In this asymptomatic population, a characteristic finding such as syringomyelia or scoliosis is generally required for surgical intervention to be indicated.

In a symptomatic patient with a symptom complex that is consistent with posterior fossa compression, surgical decompression is very likely to improve the condition. Similarly, children with CM1 and syringomyelia should generally be considered for surgical intervention regardless of their presenting symptoms.

Selection of the most appropriate surgical technique for CM1 is not yet guided by evidence that is stronger than level IIb and the balance of the evidence is level III. Consistent with this, there is considerable debate regarding which operative technique is most appropriate for children with CM1. Hindbrain decompression through suboccipital craniectomy and removal of the dorsal arch of the atlas is the current first-line treatment for CM1. This has most commonly been accompanied by dural opening and duraplasty. There is, however, debate regarding when duraplasty is most appropriate. Current data leave the treating surgeon to choose between a procedure that is more likely to require reoperation (PFD) and one that is more likely to result in perioperative CSF-related complications (PFDD). The frequency of these suboptimal outcomes (12.6% and 18.5%, respectively, in Durham and Fjeld-Olenec's meta-analysis [12]) does little to clarify which approach is most appropriate for a given patient. Furthermore, wide ranges of clinical efficacy and complications have been reported.

Lastly, the spectrum of presentation in children with CM1 extends from asymptomatic to potentially life-threatening symptomatology. It is therefore not surprising that no single surgical approach is universally recommended. As such, if a particular neurosurgeon has significant problems with dural opening then PFD is an attractive option. If, however, PFDD is associated with hospital discharge in less than 3 days and a very low reoperation rate (<1%) then adding the additional steps of opening the dura, looking for fourth ventricular outlet obstruction, and grafting the dura to prevent chemical meningitis has great appeal.

Recommendations	Evidence level
◆ Posterior fossa decompression with or without dural opening (PFD or PFDD) is the most effective first-line surgical treatment for patients with CM1 without hydrocephalus.	III/B
◆ PFDD has a lower rate of reoperation than PFD.	IIb/B
◆ PFD has a lower rate of CSF-related complications than PFDD.	IIb/B
◆ With regard to clinical improvement and syrinx resolution, no significant difference between PFD and PFDD has been demonstrated.	IIb/B
◆ PFDD is the most common first-line surgical technique for CM1 without hydrocephalus.	IV/C
◆ Repeat PFD with or without duraplasty is an effective second-line treatment for patients with persistent or recurrent signs or symptoms of CM1.	III/B

Chapter 22

References

1. Aitken LA, Lindan CE, Sidney S, *et al*. Chiari type I malformation in a pediatric population. *Pediatr Neurol* 2009; 40: 449-54.

2. Hankinson TC, Klimo P Jr, Feldstein NA, Anderson RC, Brockmeyer D. Chiari malformations, syringohydromyelia and scoliosis. *Neurosurg Clin N Am* 2007; 18: 549-68.

3. Tubbs RS, McGirt MJ, Oakes WJ. Surgical experience in 130 pediatric patients with Chiari I malformations. *J Neurosurg* 2003; 99: 291-6.

4. Hayhurst C, Osman-Farah J, Das K, Mallucci C. Initial management of hydrocephalus associated with Chiari malformation type I - syringomyelia complex via endoscopic third ventriculostomy: an outcome analysis. *J Neurosurg* 2008; 108: 1211-4.

5. Fischer EG. Posterior fossa decompression for Chiari I deformity, including resection of the cerebellar tonsils. *Childs Nerv Syst* 1995; 11: 625-9.

6. Galarza M, Sood S, Ham S. Relevance of surgical strategies for the management of pediatric Chiari type I malformation. *Childs Nerv Syst* 2007; 23: 691-6.

7. Krieger MD, McComb JG, Levy ML. Toward a simpler surgical management of Chiari I malformation in a pediatric population. *Pediatr Neurosurg* 1999; 30: 113-21.

8. Navarro R, Olavarria G, Seshadri R, Gonzales-Portillo G, McLone DG, Tomita T. Surgical results of posterior fossa decompression for patients with Chiari I malformation. *Childs Nerv Syst* 2004; 20: 349-56.

9. Tubbs RS, Smyth MD, Wellons JC 3rd, Oakes WJ. Arachnoid veils and the Chiari I malformation. *J Neurosurg* 2004; 100: 465-7.

10. Haroun RI, Guarnieri M, Meadow JJ, Kraut M, Carson BS. Current opinions for the treatment of syringomyelia and Chiari malformations: survey of the Pediatric Section of the American Association of Neurological Surgeons. *Pediatr Neurosurg* 2000; 33: 311-7.

11. Schijman E, Steinbok P. International survey on the management of Chiari I malformation and syringomyelia. *Childs Nerv Syst* 2004; 20: 341-8.

12. Durham SR, Fjeld-Olenec K. Comparison of posterior fossa decompression with and without duraplasty for the surgical treatment of Chiari malformation type I in pediatric patients: a meta-analysis. *J Neurosurg Pediatr* 2008; 2: 42-9.

13. McGirt M, Attenello F, Chaichana K, Weingart JD, Carson BS, Jallo GI. Duraplasty versus cranial decompression alone reduces treatment failure for pediatric Chiari I malformation patient with tonsillar herniation caudal to C1 but does not effect outcome in patients with tonsillar herniation rostral to C1. *Neurosurgery* 2007; 61: 208 (abstr. 843).

14. Munshi I, Frim D, Stine-Reyes R, Weir BK, Hekmatpanah J, Brown F. Effects of posterior fossa decompression with and without duraplasty on Chiari malformation-associated hydromyelia. *Neurosurgery* 2000; 46: 1384-9; discussion 1389-90.

15. Ventureyra EC, Aziz HA, Vassilyadi M. The role of cine flow MRI in children with Chiari I malformation. *Childs Nerv Syst* 2003; 19: 109-13.

16. Limonadi FM, Selden NR. Dura-splitting decompression of the craniocervical junction: reduced operative time, hospital stay, and cost with equivalent early outcome. *J Neurosurg* 2004; 101: 184-8.

17. Yeh DD, Koch B, Crone KR. Intraoperative ultrasonography used to determine the extent of surgery necessary during posterior fossa decompression in children with Chiari malformation type I. *J Neurosurg* 2006; 105: 26-32.

18. Attenello FJ, McGirt MJ, Gathinji M, *et al*. Outcome of Chiari-associated syringomyelia after hindbrain decompression in children: analysis of 49 consecutive cases. *Neurosurgery* 2008; 62: 1307-13.

19. McGirt MJ, Attenello FJ, Datoo G, *et al*. Intraoperative ultrasonography as a guide to patient selection for duraplasty after suboccipital decompression in children with Chiari malformation type I. *J Neurosurg Pediatr* 2008; 2: 52-7.

20. Zamel K, Galloway G, Kosnik EJ, Raslan M, Adeli A. Intraoperative neurophysiologic monitoring in 80 patients with Chiari I malformation: role of duraplasty. *J Clin Neurophysiol* 2009; 26: 70-5.

21. Anderson RC, Dowling KC, Feldstein NA, Emerson RG. Chiari I malformation: potential role for intraoperative electrophysiologic monitoring. *J Clin Neurophysiol* 2003; 20: 65-72.

22. Anderson RC, Emerson RG, Dowling KC, Feldstein NA. Improvement in brainstem auditory evoked potentials after suboccipital decompression in patients with Chiari I malformations. *J Neurosurg* 2003; 98: 459-64.

23. Caldarelli M, Novegno F, Vassimi L, Romani R, Tamburrini G, Di Rocco C. The role of limited posterior fossa craniectomy in the surgical treatment of Chiari malformation type I: experience with a pediatric series. *J Neurosurg* 2007; 106: 187-95.

24. Genitori L, Peretta P, Nurisso C, Macinante L, Mussa F. Chiari type I anomalies in children and adolescents: minimally invasive management in a series of 53 cases. *Childs Nerv Syst* 2000; 16: 707-18.

25. Wetjen NM, Heiss JD, Oldfield EH. Time course of syringomyelia resolution following decompression of Chiari malformation type I. *J Neurosurg Pediatr* 2008; 1: 118-23.

26. Attenello FJ, McGirt MJ, Atiba A, *et al*. Suboccipital decompression for Chiari malformation-associated scoliosis: risk factors and time course of deformity progression. *J Neurosurg Pediatr* 2008; 1: 456-60.

27. Alzate JC, Kothbauer KF, Jallo GI, Epstein FJ. Treatment of Chiari I malformation in patients with and without syringomyelia: a consecutive series of 66 cases. *Neurosurg Focus* 2001; 11: E3.

28. Danish SF, Samdani A, Hanna A, Storm P, Sutton L. Experience with acellular human dura and bovine collagen matrix for duraplasty after posterior fossa decompression for Chiari malformations. *J Neurosurg* 2006; 104: 16-20.

29. Ellenbogen RG, Armonda RA, Shaw DW, Winn HR. Toward a rational treatment of Chiari I malformation and syringomyelia. *Neurosurg Focus* 2000; 8: E6.

30. Feldstein NA, Choudhri TF. Management of Chiari I malformations with holocord syringohydromyelia. *Pediatr Neurosurg* 1999; 31: 143-9.

31. Hoffman CE, Souweidane MM. Cerebrospinal fluid-related complications with autologous duraplasty and arachnoid sparing in type I Chiari malformation. *Neurosurgery* 2008; 62: 156-60; discussion 160-1.

32. Park JK, Gleason PL, Madsen JR, Goumnerova LC, Scott RM. Presentation and management of Chiari I malformation in children. *Pediatr Neurosurg* 1997; 26: 190-6.

33. Attenello FJ, McGirt MJ, Garces-Ambrossi GL, Chaichana KL, Carson B, Jallo GI. Suboccipital decompression for Chiari I malformation: outcome comparison of duraplasty with expanded polytetrafluoroethylene dural substitute versus pericranial autograft. *Childs Nerv Syst* 2009; 25: 183-90.

34. Tubbs RS, Webb DB, Oakes WJ. Persistent syringomyelia following pediatric Chiari I decompression: radiological and surgical findings. *J Neurosurg* 2004; 100: 460-4.

35. Doughty KE, Tubbs RS, Webb D, Oakes WJ. Delayed resolution of Chiari I-associated hydromyelia after posterior fossa decompression: case report and review of the literature. *Neurosurgery* 2004; 55: 711.

36. Tubbs RS, Doyle S, Conklin M, Oakes WJ. Scoliosis in a child with Chiari I malformation and the absence of syringomyelia: case report and a review of the literature. *Childs Nerv Syst* 2006; 22: 1351-4.

37. Huebert HT, MacKinnon WB. Syringomyelia and scoliosis. *J Bone Joint Surg Br* 1969; 51: 338-43.

38. Isu T, Chono Y, Iwasaki Y, *et al*. Scoliosis associated with syringomyelia presenting in children. *Childs Nerv Syst* 1992; 8: 97-100.

39. Williams B. Orthopaedic features in the presentation of syringomyelia. *J Bone Joint Surg Br* 1979; 61-B: 314-23.

40. Brockmeyer D, Gollogly S, Smith JT. Scoliosis associated with Chiari I malformations: the effect of suboccipital decompression on scoliosis curve progression: a preliminary study. *Spine* (Phila Pa 1976) 2003; 28: 2505-9.

41. Eule JM, Erickson MA, O'Brien MF, Handler M. Chiari I malformation associated with syringomyelia and scoliosis: a twenty-year review of surgical and nonsurgical treatment in a pediatric population. *Spine* (Phila Pa 1976) 2002; 27: 1451-5.

42. Farley FA, Puryear A, Hall JM, Muraszko K. Curve progression in scoliosis associated with Chiari I malformation following suboccipital decompression. *J Spinal Disord Tech* 2002; 15: 410-4.

43. Flynn JM, Sodha S, Lou JE, *et al*. Predictors of progression of scoliosis after decompression of an Arnold Chiari I malformation. *Spine* (Phila Pa 1976) 2004; 29: 286-92.

44. Ghanem IB, Londono C, Delalande O, Dubousset JF. Chiari I malformation associated with syringomyelia and scoliosis. *Spine* (Phila Pa 1976) 1997; 22: 1313-7; discussion 1318.

45. Hida K, Iwasaki Y, Koyanagi I, Abe H. Pediatric syringomyelia with Chiari malformation: its clinical characteristics and surgical outcomes. *Surg Neurol* 1999; 51: 383-90; discussion 390-1.

46. Muhonen MG, Menezes AH, Sawin PD, Weinstein SL. Scoliosis in pediatric Chiari malformations without myelodysplasia. *J Neurosurg* 1992; 77: 69-77.

47. Özerdemoglu RA, Transfeldt EE, Denis F. Value of treating primary causes of syrinx in scoliosis associated with syringomyelia. *Spine* (Phila Pa 1976) 2003; 28: 806-14.

48. Sengupta DK, Dorgan J, Findlay GF. Can hindbrain decompression for syringomyelia lead to regression of scoliosis? *Eur Spine J* 2000; 9: 198-201.

Chapter 22

Chiari I malformation in children

Chapter 23

Surgical treatment of hydrocephalus in children

Shobhan Vachhrajani MD, Neurosurgery Resident

James M Drake MBBCh MSc FRCSC, Professor and Neurosurgeon-in-Chief

Abhaya V Kulkarni MD PhD FRCSC, Associate Professor and Neurosurgeon

DIVISION OF NEUROSURGERY, HOSPITAL FOR SICK CHILDREN,
UNIVERSITY OF TORONTO, TORONTO, ONTARIO, CANADA

Introduction

Hydrocephalus remains a large source of morbidity and mortality for children worldwide. In the developed world, the incidence of hydrocephalus has been progressively decreasing as maternal folate supplementation has reduced the frequency of neural tube defects, and improved antenatal screening and perinatal care have resulted in a decreased incidence of intraventricular hemorrhage associated with prematurity [1]. Hydrocephalus continues to pose a major threat to life in developing countries, however, where differences in etiology and markedly limited access to care have stimulated the use of novel management techniques [2].

Since the introduction of the first ball valve by Nulsen and Spitz in 1952, a variety of new valve mechanisms, including pressure- and flow-regulated valves, externally programmable valves, and antisiphon devices, have become available [3]. The use of antibiotic-impregnated shunt catheters (AIS) and endoscopic third ventriculostomy (ETV) is also now quite common. Despite these changes, shunt failure and shunt infection continue to be problematic and recent reports of the delayed acute sudden deaths of children with prior ETVs serve to underline its imperfection as a treatment modality [4, 5].

This chapter focuses on four key issues in the surgical management of pediatric hydrocephalus:

- Shunt valve design.
- The use of AIS.
- The importance of proximal catheter location and technique of placement.
- The comparison of outcomes between ETV and shunt placement in this patient population.

Methodology

Medline, EMBASE, and the Cochrane Collaboration databases were searched using terms including 'hydrocephalus,' 'cerebrospinal fluid shunt,' 'pediatric,' 'antibiotic-impregnated,' 'endoscopic,' and 'endoscopic third ventriculostomy.' The available evidence for each of these treatment scenarios has been summarized and we provide some guidance as to the optimal strategy for each, within the confines of the often-limited literature.

The influence of shunt valve design

The debate concerning the choice of shunt valve design has been ongoing for many years. Typical mechanisms include ball-in-spring, diaphragm, miter, and slit designs. Most commonly used valves open at a fixed differential pressure generated across the valve although, in recent years, externally programmable valves for which the pressure can be manipulated across a range of values have been used more frequently in selected patients. Antisiphon devices have also been incorporated into valve design in an attempt to reduce the gravitational effects of cerebrospinal fluid (CSF) overdrainage encountered with upright posture. Naturally following this discussion is a simple question: does any particular valve design afford increased longevity in shunt function or an overall decrease in the chance of shunt malfunction?

Randomized trials

Arguably the most compelling evidence regarding shunt valve design is found in the Shunt Design Trial published by Drake *et al* in 1998 [6]. In this randomized trial comparing standard fixed-pressure valves, Delta, and Orbis-Sigma valves, 344 patients were included from 12 centers in an attempt to show a reduction in the incidence of shunt failure from 40% to 20% at 1 year after insertion. Children younger than 18 years undergoing first-time shunt insertion were eligible, and were followed for 3 years after shunt placement. A particular strength of this trial is the detailed definition of shunt malfunction, which was subdivided into obstruction, overdrainage, loculated ventricles, and infection [7]. Most patients were infants or neonates at the time of shunt insertion, and the etiologies of intraventricular hemorrhage or myelomeningocele were most prominent in the group. Pressure settings within the type of valve allocated were left to the surgeon's preference: those placing standard valves most commonly opted for medium pressure, while those placing Delta valves chose level 1 pressure settings. Almost all patients received perioperative prophylactic antibiotics.

Overall, 150 patients (43.6%) experienced shunt failure, with most suffering shunt obstruction (n=108;

31.4%). Overdrainage was seen in 12 patients (3.5%), loculated compartments were seen in two patients (0.6%), and 28 patients (8.1%) suffered shunt infection. No differences were seen in the frequency of shunt malfunction between the allocated groups. Similarly, 61% of patients at 1 year and 47% of patients at 2 years had not suffered shunt malfunction, with median shunt survival of 656 days in the overall cohort. No differences in shunt survival were observed across the three treatment groups (p=0.24, log-rank) (Figure 1) [6]. The results of the trial appeared durable in long-term follow-up, with 41% of patients having functioning shunts at 4 years after insertion and no difference in shunt survival among the three valve designs [8]. Further analysis also demonstrated no effect of surgeon experience on shunt survival [9]. Valve design does not appear to influence the incidence of shunt survival or shunt failure **(Ib/A)**.

A randomized trial by Pollack *et al* rendered similar findings although with a different valve design under study [10]. This group randomized 377 patients younger than 18 years to a Codman Hakim-Medos programmable valve or to a fixed-pressure valve of the treating surgeon's choice; the latter group also included Delta and Orbis-Sigma valves. The trial was designed to detect a 1.5-fold change in the shunt failure rate between the two treatment groups, assuming a baseline failure of 65% in the first year with a fixed-pressure valve. During the 2-year follow-up, 48% of shunts did not fail overall, and no statistically significant difference was seen between the programmable valve and the fixed-pressure valve groups for either primary or revised shunts (52% vs. 50%; p>0.05; Chi-square). Similarly, there was no statistically significant difference in the incidence of shunt infection between the two groups (10.8% vs. 8.7%; p>0.05; Chi-square). Once again, this study indicates that shunt valve design does not appear to influence the incidence of shunt failure **(Ib/A)**.

The final randomized trial on this issue emanates from Uganda, in which a comparison of 90 patients randomized to the Codman Hakim Micro Precision valve system or Chhabra proximal slit-in-spring valve was performed [11]. The primary outcome in this study was repeated operation for shunt failure, infection, or wound complications. Sample size was determined

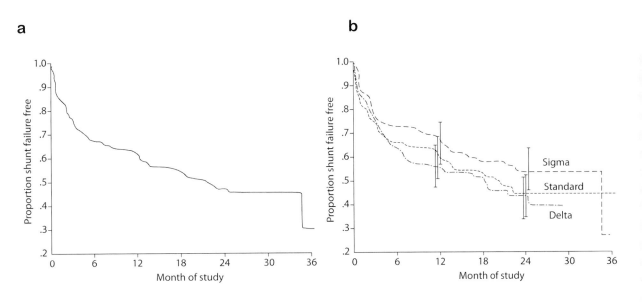

Figure 1. Kaplan-Meier survival curve from the Shunt Design Trial of shunt survival against time after insertion for a) the overall cohort and b) each of the three valve types. There were no statistically significant differences in shunt survival (p=0.24, log-rank). *Reproduced with permission from the Congress of Neurological Surgeons and Wolters Kluwer Health, © 1998. Drake JM, et al* [6].

based on the availability of the two shunt systems, rather than known baseline estimates of shunt failure. Patients were deemed eligible based on their need for shunt placement. Follow-up of these patients was difficult given pretreatment socioeconomic conditions in Uganda, but only 11 out of 90 patients were lost to follow-up at 1 year after shunt placement. No differences were observed in any primary outcome parameter between the Codman and Chhabra groups, including shunt failure, infection, or mortality (all p>0.05).

Non-randomized studies

Prospective non-randomized studies of valve design have shown similar results. Jain *et al* published a report of 50 patients undergoing new shunt placement [12]. The patients were assigned to either standard differential pressure valves (n=23) or Delta valves (n=27) according to the surgeon's preference. The average time to shunt failure was no different between groups, with standard valves failing at 37.1 months and Delta valves at 34.6 months (p=0.72;

Student's t-test). The proportion of shunt failure was similar in both groups (39.1% vs. 40.7%), although no statistical comparison was reported. The distribution of failure causes differed between the groups, with shunt obstruction and overdrainage more common in the standard group compared with the Delta valve group, and obstruction and infection were more common in the latter. Despite a non-randomized design, no difference in clinical outcome was seen between these two valve designs.

Kestle *et al* conducted a multicenter prospective cohort study examining the function of the Strata valve in 315 patients [13]. Patients either underwent new shunt placement (n=201) or shunt revision (n=114). Overall shunt failure was 33% at 1 year in the first group, with obstruction and infection comprising the largest subgroups at 17% and 11%, respectively. Overdrainage and loculation were responsible for 1.5% and 2% of failures, respectively. In the revision group, 29% of shunts failed at 1 year, with failures due to obstruction in 20%, infection in 6%, and overdrainage in 4%.

Chapter 23

Retrospective case series

Several retrospective case series either reviewing single-valve designs or comparing multiple-valve designs have yielded similar results. McGirt et al reviewed data from 279 patients who were treated with fixed-pressure valves, or with Codman Hakim-Medos or Strata valves [14]. Overall, 24% of patients suffered proximal shunt obstruction, although the placement of a programmable valve appeared to be protective against the need for shunt revision (relative risk [RR] 0.39; 95% confidence interval [CI], 0.27-0.80). Of the programmable valves, the Codman Hakim-Medos valves were less likely to require revision compared with Strata valves, although this difference was not statistically significant (RR 0.38; 95% CI, 0.18-1.11). Another study by Mangano et al retrospectively reviewed data from 100 patients who had received either Codman Hakim-Medos or Strata valves and compared these with data from 89 patients who had received fixed-pressure valves [15]. Shunt failure was observed in 35% of patients with programmable valves, compared with 20.2% in the fixed-pressure valve group. Infection rates were low in both groups, at 3% in the programmable valve group and 1.1% in the fixed-pressure valve group over 26 months of follow-up. Finally, a more recent comparative retrospective review of programmable, fixed differential pressure, and other unknown valve designs in 253 children found no significant differences in shunt survival (p=0.11; log-rank) or the number of revisions needed (p=0.06; Student's t-test) [16]. Younger patients and those with intraventricular hemorrhage or myelomeningocele experienced faster times to failure, regardless of the type of shunt valve placed.

Reviews of single-valve designs have also contributed to the body of evidence on this topic, largely by providing baseline estimates of shunt failure upon which inferential studies can be launched. Zemack et al reviewed data from 153 children undergoing placement of Codman Hakim-Medos programmable valves [17]. Shunt survival was 60.5% at 1 year, 47.1% at 2 years, and 43.9% at 3 years after placement. In an older study by Reinprecht et al, 46 patients underwent primary shunt placement with the same valve. Over a median follow-up of 26.5 months, 39.1% of patients experienced shunt failure; 12 of 18

patients in this group experienced infection, proximal catheter obstruction, or valve obstruction [18]. A report from Rohde et al in which the valve was placed in 60 children demonstrated that 50% of children experienced either shunt obstruction or infection over 2 years of follow-up [19].

Reports on Strata valves have revealed similar figures. In a study of 53 children receiving Strata valves, 32.8% of shunts had failed at 1 year after placement [20]. Martinez-Lage et al prospectively studied the programmable Sophy (n=86) and Polaris valves (n=14) in a group of 100 consecutive neonates younger than 2 months [21]. Over a mean follow-up of 55 months, proximal obstruction was observed in 20% of patients and infection occurred in 5%. No subgroup analysis was provided for each valve type.

Finally, a retrospective review of various fixed differential pressure valves in a group of 200 infants younger than 1 year revealed different shunt survival figures based on the pressure settings used. Follow-up data were available for 158 patients over a mean period of 39.8 months. Shunt failure in no- or low-pressure valves occurred in 58% and 72% of patients at 1 and 5 years, respectively, compared with 31% and 47% for those receiving medium- or high-pressure valves (p=0.0005; Wilcoxon rank-sum) [22]. In addition, the requirement for revision was much higher in the low-pressure valve patients compared with medium or high pressure; only 38% of patients with low-pressure valves were revision-free in the first 6 months after implantation, compared with 78% with high-pressure valves. Extrapolation to older patients, however, is difficult.

Flow-regulated and gravity-assisted valves

Attempts to improve outcomes with flow-regulated and gravity-assisted valves have not shown convincing differences in outcomes compared with the published experience with other valve types, in either prospective or retrospective study. A prospective study of 557 adults and children undergoing Orbis-Sigma II valve placement revealed no difference in shunt survival between adults and

Table 1. Summary of evidence outlining the influence of valve design on shunt failure. *Continued overleaf.*

Author	Study design	n	Treatment	Results
Drake et al, 1998 [6]	RCT	115 114 115	Delta valve Standard valve Orbis-Sigma valve	Overall shunt failure rate: 31.4% (1 year) No difference in survival among the three groups (p=0.24)
Kestle et al, 2000 [8]	RCT	115 114 115	Delta Standard valve Orbis-Sigma valve	Overall shunt failure rate: 51% (3 years) No difference in survival among the three groups (p-value not specified)
Pollack et al, 1999 [10]	RCT	194 183	Codman Hakim-Medos programmable valve Standard valve	Proximal obstruction: 56% (Codman) vs. 57% (standard) No statistically significant difference in shunt survival
Warf, 2005 [11]	RCT	90 105	Codman or Chhabra shunt Chhabra shunt after ETV failure	No difference in shunt failure, mortality, or infection
Jain et al, 2000 [12]	Prospective cohort	27 23	Delta Standard valve	Obstruction: 18.5% (Delta) vs. 21.7% (standard) Mean time to failure: 34.6 (Delta) vs. 37.1 months (standard) p>0.05 for all outcomes
Hanlo et al, 2003 [23]	Prospective cohort	557 (adults and children)	Orbis-Sigma Valve II	No difference in shunt survival for adults vs. children Higher failure in those aged <6 vs. >6 months
Meling et al, 2005 [26]	Prospective cohort	32	Paedi-GAV	Failure rate: 46.9% (1 year), 55.1% (2 years) Mean time to failure: 123 days
Kestle et al, 2005 [13]	Prospective cohort	201 114	Strata valve, primary insertion Strata valve, revision	Failure rate (1 year): 33% (primary insertion), 29% (revision)
Haberl et al, 2009 [25]	Prospective cohort	182	Paedi-GAV	Shunt failure: 27.4% (1 year), 40% (2 years)
Rohde et al, 2009 [27]	Prospective cohort	53	ProGAV	Shunt failure: 24.5% (mean follow-up 15.2 months)
Serlo et al, 1995 [24]	Retrospective review	80	Orbis-Sigma valve	Failure rate: 43% (5 years)

Table 1. Summary of evidence outlining the influence of valve design on shunt failure. *Continued.*

Author	Study design	n	Treatment	Results
Reinprecht et al, 1997 [18]	Retrospective review	46	Codman Hakim Medos valve, primary insertion	Failure rate (2 years): 39.1% (primary insertion), 15.6% (revision)
		32	Codman Hakim-Medos valve, revision	
Rohde et al, 1998 [19]	Retrospective review	60	Codman Hakim-Medos valve	Failure rate: 50% (2 years)
Robinson et al, 2002 [22]	Retrospective review	158	No valve Low pressure Medium pressure High pressure	Failure rate (no/low pressure): 58% (1 year), 72% (5 years) Failure rate (medium/high pressure): 31% (1 year), 47% (5 years)
Zemack et al, 2003 [17]	Retrospective review	158	Codman Hakim-Medos valve	Failure rate: 39.5% (1 year), 52.9% (2 years), 56.1% (3 years)
Mangano et al, 2005 [15]	Retrospective review	100	Codman Hakim-Medos valve	Failure rate (2 years): 35% (Codman) vs. 20.2% (standard)
		89	Standard fixed-pressure valve	
Ahn et al, 2007 [20]	Retrospective review	53	Strata valve	Failure rate: 32.8% (1 year)
McGirt et al, 2007 [14]	Retrospective review	78	Codman Hakim-Medos or Strata programmable valve	Relative risk 0.54 for revision, 0.35 for proximal obstruction of programmable valve compared with fixed-pressure
		201	Fixed-pressure valves	
Martinez-Lage et al, 2008 [21]	Retrospective review	86	Sophy valve	Overall shunt failure rate: 27% (4.5 years)
		14	Polaris valve	
Weinzierl et al, 2008 [58]	Retrospective review	15	Codman Hakim-Medos valve	Failure rate: 6.6% (2.5 years)
Notarianni et al, 2009 [16]	Retrospective review	160	Standard fixed-pressure	Overall shunt failure rate: 78%
		73	Programmable valve	No significant difference in rates between the three valve types (p=0.11)
		20	Unknown/other valve	

ETV = endoscopic third ventriculostomy; RCT = randomized controlled trial children, although specific survival figures were not provided for each group [23]. Patients younger than 6 months at the time of shunt insertion were reported to experience a higher proportion of shunt failure compared with those older than 6 months (45% vs. 37%; p>0.05; Chi-square). In another study of 80 children receiving Orbis-Sigma valves for primary insertions and shunt revisions, 43% of shunts had failed at 5 years after insertion, and valve malfunction was estimated at 30%. Children younger than 1 year were at higher risk for malfunction [24].

A study of 182 children with Paedi-GAV implantation revealed 27.4% and 40% shunt failure at 1 and 2 years, respectively [25]. An older study of 32 children receiving the Paedi-GAV in shunt revisions revealed shunt failure rates of 46.9% and 55.1% at 1 and 2 years, respectively [26]. The median survival was 388 days, and obstruction was responsible for 37.5% of failures, with infection accounting for 3.1%. A smaller study of the proGAV in 53 children showed shunt failure to be 24.5% at 1 year after insertion [27].

Table 1 summarizes the evidence on the impact of valve design on outcomes in pediatric hydrocephalus. The data obtained from randomized trials suggest no benefit of one particular shunt valve design over any other; similar outcome figures have been obtained from other non-randomized prospective and retrospective studies (Ib/A).

Antibiotic-impregnated catheters and shunt infection

Shunt infection continues to pose a major problem for children with shunted hydrocephalus. The estimated incidence hovers at around 8%, as reported in early prospective studies, and this has since been confirmed by others [1, 6, 10, 13, 28]. Use of perioperative prophylactic antibiotics has managed to decrease the incidence of shunt infection, and identification and possible control of risk factors such as patient age, holes in surgical gloves, and postoperative CSF leak are important in preventing CSF infection after shunt placement [29-31].

AIS may be another useful adjunct in an effort to reduce shunt infection in children. The only Cochrane Collaboration review on this topic, published in 2006, suggests a significant benefit to the use of AIS [32]. However, two important caveats must be considered:

- First, neither of the two included trials was exclusively conducted in the pediatric population; therefore, the mixing of adult patients will undoubtedly change the estimates of infection outcome.
- Second, the authors of the review considered the placement of external ventricular drains (EVDs) to be equivalent to the placement of an internalized shunt; therefore, one of the trials applies to an entirely different population.

Overall, the meta-analysis found a significant benefit to the use of AIS in the reduction of shunt infection (RR 0.21; 95% CI, 0.08-0.55). This benefit was incurred entirely from the EVD patients, given their stronger effect size (RR 0.13; 95% CI, 0.03-0.60) and 60.8% weighting in the meta-analysis [32, 33]. By contrast, the study comparing internalized AIS with standard components did not yield any statistical benefit to the use of AIS, although a trend was evident (RR 0.32; 95% CI, 0.08-1.23) [34]. Application of these results to the pediatric population is difficult, given the heterogeneous population and lack of specific subgroup analysis.

A smaller randomized trial published afterwards may demonstrate more applicable results for shunt infection outcomes in children. Eymann *et al* randomized 48 children undergoing primary shunt insertion to receive either AIS or non-AIS components; the allocation was to a group of surgeons who exclusively used one type of shunt hardware [35]. Only one of 26 children (3.8%) in the AIS group developed shunt infection (with *Staphylococcus aureus*) 57 days after shunt implantation, while three of 22 children (13.6%) in the control group developed *S. epidermidis* infection at 10, 32, and more than 60 days after shunt insertion. The children were part of a larger study population comprising 317 adults and children, and there was an overall reduction in the incidence of shunt infection among all patients (from 5.8% to 1%; p=0.0145). No pediatric subgroup statistical analysis was presented, but there was a suggestion of a possible decreased shunt infection incidence in children with the use of AIS (Ib/A).

Chapter 23

Table 2. Summary of evidence on the effect of antibiotic-impregnated shunt catheters in reducing shunt infection.

Author	Study design	n	Treatment allocation	Infection rate (%)
Ratilal et al, 2006 [32]	Cochrane review (two studies)	199 199	AIS Standard	2.5 11.6 RR 0.21 (95% CI, 0.08-0.55)
Eymann et al, 2008 [35]	Randomized trial	26 22	AIS Standard	3.8 13.6
Pattavilakom et al, 2007 [42]	Prospective cohort	102	AIS with ceftriaxone prophylaxis	2.9
Sciubba et al, 2008 [38]	Prospective cohort	108	AIS	4.6
Aryan et al, 2005 [40]	Retrospective review	32 46	AIS Standard	3.1 15.2
Sciubba et al, 2005 [37]	Retrospective review	145 208	AIS (after 2002) Standard (before 2002)	1.4 12 RR 0.41 (95% CI, 0.32-0.52)
Kan et al, 2007 [41]	Retrospective review	80 80	AIS Standard	5.0 8.8 Odds ratio 0.353 (95% CI, 0.04-3.00)
Sciubba et al, 2007 [39]	Retrospective review	262	AIS	3.82
Hayhurst et al, 2008 [43]	Retrospective review	214 77	AIS Standard	9.8 10.4
Parker et al, 2009 [36]	Retrospective review	502 570	AIS (after 2002) Standard (before 2002)	3.2 11.2 Hazard ratio 3.18 (95% CI, 2.05-4.93)

AIS = antibiotic-impregnated shunt catheter; CI = confidence interval; RR = relative risk

Several comparative retrospective reviews have shown benefits of AIS over standard catheters in reducing shunt infections. Parker et al published a recent report on this question, reviewing data from 544 children who underwent 1,072 shunt procedures [36]. All shunts placed prior to 2002 comprised standard catheters (n=570), whereas all shunts placed after 2002 utilized AIS components. Survival analysis revealed a significant benefit in the AIS group compared with the non-AIS group (infection in 3.2% vs. 11.2%, respectively; hazard ratio [HR] 3.18; 95% CI, 2.05-4.93). This benefit was maintained in all high-risk patient subgroups including, prematurity, post-meningitis, prolonged hospital stay, and those being converted from EVD to internalized shunt systems. Given that the use of AIS was not randomized, and that the change in treatment protocol occurred at a single time point, it is impossible to glean whether other concurrent changes in surgical technique or surgeon experience may have contributed to the observed benefits.

This report builds on previous retrospective analyses, including many of the same patients, from the same institution. Sciubba et al reported on 211 patients undergoing 353 shunt procedures, and found a significant reduction in shunt infection incidence from 12% in the non-AIS group to 1.4% in the AIS group over the first 6 months following shunt placement (adjusted RR 0.41; 95% CI, 0.32-0.52) [37]. The high baseline rate of shunt infection in the control group exaggerates this difference. Another prospective cohort study by the same author found an infection rate of 4.6% in infants younger than 1 year receiving AIS components for primary shunt placement or shunt revisions, or after having received previous reservoirs for ventricular access [38]. A large proportion of this group had suffered prior intraventricular hemorrhage associated with prematurity. Finally, a retrospective review of 262 children undergoing AIS implantation revealed a shunt infection incidence of 3.8%, with all infections occurring in the first 6 months after shunt placement [39].

Other institutions have reported similar shunt infection figures associated with the use of AIS components. Aryan et al reported on 31 patients who received AIS components and compared them with a historical unmatched control group of 46 patients [40]. There was a trend toward decreased incidence of shunt infection in the AIS group (3.1% vs. 15.2%), although this difference was not statistically significant. A similar review by Kan and Kestle compared 80 AIS procedures with 80 standard procedures, and found a non-significant difference in shunt infection rates (5.0% vs. 8.8%; adjusted odds ratio [OR] 0.353; 95% CI, 0.0414-3.00) [41]. An Australian study reported shunt infection in 2.9% of 102 children receiving AIS components [42]. Again, this patient group was part of a larger mixed adult and pediatric cohort, where the authors compared with a historical control group; however, no pediatric specific comparisons were provided. Finally, a report by

Hayhurst et al showed a no reduction in the incidence of shunt infection between a group of 150 children receiving AIS catheters and a historical control group of 65 children (9.8% vs. 10.4%; p=0.884; Chi-square) [43]. No differences were observed in any of the shunt placement subgroups: de novo shunt placement, non-infected revision, conversion from sterile EVD to internalized shunt, and conversion from infected EVD to internalized shunt.

The body of evidence on the use of AIS suggests a possible benefit in reducing shunt infections. However, much of the evidence is retrospective and uncontrolled, and this area would benefit from studies with stronger methodological rigor. The randomized trials on this topic do appear to favor the use of AIS, but their results must be interpreted with caution (Ib/A). Table 2 summarizes the evidence on AIS in the treatment of pediatric hydrocephalus.

Proximal catheter placement: location and technique

In addition to valve design and catheter components, the technique of shunt placement may also influence outcome. Two specific factors should be assessed when evaluating this question:

* The location of proximal catheter placement.
* The use of navigational adjuncts such as endoscopy or computerized neuronavigation systems.

Proximal catheter location

The evidence regarding the influence of proximal catheter location on outcome is scant and dates back to the late 1990s. Of many analyses performed upon data emerging from the previously discussed Shunt Design Trial, one entailed a post hoc analysis of catheter location and position within the ventricle as a determinant of shunt survival [6]. Multivariate analysis demonstrated that occipital placement had the lowest chance of shunt failure (HR 0.45; 95% CI, 0.28-0.74), followed by frontal placement (HR 0.60; 95% CI, 0.39-0.91), when compared with other locations of proximal catheter placement [44]. Similarly, catheter tips surrounded by CSF were most likely to survive (HR 0.21; 95% CI, 0.094-0.45), followed by catheter tips touching the brain (HR 0.33; 95% CI, 0.21-0.51), when compared with catheter tips completely surrounded by brain **(IIa/B)**.

Post hoc graphical analysis from the Endoscopic Shunt Insertion Trial (ESIT) demonstrated improved shunt survival curves in cases where proximal catheter tips were shown to be positioned away from the choroid plexus on postoperative CT scan (Figure 2) [28]. No formal statistical analysis for this subgroup was provided, however. A retrospective analysis by

Albright *et al* displayed a significant survival benefit for 62 frontally placed shunts compared with 52 parietally placed shunts (p=0.008, Wilcoxon) [45]. CT scan follow-up was available in 83 patients, and placement was graded as good if the catheter was in the ipsilateral ventricle ventral to the foramen of Monro, fair if it was in the contralateral frontal horn or near the choroid plexus, and poor if it was located in the brain parenchyma. Patients with good placement through a frontal approach experienced 70% shunt survival over 5 years, compared with 40% of well-placed parietal shunts. There were no significant differences in baseline characteristics between the patients receiving frontal or parietal shunts **(III/B)**.

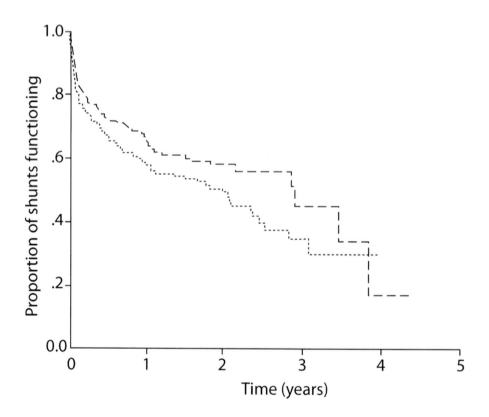

Figure 2. Kaplan-Meier survival curve from the Endoscopic Shunt Insertion Trial of shunt survival against time after shunt insertion. The dotted line represents endoscopically inserted shunts, while the dashed line represents shunts inserted using standard techniques. There were no statistically significant differences in shunt survival (p=0.09, log-rank) [28]. *Reproduced with permission from the American Association of Neurological Surgeons and JNS Publishing Group, © 2003. Kestle JR, et al* [28].

Table 3. Summary of evidence on the influence of proximal catheter placement on shunt failure.

Author	Study design	n	Treatment allocation	Results
Tuli *et al*, 1999 [44]	Prospective (post hoc analysis of RCT)	344	Delta valve Standard valve Orbis-Sigma valve	Occipital location: HR 0.45 (95% CI, 0.28-0.74) Frontal location: HR 0.60 (95% CI, 0.39-0.91) Ventricular tip surrounded by CSF: HR 0.21 (95% CI, 0.09-0.45) Ventricular tip catheter touching brain: HR 0.33 (95% CI, 0.21-0.51)
Kestle *et al*, 2003 [28]	Prospective (post hoc analysis of RCT)	173 113	Catheter position away from choroid plexus Catheter near the choroid plexus	Shunt failure less common when catheter positioned away from choroid plexus (statistical analysis not presented)
Albright *et al*, 1988 [45]	Retrospective review	62 52	Frontal placement Parietal placement	Failure rate (5 years): 30% (frontal) vs. 60% (parietal)

CI = confidence interval; CSF = cerebrospinal fluid; HR = hazard ratio; RCT = randomized controlled trial

Table 3 summarizes this evidence. A randomized trial may be the best vehicle by which to answer the question of optimal proximal catheter placement, although variations in ventricular anatomy may make patient randomization difficult.

Endoscopically-assisted shunt placement

Technological adjuncts to optimize proximal catheter placement have been trialed with little success. The most convincing evidence showing lack of benefit for the use of endoscopy in proximal shunt catheter placement comes from the ESIT. Patients undergoing primary shunt placement were randomized to endoscopically-assisted shunt placement, aimed at positioning the tip of the proximal catheter away from the choroid plexus (n=194), or to shunt insertion by standard techniques (n=199) [28]. The study was designed to detect a 10-15% absolute reduction in the shunt failure rate at 1 year after insertion, and was conducted at 16 pediatric neurosurgery centers. Patients were evenly distributed across both groups, including the type of

valve used at the time of shunt placement. Overall, shunt failure was seen in 38% of patients at 1 year after surgery and in 47% at 2 years after insertion. More importantly, however, there was no significant difference in the time to shunt failure or in the proportion of patients experiencing failure between the endoscopic and non-endoscopic groups (42% vs. 34%; p=0.09; log-rank). Much of this may be attributable to the inability of endoscopy to reliably place the ventricular catheter; postoperative imaging revealed that the catheter tip was positioned away from the choroid plexus in only 67% of patients. Based on these randomized trial data, endoscopic placement of proximal ventricular catheters does not appear to improve shunt survival **(Ib/A)**.

The ESIT results mirror findings from other smaller retrospective case series examining the use of endoscopy in shunt placement. A review of endoscopically placed shunts revealed that 49% required revision within the first year, compared with 67% of non-endoscopic controls [46]. No statistical comparison was presented and, interestingly, 90% of shunts were reported to be positioned at the correct

Table 4. Summary of evidence for the influence of navigation-assisted proximal catheter placement on shunt failure.

Author	Study design	n	Treatment allocation	Results
Kestle et al, 2003 [28]	Randomized controlled trial	194	Endoscopic proximal catheter placement	Failure rate (1 year): 42% (endoscopic) vs. 34% (standard)
		199	Standard placement	Overall failure rate: 38% (1 year), 47% (2 years)
Gil et al, 2002 [49]	Prospective cohort	9	Frameless neuronavigation	All patients improved over 8 months' follow-up
Manwaring 1992 [46]	Retrospective review	200	Endoscopic proximal catheter placement	Failure rate: 49% (1 year) 90% positioning at selected site
Taha et al, 1996 [47]	Retrospective review	100	Endoscopic proximal catheter placement	Failure rate: 13% 98% catheter placement away from choroid
Villavicencio et al, 2003 [48]	Retrospective review	605	Endoscopic proximal catheter placement	Overall shunt failure rate: 53% Hazard ratio 1.08 (95% CI, 0.84-1.41) for endoscopy
		360	Standard proximal catheter placement	

CI = confidence interval

site. Taha and Crone presented a series of 100 patients who underwent endoscopically-assisted shunt placement [47]. Of these, 68 patients underwent placement performed using a large endoscope with standard techniques, while 32 patients had an endoscope placed through the lumen of the proximal catheter. The authors reported that 98% of catheters were positioned away from the choroid, and found a 13% shunt failure rate over a mean 2.5-year follow-up. Finally, Villavicencio et al reported a comparative series of 605 endoscopically placed shunts and 360 non-endoscopically placed shunts [48]. Overall, 53% of shunts failed during the study, although the follow-up period was unclear, and neuroendoscopy did not independently influence shunt survival (HR 1.08; 95% CI, 0.84-1.41). In those shunts that did fail, however, the use of endoscopy decreased the likelihood of proximal malfunction (OR 0.56; 95% CI, 0.32-0.93). The use of endoscopy did not demonstrate any effect on the incidence of shunt infection (OR 1.42; 95% CI, 0.78-2.61).

Other shunt placement adjuncts

It should be noted that the literature on the use of other adjuncts in shunt placement is limited. No published sources outlining the impact of ultrasound were found, and only one paper has been published detailing the use of frameless neuronavigation for pediatric shunt placement. Gil et al reported on a prospective cohort of nine children in whom neuronavigation was used to place either primary or revision shunts [49]. During a mean follow-up of 8 months, all patients improved symptomatically and no shunt revisions were required. Unfortunately, the authors did not comment on the level of satisfaction with catheter placement or any potential radiographic confirmation.

The body of evidence on the use of technical adjuncts for pediatric shunt placement, summarized in Table 4, does not show any benefit to their use. Of these, endoscopy is the most well studied and a well-conducted randomized trial did not show any benefit to its use in proximal catheter placement **(Ib/A)**.

The use of ETV versus traditional CSF shunts

Renewed interest in the use of ETV, particularly in patients with obstructive hydrocephalus, has led many to compare ETV with the placement of CSF shunts in the treatment of pediatric hydrocephalus. The use of ETV dates back to the 1920s, although the introduction of CSF shunts in the 1950s significantly decreased the use of ETV as a treatment modality. With the passage of time, neurosurgeons became increasingly aware of the ongoing complications associated with CSF shunts. This, coupled with improvements in endoscopic technology and imaging to better identify patients who may be suitable candidates, has led to increasing use of ETV [1]. A large multicenter Canadian review has suggested that age is the major determinant of outcome, with neonates having the greatest risk of ETV failure [50]. Other studies have detailed the roles of both age and etiology in the success of ETV, and an ETV success prediction model and success score published in 2009 may help to better select those patients most suited for ETV [51].

Comparative literature on the use of ETV versus CSF shunting has primarily considered two outcomes: failure to control hydrocephalus and quality of life.

Failure to control hydrocephalus

Garton *et al* conducted a case-control study with 28 patients undergoing ETV matched to patients receiving CSF shunts based on age and etiology of hydrocephalus [52]. The treatment used in each patient was based on the predominant practice patterns of the time. In the ETV group, 46% of patients failed treatment over a median follow-up of 34.7 months. Most failures (10/13) occurred in the first 6 months, with one hydrocephalus-related death. By contrast, 60% of shunts failed over the same time period; however, no statistical comparison was provided. As an aside, ETV, despite its apparent benefit in treating hydrocephalus, was not more cost-effective due to the increased frequency of early complications when compared with the shunt group **(IIa/B)**.

A prospective cohort study did not reveal a benefit for either treatment modality in 242 patients, although the sample was weighted heavily toward shunt patients (n=210) [53]. All patients were suffering from obstructive hydrocephalus due to either aqueductal stenosis or tumor prior to their first CSF diversion procedure. No crude difference in median survival was seen between the shunt and ETV groups (1,055 vs. 1,302 days; p=0.87; log-rank). This lack of difference was evident even after adjusted analysis for sex, age, etiology, and prior placement of EVD (HR 1.19; 95% CI, 0.55-2.56) **(IIb/B)**.

A Swiss retrospective study yielded similar findings in 55 patients receiving initial treatment for hydrocephalus [54]. In this group, 31 patients underwent shunt placement and 24 had ETV; eight of 24 patients (33%) in the ETV group required a revision procedure compared with 16 of 31 patients (52%) in the shunt group. Neither this nor the number of revisions per patient were statistically different between the two groups (p=0.06; Student's t-test). Similarly, the median time to revision was no different between the groups (24 vs. 19 months; p=0.75; log-rank).

At least from these comparative studies, the use of ETV confers no advantage over CSF shunting in selected patients. Most of this literature, however, does not discuss at length the differential risk of complications between the two procedures, and this must be taken this into account during clinical decision-making.

Quality of life and neurodevelopment

The impact of ETV versus shunt placement on post-treatment quality of life and neurodevelopment in children with hydrocephalus is somewhat more equivocal. A Japanese study of 25 patients receiving shunt or ETV suggested that neurodevelopmental outcome was improved in patients who were shunted with abnormal cortical development [55]. This study was grossly flawed, however. Investigators arbitrarily placed CSF shunts when they felt that ETV had not provided any beneficial outcome. Subsequent follow-up revealed that the ETV was non-functioning in the vast majority of patients.

Table 5. Summary of evidence comparing outcomes after ETV versus CSF shunting.

Author	Study design	n	Treatment allocation	Results
Garton et al, 2002 [52]	Matched case-control	28 28	ETV Shunt	Failure rate: 46.4% (ETV) vs. 60% (shunt)
Tuli et al, 1999 [53]	Prospective cohort	32 210	ETV Shunt	Median time to failure: 1,302 (ETV) vs. 1,055 days (shunt) Hazard ratio 1.19 (95% CI, 0.55-2.56)
Takahashi et al, 2006 [55]	Prospective cohort	25	ETV, shunt, or both	Improved outcome with shunting and abnormal cortical development
de Ribaupierre et al, 2007 [54]	Retrospective review	24 31	ETV Shunt	Failure rate: 33% (ETV) vs. 52% (shunt) Average time to revision: 19 (ETV) vs. 24 months (shunt)
Drake et al, 2009 [56]	Decision analysis	1105	ETV or shunt	Higher net quality-adjusted life-years for ETV vs. shunt
Kulkarni et al, 2010 [57]	Cross-sectional study	24 23	ETV Shunt	No significant difference in quality of life or IQ between groups

CI = confidence interval; CSF = cerebrospinal fluid; ETV = endoscopic third ventriculostomy

A subsequent decision analysis by Drake et al showed that a small higher net quality-adjusted life-year (QALY) difference was obtained in patients undergoing ETV compared with shunting [56]. This study utilized patient data gathered in the previously discussed ESIT and Shunt Design Trial and, given that the QALY difference was small, the authors considered the two groups to be similar. Two factors primarily influenced the results based on sensitivity analysis. First, the threshold for a severe adverse outcome after ETV was 7%; if this threshold value was exceeded, CSF shunting became superior. Second, the utility score (the value assigned to a health state, with increasing values indicating better states of health), had to be above 0.923 for a functioning ETV or above 0.926 for a functioning shunt. Utility scores below those thresholds conferred a net benefit on the competing modality. Lastly, a study on quality of life after ETV or shunt for obstructive hydrocephalus published in 2010 found no difference in outcomes using the Health Utilities Index Mark 3 and the Hydrocephalus Outcome Questionnaire (p>0.09 for all measures) [57]. In this study, 24 patients had undergone ETV as their primary treatment for hydrocephalus compared with 23 children who received a shunt. A subset of ETV patients (n=6) and shunt (n=5) patients were assessed on the Wechsler Intelligence Scale for Children; there were no significant differences in full-scale, verbal, or non-verbal IQ (all p>0.11).

Although limited in its scope, the literature on quality of life after treatment of hydrocephalus does not seem to suggest a benefit for ETV over CSF shunting (**IIa/B**). Table 5 provides a summary of the evidence.

Conclusions

The optimal surgical treatment of pediatric hydrocephalus remains a topic of debate, at least as it pertains to the topics addressed in this chapter. The evidence suggests that:

- Rates of shunt failure are not influenced by the type of valve used in the shunt system.
- Although there appears to be a trend, there is not convincing evidence that the use of AIS reduces the incidence of shunt infection in children.
- Endoscopically-assisted placement of proximal catheters is not helpful in reducing the incidence of shunt failure.

- Proximal catheters completely surrounded by CSF have the greatest chance of shunt survival.
- ETV does not confer a convincing advantage over CSF shunting for either shunt failure or quality of life outcomes in patients with obstructive hydrocephalus.

Further study is undoubtedly necessary to more definitively answer some of these questions. Until such time, the evidence presented here will hopefully guide pediatric neurosurgeons to provide the best evidence-based treatment for their patients with hydrocephalus.

Chapter 23

Recommendations	Evidence level
No shunt valve design has been shown to be superior to any other in reducing the rate of shunt failure.	Ib/A
There is no convincing evidence that AIS reduces the incidence of shunt infection in children.	Ib/A
Endoscopic assistance in placing proximal catheters is not beneficial in reducing the risk of shunt failure.	Ib/A
Positioning proximal catheters away from the choroid plexus and brain parenchyma is beneficial in improving shunt survival.	IIa/B
The use of ETV over traditional CSF shunting does not improve shunt survival or quality of life in children with obstructive hydrocephalus.	IIa/B

References

1. Drake JM. The surgical management of pediatric hydrocephalus. *Neurosurgery* 2008; 62(Suppl. 2): 633-40; discussion 40-2.
2. Warf BC, Mugamba J, Kulkarni AV. Endoscopic third ventriculostomy in the treatment of childhood hydrocephalus in Uganda: report of a scoring system that predicts success. *J Neurosurg Pediatr* 2010; 5(2): 143-8.
3. Nulsen FE, Spitz EB. Treatment of hydrocephalus by direct shunt from ventricle to jugular vein. *Surg Forum* 1952; 3: 399-403.
4. Hader WJ, Drake J, Cochrane D, Sparrow O, Johnson ES, Kestle J. Death after late failure of third ventriculostomy in children. Report of three cases. *J Neurosurg* 2002; 97(1): 211-5.
5. Drake J, Chumas P, Kestle J, *et al*. Late rapid deterioration after endoscopic third ventriculostomy: additional cases and

review of the literature. *J Neurosurg* 2006; 105(2 Suppl.): 118-26.
6. Drake JM, Kestle JR, Milner R, *et al*. Randomized trial of cerebrospinal fluid shunt valve design in pediatric hydrocephalus. *Neurosurgery* 1998; 43(2): 294-303; discussion 303-5.
7. Drake JM, Kestle J. Determining the best cerebrospinal fluid shunt valve design: the pediatric valve design trial. *Neurosurgery* 1996; 38(3): 604-7.
8. Kestle J, Drake J, Milner R, *et al*. Long-term follow-up data from the Shunt Design Trial. *Pediatr Neurosurg* 2000; 33(5): 230-6.
9. Kestle J, Milner R, Drake J. The Shunt Design Trial: variation in surgical experience did not influence shunt survival. *Pediatr Neurosurg* 1999; 30(6): 283-7.
10. Pollack IF, Albright AL, Adelson PD. A randomized, controlled study of a programmable shunt valve versus a conventional valve for patients with hydrocephalus. Hakim-Medos

Investigator Group. *Neurosurgery* 1999; 45(6): 1399-408; discussion 408-11.

11. Warf BC. Comparison of 1-year outcomes for the Chhabra and Codman-Hakim Micro Precision shunt systems in Uganda: a prospective study in 195 children. *J Neurosurg* 2005; 102(4 Suppl.): 358-62.

12. Jain H, Sgouros S, Walsh AR, Hockley AD. The treatment of infantile hydrocephalus: 'differential-pressure' or 'flow-control' valves: a pilot study. *Childs Nerv Syst* 2000; 16(4): 242-6.

13. Kestle JRW, Walker ML, Strata I. A multicenter prospective cohort study of the Strata valve for the management of hydrocephalus in pediatric patients. *J Neurosurg* 2005; 102(2 Suppl.): 141-5.

14. McGirt MJ, Buck DW 2nd, Sciubba D, et al. Adjustable vs. set-pressure valves decrease the risk of proximal shunt obstruction in the treatment of pediatric hydrocephalus. *Childs Nerv Syst* 2007; 23(3): 289-95.

15. Mangano FT, Menendez JA, Habrock T, et al. Early programmable valve malfunctions in pediatric hydrocephalus. *J Neurosurg* 2005; 103(6 Suppl.): 501-7.

16. Notarianni C, Vannemreddy P, Caldito G, et al. Congenital hydrocephalus and ventriculoperitoneal shunts: influence of etiology and programmable shunts on revisions. *J Neurosurg Pediatr* 2009; 4(6): 547-52.

17. Zemack G, Bellner J, Siesjo P, Stromblad L-G, Romner B. Clinical experience with the use of a shunt with an adjustable valve in children with hydrocephalus. *J Neurosurg* 2003; 98(3): 471-6.

18. Reinprecht A, Dietrich W, Bertalanffy A, Czech T. The Medos Hakim programmable valve in the treatment of pediatric hydrocephalus. *Childs Nerv Syst* 1997; 13(11-12): 588-94.

19. Rohde V, Mayfrank L, Ramakers VT, Gilsbach JM. Four-year experience with the routine use of the programmable Hakim valve in the management of children with hydrocephalus. *Acta Neurochirurgica* 1998; 140(11): 1127-34.

20. Ahn ES, Bookland M, Carson BS, Weingart JD, Jallo GI. The Strata programmable valve for shunt-dependent hydrocephalus: the pediatric experience at a single institution. *Childs Nerv Syst* 2007; 23(3): 297-303.

21. Martinez-Lage JF, Almagro M-J, Del Rincon IS, et al. Management of neonatal hydrocephalus: feasibility of use and safety of two programmable (Sophy and Polaris) valves. *Childs Nerv Syst* 2008; 24(5): 549-56.

22. Robinson S, Kaufman BA, Park TS. Outcome analysis of initial neonatal shunts: does the valve make a difference? *Pediatr Neurosurg* 2002; 37(6): 287-94.

23. Hanlo PW, Cinalli G, Vandertop WP, et al. Treatment of hydrocephalus determined by the European Orbis Sigma Valve II survey: a multicenter prospective 5-year shunt survival study in children and adults in whom a flow-regulating shunt was used. *J Neurosurg* 2003; 99(1): 52-7.

24. Serlo W. Experiences with flow-regulated shunts (Orbis-Sigma valves) in cases of difficulty in managing hydrocephalus in children. *Childs Nerv Syst* 1995; 11(3): 166-9.

25. Haberl EJ, Messing-Juenger M, Schuhmann M, et al. Experiences with a gravity-assisted valve in hydrocephalic children. *J Neurosurg Pediatr* 2009; 4(3): 289-94.

26. Meling TR, Egge A, Due-Tonnessen B. The gravity-assisted Paedi-Gav valve in the treatment of pediatric hydrocephalus. *Pediatr Neurosurg* 2005; 41(1): 8-14.

27. Rohde V, Haberl E-J, Ludwig H, Thomale U-W. First experiences with an adjustable gravitational valve in childhood hydrocephalus. *J Neurosurg Pediatr* 2009; 3(2): 90-3.

28. Kestle JR, Drake JM, Cochrane DD, et al. Lack of benefit of endoscopic ventriculoperitoneal shunt insertion: a multicenter randomized trial. *J Neurosurg* 2003; 98(2): 284-90.

29. Kulkarni AV, Drake JM, Lamberti-Pasculli M. Cerebrospinal fluid shunt infection: a prospective study of risk factors. *J Neurosurg* 2001; 94(2): 195-201.

30. Haines SJ, Walters BC. Antibiotic prophylaxis for cerebrospinal fluid shunts: a metanalysis. *Neurosurgery* 1994; 34(1): 87-92.

31. Langley JM, LeBlanc JC, Drake J, Milner R. Efficacy of antimicrobial prophylaxis in placement of cerebrospinal fluid shunts: meta-analysis. *Clin Infect Dis* 1993; 17(1): 98-103.

32. Ratilal B, Costa J, Sampaio C. Antibiotic prophylaxis for surgical introduction of intracranial ventricular shunts. *Cochrane Database Syst Rev* 2006; 3: CD005365.

33. Zabramski JM, Whiting D, Darouiche RO, et al. Efficacy of antimicrobial-impregnated external ventricular drain catheters: a prospective, randomized, controlled trial. *J Neurosurg* 2003; 98(4): 725-30.

34. Govender ST, Nathoo N, van Dellen JR. Evaluation of an antibiotic-impregnated shunt system for the treatment of hydrocephalus. *J Neurosurg* 2003; 99(5): 831-9.

35. Eymann R, Chehab S, Strowitzki M, Steudel W-I, Kiefer M. Clinical and economic consequences of antibiotic-impregnated cerebrospinal fluid shunt catheters. *J Neurosurg Pediatr* 2008; 1(6): 444-50.

36. Parker SL, Attenello FJ, Sciubba DM, et al. Comparison of shunt infection incidence in high-risk subgroups receiving antibiotic-impregnated versus standard shunts. *Childs Nerv Syst* 2009; 25(1): 77-83; discussion 85.

37. Sciubba DM, Stuart RM, McGirt MJ, et al. Effect of antibiotic-impregnated shunt catheters in decreasing the incidence of shunt infection in the treatment of hydrocephalus. *J Neurosurg* 2005; 103(2 Suppl.): 131-6.

38. Sciubba DM, Noggle JC, Carson BS, Jallo GI. Antibiotic-impregnated shunt catheters for the treatment of infantile hydrocephalus. *Pediatr Neurosurg* 2008; 44(2): 91-6.

39. Sciubba DM, McGirt MJ, Woodworth GF, Carson B, Jallo GI. Prolonged exposure to antibiotic-impregnated shunt catheters does not increase incidence of late shunt infections. *Childs Nerv Syst* 2007; 23(8): 867-71.

40. Aryan HE, Meltzer HS, Park MS, Bennett RL, Jandial R, Levy ML. Initial experience with antibiotic-impregnated silicone catheters for shunting of cerebrospinal fluid in children. *Childs Nerv Syst* 2005; 21(1): 56-61.

41. Kan P, Kestle J. Lack of efficacy of antibiotic-impregnated shunt systems in preventing shunt infections in children. *Childs Nerv Syst* 2007; 23(7): 773-7.

Chapter 23

42. Pattavilakom A, Xenos C, Bradfield O, Danks RA. Reduction in shunt infection using antibiotic impregnated CSF shunt catheters: an Australian prospective study. *J Clin Neurosci* 2007; 14(6): 526-31.

43. Hayhurst C, Cooke R, Williams D, Kandasamy J, O'Brien DF, Mallucci CL. The impact of antibiotic-impregnated catheters on shunt infection in children and neonates. *Childs Nerv Syst* 2008; 24(5): 557-62.

44. Tuli S, O'Hayon B, Drake J, Clarke M, Kestle J. Change in ventricular size and effect of ventricular catheter placement in pediatric patients with shunted hydrocephalus. *Neurosurgery* 1999; 45(6): 1329-33; discussion 1333-5.

45. Albright AL, Haines SJ, Taylor FH. Function of parietal and frontal shunts in childhood hydrocephalus. *J Neurosurg* 1988; 69(6): 883-6.

46. Manwaring KH. Endoscopic-guided placement of the ventriculoperitoneal shunt. In: *Neuroendoscopy*. Manwaring KH, Crone KR, Eds. New York: Mary Ann Liebert, 1992; 29-40.

47. Taha JM, Crone KR. Endoscopically guided shunt placement. *Techn Neurosurg* 1996; 1: 159-67.

48. Villavicencio AT, Leveque J-C, McGirt MJ, Hopkins JS, Fuchs HE, George TM. Comparison of revision rates following endoscopically versus nonendoscopically placed ventricular shunt catheters. *Surg Neurol* 2003; 59(5): 375-9; discussion 379-80.

49. Gil Z, Siomin V, Beni-Adani L, Sira B, Constantini S. Ventricular catheter placement in children with hydrocephalus and small ventricles: the use of a frameless neuronavigation system. *Childs Nerv Syst* 2002; 18(1-2): 26-9.

50. Drake JM. Endoscopic third ventriculostomy in pediatric patients: the Canadian experience. *Neurosurgery* 2007; 60(5): 881-6.

51. Kulkarni AV, Drake JM, Mallucci CL, et al. Endoscopic third ventriculostomy in the treatment of childhood hydrocephalus. *J Pediatr* 2009; 155(2): 254-9.e1.

52. Garton HJL, Kestle JRW, Cochrane DD, Steinbok P. A cost-effectiveness analysis of endoscopic third ventriculostomy. *Neurosurgery* 2002; 51(1): 69-77; discussion 77-8.

53. Tuli S, Alshail E, Drake J. Third ventriculostomy versus cerebrospinal fluid shunt as a first procedure in pediatric hydrocephalus. *Pediatr Neurosurg* 1999; 30(1): 11-5.

54. de Ribaupierre S, Rilliet B, Vernet O, Regli L, Villemure JG. Third ventriculostomy vs. ventriculoperitoneal shunt in pediatric obstructive hydrocephalus: results from a Swiss series and literature review. *Childs Nerv Syst* 2007; 23(5): 527-33.

55. Takahashi Y. Long-term outcome and neurologic development after endoscopic third ventriculostomy versus shunting during infancy. *Childs Nerv Syst* 2006; 22(12): 1591-602.

56. Drake JM, Kulkarni AV, Kestle J. Endoscopic third ventriculostomy versus ventriculoperitoneal shunt in pediatric patients: a decision analysis. *Childs Nerv Syst* 2009; 25(4): 467-72.

57. Kulkarni AV, Hui S, Shams I, Donnelly R. Quality of life in obstructive hydrocephalus: endoscopic third ventriculostomy compared to cerebrospinal fluid shunt. *Childs Nerv Syst* 2010; 26(1): 75-9.

58. Weinzierl MR, Rohde V, Gilsbach JM, Korinth M. Management of hydrocephalus in infants by using shunts with adjustable valves. *J Neurosurg Pediatr* 2008; 2(1): 14-8.

Chapter 23

Chapter 24

Myelomeningocele

Jeffrey P Blount MD

Associate Professor

SECTION OF PEDIATRIC NEUROSURGERY, CHILDREN'S OF ALABAMA,
UNIVERSITY OF ALABAMA AT BIRMINGHAM, BIRMINGHAM, ALABAMA, USA

Introduction

Myelomeningocele (MMC) is the most common and complex congenital anomaly affecting the central nervous system. Although the overall incidence of the disease has been steadily declining in Western cultures, it can still be reasonably anticipated that approximately 1,500 children born in the USA each year will have MMC (five cases per 10,000 births). In lay parlance, MMC is often referred to as spina bifida. However, 'spina bifida' is an overly general term that incorporates the full spectrum of neural tube defects, including lipomyelomeningocele, meningocele, diastematomyelia and dermal sinus tracts, in addition to the more common and more serious MMC. 'Spina bifida aperta' or 'spina bifida cystica' properly refers to classic 'open' MMC, while 'spina bifida occulta' refers to a family of related disorders in which the overlying skin is intact.

In MMC, the caudal end of the developing neural tube fails to assume its normal tubular structure during the sixth to eighth week of embryonic life. The neural tube remains as a flattened plate or placode of tissue that retains lateral connectivity with the skin and is therefore not skin covered. The spinal fluid characteristically accumulates in a large cisternal space beneath the exposed neural placode and can deflect the placode above the edges of the adjacent skin (Figure 1). The exposed neural tissue is rendered non-functional, but the exact mechanism by which this occurs remains controversial and incompletely

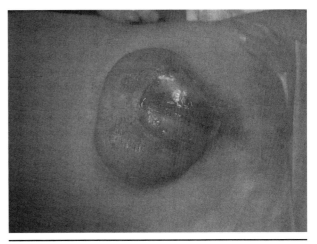

Figure 1. Lumbar myelomeningocele in a newborn infant. Note the flattened placode at the inferior edge of the defect. The dorsal projection and blister-like appearance of the tissue arises from the cistern of cerebrospinal fluid below the placode.

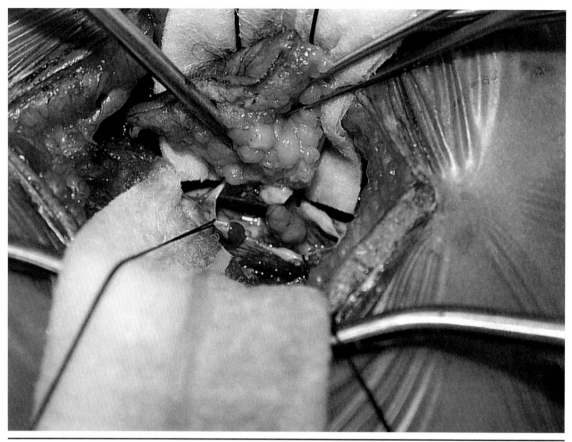

Figure 2. Dermal sinus tract. In this intraoperative photograph, the fatty-fibrous stalk has been further dissected and its route through the opened dura is visible. Note the fatty-fibrous connection immediately to the surface of the underlying spinal cord. *Photograph courtesy of Curtis J Rozelle MD.*

understood. By contrast, occult neural tube defects are characterized by less severe forms of caudal neural tube non-disjunction. In each of the variant forms of occult dysraphism, a component of the cutaneous ectoderm fails to properly separate from the neural ectoderm. The skin is thus intact but the underlying cord is progressively at risk for insult from tether. Tethering is the central event in the pathophysiology of occult neural tube defects. In the dermal sinus tract (Figure 2), a thin tract of ectoderm-derived tissue connects the skin and the caudal spinal cord, which it tethers. The lipomyelomeningocele (Figure 3) or spinal lipoma is characterized by an accumulation of fatty-fibrous tissue that may be evident as a painless subcutaneous mass under the uncompromised skin. The fatty-fibrous tissue characteristically adheres to the conus medullaris and

tethers the cord as it tracks rostrally during normal development. Such tethering typically leads to pain and progressive loss of lower extremity and sphincter function and may, if accompanied by a syrinx, also threaten upper extremity and bulb function. The terminology of neural tube defects is often further confused in the use of the term 'spina bifida occulta.' This term is often used to refer to the whole family of skin-covered occult neural tube defects, whereas it in fact most precisely applies to the least serious form in which the posterior elements of the bony spine fail to fuse, but the neural elements are normal in function and structure and the spinal cord is not tethered.

MMC is the most common and serious form of neural tube defect. It requires continued neurosurgical management and typically multiple interventions

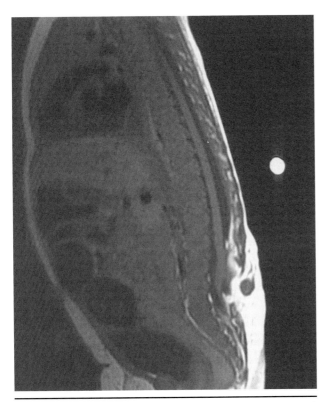

Figure 3. Sagittal MRI demonstrating spinal lipoma or lipomyelomeningocele. The hyperdense (white) tissue underlying the skin can be seen to enter the spinal canal and attach to the caudal spinal cord. This characteristically gives rise to tethered spinal cord syndrome.

throughout the lifespan of the patient. As a result, this review focuses on the best available medical evidence for the treatment of MMC. The three central, core, recurring neurosurgical issues are:

* Hydrocephalus.
* Chiari malformation type II (CM2).
* Tethered spinal cord (TSC).

The primary causes of childhood death in patients with MMC are un- or under-recognized hydrocephalus and CM2-related brainstem failure. (The most common non-neurologic cause of death is urosepsis.) Additional issues include consideration of the route of delivery (vaginal versus Cesarean section) and the timing of and closure technique for the open MMC. Each of these issues is addressed as it might arise chronologically in the lifespan of an affected infant.

Methodology

A National Library of Medicine (PubMed) search was performed for English-language references published from 1966 through February 2010 with the medical subject heading 'myelomeningocele' in combination with 'hydrocephalus, Chiari II malformation' and 'tethered spinal cord,' (separately) yielding a total of 1,340 abstracts for review. The bibliographies of selected chapters from current textbooks were also reviewed to identify other pertinent articles. Articles pertaining to management strategies and controversies surrounding closure, hydrocephalus, Chiari II malformation, and the tethered cord were subselected and carefully reviewed with regard to principles of evidence-based medicine. Approximately 80 such papers form the basis of review for this chapter.

Intrauterine closure

The central premise supporting intrauterine closure (IUC) is that neurologic function is progressively lost during embryonic life for a fetus harboring an MMC, and it has been hypothesized that repair of the defect may minimize or reverse ongoing damage to neural elements [1, 2]. This concept is unproven, but arose initially from anecdotal observations from early ultrasound studies in which movements of the lower extremities were noted early in the pregnancy but not in later gestation. Large animal-model MMC studies and pathologic studies of postmortem infants with MMC gave further support to the hypothesis that ongoing damage in MMC was secondary and was perhaps due to exposure of the placode to amniotic fluid [3, 4]. If this were true then IUC could potentially arrest ongoing decline and result in a newborn with greater retained neurologic function.

The first attempts at IUC were conducted in 1994. Early retrospective case series suggested that patients undergoing IUC showed a lower incidence of shunt dependency and CM2 (so-called 'hindbrain hernia') [1, 5], although urologic status appeared unchanged [6]. Bruner *et al* demonstrated a statistically significant decrease in the incidence of need for ventriculoperitoneal (VP) shunt in a retrospective case-control study of 29 patients treated with IUC [1] **(III/B)**. The incidence of 'hindbrain hernia' was also less (IUC 38%, control 95%) [1] **(III/B)**. Identified fetal risks included direct neurologic injury, placental abruption, and premature delivery, and the risks for oligohydramnios were significantly elevated [1, 7]. Maternal risks included infection, infertility, amniotic fluid leak, and bleeding.

Despite these risks and limited power of the supporting evidence, the promising outcomes reported in initial papers led to an explosion of interest in IUC. By 2003, it was estimated that more than 400 IUC procedures had been performed worldwide [2-6]. In an effort to better define the contribution of IUC, the US National Institute of Child Health and Human Development sponsored a prospective, randomized clinical trial to evaluate outcomes [8, 9]. This trial (the Management of Myelomeningocele Study or MOMS trial) aimed to enroll 200 women aged 18 years or older who were pregnant with a child with MMC, and randomize them to treatment with IUC or conventional postnatal closure (PNC) [8]. Simultaneously, fetal surgery and pediatric neurosurgery centers agreed a moratorium on further IUC studies that were not part of the MOMS trial. The recent publication of the MOMS trial [8] has revolutionized and reinvigorated the entire field of MMC management in neurosurgery through the extent and degree of the reported findings and the quality of the underlying evidence **(Ib/A)**.

The MOMS trial

Enrollment for the MOMS trial began in 2003. Three geographically diverse institutions (the Children's Hospital of Philadelphia, the University of California at San Francisco, and Vanderbilt University) functioned as study centers and data were compiled, stored, and managed at the George Washington University Biostatistics Center. The study was initially powered to require 100 patients in each of two treatment arms (IUC or PNC) and aimed to complete enrollment within 5 years. However, the study was halted in 2010 after enrollment of 183 patients because ongoing analysis demonstrated significantly better outcomes in patients treated with IUC.

Maternal eligibility criteria at the initial screening included the following:

- Age 18 years or older.
- A single pregnancy between 19 and 25.9 weeks' gestation, with the fetus affected by MMC.
- Absence of obesity (BMI <35kg/m^2).

Obstetric exclusion criteria included a history of preterm delivery or risk thereof (short or incompetent cervix) and evidence of placental abruption. Fetal exclusion criteria included an abnormal karyotype, kyphoscoliosis, or evidence of any other anomaly beyond MMC. Additional maternal exclusions related to social and economic factors such as the presence of a partner and the ability to continue all care at the study center where care was initially provided. A total of 1,087 women were initially screened, but only 27.5% were referred to a center to be considered for inclusion. After further screening at the study centers and detailed informed consent discussions, 183 patients were ultimately enrolled (91 IUC, 92 PNC). White women were disproportionately represented (>92% in each treatment arm). Data were available from 158 patients at the time of analysis, with 30-month follow-up data from 134 patients. This represents approximately 15% of the original cohort that underwent screening.

Women randomized to IUC underwent surgery before 26 weeks of gestation. A hysterotomy was performed with the mother under general anesthesia. The fetus was further anesthetized then turned to expose the MMC, and a multilayer closure was performed. Tocolytics and antibiotics were administered per protocol. Fetal wellbeing was assessed via standard protocols, including ultrasound imaging. Preterm labor was treated with tocolytics and patients not responsive to tocolytics were delivered urgently via Cesarean section. Otherwise, routine Cesarean delivery was performed at 37 weeks via the same incision.

Women randomized to PNC returned to their home institution until delivery, when they returned to their study centre for a Cesarean section. PNC was performed by the same team who performed IUC for those women randomized to IUC, utilizing standardized techniques.

Primary outcome measures included neonatal death or placement of a VP shunt. The decision to shunt was made by a blinded panel of experienced pediatric neurosurgeons employing standardized criteria. Secondary outcomes included surgical and pregnancy complications, neonatal morbidity and mortality, extent of hindbrain herniation (as defined by MRI interpretation by radiologists blinded to the treatment group), time to first shunt, locomotion capabilities, and assessment of disability. Additional secondary outcomes included performance on a battery of standardized scales of development (Bayley Scales of Infant Development II and the Peabody Developmental Motor Scales).

There was a statistically significant difference between the groups in the primary outcome measure. The group treated with PNC had a 98% likelihood of neonatal death or placement of a VP shunt, compared with 68% in the IUC group (p<0.001). This was entirely due to a significant difference in the rate of VP shunt placement between the two groups. Mortality was identical. At 12 months' follow-up, 82% of patients in the PNC group required a shunt, compared with only 40% in the IUC group (p<0.001) **(Ib/A)**. In addition, the extent of hindbrain hernia was reduced in the IUC group (64% of patients) compared with the PNC group (98%) **(Ib/A)**.

The incidence of maternal and fetal complications was higher in the IUC group, with the only cases of chorioamniotic membrane separation (p<0.0001) or premature spontaneous rupture of membranes seen in this group. Rates of premature delivery were also markedly higher in the IUC group (p<0.001) with 13% of this group delivering before 30 weeks and 26% by 34 weeks. Overall, 79% of the IUC group and 15% of the PNC group delivered before the targeted 37 weeks' gestation. The only mortality in the IUC group was due to prematurity.

Although the MOMS trial produced important class I evidence, it has several important limitations. The

most immediate of these pertains to the applicability of the data. The sample studied was a highly selected group that featured almost exclusively white, non-obese women. Indeed, only around 15% of the original group screened for candidacy was ultimately enrolled in the study [10]. In addition, the initial report does not present data on urologic outcomes or any consideration of TSC [10-12]. It will be essential for future reports from these centers to include these important data, as well as longitudinal data incorporating standardized assays of neuropsychological development for comprehensive analysis of the effectiveness of IUC.

Route of delivery for MMC patients

An area of debate in the management of MMC patients is the method of delivery at birth. Because of the structural defect and incompetent skin overlying the delicate neural tissue, there is often an intuitive inclination on the part of providers to recommend Cesarean delivery. Studies show mixed results with regard to the necessity for Cesarean (or abdominal) delivery versus normal spontaneous vaginal delivery (NSVD) for the child antenatally diagnosed with MMC. Perhaps the strongest clinical indication for Cesarean delivery is cephalopelvic disproportion arising from fetal macrocephaly from hydrocephalus. In the absence of antenatal macrocephaly, review of approximately a dozen papers in the medical literature reveals few compelling data differentiating the two delivery approaches **(III/B)**.

Cochrane *et al* reviewed data from 200 children with MMC delivered at a single institution in an attempt to better identify risk factors for poor outcomes in delivery [13]. The group found an increased likelihood of neurologic impairment if the baby presented breech, but no difference between NSVD and Cesarean delivery for infants presenting vertex. Even those infants with MMC who were delivered breech via NSVD and demonstrated neurologic impairment showed sufficient improvements over 2 years that no difference was noted at 2-year follow-up **(III/B)**. Sakala and Andree reviewed 35 patients and found no difference in sac disruption, VP shunt incidence, urologic outcome, seizures, or meningitis between groups delivered via NSVD (n=20) or Cesarean delivery (n=15) [14] **(III/B)**. Merrill *et al* similarly found no difference in neurologic outcome, neonatal mortality, birth weight, or other morbidities between infants delivered via NSVD versus Cesarean delivery in a retrospective single-institution review covering 1971-1995 [15] **(III/B)**. Lewis *et al* found better ambulatory capability in a retrospective cohort study of infants delivered via NSVD compared with Cesarean delivery at both 2- and 10-year follow-up [16]. However, logistic regression analysis eliminated any statistical significance between the groups and the authors concluded there is no convincing case to be made for a preference for either method of delivery **(III/B)**. By contrast, Luthy *et al* reported significantly better motor performance for infants delivered by Cesarean section before the onset of labor. Interestingly, the benefit was not as great if the mothers were permitted to begin labor and then were converted to Cesarean section [17] **(III/B)**. This widely quoted study (n=200) from the *New England Journal of Medicine* is probably the most influential report on this topic.

Closure of the MMC

While subtle methodologic differences may exist between pediatric neurosurgeons in the techniques utilized to close the MMC, the central concepts surrounding the actual closure of the back defect are generally well accepted with minimal controversy [18-21]. Similar techniques that are practiced between centers have evolved without guidelines and have not been subjected to rigorous evaluation. Fundamentally, the closure of the back defect serves to 'un-do' part of the embryopathy in that it surgically separates the cutaneous ectoderm (skin edge) from the neuroectoderm (placode edge) as its first maneuver [22]. Each of the normal layers (pia, dura, fascia, and skin) are identified and surgically developed as a separate layer. Each is then closed sequentially to allow skin coverage and containment of the CSF. Successful operations often include identifying ventral and superior tethering bands and wide release of the skin from the underlying fascia [18]. Much of the data supporting these methodologies are derived from anecdotal reports of shared wisdom from

experienced neurosurgeons [23-26] **(IV/C)**. A variety of flaps have been described in the plastic surgery literature that may be valuable in closing very large defects, but all similarly arise from accumulated experience and comparative evaluations of techniques are lacking [23, 25].

Hydrocephalus

Overview

For the neurosurgeon treating patients with MMC, a primary concern is the ongoing management of hydrocephalus. Historically, approximately 85% of patients with MMC develop hydrocephalus that requires surgical management [25, 26]. Most patients are treated with placement of a shunt, although increasing attention is being paid to the utilization of alternative methods of CSF diversion, including endoscopic third ventriculostomy (ETV) and – in some cases – concomitant choroid plexus cauterization (CPC) to reduce CSF production [27, 28]. Substantial controversy exists regarding the management of hydrocephalus in the child with MMC.

Criteria for shunt insertion

Traditional criteria for insertion of a VP shunt are either of the following [29] **(III/B)**:

- Progressive head and ventricular enlargement disproportionate to body growth following MMC closure.
- Leakage from the site of closure on the back.

CSF shunts have an established performance record of controlling head growth, reducing ventricular size, and preventing leakage from the closure site. However, the management of hydrocephalus in patients with MMC is often multifactorial and complex. MMC patients characteristically have 'brittle' hydrocephalus in which severe manifestations of shunt malfunction may become evident in short periods of time. MMC patients often undergo multiple revisions and frequently have extended hospital stays secondary to their numerous medical issues.

As a consequence of the complications inherent to shunts in this population, there has been recent consideration by some groups as to whether the initial criteria for shunt placement should be more rigorous, with the expected result being that the overall incidence of shunts would decrease in patients with MMC [26, 30]. Bowman et al have limited the criteria for shunt insertion to wound leakage or progressive macrocephaly and in so doing have reduced the incidence of shunt placement to 50% [30]. To date, these patients have demonstrated stable and good neurologic development. It is unknown whether the trade-off in lower shunt complications (presumed due to a lower incidence of shunt placement) will be offset by cognitive changes from sustained ventricular dilation.

Timing of shunt insertion

The timing of shunt placement remains contentious and there are limited data to guide management. Options include placing a shunt at the time of MMC closure, or staging procedures by placing the shunt in a separate operation at a later date. Simultaneous shunt placement with MMC closure is efficient and protects the fresh closure from leaking CSF (assuming adequate shunt function is realized). In contrast, some authors contend that the risk for infection of the CSF shunt is higher because of potential contamination of the CSF from the open defect. Several papers have addressed this controversy, but all are limited as they consist of retrospective case series.

Hubballah and Hoffman reported good outcomes in nine of 10 patients shunted at the time of MMC closure in an early case series [31] **(III/B)**. Miller et al reported on 69 consecutive patients treated with simultaneous MMC closure and shunt insertion and found no difference in shunt infection, overall shunt complications, or symptomatic CM2 between the 21 patients who underwent simultaneous shunt insertion and the 48 patients who were staged [32] **(III/B)**. Group designation was based singularly upon surgeon preference and the groups did not differ significantly in head size or other preoperative morbidity. The rate of wound leakage was higher and the hospital stay

longer in the group undergoing staged shunt insertion [32]. Similarly Machado and Santos de Oliveira reported no difference in complications between groups undergoing simultaneous or delayed shunt placement [33] **(III/B)**.

It is interesting to note that this topic remains debated and surgeons appear divided, despite a preponderance of reports indicating minimal or no additional risk with simultaneous shunt placement. Potential explanations include the possibility that surgeons hope to avoid shunt placement unless absolutely necessary (possible with a longer confirmatory period of observation with staged operations), limited acceptance of the existing data due to the lack of high-quality evidence (all are retrospective series), or concerns that many neurosurgeons harbor about taking any action that may increase the rate of shunt infection.

Role of endoscopic third ventriculostomy instead of a VP shunt

An alternative procedure that has received much attention and acclaim for the treatment of hydrocephalus is ETV. In this procedure, a hole is made in the floor of the third ventricle allowing the ventricular CSF to drain directly into the adjacent cisternal space, where it gains access to the arachnoid granulations and may be reabsorbed. The need for a shunt is eliminated, obviating many of the risks associated with implanted hardware (e.g., infection, obstruction). A large multicenter Canadian ETV study indicated 1- and 5-year rates of success of 65% and 52%, respectively, for children with hydrocephalus from a variety of different etiologies [34]. These encouraging results are tempered in the setting of patients with MMC, as stratification of patients by etiology in this study (and others) revealed a significantly lower success rate and higher complication rate for patients with hydrocephalus associated with MMC [34] **(III/B)**. Age was a more powerful determinant of poor outcome, with the youngest children faring the worst.

Balanced against these larger studies are individual reports demonstrating very high rates of success in using ETV to control hydrocephalus. Teo and Jones reported a 72% success rate in long-term control of hydrocephalus in a group of patients with MMC [35] **(III/B)**. They noted that the success rate increased to 80% if young patients were removed from the series. Warf and Campbell reported the largest experience to date in 2009 with their prospective trial of 115 patients from East Africa treated with ETV in conjunction with CPC [27]. CPC reduces the production capability for CSF and is an important adjuvant to ETV in the experience of these providers [27, 28] **(III/B)**. The data analysis was also different in this study. Data were compiled and analyzed via life-table analysis utilizing an intent-to-treat paradigm. Predictors for failure were evaluated with multivariate logistic regression. Utilizing these techniques, Warf and Campbell demonstrated that 72% of patients with hydrocephalus from MMC could be successfully treated with ETC/CPC. Scarring of the cisterns or choroid plexus were predictors of failure, but age alone was not [27, 28].

Despite the strength of this evidence, many neurosurgeons are currently reluctant to embrace ETV for hydrocephalus from MMC. This is presumably due to concerns that the successful execution of ETV in MMC patients with complex anatomy can be challenging, leading to potential increased risk and decreased success in centers with a lower volume of MMC patients.

Role of hydrocephalus in unmasking symptoms of other comorbidities

Another controversy surrounding hydrocephalus in MMC relates to the overall contribution that subtle perturbations in hydrocephalus control may exert on the clinical manifestations of other MMC comorbidities such as CM2 or TSC. The rationale behind this view holds that there is a multitude of fundamental cellular and neuroanatomic abnormalities in the patient with MMC. As such, the entire central nervous system is compromised to a variable degree. Many patients exist with reduced margins for stress to the nervous system and thus more readily become symptomatic when presented with other physiologic challenges. The classic example is CM2 in the neonate [36, 37]. Because alterations in CSF dynamics are the major potential stressors to the already compromised nervous system, CSF problems must be avoided to maintain good neurologic function. This hypothesis provides a conceptual framework to understand how shunt failure may cause an increase in symptoms of either a compromised brain stem or posterior fossa, CM2, or TSC [36-39] **(III/B)**. The number of papers directly addressing this phenomenon is limited and the evidence is all level III, but practice appears to be gradually evolving toward implicating shunt failure as a potential important causative etiology for multiple different symptoms in the patient with MMC. As such, assurance of shunt function becomes foremost in addressing the symptomatic patient with MMC and hydrocephalus **(III/B)**.

Assurance of adequate shunt function is itself another topic of uncertainty and controversy in the MMC population. Most experienced pediatric neurosurgeons hold surgical exploration of the shunt as the 'gold standard' to determine adequacy of flow and function. This position is derived in part from the well-described phenomenon of shunt failure without evidence of change in ventricular size on imaging studies [39]. Consequently, the threshold for operative exploration of the shunt in MMC patients has diminished in many pediatric neurosurgery groups, and operative exploration should be considered in the setting of the symptomatic patient without an obvious alternative explanation for the presenting symptoms [37, 39].

Chiari II malformation

CM2 includes a constellation of anatomic abnormalities within the posterior fossa and incorporates changes in the brainstem, cerebellum, skull, spinal cord, and rostral bony spine [37, 39]. Widespread utility of MRI has allowed careful delineation of hallmark abnormalities, which include caudal descent of the brainstem with elongation and abnormal angulation with respect to the midbrain [40] (Figure 4). The caudal medulla is elongated and

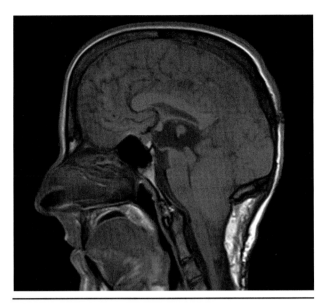

Figure 4. Sagittal MRI from a patient with MMC demonstrating characteristic findings for the Chiari malformation type II (CM2). These include caudal descent of the brainstem with elongation and abnormality angulation with respect to the midbrain. The caudal medulla is elongated and migrated further caudally and often resides disproportionately below the foramen magnum. The posterior fossa is characteristically reduced in size and the tentorium cerebelli is steeply angled and originates immediately above the foramen magnum. This abnormality often caudally displaces the torcula so that opening of the dura if CM2 decompression is undertaken may risk catastrophic inadvertent intrusion into the torcula.

migrated caudally, often disproportionately below the foramen magnum. The posterior fossa is characteristically reduced in size, frequently in conjunction with steep angulation of the tentorium cerebelli. This abnormality often caudally displaces the torcula so that it may lie at or immediately above the foramen magnum. Overall, the posterior fossa appears markedly elongated, stretched, and crowded [40].

A number of different theories have been proposed to account for the observed anatomic anomalies, including those that hypothesize hydrodynamic abnormalities, traction from distal tethering, and dysgenesis of the posterior fossa [40, 41]. Many children

with MMC will present with symptoms referable to dysfunction of neural elements in the posterior fossa or cervicomedullary junction. Worley *et al* observed a 1% incidence of the development of brainstem symptoms in a cohort of 63 patients with MMC who were serially observed [42]. Surgical decompression of CM2 has been utilized in an attempt to relieve pressure on the compromised, compressed neural elements and allow better perfusion and flow of CSF across the craniocervical junction [41, 43, 44].

The extent, urgency, and overall value of surgical decompression remain controversial [37, 39, 41-46]. Surgical decompression of the posterior fossa contributed little toward preventing mortality in those with early manifestations of brainstem dysfunction in the series by Worley *et al* [42] **(III/B)**. In contrast, Pollack *et al* published a comprehensive 14-year review in which they identified 25 patients with MMC who developed signs and symptoms of brainstem dysfunction [41]. They defined two groups that differed by age (neonates and children). Neonates declined more abruptly and both groups declined relentlessly until posterior fossa decompression was undertaken. Single and multivariate analysis demonstrated that outcome was dependent upon preoperative neurologic status. Neonates had more profound deficits, which the authors attributed to preoperative decline and they found that age was not a predictor of outcome. They concluded that prompt aggressive decompression is warranted to optimize neurologic outcomes **(III/B)**.

There appears to have been a gradual evolution in management principles away from immediate and aggressive decompression. Most centers at least initially advocate careful and comprehensive evaluation of shunt function. There is variability between centers as to what this means. Surgical exploration may be considered with or without evidence of ventricular change on radiographic studies. At present, no disease-specific outcome measure has been developed to facilitate comparison of outcomes; in addition, comparative effectiveness trials have not been conducted to investigate shunt exploration from CM2 surgical decompression.

Tethered spinal cord

Management of TSC is a key component of patient care. Cord tethering is thought to arise as a result of scar formation between the surgically closed placode and the surrounding dura. Technical details at the time of closure, such as ensuring that pial surfaces face the dura, may reduce the incidence and severity of tethering. At present, however, there are no widely accepted methods that eliminate TSC.

Despite substantial efforts, much remains unknown about the pathophysiology of TSC [47]. Perhaps the most obvious example of this is that TSC is not a uniform finding in MMC patients. While some degree of scarring and anatomic re-tether must take place in all patients, only approximately 30-35% of patients with MMC will demonstrate symptomatic TSC [47-50]. All patients who have had an MMC closed have a low-lying conus, whether or not they demonstrate symptomatic TSC [51-53].

The most common symptoms of TSC are back pain, progressive scoliosis, and progressive neurologic deficit involving the lower extremities [51, 54, 55]. Surgical untethering aims to identify any areas of scar that cause adherence between the distal cord or placode and the surrounding dura, with the goal of reducing or reversing these symptoms. Bowman *et al* have conducted the most comprehensive, long-term population studies of TSC in MMC [55]. Between 1975 and 2008, 502 newborns with MMC were closed at the Children's Memorial Hospital, Chicago. Approximately a quarter (n=114; 24%) required surgical release of TSC at an average age of 7 years, and 71% of patients required only a single release. Nine percent required two untetherings and only 3% required more than two untetherings. Nearly all had hydrocephalus and had required a VP shunt. Indications for surgery included a change in manual motor testing on routine examination in conjunction with symptoms. Urodynamics were uniformly obtained and defined a baseline level of function; they may be helpful in certain equivocal cases. The incidence of neurologic decline following TSC release was 3.5% [55] **(III/B)**.

Perhaps the greatest controversy surrounding TSC is the degree to which aggressive untethering should be undertaken. Few conclusive data exist to establish management guidelines. Most practice is now driven by single-institution experience and individual practice. Drake has written eloquently on this controversy and has urged caution in embracing prophylactic surgery [56] **(IV/C)**.

Quality of evidence

Despite a paucity of high-quality evidence available to guide the surgical management of MMC, patients have demonstrably experienced longer lifespans with reduced morbidity over the past several decades [57-60]. Early studies reported single-institution or single-provider experiences. Insights were shared as clinical pearls and observations were minimally analyzed. Later studies often involved larger groups, more precise definitions, more comprehensive evaluation of data, and more sophisticated statistical analysis. Very limited numbers of prospective studies have been performed and the MOMS trial is the only prospective randomized controlled trial within the field.

Recognition of the importance of evidence-based medicine by important advocacy and support organizations such as the Spina Bifida Association (SBA) and government agencies such as the Centers for Disease Control and Prevention (CDC) and the Agency for Healthcare Research and Quality (AHRQ) is driving improved research in this population. As early as the mid-1990s, the SBA formally recognized the importance of developing an evidence-based medicine approach to the multidisciplinary care of children with MMC. In 2002, the SBA Professional Advisory Council was instituted to develop a core research agenda. This effort culminated in a multidisciplinary symposium sponsored by the CDC, National Institutes of Health (NIH), Child Health and Human Development, National Center for Medical Rehabilitation Research, Interagency Committee of Disability Research, Interagency Committee on Disability Research, AHRQ, NIH Office of Rare Diseases, and SBA. Initial comments at this meeting acknowledged that "the evidence base for current care is shaky at best" [51]. The result of the symposium was a monograph entitled *Evidence-Based Practice in Spina Bifida: Developing a Research Agenda*. Neurosurgical topics included hydrocephalus, Chiari malformation, TSC, tethering in adults, syringomyelia, neurosurgical causes of scoliosis, and the reliability of adjunctive tests of neurologic functioning. The following research priorities were identified in neurosurgery:

♦ Assessment and treatment of hydrocephalus in patients with MMC.
♦ The role of TSC in the long-term management of patients with MMC.
♦ The long-term neurologic priorities, challenges, complications, and treatments for adults with MMC.
♦ Identification of patients with neurologic deterioration from hydrocephalus, shunt malfunction, tethering, Chiari malformation, and syringomyelia.
♦ The role of neurosurgical causes of scoliosis in people with MMC.

Looking to the future

The SBA is now attempting to foster development of evidence-based guidelines for the treatment for patients with MMC. Three new initiatives have been developed since 2003 to further the quality of the evidence available for analysis, studies, and observations. These include the following:

♦ Development of an electronic medical record-based patient registry.
♦ Development of a classification and registry of clinics.
♦ Organization and sponsorship of an international, multidisciplinary research meeting (world congress) addressing recent developments and challenges in research related to MMC.

The patient registry initiative is designed to centrally compile a progressively larger amount of patient data in a manner compliant with the Health Insurance Portability and Accountability Act and institutional review boards. The clinic classification and registration initiative strives to organize the wide variety of clinics that are providing care for patients with MMC.

Historical studies, while often methodologically limited, have served to pioneer successful treatment algorithms and highlight areas of controversy that span the entire spectrum of neurosurgical management of MMC. Ongoing research is focused on evidence-based studies supported by the rigorous and comprehensive collection of data relevant to improving the treatment of patients with MMC.

Conclusions

MMC remains the most complex and most common congenital anomaly of the human central nervous system. Clinical controversies surround the management of hydrocephalus, CM2 and TSC. Level III and IV evidence informed all clinical decision-making until the recent publication of the MOMS trial **(Ib/A)**, which demonstrated a reduced need for VP shunt and a reduced incidence of hindbrain hernia when IUC was undertaken. These advantages must be weighed against a higher incidence of premature delivery and other maternal and fetal complications. The applicability of the trial to broad populations must also be questioned given the narrow inclusion criteria employed. Nonetheless the publication of the MOMS trial represents a landmark accomplishment in evidence-based medicine in MMC.

Recommendations	Evidence level
◆ IUC of MMC is associated with a statistically significant reduction in the need for a VP shunt and a lower incidence of radiographic hindbrain hernia. However, prematurity and maternal and fetal complications such as premature rupture of membranes and chorioamniotic membrane separation are increased with IUC.	Ib/A
◆ Layered, surgical closure of MMC is warranted to cover exposed neural tissue, retain and control CSF, and minimize the risk of developing TCS.	IV/C
◆ For antenatally diagnosed MMC, Cesarean delivery is more common but unproven to be superior to NSVD.	III/B
◆ Shunt insertion is necessary and useful in controlling hydrocephalus in 85% of children with MMC.	III/B
◆ CSF leakage from MMC closure, signs of symptomatic CM2, and progressive macrocephaly (with ventriculomegaly) are criteria for VP shunt insertion.	III/B
◆ Shunt insertion at the time of MMC closure does not result in a higher infection rate than delayed shunt insertion.	III/B
◆ ETV shows higher rates of failure and complications in patients with MMC than other etiologies of hydrocephalus.	III/B
◆ ETV with choroid plexus coagulation may be a superior technique to control hydrocephalus in patients with MMC.	III/B
◆ Relaxing the criteria for insertion of a VP shunt reduces the incidence of shunts and appears well tolerated in limited series.	III/B

References

1. Bruner JP, Tulipan N, Paschall RL, *et al*. Fetal surgery for myelomeningocele and the incidence of shunt-dependent hydrocephalus. *JAMA* 1999; 282: 1819-25.

2. Olutoye OO, Adzick NS. Fetal surgery for myelomeningocele. *Semin Perinatol* 1999; 23: 462-73.

3. Meuli M, Meuli-Simmen C, Hutchins GM, *et al*. The spinal cord lesion in human fetuses with myelomeningocele: implications for fetal surgery. *J Pediatr Surg* 1997; 32: 448-52.

4. Sutton LN. Fetal surgery for neural tube defects. *Best Pract Res Clin Obstet Gynaecol* 2008; 22: 175-88.

5. Tulipan N, Bruner JP, Hernanz-Schulman M, *et al*. Effect of intrauterine myelomeningocele repair on central nervous system structure and function. *Pediatr Neurosurg* 1999; 31: 183-8.

6. Holmes NM, Nguyen HT, Harrison MR, *et al*. Fetal intervention for myelomeningocele: effect on postnatal bladder function. *J Urol* 2001; 166: 2383-6.

7. Barini R, Barreto MW, Cursino K, *et al*. Abruptio placentae during fetal myelomeningocele repair. *Fetal Diagn Ther* 2006; 21: 115-7.

8. Adzick NS, Thom EA, Spong CH, *et al*. A randomized trial of prenatal versus postnatal repair of myelomeningocele. *N Engl J Med* 2011; 364: 993-1004.

9. Sutton LN, Adzick NS, Johnson MP. Fetal surgery for myelomeningocele. *Childs Nerv Syst* 2003; 19: 587-91.

10. Bauer SB. Prenatal vs. postnatal repair of myelomeningocele. *N Engl J Med* 2011; 364: 2554 [Letter to the editor].

11. Reefhuis J, Rasmussen SA, Honein MA. Prenatal vs. postnatal repair of myelomeningocele. *N Engl J Med* 2011; 364: 2555 [Letter to the editor].

12. Heep A, Cremer R, Sival D. Prenatal vs. postnatal repair of myelomeningocele. *N Engl J Med* 2011; 364: 2555 [Letter to the editor].

13. Cochrane D, Aronyk K, Sawatzky B, Wilson D, Steinbok P. The effects of labor and delivery on spinal cord function and ambulation in patients with meningomyelocele. *Childs Nerv Syst* 1991; 7: 312-5.

14. Sakala EP, Andree I. Optimal route of delivery for meningomyelocele. *Obstet Gynecol Surv* 1990; 45: 209-12.

15. Merrill DC, Goodwin P, Burson JM, *et al*. The optimal route of delivery for fetal meningomyelocele. *Am J Obstet Gynecol* 1998; 179: 235-40.

16. Lewis D, Tolosa JE, Kaufmann M, *et al*. Elective Cesarean delivery and long-term motor function or ambulation status in infants with meningomyelocele. *Obstet Gynecol* 2004; 103: 469-73.

17. Luthy DA, Wardinsky T, Shurtleff DB, *et al*. Cesarean section before the onset of labor and subsequent motor function in infants with meningomyelocele diagnosed antenatally. *N Engl J Med* 1991; 324: 662-6.

18. Shurtleff DB, Gordon L, Foltz EL, *et al*. Hydrocephalus and meningomyelocele: practical considerations. *GP* 1965; 32: 101-12.

19. Ransohoff J, Mathews ES. Neurosurgical management of patients with spina bifida and myelomeningocele. *Med Clin North Am* 1969; 53: 493-6.

20. McCullough DC, Johnson DL. Myelomeningocele repair: technical considerations and complications. 1988. *Pediatr Neurosurg* 1994; 21: 83-9; discussion 90.

21. Guthkelch AN, Pang D, Vries JK. Influence of closure technique on results in myelomeningocele. *Childs Brain* 1981; 8: 350-5.

22. Iskandar BJ, McLaughlin C, Oakes WJ. Split cord malformations in myelomeningocele patients. *Br J Neurosurg* 2000; 14: 200-3.

23. Shurtleff DB. 44 years experience with management of myelomeningocele: presidential address Society for Research into Hydrocephalus and Spina Bifida. *Eur J Pediatr Surg* 2000; 10(Suppl. 1): 5-8.

24. Epstein F. Meningomyelocele: 'pitfalls' in early and late management. *Clin Neurosurg* 1983; 30: 366-84.

25. McLone DG. Continuing concepts in the management of spina bifida. *Pediatr Neurosurg* 1992; 18: 254-6.

26. Bowman RM, McLone DG, Grant JA, *et al*. Spina bifida outcome: a 25-year prospective. *Pediatr Neurosurg* 2001; 34: 114-20.

27. Warf BC, Campbell JW. Combined endoscopic third ventriculostomy and choroid plexus cauterization as primary treatment of hydrocephalus for infants with myelomeningocele: long-term results of a prospective intent-to-treat study in 115 East African infants. *J Neurosurg Pediatr* 2008; 2: 310-6.

28. Warf BC, Wright EJ, Kulkharni AV. Factors affecting survival of infants with myelomeningocele in southeastern Uganda. *J Neurosurg Pediatr* 2011; 7: 127-33.

29. Rekate HL. To shunt or not to shunt: hydrocephalus and dysraphism. *Clin Neurosurg* 1985; 32: 593-607.

30. Bowman RM, Boshnjaku V, McLone DG. The changing incidence of myelomeningocele and its impact on pediatric neurosurgery: a review from the Children's Memorial Hospital. *Childs Nerv Syst* 2009; 25: 801-6.

31. Hubballah MY, Hoffman HJ. Early repair of myelomeningocele and simultaneous insertion of ventriculoperitoneal shunt: technique and results. *Neurosurgery* 1987; 20: 21-3.

32. Miller PD, Pollack IF, Pang D, *et al*. Comparison of simultaneous versus delayed ventriculoperitoneal shunt insertion in children undergoing myelomeningocele repair. *J Child Neurol* 1996; 11: 370-2.

33. Machado HR, Santos de Oliveira R. Simultaneous repair of myelomeningocele and shunt insertion. *Childs Nerv Syst* 2004; 20: 107-9.

34. Drake JM; Canadian Pediatric Neurosurgery Study Group. Endoscopic third ventriculostomy in pediatric patients: the Canadian experience. *Neurosurgery* 2007; 60: 881-6.

35. Teo C, Jones R. Management of hydrocephalus by endoscopic third ventriculostomy in patients with myelomeningocele. *Pediatr Neurosurg* 1996; 25: 57-63.

36. Rath GP, Bithal PK, Chaturvedi A. Atypical presentations in Chiari II malformation. *Pediatr Neurosurg* 2006; 42: 379-82.

37. Cai C, Oakes WJ. Hindbrain herniation syndromes: the Chiari malformations (I and II). *Semin Pediatr Neurol* 1997; 4: 179-91.

38. Lee TT, Uribe J, Ragheb J, *et al*. Unique clinical presentation of pediatric shunt malfunction. *Pediatr Neurosurg* 1999; 30: 122-6.

39. Blount JP. Symptoms of the Chiari 2 malformation. In: *The Chiari Malformations*. Oakes WJ, Tubbs RS, Eds. Elsevier; in press.

40. Rossi A, Cama A, Piatelli G, *et al*. Spinal dysraphism: MR imaging rationale. *J Neuroradiol* 2004; 31: 3-24.

41. Pollack IF, Pang D, Albright AL, Krieger D. Outcome following hindbrain decompression of symptomatic Chiari malformations in children previously treated with myelomeningocele closure and shunts. *J Neurosurg* 1992; 77: 881-8.

42. Worley G, Schuster JM, Oakes WJ. Survival at 5 years of a cohort of newborn infants with myelomeningocele. *Dev Med Child Neurol* 1996; 38: 816-22.

43. McLone DG, Dias MS. The Chiari II malformation: cause and impact. *Childs Nerv Syst* 2003; 19: 540-50.

44. Pollack IF, Kinnunen D, Albright AL. The effect of early craniocervical decompression on functional outcome in neonates and young infants with myelodysplasia and symptomatic Chiari II malformations: results from a prospective series. *Neurosurgery* 1996; 38: 703-10.

45. McLone DG, Knepper PA. The cause of Chiari II malformation: a unified theory. *Pediatr Neurosci* 1989; 15: 1-12.

46. Rahman M, Perkins LA, Pincus DW. Aggressive surgical management of patients with Chiari II malformation and brainstem dysfunction. *Pediatr Neurosurg* 2009; 45: 337-44.

47. Yamada S, Won DJ, Yamada SM. Pathophysiology of tethered cord syndrome: correlation with symptomatology. *Neurosurg Focus* 2004; 16: E6.

48. Yamada S, Knerium DS, Mandybur GM, *et al*. Pathophysiology of tethered cord syndrome and other complex factors. *Neurol Res* 2004; 26: 722-6.

49. Yamada S, Won DJ, Siddiqi J, *et al*. Tethered cord syndrome: overview of diagnosis and treatment. *Neurol Res* 2004; 26: 719-21.

50. Hudgins RJ, Gilreath CL. Tethered spinal cord following repair of myelomeningocele. *Neurosurg Focus* 2004; 16: E7.

51. Tamaki N, Shirataki K, Kojima N, *et al*. Tethered cord syndrome of delayed onset following repair of myelomeningocele. *J Neurosurg* 1988; 69: 393-8.

52. Just M, Ermert J, Higer HP, *et al*. Magnetic resonance imaging of postrepair-myelomeningocele - findings in 31 children and adolescents. *Neurosurg Rev* 1987; 10: 47-52.

53. Balasubramaniam C, Laurent JP, McCluggage C, *et al*. Tethered-cord syndrome after repair of meningomyelocele. *Childs Nerv Syst* 1990; 6: 208-11.

54. Herman JM, McLone DG, Storrs BB, *et al.* Analysis of 153 patients with myelomeningocele or spinal lipoma reoperated upon for a tethered cord. Presentation, management and outcome. *Pediatr Neurosurg* 1993; 19: 243-9

55. Bowman RM, Mohan A, Ito J, *et al.* Tethered cord release: a long-term study in 114 patients. *J Neurosurg Pediatr* 2009; 3: 181-7

56. Drake JM. Surgical management of the tethered spinal cord - walking the fine line. *Neurosurg Focus* 2007; 23: E4

57. Liptak GS. Introductory comments. In: *Evidence-Based Medicine in Spina Bifida; Toward a Research Agenda.* Washington: Spina Bifida Association of America, 2003; 4-6.

58. Rekate HL. Pediatric neurosurgical patient: the challenge of growing up. *Semin Paediatr Neurol* 2009; 16: 2-8.

59. Piatt JH Jr. Treatment of myelomeningocele: a review of outcomes and continuing neurosurgical considerations in adults. *J Neurosurgery Pediatr* 2010; 6: 515-25.

60. Alriksson-Schmidt A. Transition in young people with myelomeningocele. *Dev Med Child Neurol* 2011; 53: 581-2.

Chapter 25

Medulloblastoma

Paul Klimo Jr MD MPH, Neurosurgeon 1, 2
Samuel Adediran BS, Medical Student 3
Nicholas Wetjen MD, Assistant Professor, Neurosurgeon 4
Corey Raffel MD, Neurosurgeon 5

1 Semmes-Murphey Neurologic & Spine Clinic, Memphis, Tennessee, USA
2 St Jude Children's Research Hospital, Memphis, Tennessee, USA
3 Wright State University Medical School, Dayton, Ohio, USA
4 Mayo Clinic, Rochester, Minnesota, USA
5 Nationwide Children's Hospital, Columbus, Ohio, USA

Introduction

Medulloblastoma accounts for 20% of all childhood central nervous system tumors and 40% of posterior fossa tumors [1]. Incidence peaks between the ages of 3 and 5 years and is slightly more predominant in males [2]. In adults, it is a rare tumor with an incidence rate of 0.5 per million per year, accounting for 1-2% of all adult brain tumors [3].

Treatment of medulloblastoma includes surgical resection, radiation therapy, and chemotherapy. As a result of advances in treatment efficacy (including more effective management of related conditions such as hydrocephalus), event-free survival has dramatically increased in children with medulloblastoma over the past 20 years. Improvements in prognostic accuracy have paralleled these therapeutic advances. Clinical findings that have been found to serve as negative prognostic variables include the presence of residual tumor after resection, the presence of cerebrospinal fluid (CSF) dissemination, and age younger than 3 years at the time of treatment. Molecular and histological factors have also been studied to help in disease prognostication.

Methodology

A National Library of Medicine computerized literature search of PubMed was performed of publications from 1990 to 2010, using the following search terms alone and in combination: 'medulloblastoma,' 'pediatric,' 'classification,' 'hydrocephalus,' and 'endoscopic third ventriculostomy.' The titles and abstracts of the returned articles were reviewed and articles that were appropriate for an evidence-based review were selected. The bibliographies of these selected articles were also reviewed for other possible inclusions.

Diagnostic imaging

Computed tomography

Because most patients with medulloblastoma obtain the initial diagnosis following presentation to the emergency department, CT is usually the first imaging test obtained. On CT, medulloblastomas commonly appear as a solid, hyperdense cerebellar mass, often with surrounding vasogenic edema and frequently with evidence of obstructive hydrocephalus [4]. Enhancement following contrast is the norm (Nelson *et al* reported enhancement in 95% of 233 patients) and the tumors are usually well-circumscribed (found in 93% of studies from this series) (Figure 1) [5]. While most medulloblastomas are midline and within the fourth ventricle, one large series reported atypical locations, such as the cerebellar hemisphere (15%) and cerebellopontine angle (3.5%), in a notable minority of cases. Calcifications or cysts may be present in about half of cases. Hypodensity and non-enhancement are rare, but have been reported in very few patients [6].

While the vast majority of medulloblastomas occur in children, it is important to note that adult lesions may have distinct imaging characteristics. Adult medulloblastoma predominantly presents as a cerebellar hemispheric mass with poorly defined margins, cysts, and areas of necrotic degeneration [7, 8].

Magnetic resonance imaging

Contrast-enhanced cranial and full spine MRI is the study of choice for the surgical planning and staging of medulloblastoma. MRI shows in detail the location, size, and extent of the tumor, as well as the degree of ventricular obstruction. The tumor classically appears as a region of hypointensity on T1-weighted images, a region of iso- or hyperintensity on T2-weighted images, and with heterogeneous enhancement on contrast T1-weighted images (Figure 2) [9]. The composition of medulloblastoma – hypercellular with little extracellular water – accounts for its appearance on T2-weighted imaging, restricted diffusion on diffusion-weighted imaging, and increased ratios of choline to creatine and choline to N-acetyl aspartate [10-12].

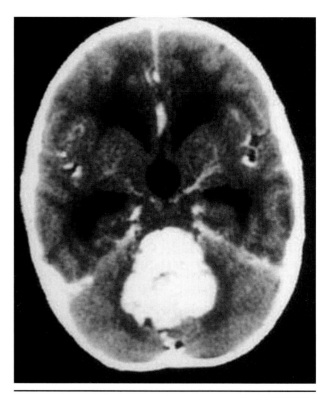

Figure 1. An axial contrast-enhanced CT image showing a midline fourth ventricular homogenously enhancing mass in the posterior fossa with obstructive hydrocephalus.

Although uncommon, intratumoral cysts, calcification, and vascular flow voids have been reported on MRI. Foraminal extension (in which tumor grows out the foramen of Luschka) – classically ascribed to ependymoma – is seen in approximately 14% of children with medulloblastoma [13].

Studies have shown contrast-enhanced MRI to be more sensitive in detecting spinal metastases than other diagnostic procedures (Figure 3). Preoperative spinal MRI establishes if there is spinal dissemination, which typically appears as nodular enhancement of the spinal cord surface or nerve roots, clumped nerve roots, or diffuse enhancement of the surface of the spinal cord or intracranial subarachnoid space ('sugar-coating') [4]. For postoperative staging, spinal MRI should be delayed until 2-3 weeks post-resection; blood can be difficult to distinguish from true CSF dissemination on MRI immediately after resection [9].

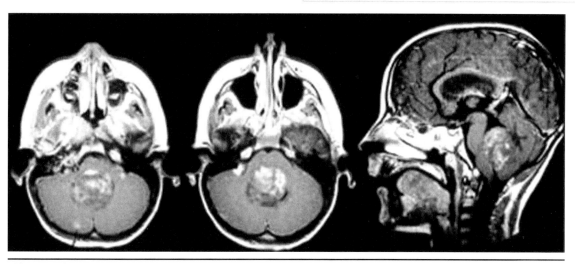

Figure 2. Axial and sagittal T1-weighted MRI with contrast, showing a heterogeneously enhancing mass within the fourth ventricle. Note the ventral shift of the pontomedullary region of the brainstem due to the tumor.

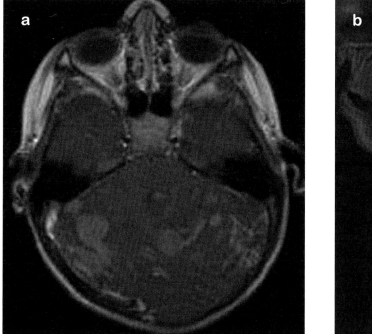
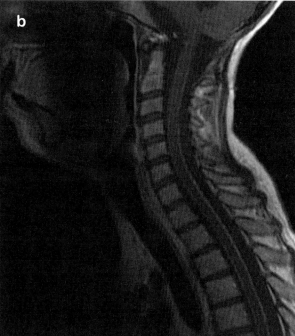

Figure 3. Contrast-enhanced MRI, demonstrating a) disseminated disease throughout the posterior fossa and b) leptomeningeal metastases coating the spinal cord.

Cerebrospinal fluid cytology

Spinal metastasis through leptomeningeal dissemination is frequent in medulloblastoma, being present in about 32% of patients at the time of diagnosis [4]. CSF sampling to detect leptomeningeal disease is best performed through a lumbar puncture (as opposed to a shunt tap or an external ventricular drain [EVD]). CSF analysis has, however, been shown to be less sensitive in detecting spinal metastases than spinal MRI. Meyers *et al* reported 86% sensitivity with MRI versus 60% with CSF study for the detection of tumor dissemination [14]. With multiple CSF cytological examinations, the sensitivity improved to 78%. In another study of 106 patients, nine had positive MRI but negative CSF findings; 12 had positive CSF but negative MRI findings [15]. The study concluded that spinal dissemination would be missed in 14-18% of patients with the use of either CSF cytology or spinal MRI alone **(III/B)**. Although MRI has better sensitivity, it still has the tendency to miss some metastases that may be positive with CSF cytology. Therefore, both diagnostic procedures are employed to minimize the number of patients with metastases who go undiagnosed.

Sampling should ideally be performed preoperatively, although this is sometimes not possible (depending on clinical status at presentation, including the possible presence of significant obstructive hydrocephalus precluding a safe tap). If done after resection, lumbar puncture should be performed 2-3 weeks postoperatively when there is no residual mass effect within the posterior fossa and the CSF is clear of surgical debris and blood products [15, 16].

Staging

Chang system

Medulloblastoma patients were traditionally classified by the Chang staging system, which is based on the extent of tumor dissemination – the M stage – and the size of the tumor – the T stage [17]. Several studies have shown that the M stage is far more important in determining the patient's prognosis than the T stage. In a prospective randomized trial that included 233 patients aged 3-16 years, 42 patients were stage M1-3 and 191 were M0. The rate of 5-year event-free survival was higher for M0 than for M1-3 patients (59% vs. 36%, respectively; p<0.003) [18] **(Ib/A)**. Zeltzer *et al* further confirmed the predictive value of M staging on prognosis, with reported mean (±standard deviation [SD]) 5-year progression-free survival (PFS) rates of 70±5%, 57±10%, and 40±8% in patients with M0, M1, and M2 disease, respectively [19]. There was no statistically significant difference in survival rates based on the method of detection of dissemination – rates were the same for patients with positive CSF cytology and those with evidence of radiographic dissemination. T staging has no predictive value on its own, but does complement M staging to determine prognosis [19].

Current risk evaluation

Over time the Chang system has been simplified to a high/average-risk categorization, with the inclusion of age as an additional risk factor. Zeltzer *et al* reported that children younger than 3 years had lower 5-year PFS rates than children of 3 years or older (mean±SD 32±10% vs. 58±4%, respectively; p=0.0014) [19] **(Ib/A)**. Complicating the analysis, however, is that children younger than 3 years received a lower radiation dose, both local boost and craniospinal, than older children. Recent treatment protocols call for no craniospinal radiation in patients younger than 3 years. In a review of the published literature, Packer *et al* noted that many of the studies evaluating age were published prior to the recognition of a subgroup of very young patients thought to have medulloblastoma [17]. These patients may in fact have had atypical teratoid or rhabdoid tumors, which have a worse prognosis.

Although age younger than 3 years is still considered a negative prognostic variable, the different regimen of treatment given to each group makes it difficult to determine the true impact of age on prognosis. Overall, a patient with gross total resection with no radiographic or CSF evidence of leptomeningeal dissemination, who is over the age of 3 years, is considered average risk. If any one of the three factors is present (subtotal resection, disseminated disease, or age younger than 3 years), the patient is in the high-risk category.

Management of preoperative hydrocephalus

Hydrocephalus is present in approximately 82-91% of medulloblastoma patients at the time of diagnosis and contributes to the overall morbidity and mortality in this population [20]. Tumor resection with opening of normal CSF pathways results in resolution of hydrocephalus in a majority of patients **(IIb/B)**. Fritsch *et al* retrospectively reviewed data from 52 patients with hydrocephalus secondary to posterior fossa tumors, 17 of which were medulloblastomas [21]. All patients underwent early tumor resection within 2 days of hospital admission and five patients required an EVD. The mean follow-up was 25 months. Only 11.5% of patients (6/52) required a shunt or endoscopic third ventriculostomy (ETV) post-resection. Only two of the six patients who required postoperative ETV had medulloblastoma. If ETV was routinely performed to manage hydrocephalus preoperatively, 88.5% of the patients would have been unnecessarily exposed to the complications of

the procedure **(III/B)**. Tamburrini *et al* reported that surgical resection along with EVD resolved hydrocephalus in 66.7% of patients with medulloblastoma [22] **(IIb/B)**. Overall, these data suggest that the majority of patients who present with obstructive hydrocephalus and medulloblastoma will experience successful resolution of their hydrocephalus without the need for permanent shunting.

Endoscopic third ventriculostomy

The approach to managing hydrocephalus prior to tumor resection has evolved over time, with ETV increasingly replacing ventriculoperitoneal (VP) shunting. This is because of the intraventricular/obstructive etiology of the hydrocephalus, which presents an ideal indication for an ETV, and the many complications associated with VP shunts.

A retrospective review of 206 patients with posterior fossa tumors compared 67 patients who underwent ETV before resection with 82 patients who were given steroids and had early surgery with EVD

Table 1. ETV procedure performed before the resection of a posterior fossa tumor, including medulloblastoma.

Reference	Study period, years	Patients operated on for a posterior crania fossa tumor associated with hydrocephalus, n	Patients treated with preoperative ETV, n	Success rate, %	Patients with complications, n (%)
Sainte-Rose *et al*, 2001 [23]	4	159	67 (31 medulloblastoma)	97	4 (6)
Morelli *et al*, 2005 [25]	15	114	14	79	2 (14)
Ruggiero *et al*, 2004 [26]	3	46	20 (seven medulloblastoma)	80	1 (5)
Bhatia *et al*, 2009 [27]	8	59	37	87	3 (8)

ETV = endoscopic third ventriculostomy

placement [23]. Although there was no randomization, the groups were relatively homogenous with respect to tumor location, tumor types, and extent of resection. A total of 94 patients had medulloblastoma, 81 of whom presented with preresection hydrocephalus. Only 6% of those treated with ETV preresection developed persistent postoperative hydrocephalus that required further treatment, compared with 26.8% of those with no preresection ETV [23] **(III/B)**. ETV is not, however, without complications. Infection, bleeding, neurological injury, fever, vomiting, and delayed occlusion of the stoma have all been reported. Hopf *et al* identified an overall complication rate of 6% [24]. Whether to pursue early surgical resection or to perform routine preoperative ETV is still a subject of debate. The studies to date are summarized in Table 1 [23, 25-27].

Risk factors prognostic of persistent hydrocephalus

Many studies have been conducted with a view to identifying factors predictive of postoperative hydrocephalus, as this knowledge would help guide therapeutic decision-making. Despite the lack of

consensus these studies suggest some commonalities [20, 28]:

* Age younger than 3 years.
* Partial or subtotal resection.
* Long duration of EVD use.
* CSF dissemination.
* Moderate or severe hydrocephalus on presentation.

In a prospective cohort study, Riva-Cambrin *et al* studied 454 children with the goal of using identifiable presenting characteristics as variables that could be used to formulate a score to help predict the risk of persistent hydrocephalus. The variables most predictive of persistent hydrocephalus are shown in Table 2 [29]. Patients with scores of 5 or greater were deemed high risk (Table 3) **(IIb/B)**.

Table 2. Canadian Preoperative Prediction Rule for Hydrocephalus in children with posterior fossa neoplasm [29]. *Reprinted with permision from the Journal of Neurosurgery Publishing Group.*

Predictor	Score
Age <2 years	3
Papilledema	1
Moderate/severe hydrocephalus	2
Cerebral metastases	3
Medulloblastoma	1
Total possible score	**10**

Table 3. Predicted probability of hydrocephalus at 6 months after resection on the Canadian Preoperative Prediction Rule for Hydrocephalus [29]. *Reprinted with permision from the Journal of Neurosurgery Publishing Group.*

Score	Probability of hydrocephalus
0	0.071
1	0.118
2	0.191
3	0.293
4	0.422
5	0.562
6	0.693
7	0.799
8	0.875
9	0.925
10	0.956

Management of postoperative hydrocephalus

After resection of medulloblastoma, hydrocephalus persists in 22-63% of patients [20]. In addition to the risk factors discussed previously, intra- and perioperative issues such as subarachnoid hemorrhage and cerebellar swelling may precipitate post-resection hydrocephalus [23]. VP shunt has been the predominant procedure in the management of postoperative hydrocephalus. However, studies have reported reduced survival rates in patients who undergo VP shunt placement [30]. In addition to the risks inherent to any shunted patient with hydrocephalus (e.g., infection, need for repeated operation), a concern unique with tumor patients is the risk of seeding the distal shunt site with metastases.

In a review of published studies, Rochkind et al reported 34 possible cases of metastases related to VP shunt placement in patients treated for medulloblastoma in 16 studies conducted between 1963 and 1984 [31]. Extracranial metastases were seen earlier in patients with VP shunt (13 months) than in those without VP shunt (24 months). In contrast, Berger et al found extracranial metastases occurred later in patients with VP shunt (25 months) than in those without (15 months). There was also no significant difference in extracranial metastases in those with shunt or without placement [32]. The authors therefore concluded that CSF shunts, regardless of type, did not predispose patients to extraneural metastases. While case reports of shunts causing the spread of malignancy outside of the craniospinal axis exist, the actual risk remains unclear (although presumably quite low) [33-35]. In response to the acknowledged risks of shunt placement, there has been growing enthusiasm by some for increased utilization of ETV as a management modality for tumor-related hydrocephalus. The results of these efforts are summarized in Table 4 [21, 23, 25, 26, 36, 37] **(III/B)**.

Table 4. ETV procedures performed after surgical resection of posterior fossa neoplasm including medulloblastoma.

Reference	Period of study, years	Patients operated on for a posterior crania fossa tumor associated with hydrocephalus, n	Patients with persisting hydrocephalus, n	Patients treated by postoperative ETV, n	Success rate of postoperative ETV, %
Sainte-Rose et al, 2001 [23]	4	159	26	9	100
Ruggiero et al, 2004 [26]	3	46	6	4	50
Fritsch et al, 2005 [21]	4	52	6	2	100
Morelli et al, 2005 [25]	15	114	17	8	100
Due-Tønnessen and Helseth, 2007 [36]	13	69	34	2	100
Tamburrini et al, 2008 [37]	6	104	30	30	90

ETV = endoscopic third ventriculostomy

Tumor treatment

Surgery

The impact of maximal tumor resection – the ideal goal of surgery for medulloblastoma – on prognosis has being the subject of debate for a long time. Radical resection reduces tumor bulk and rids the tumor of necrosis, possibly improving the efficacy of radiation therapy. Since all patients will receive adjuvant therapy, overly aggressive resection of tumors in critical areas (particularly the brainstem) is often ill-advised. It has been more than 30 years since Raimondi and Tomita showed that radical or complete resection increased survival, and more recent analyses have demonstrated that the quantity of residual tumor is the more important variable [38].

Albright *et al* reported that imaging was a more effective method of determining the degree of postoperative residual tumor than surgeon reporting [39]. More importantly, they found that, in children older than 3 years with no evidence of tumor dissemination (M0), 5-year PFS was better in those with residual tumor of less than $1.5cm^2$ than in children with residual tumor of more than $1.5cm^2$ (77% vs. 53%; p=0.03) [39] **(IIb/B)**. A study of 203 patients also demonstrated better prognosis in those with decreased postoperative tumor mass. Mean (±SD) 5-year PFS was 78±6% in M0 patients with less than $1.5cm^2$ residual tumor versus 54±11% in those with more than $1.5cm^2$ residual tumor (p=0.023) [19]. The prognostic advantage of maximal cytoreductive surgery ($<1.5cm^2$) was eliminated if the patient had metastatic disease. Thus, in patients with newly diagnosed medulloblastoma and disseminated disease, surgery should still be performed to relieve mass effect and re-establish CSF pathways, but aggressive resection at the risk of causing neurologic deficits is not justified. (It is, however, important to note that neurologic deficit can sometimes occur even in the setting of limited resection.)

Radiation and chemotherapy

Medulloblastoma can recur locally, throughout the neuraxis, and, rarely, outside the central nervous system. Because of its propensity for recurrence within the central nervous system, radiation delivered to the posterior fossa as well as the craniospinal axis has been a mainstay of adjuvant therapy. Radiation doses of 35-40Gy to the neuraxis and 50-60Gy to the posterior fossa have typically been used. In 1990, Evans *et al* was the first to report a randomized trial demonstrating the benefits of chemotherapy in conjunction with irradiation versus irradiation alone [18] **(Ib/A)**. Since then, numerous trials have examined various chemotherapy regimens before, during, and after radiotherapy [40-43].

The general consensus is that chemotherapy has improved survival for children with medulloblastoma. Typical chemotherapeutic agents include lomustine (CCNU), vincristine, cisplatin, and cyclophosphamide. Currently, the 5-year survival rates are 80-85% and 60% for average- and high-risk patients, respectively, with adjuvant chemo- and radiotherapy following aggressive resection. The addition of chemotherapy has allowed a reduction in the average dose of craniospinal irradiation to 23.4Gy while maintaining an 80% 5-year survival rate [41] **(Ib/A)**. Although better than radiation alone, preradiation chemotherapy is not as effective as immediate postoperative radiotherapy and concomitant chemotherapy [40, 44, 45] **(Ib/A)**. More recently, high-dose myeloablative chemotherapy with autologous stem-cell rescue has garnered interest. It is usually reserved for patients who cannot undergo the more standard chemo-radiotherapy regimens (young children) or those with recurrent disease [46-48]. Myeloablative chemotherapy has not been shown to be more effective than standard regimens in the treatment of *de novo* patients older than 3 years [43] **(IIb/B)**.

Radiation to the brain is not without long-term risks of cognitive decline, endocrine abnormalities, vascular complications, and secondary malignancies. As a result, much effort has been made over the years to either reduce the amount of radiation administered or eliminate it completely. After 36Gy, children between the ages of 3-7 years can experience a 20-30 point drop in their IQ [49]. Even with reduced craniospinal radiation (to 23.4Gy), a decrease of 10-15 points may occur. Conformal proton-beam therapy has also been investigated as an alternative to conventional electron radiotherapy in children with medulloblastoma because less radiation is administered to both the target and surrounding normal tissue [50] **(III/B)**.

The damaging effects of radiation are much more pronounced in children younger than 5 years. Thus, many have investigated treating these patients with chemotherapy alone initially and delaying radiation for as long as possible [51-54]. Unfortunately chemotherapy itself can have long-term consequences, such as cisplatin-induced hearing loss and vincristine-associated neuropathy [55].

Surveillance

Surveillance imaging is conducted to detect residual tumor, metastases, and tumor recurrence, and evaluate response to therapy [56, 57]. A commonly accepted protocol has been to perform a postoperative MRI within 2 days after surgical resection, again at 3 months, then every 6 months for 2 years, and annually thereafter. Most recurrences occur within the first 2 years. The therapeutic options for recurrence are similar to those at initial diagnosis, including chemotherapy, radiotherapy, and reoperation.

The value of surveillance imaging in medulloblastoma has been debated by some groups. Recurrent medulloblastoma carries a very high risk of subsequent death. Critics cite cases of recurrence not found by surveillance imaging. In addition, the purported survival benefit may be due to lead-time bias **(III/B)**. Importantly, there are no randomized trials to confirm the benefit of surveillance imaging. Adding to the controversy, the authors of a limited number of retrospective studies have reported relatively similar outcomes, but different conclusions. Saunders et al retrospectively studied surveillance MRIs of 107 patients followed for 5 years [58]. There were 53 recurrences, 15 of which were identified by surveillance imaging. They reported a median survival time of 17 months after surveillance-detected recurrence and 4 months after symptomatic tumor recurrence. They concluded that such a significant increase in survival time after surveillance-detected

recurrence proves the benefit of continuous postoperative surveillance imaging. In contrast, a report by Torres et al concluded that screening was of little value [59]. Their study population contained 23 recurrences among 86 patients who underwent treatment after surgical resection. The average survival time was 20 months in four patients after surveillance-detected recurrence, and 5 months in the 19 patients with symptomatic recurrence. Although the difference between the two groups was substantial, the authors accorded the difference to lead-time bias, length of time bias, or inadequate sensitivity of the MRI and CT scans used at the time. A major limitation of this study, however, is its age. It is nearly two decades old and does not reflect the potential benefits of modern adjuvant therapies and neuroimaging technology.

Biological factors of prognostic significance

Recent advances in molecular genetic techniques have spurred interest in applying these technologies to enhance the accuracy of risk stratification in medulloblastoma patients [60]. The presence of specific molecular and genetic markers in tumor specimens has been found to have some correlation with survival in limited studies. For example, increased expression of TrkC, the neurotrophin-3-receptor, and beta-catenin in medulloblastomas has been associated with better survival, whereas ERBB2, survivin, PDGF-RA, and p53 have been associated with metastasis and poorer survival [49]. Expression levels of certain species of mRNA have also been associated with patient outcome. Increased expression of c-Myc mRNA has been associated with a poorer prognosis, while increased expression of TrkC mRNA correlates with an improved prognosis [61]. Rutkowski et al found increased c-Myc to significantly portend a worse prognosis only in those with postoperative residual tumor, while increased TrkC conveyed better prognosis only in those with complete resection [62].

A major development over the last several years has been the molecular classification of medulloblastomas [63]. The four principal subgroups are Wnt, Shh, group 3 (non-Wnt, non-Shh) and group

4. Wnt and Shh (sonic hedgehog) were named for the signaling pathways thought to play prominent roles in the pathogenesis of the first two groups, but less is known for groups 3 and 4. Prognosis is excellent for patients with Wnt tumors, intermediate for those with Shh and group 4 tumors, and poor for those with group 3 disease.

Evidence on anaplasia, desmoplasia, and extent of nodularity

The contribution of histopathology to the clinical stratification of medulloblastoma, although promising, has been fraught with conflicting outcomes. Traditional histopathologic subtypes are based on morphology (histopathology) and include desmoplastic/nodular, medulloblastoma with extensive nodularity (MBEN), classic medulloblastoma, large cell, and anaplastic medulloblastoma. Anaplastic tumors carry a poor prognosis compared to classic or desmoplastic. Ozer et al, among others, have demonstrated that anaplasia correlates with an unfavorable prognosis [64]. A study by the Pediatric Oncology Group evaluated the extent of anaplasia in tumor specimens, and found that increasing degrees of anaplasia strongly correlated with progressively worse clinical outcomes [65]. There was, however, no increasing association between anaplasia grades and M stages. In contrast, alternative studies found no statistically significant association between anaplasia and worse prognosis (although there was a trend toward an association) [66].

Desmoplasia (found more commonly in adult medulloblastomas) has historically been associated with better prognosis; a reason, it was thought, why adults with medulloblastoma have better survival than children. More recent studies cast doubt on this assertion. In a study of 330 patients, Eberhart et al found no association between longer survival and the presence of desmoplasia [65].

Another potential prognostic factor that has been debated is the presence of nodularity on pathologic examination. Ozer et al found that extensive nodularity was associated with better outcomes on univariate analysis, but not on multivariate analysis [64]. Eberhart et al showed better outcomes with the presence of extensive nodularity, but found that grading of nodularity did not provide any additional use in risk stratification [65].

The continued research into predictive radiographic, pathologic, and molecular prognostic markers of medulloblastoma behavior will serve to improve the treatment of patients afflicted with these tumors.

Conclusions

Clear evidence supports the following:

* Age, spinal dissemination, and extent of residual tumor are the most important prognostic factors for survival.
* MRI and CSF studies are required diagnostic procedures for the identification of spinal dissemination.
* Age, moderate/severe hydrocephalus, metastases, papilledema, and tumor type are predictive of postoperative hydrocephalus.
* Adjuvant chemotherapy and radiation improve survival.
* According to molecular analysis studies, there are four distinct populations of medulloblastomas. This molecular subgrouping has proved useful for risk stratification and will serve as a means to develop targeted chemotherapy.

Controversy exists over the following:

* Whether the use of ETV or early surgical resection decreases the risk of postoperative persistent hydrocephalus.
* The risk of extraneural spread of the tumor with a shunt.
* Whether postoperative ETV adequately treats persistent hydrocephalus.
* Whether surveillance imaging is of benefit.

Recommendations	Evidence level
◆ Both CSF cytology and MRI are required to ensure the detection of spinal dissemination.	III/B
◆ Children older than 3 years have superior 5-year PFS and, with little residual disease after resection and no CSF dissemination, are considered average risk. Children younger than 3 years have an inferior 5-year PFS and are considered high risk.	Ib/A
◆ Early surgical resection resolves hydrocephalus in most patients with medulloblastoma.	IIb/B
◆ Fewer patients with preresection ETV have persistent hydrocephalus compared with no preresection ETV. Whether to treat hydrocephalus with early surgical resection or routine ETV is still controversial.	III/B
◆ Age less than 2 years, presence of papilledema, moderate/severe hydrocephalus, cerebral metastases, and tumor type are predictive of postoperative hydrocephalus.	IIb/B
◆ The use of ETV as an alternative to CSF shunt in the treatment of post-resection hydrocephalus has a high success rate.	III/B
◆ Radical tumor resection (<1.5cm^2) correlates with better prognosis. No evidence supports the benefit of total radical resection in patients with a disseminated tumor.	IIb/B
◆ Chemotherapy in conjunction with irradiation improves survival compared with irradiation alone.	Ib/A
◆ For the treatment of average-risk medulloblastoma, a reduced craniospinal irradiation dose of 23.4Gy is now considered feasible.	Ib/A
◆ Preradiation chemotherapy is not as effective as immediate postoperative radiotherapy and concomitant chemotherapy.	Ib/A
◆ High-dose myeloablative chemotherapy and stem-cell rescue have not been demonstrated to be superior to a standard chemotherapy regimen.	IIb/B
◆ Proton-beam therapy is an attractive alternative to conventional irradiation, because it exposes less radiation to the posterior fossa, craniospinal axis, and surrounding normal tissue.	III/B
◆ The benefit of surveillance imaging in terms of survival is controversial.	III/B

References

1. Mueller S, Chang S. Pediatric brain tumors: current treatment strategies and future therapeutic approaches. *Neurotherapeutics* 2009; 6: 570-86.
2. Kaderali Z, Lamberti-Pasculli M, Rutka JT. The changing epidemiology of paediatric brain tumours: a review from the Hospital for Sick Children. *Childs Nerv Syst* 2009; 25: 787-93.
3. Lai R. Survival of patients with adult medulloblastoma: a population-based study. *Cancer* 2008; 112: 1568-74.
4. Koeller KK, Rushing EJ. From the archives of the AFIP: medulloblastoma: a comprehensive review with radiologic-pathologic correlation. *Radiographics* 2003; 23: 1613-37.
5. Nelson M, Diebler C, Forbes WS. Paediatric medulloblastoma: atypical CT features at presentation in the SIOP II trial. *Neuroradiology* 1991; 33: 140-2.
6. Kumar R, Achari G, Banerjee D, Chhabra DK. Uncommon presentation of medulloblastoma. *Childs Nerv Syst* 2001; 17: 538-42; discussion 543.
7. Bourgouin PM, Tampieri D, Grahovac SZ, *et al.* CT and MR imaging findings in adults with cerebellar medulloblastoma: comparison with findings in children. *AJR Am J Roentgenol* 1992; 159: 609-12.
8. de Carvalho Neto A, Gasparetto EL, Ono SE, *et al.* Adult cerebellar medulloblastoma: CT and MRI findings in eight cases. *Arq Neuropsiquiatr* 2003; 61: 199-203.

Chapter 25

9. Blaser SI, Harwood-Nash DC. Neuroradiology of pediatric posterior fossa medulloblastoma. *J Neurooncol* 1996; 29: 23-34.

10. Provenzale JM, Mukundan S, Barboriak DP. Diffusion-weighted and perfusion MR imaging for brain tumor characterization and assessment of treatment response. *Radiology* 2006; 239: 632-49.

11. Yamashita Y, Kumabe T, Higano S, et al. Minimum apparent diffusion coefficient is significantly correlated with cellularity in medulloblastomas. *Neurol Res* 2009; 31: 940-6.

12. Kan P, Liu JK, Hedlund G, et al. The role of diffusion-weighted magnetic resonance imaging in pediatric brain tumors. *Childs Nerv Syst* 2006; 22: 1435-9.

13. Tortori-Donati P, Fondelli MP, Rossi A, et al. Medulloblastoma in children: CT and MRI findings. *Neuroradiology* 1996; 38: 352-9.

14. Meyers SP, Wildenhain SL, Chang JK, et al. Postoperative evaluation for disseminated medulloblastoma involving the spine: contrast-enhanced MR findings, CSF cytologic analysis, timing of disease occurrence, and patient outcomes. *AJNR Am J Neuroradiol* 2000; 21: 1757-65.

15. Fouladi M, Gajjar A, Boyett JM, et al. Comparison of CSF cytology and spinal magnetic resonance imaging in the detection of leptomeningeal disease in pediatric medulloblastoma or primitive neuroectodermal tumor. *J Clin Oncol* 1999; 17: 3234-7.

16. Gajjar A, Fouladi M, Walter AW, et al. Comparison of lumbar and shunt cerebrospinal fluid specimens for cytologic detection of leptomeningeal disease in pediatric patients with brain tumors. *J Clin Oncol* 1999; 17: 1825-8.

17. Packer RJ, Rood BR, MacDonald TJ. Medulloblastoma: present concepts of stratification into risk groups. *Pediatr Neurosurg* 2003; 39: 60-7.

18. Evans AE, Jenkin RD, Sposto R, et al. The treatment of medulloblastoma. Results of a prospective randomized trial of radiation therapy with and without CCNU, vincristine, and prednisone. *J Neurosurg* 1990; 72: 572-82.

19. Zeltzer PM, Boyett JM, Finlay JL, et al. Metastasis stage, adjuvant treatment, and residual tumor are prognostic factors for medulloblastoma in children: conclusions from the Children's Cancer Group 921 randomized Phase III study. *J Clin Oncol* 1999; 17: 832-45.

20. Kombogiorgas D, Natarajan K, Sgouros S. Predictive value of preoperative ventricular volume on the need for permanent hydrocephalus treatment immediately after resection of posterior fossa medulloblastomas in children. *J Neurosurg Pediatr* 2008; 1: 451-5.

21. Fritsch MJ, Doerner L, Kienke S, et al. Hydrocephalus in children with posterior fossa tumors: role of endoscopic third ventriculostomy. *J Neurosurg* 2005; 103(Suppl.): 40-2.

22. Tamburrini G, Massimi L, Caldarelli M, et al. Antibiotic impregnated external ventricular drainage and third ventriculostomy in the management of hydrocephalus associated with posterior cranial fossa tumours. *Acta Neurochir* (Wien) 2008; 150: 1049-55; discussion 1055-6.

23. Sainte-Rose C, Cinalli G, Roux FE, et al. Management of hydrocephalus in pediatric patients with posterior fossa tumors: the role of endoscopic third ventriculostomy. *J Neurosurg* 2001; 95: 791-7.

24. Hopf NJ, Grunert P, Fries G, et al. Endoscopic third ventriculostomy: outcome analysis of 100 consecutive procedures. *Neurosurgery* 1999; 44: 795-804; discussion 804-6.

25. Morelli D, Pirotte B, Lubansu A, et al. Persistent hydrocephalus after early surgical management of posterior fossa tumors in children: is routine preoperative endoscopic third ventriculostomy justified? *J Neurosurg* 2005; 103(Suppl.): 247-52.

26. Ruggiero C, Cinalli G, Spennato P, et al. Endoscopic third ventriculostomy in the treatment of hydrocephalus in posterior fossa tumors in children. *Childs Nerv Syst* 2004; 20: 828-33.

27. Bhatia R, Tahir M, Chandler CL. The management of hydrocephalus in children with posterior fossa tumours: the role of pre-resectional endoscopic third ventriculostomy. *Pediatr Neurosurg* 2009; 45: 186-91.

28. Schmid UD, Seiler RW. Management of obstructive hydrocephalus secondary to posterior fossa tumors by steroids and subcutaneous ventricular catheter reservoir. *J Neurosurg* 1986; 65: 649-53.

29. Riva-Cambrin J, Detsky AS, Lamberti-Pasculli M, et al. Predicting postresection hydrocephalus in pediatric patients with posterior fossa tumors. *J Neurosurg Pediatr* 2009; 3: 378-85.

30. Sun LM, Yeh SA, Wang CJ, et al. Postoperative radiation therapy for medulloblastoma - high recurrence rate in the subfrontal region. *J Neurooncol* 2002; 58: 77-85.

31. Rochkind S, Blatt I, Sadeh M, et al. Extracranial metastases of medulloblastoma in adults: literature review. *J Neurol Neurosurg Psychiatry* 1991; 54: 80-6.

32. Berger MS, Baumeister B, Geyer JR, et al. The risks of metastases from shunting in children with primary central nervous system tumors. *J Neurosurg* 1991; 74: 872-7.

33. Magtibay PM, Friedman JA, Rao RD, et al. Unusual presentation of adult metastatic peritoneal medulloblastoma associated with a ventriculoperitoneal shunt: a case study and review of the literature. *Neuro Oncol* 2003; 5: 217-220.

34. Jamjoom ZA, Jamjoom AB, Sulaiman AH, et al. Systemic metastasis of medulloblastoma through ventriculoperitoneal shunt: report of a case and critical analysis of the literature. *Surg Neurol* 1993; 40: 403-10.

35. Loiacono F, Morra A, Venturini S, et al. Abdominal metastases of medulloblastoma related to a ventriculoperitoneal shunt. *AJR Am J Roentgenol* 2006; 186: 1548-50.

36. Due-Tønnessen BJ, Helseth E. Management of hydrocephalus in children with posterior fossa tumors: role of tumor surgery. *Pediatr Neurosurg* 2007; 43: 92-6.

37. Tamburrini G, Pettorini BL, Massimi L, et al. Endoscopic third ventriculostomy: the best option in the treatment of persistent hydrocephalus after posterior cranial fossa tumour removal? *Childs Nerv Syst* 2008; 24: 1405-12.

38. Raimondi AJ, Tomita T. Medulloblastoma in childhood. *Acta Neurochir* (Wien) 1979; 50: 127-38.

39. Albright AL, Wisoff JH, Zeltzer PM, Boyett JM, Rorke LB, Stanley P. Effects of medulloblastoma resections on outcome

in children: a report from the Children's Cancer Group. *Neurosurgery* 1996; 38: 265-71.

40. Taylor RE, Bailey CC, Robinson K, *et al.* Results of a randomized study of preradiation chemotherapy versus radiotherapy alone for nonmetastatic medulloblastoma: The International Society of Paediatric Oncology/United Kingdom Children's Cancer Study Group PNET-3 Study. *J Clin Oncol* 2003; 21: 1581-91.

41. Packer RJ, Gajjar A, Vezina G, *et al.* Phase III study of craniospinal radiation therapy followed by adjuvant chemotherapy for newly diagnosed average-risk medulloblastoma. *J Clin Oncol* 2006; 24: 4202-8.

42. Thomas PR, Deutsch M, Kepner JL, *et al.* Low-stage medulloblastoma: final analysis of trial comparing standard-dose with reduced-dose neuraxis irradiation. *J Clin Oncol* 2000; 18: 3004-11.

43. Gajjar A, Chintagumpala M, Ashley D, *et al.* Risk-adapted craniospinal radiotherapy followed by high-dose chemotherapy and stem-cell rescue in children with newly diagnosed medulloblastoma (St Jude Medulloblastoma-96): long-term results from a prospective, multicentre trial. *Lancet Oncol* 2006; 7: 813-20.

44. Kuhl J, Muller HL, Berthold F, *et al.* Preradiation chemotherapy of children and young adults with malignant brain tumors: results of the German pilot trial HIT'88/'89. *Klin Padiatr* 1998; 210: 227-33.

45. Bailey CC, Gnekow A, Wellek S, *et al.* Prospective randomised trial of chemotherapy given before radiotherapy in childhood medulloblastoma. International Society of Paediatric Oncology (SIOP) and the (German) Society of Paediatric Oncology (GPO): SIOP II. *Med Pediatr Oncol* 1995; 25: 166-78.

46. Rosenfeld A, Kletzel M, Duerst R, *et al.* A Phase II prospective study of sequential myeloablative chemotherapy with hematopoietic stem cell rescue for the treatment of selected high risk and recurrent central nervous system tumors. *J Neurooncol* 2010; 97: 247-55.

47. Butturini AM, Jacob M, Aguajo J, *et al.* High-dose chemotherapy and autologous hematopoietic progenitor cell rescue in children with recurrent medulloblastoma and supratentorial primitive neuroectodermal tumors: the impact of prior radiotherapy on outcome. *Cancer* 2009; 115: 2956-63.

48. Marachelian A, Butturini A, Finlay J. Myeloablative chemotherapy with autologous hematopoietic progenitor cell rescue for childhood central nervous system tumors. *Bone Marrow Transplant* 2008; 41: 167-72.

49. Packer RJ, Vezina G. Management of and prognosis with medulloblastoma: therapy at a crossroads. *Arch Neurol* 2008; 65: 1419-24.

50. Yuh GE, Loredo LN, Yonemoto LT, *et al.* Reducing toxicity from craniospinal irradiation: using proton beams to treat medulloblastoma in young children. *Cancer J* 2004; 10: 386-90.

51. Duffner PK, Horowitz ME, Krischer JP, *et al.* Postoperative chemotherapy and delayed radiation in children less than three years of age with malignant brain tumors. *N Engl J Med* 1993; 328: 1725-31.

52. Dhall G, Grodman H, Ji L, *et al.* Outcome of children less than three years old at diagnosis with non-metastatic medulloblastoma treated with chemotherapy on the 'Head Start' I and II protocols. *Pediatr Blood Cancer* 2008; 50: 1169-75.

53. Rutkowski S, Gerber NU, von Hoff K, *et al.* Treatment of early childhood medulloblastoma by postoperative chemotherapy and deferred radiotherapy. *Neuro Oncol* 2009; 11: 201-10.

54. Rutkowski S, Bode U, Deinlein F, *et al.* Treatment of early childhood medulloblastoma by postoperative chemotherapy alone. *N Engl J Med* 2005; 352: 978-86.

55. Kolinsky DC, Hayashi SS, Karzon R, *et al.* Late onset hearing loss: a significant complication of cancer survivors treated with cisplatin containing chemotherapy regimens. *J Pediatr Hematol Oncol* 2010; 32: 119-23.

56. Mendel E, Levy ML, Raffel C, *et al.* Surveillance imaging in children with primitive neuroectodermal tumors. *Neurosurgery* 1996; 38: 692-4; discussion 694-5.

57. Steinbok P, Hentschel S, Cochrane DD, *et al.* Value of postoperative surveillance imaging in the management of children with some common brain tumors. *J Neurosurg* 1996; 84: 726-32.

58. Saunders DE, Hayward RD, Phipps KP, *et al.* Surveillance neuroimaging of intracranial medulloblastoma in children: how effective, how often, and for how long? *J Neurosurg* 2003; 99: 280-6.

59. Torres CF, Rebsamen S, Silber JH, *et al.* Surveillance scanning of children with medulloblastoma. *N Engl J Med* 1994; 330: 892-5.

60. Gajjar A, Hernan R, Kocak M, *et al.* Clinical, histopathologic, and molecular markers of prognosis: toward a new disease risk stratification system for medulloblastoma. *J Clin Oncol* 2004; 22: 984-93.

61. Grotzer MA, Hogarty MD, Janss AJ, *et al.* MYC messenger RNA expression predicts survival outcome in childhood primitive neuroectodermal tumor/medulloblastoma. *Clin Cancer Res* 2001; 7: 2425-33.

62. Rutkowski S, von Bueren A, von Hoff K, *et al.* Prognostic relevance of clinical and biological risk factors in childhood medulloblastoma: results of patients treated in the prospective multicenter trial HIT'91. *Clin Cancer Res* 2007; 13: 2651-7.

63. Taylor MD, Northcott PA, Korshunov A, *et al.* Molecular subgroups of medulloblastoma: the current consensus. *Acta Neuropathol* 2012; 123: 465-72.

64. Ozer E, Sarialioglu F, Cetingoz R, *et al.* Prognostic significance of anaplasia and angiogenesis in childhood medulloblastoma: a Pediatric Oncology Group study. *Pathol Res Pract* 2004; 200: 501-9.

65. Eberhart CG, Kepner JL, Goldthwaite PT, *et al.* Histopathologic grading of medulloblastomas: a Pediatric Oncology Group study. *Cancer* 2002; 94: 552-60.

66. Shim KW, Joo SY, Kim SH, *et al.* Prediction of prognosis in children with medulloblastoma by using immunohistochemical analysis and tissue microarray. *J Neurosurg Pediatr* 2008; 1: 196-205.

Medulloblastoma

Introduction

Vascular neurosurgery

H Hunt Batjer MD FACS FAANS, Michael J Marchese Professor and Chair
Rudy J Rahme MD, Postdoctoral Research Fellow
Bernard R Bendok MD FACS FAANS FAHA, Associate Professor

DEPARTMENT OF NEUROLOGICAL SURGERY, NORTHWESTERN UNIVERSITY FEINBERG SCHOOL OF MEDICINE AND McGAW MEDICAL CENTER, CHICAGO, ILLINOIS, USA

"I firmly believe that if the whole materia medica could be sunk to the bottom of the sea, it would be all the better for mankind and all the worse for the fishes." With these words, spoken in 1860 in front of the Massachusetts Medical Society, Oliver Wendell Holmes Sr perhaps unknowingly set the foundation for the modern concept of evidence-based medicine (EBM). The basis of this approach is to doubt any given information until it is proven true by rigid scientific methods.

While level I evidence is considered the gold standard for guiding clinical practice, 'lesser' levels of evidence must also be thoughtfully analyzed and integrated into decision-making. The reasons for this are several. First, for any given question, a randomized trial may not be feasible, practical, or even ethical. The question of treating an epidural hematoma with brainstem signs is a clear example of this. Ventriculostomy for acute hydrocephalus is another. Second, even randomized trials cannot fully answer all aspects of a clinical question. Selection bias and other issues with internal and external validity are in part the reason for this. While ruptured aneurysms of less than 7mm in the anterior circulation

constitute the bread and butter of cerebrovascular practice, the International Study of Unruptured Intracranial Aneurysms suggested that most of these aneurysms should never rupture [1]! Third, intuition and wisdom constitute a complex summation of real-world experience, the digestion of complex and often conflicting 'knowledge' from the literature, and insight gained from peers. This last category is the most difficult to quantify and analyze, but often the easiest to appreciate when we see it in action. We can often tell when a neurosurgeon has good intuition and wisdom, but we have difficulty describing it.

On the other hand, many questions in neurosurgery can be answered with randomized trials and this form of scientific inquiry should be pursued and embraced where the stakes are worthwhile. Should an intraventricular lytic agent be administered in the setting of intraventricular hemorrhage is one such question. Should intravenous or intra-arterial tissue plasminogen activator be used in the first 3 hours after stroke for large-vessel occlusions is another. It should be kept in mind that a randomized trial is subject to scientific limitations, just like any other form of scientific inquiry. We should not necessarily blindly accept the results from a randomized trial merely because of the methodology. The results of randomized trials should be assessed on a number of factors, including the methods, bias, and both internal and external validity. Unfortunately, the mainstream media has contributed to the occasional over-reaction and carte-blanche acceptance of results from randomized trials via sensationalism, while often ignoring important scientific contexts.

In the past two decades the field of vascular neurosurgery has been enriched by a number of randomized trials, which have had varying impacts on clinical practice. The North American Symptomatic Carotid Endarterectomy Trial (NASCET) has had a profound impact on the management of symptomatic carotid disease and validated endarterectomy for select patients. The bypass trial (The International Cooperative Study of Extracranial/Intracranial Arterial Anastomosis), on the other hand, clearly blunted the practice of bypass for brain ischemic states but also ushered in a new era of hemodynamic assessment and arguably helped refine our understanding of bypass surgery and approaches to patient selection. The International Subarachnoid Aneurysm Trial (ISAT) continues to be debated and seems to have altered practice patterns at some institutions, but has raised questions regarding study design and operator proficiency on the surgical side.

More recently, greater economic pressures have increased the scrutiny on industry and practitioners to prove a given treatment. Endovascular treatment of intracranial and extracranial atherosclerosis has perhaps been subject of the most such scrutiny in vascular neurosurgery. Unfortunately, trial results are not as clear-cut and categorical as often claimed. The Carotid Revascularization Endarterectomy vs. Stenting Trial (CREST) revealed that carotid angioplasty and stenting is a valid alternative to carotid endarterectomy in select cases, with variables such as personal procedural experience, anatomic features, patient age, and comorbidities all playing key parts in the decision-making process [2, 3]. However, the strict criteria for operator experience in CREST have raised concerns about the generalizability of the results. Similarly, the conclusion of the Stenting and Aggressive Medical Management for Preventing

Recurrent stroke in Intracranial Stenosis (SAMMPRIS) trial – that medical management alone is superior to stenting plus medical management – seems warranted based on the data alone, but one has to consider several issues to reach more nuanced conclusions [4, 5]. Questions have been raised about patient selection criteria and the external validity of the trial, leading to concerns about its generalizability. Finally, the Carotid Occlusion Surgery Study (COSS), which was designed to determine the safety and efficacy of extracranial-intracranial bypass in carotid occlusion, was marred by statistical errors that led to its early termination [6].

In neurosurgery, small numbers of patients with heterogeneous diseases often make clinical trials difficult. Revascularization for Moyamoya disease and sinus thrombosis are two such examples. Furthermore, large trials require substantial funding, which is becoming more scant. Ethical issues often hinder randomization. An example of the discord created by such issues is the denial by some insurance companies of reimbursement for large-vessel intracranial thrombolysis, citing lack of level I evidence. The dilemma here is that most practitioners consider randomization for this disease unethical.

EBM is an approach with both assets and liabilities for neurosurgery in general and vascular neurosurgery in particular. It is clear that regardless of the inherent limitations of EBM, neurosurgeons must become conversant in its language to thrive in the next era of neurosurgical practice. A greater appreciation of the nuances of evidence-based practice will allow neurosurgeons to shape the debate rather than react to it. This is important, since the perspective of a neurosurgeon who has agonized over the complexities and nuances of vascular diseases will be critical to avoiding fatal flaws in research design and execution.

EBM has evolved into the gold standard to determine the best care, but it is not the only 'piece of jewelry' on the shelf. Perhaps the 'diamond standard' involves incorporating many facets in addition to EBM, including but not limited to personal experience, wisdom, and lower levels of evidence where appropriate. Far from debating its utmost

Introduction

importance, our aim is to elicit the most pertinent information from the existing literature in terms of evidence, showcasing its potential critical influence on decision-making for the neurosurgical community. This section therefore discusses the most common challenges faced by vascular neurosurgeons: intracranial aneurysms, arteriovenous malformations, intracranial and extracranial arterial stenosis, vasospasm, and intraparenchymal/intraventricular hemorrhage. From there on, it is up to each physician and health care team to incorporate this evidence into their daily practice and disease management protocols in ways that serve patients with neurovascular diseases faithfully, honorably, and conscientiously.

References

1. Wiebers DO, Whisnant JP, Huston J 3rd, *et al*. Unruptured intracranial aneurysms: natural history, clinical outcome, and risks of surgical and endovascular treatment. *Lancet* 2003; 362(9378): 103-10.
2. Brott TG, Hobson RW 2nd, Howard G, *et al*. Stenting versus endarterectomy for treatment of carotid-artery stenosis. *N Engl J Med* 2010; 363(1): 11-23.
3. Rahme RJ, Aoun SG, Batjer HH, Bendok BR. Carotid revascularization after CREST. *World Neurosurg* 2011; 75(1): 2-3.
4. Chimowitz MI, Lynn MJ, Derdeyn CP, *et al*. Stenting versus aggressive medical therapy for intracranial arterial stenosis. *N Engl J Med* 2011; 365(11): 993-1003.
5. Rahme RJ, Aoun SG, Batjer HH, Bendok BR. SAMMPRIS: end of intracranial stenting for atherosclerosis or back to the drawing board? *Neurosurgery* 2011; 69(6): N16-8.
6. Powers WJ, Clarke WR, Grubb RL Jr, Videen TO, Adams HP Jr, Derdeyn CP. Extracranial-intracranial bypass surgery for stroke prevention in hemodynamic cerebral ischemia: the Carotid Occlusion Surgery Study randomized trial. *JAMA* 2011; 306(18): 1983-92.

Introduction

Vascular neurosurgery

Chapter 26

Unruptured cerebral aneurysms: observe, clip, or coil?

Andrew F Ducruet MD, Chief Resident

Robert A Solomon MD, Byron Stookey Professor of Neurosurgery; Chairman and Director of Service

DEPARTMENT OF NEUROLOGICAL SURGERY, THE NEUROLOGIC INSTITUTE OF NEW YORK, COLUMBIA UNIVERSITY, NEW YORK, USA

Introduction

Unruptured intracranial aneurysms (UIAs) are being discovered with increasing frequency, and the management of these aneurysms remains one of the most controversial topics in neurosurgery. Given the poor outcomes experienced by many patients who experience aneurysmal rupture leading to subarachnoid hemorrhage (aSAH), many UIAs have traditionally been definitively treated by surgical clip ligation and, more recently, endovascular coil embolization. An evidence-based approach to UIA treatment must take into account both the natural history of these lesions and the morbidity and long-term efficacy associated with the particular treatment strategy. Along these lines, a number of longitudinal observational studies have been undertaken in an attempt to define the natural history of UIA. However, they frequently suffer from methodologic limitations that obscure the true behavior of these lesions. In addition, although numerous case series and population-based studies have sought to define the clinical outcomes associated with the various treatment strategies for UIA, there has never been a prospective, randomized clinical trial directly comparing outcomes for clip ligation and coil embolization. Based on our interpretation of the existing literature, we present management recommendations for patients with UIA and define the quality of the evidence upon which these recommendations is based.

Methodology

A literature search was performed using the PubMed database with the following search terms: 'intracranial aneurysm,' 'unruptured,' 'clipping,' 'endovascular,' 'coil,' 'conservative management,' and 'outcome.' Of the retrieved papers, only studies from 1980 to February 2010 in the English language were considered for this review. Case series of fewer than 20 patients, studies describing treatment of ruptured cerebral aneurysms, and those without report of at least a discharge clinical outcome were excluded.

Natural history of UIA

The annual risk of rupture of UIA is controversial, and has been estimated to range from 0.1% to 8% or higher. Publication of the initial results from the International Study of Unruptured Intracranial Aneurysms (ISUIA), purporting a dramatically low risk of aSAH from aneurysms less than 10mm, incited a debate favoring observation for the majority of patients with small UIAs [1]. However, several natural history investigations have suggested a higher rate of hemorrhage [1-4]. These studies deserve careful review to understand the true natural history of UIAs (Table 1).

ISUIA is an ongoing multicenter collaboration that is attempting to delineate both the natural history and post-intervention outcomes for UIA. The first of the two publications arising from this study retrospectively assessed the natural history of these lesions [1]. The patients were divided into two groups: those without history of aSAH (n=727) and those with a previous aSAH from a different lesion (n=722). The rupture rates for UIA in these cohorts were drastically lower than in previous estimates (Table 1). The authors found that increasing size and location (posterior circulation and posterior communicating artery) were associated with rupture in those without a history of aSAH, whereas location (basilar tip) and increasing age predicted rupture in those with a previous aSAH. Although this study evaluated a large number of aneurysms across several centers, the significant selection bias secondary to investigators choosing which aneurysms to treat in a non-randomized fashion and a high rate of cross-over from conservative to definitive treatment both probably served to lower the observed rupture rate [1].

The second ISUIA publication was a prospective evaluation of the natural history of UIA [5]. In this analysis, 615 patients had a history of aSAH and 1,077 patients did not. The total risk of rupture for patients in both groups was calculated excluding those with cavernous aneurysms (Table 1). This prospective study suffered from the same selection bias as the previous ISUIA trial, and of the 1,692 patients, 534 crossed to intervention and were excluded. In a significant portion of these cross-over patients, the management strategy was probably modified because of an increase in aneurysm size or new symptoms. In addition, 193 patients (11%) died of causes other than aSAH and were excluded, including 52 who suffered intracranial hemorrhage.

Juvela et al conducted a comprehensive observational study that lacked the bias of surgical selection found in the ISUIA trials, as they examined all patients with UIA seen at their institution in Finland over a given time period [2]. This was possible because it was department policy to manage all UIAs conservatively prior to 1979, and Finland's socio-medical structure allowed 100% follow-up. The cumulative rate of aSAH is shown in Table 1. Larger aneurysm size, increasing age, and cigarette smoking were significant predictors of aSAH. Major flaws in this study include the ethnic homogeneity of the patients and the overwhelming proportion (92%) of patients with prior aSAH. Despite these flaws, the lack of a surgical selection bias and the long-term follow-up make this an invaluable contribution to our understanding of UIA bleeding rates.

Rinkel et al published an invaluable meta-analysis of the literature (1955-1996) regarding the natural history of UIA [3]. To estimate the prevalence of UIA, data were summed from 23 studies (56,304 patients). The overall prevalence of these lesions in adults with no known risk factors was 2.3%. For analysis of the bleeding rate of UIA, the authors identified nine studies including 3,907 patients (Table 1). Importantly, this same group recently performed an updated meta-analysis in 2007 that included additional natural history studies, including the ISUIA studies, for a total inclusion of 19 studies with 4,705 patients (Table 1) [4]. In univariate analysis, risk factors for rupture included age older than 60 years, female sex, Japanese/Finnish descent, aSAH size more than 5mm, posterior circulation aneurysms, and symptomatic aneurysms. The large number of patients analyzed in these papers establishes them as important investigations into the natural history of UIA.

Several factors should be considered when interpreting the literature reporting the natural history of UIA. For example, studies divide aneurysms into size categories. It is unlikely that such cut-offs will result in substantially different rupture rates. In actuality, the risk of bleeding most probably reflects a non-linear continuum of increasing risk with greater aneurysm size. In addition, it is important to realize that aneurysm size is probably not a static measure. For instance, Juvela et al found that in 36% of patients, the size of conservatively managed

Table 1. Summary of natural history studies of UIA.

Reference	Patients, n	Aneurysms, n	Mean follow-up, years	Rate of rupture
ISUIA Investigators, 1998 [1]	1,449	1,937	8.3	No previous aSAH: <10mm: 0.05%/year >10mm: 1%/year Previous aSAH: <10mm: 0.5%/year >10mm: 1%/year
Rinkel *et al*, 1998 [3]	3,907	NA	NA	Overall: 1.9%/year <10mm: 0.7%/year >10mm: 4%/year
Juvela *et al*, 2001 [7]	142	181	18.1	10.5% at 10 years 23% at 20 years 30.3% at 30 years
Wiebers *et al*, 2003 [5]	1,692	2,686	4.1	No previous aSAH: <7mm: 0%/year 7-12mm: 2.6%/year 13-24mm: 14.5%/year >25mm: 40%/year Previous aSAH: <7mm: 2.5%/year 7-12mm: 14.5%/year 13-24mm: 18.4%/year >25mm: 50%/year
Wermer *et al*, 2007 [4]	4,705	6,556	5.6	Overall: 1.2% (follow-up <5 years) 1.3% (follow-up >10 years)

ISUIA = International Study of Unruptured Intracranial Aneurysms; NA = not available; aSAH = aneurysmal subarachnoid hemorrhage; UIA = unruptured intracranial aneurysm

aneurysms increased by more than 3mm over a mean follow-up of 18.9 years [2, 6, 7]. It would be reasonable to assume that a growing aneurysm has an increased risk of rupture. Second, any estimate of rupture risk must take into account the aneurysm location. The literature indicates that posterior circulation, posterior communicating artery, and anterior communicating artery aneurysms carry the highest risk of aSAH, whereas aneurysms in the cavernous internal carotid artery carry an extremely low risk [1, 5].

Due to the variability in the existing literature, we recommend that the natural history of a given UIA should be assessed on an individual basis. Family history, smoking, excessive alcohol consumption, female sex, previous aSAH, presence of symptoms, high-risk aneurysm location, and large lesion size all predict a worse natural history [7, 8].

Table 2. Studies reporting outcomes associated with microsurgical clipping of UIA. *Continued overleaf.*

Reference	Study design	Patients, n	Outcomes
Wirth et al, 1983 [13]	Case series	107	Mortality: 0% Morbidity: 6.5%
Rice et al, 1990 [10]	Case series	167	Morbidity and mortality: 4.2%
Inagawa et al, 1992 [14]	Case series	52	Mortality: 0% Morbidity: 6%
Asari and Ohmoto, 1993 [15]	Case series	69	Mortality: 0% Morbidity: 7.2%
King et al, 1994 [16]	Meta-analysis	733	Mortality: 1.0% Morbidity: 4.1%
Solomon et al, 1994 [9]	Case series	202	Outcomes excellent 88%, good 5%, poor 3% Mortality: 3%
Khanna et al, 1996 [17]	Case series	172	Morbidity: 9.9%
Deruty et al, 1996 [18]	Case series	62	Mortality: 3% Morbidity: 3%
Raaymakers et al, 1998 [12]	Meta-analysis	2,460	Mortality: 2.6% Morbidity: 10.9%
ISUIA Investigators, 1998 [1]	Prospective, observational	996	Morbidity and mortality: No previous aSAH: 17.5% (30 days), 15.7% (1 year) Previous aSAH: 13.6% (30 days), 13.1% (1 year)
Orz et al, 2000 [19]	Case series	310	Mortality: 0.3% Outcomes excellent 84.5%, good 9.7%, fair 5.5%
Barker et al, 2003 [20]	Retrospective, population-based	3,498	Mortality: 2.1% Discharge to SNF: 3.3% Discharge to other than home: 12.8%
Moroi et al, 2005 [21]	Case series	368	Mortality: 0.3% Morbidity: 2.2%
Ogilvy and Carter, 2003 [22]	Case series	604	Mortality: 0.8% Morbidity: 15.9%

Chapter 26

Table 2. Studies reporting outcomes associated with microsurgical clipping of UIA. *Continued.*

Reference	Study design	Patients, n	Outcomes
Horn *et al*, 2004 [23]	Case series	32	Morbidity and mortality: 25%
Krisht *et al*, 2006 [24]	Case series	116	Mortality: 0.82% Morbidity: 3.44%
Nussbaum *et al*, 2007 [25]	Case series	376	Mortality: 0.27% Good outcome (6 months): 99%
Aghakhani *et al*, 2008 [26]	Case series	176	Mortality: 0% Morbidity: 2.2%
Yasunaga *et al*, 2008 [27]	Retrospective, population-based	702	mRS (at discharge): 0, 92.3%; 1, 6.3%; 2, 2.0%; 3, 0.7%; 4, 0.6%; 5, 0%

mRS = modified Rankin Scale; SNF = skilled nursing facility; UIA = unruptured intracranial aneurysm

Outcomes following treatment of UIA

No prospective, randomized, multicenter trial has directly compared surgical and endovascular treatment for UIA. The choice of a particular treatment modality must therefore take into account the size of the UIA, location, anatomic characteristics, medical comorbidities, and operator skill. The risks of intervention must be carefully weighed against the natural history of the disease. While some data exist on the relative safety and immediate angiographic efficacy of surgery and endovascular treatment, significant selection bias and heterogeneous patient populations and study designs complicate meaningful direct comparisons. While the morbidity and mortality of aneurysm treatment clearly depends on the individual neurosurgeon or interventionalist and medical center, several studies have attempted to formulate currently acceptable values.

Microsurgical clipping

A number of primarily single-center case series have accumulated in which the outcomes following microsurgical clipping of UIA have been analyzed in terms of both patient and lesion characteristics. The values reported in these studies range from 0% to 3% for death and from 2% to 16% for morbidity (Table 2) [1, 9-27]. Although these studies have employed various outcome measures and follow-up durations, several conclusions may be drawn. The risk of operative morbidity is associated with lesion size and patient age, with the best outcomes occurring for lesions smaller than 10mm in young patients [9] **(III/B)**. In addition, poor outcomes occur more frequently in patients with symptomatic or atherosclerotic/calcified aneurysms, and in those with multiple medical comorbidities [10] **(III/B)**. Furthermore, many postoperative deficits are transient and resolve upon follow-up examination [28]. Of the numerous reports of microsurgical outcomes, several best demonstrate the morbidity associated with microsurgical treatment of UIA and deserve closer analysis.

The most comprehensive analysis of outcomes following UIA microsurgery is the meta-analysis by Raaymakers *et al* [12] **(III/B)**. These authors reported 2.6% mortality and 10.9% morbidity rates in 2,460 patients. Complications were generally serious, with half of affected individuals becoming dependent for their activities of daily living. Mortality rates varied

Table 3. Studies reporting outcomes associated with endovascular coiling of UIA. *Continued overleaf.*

Reference	Study design	Patients, n	Outcomes
Malisch et al, 1997 [31]	Case series	20	Mortality: 0% Morbidity: 20%
Leber et al, 1998 [32]	Case series	45	Mortality: 4.4% Morbidity: 18%
Debrun et al, 1998 [33]	Case series	73	Mortality: 2.7% Morbidity: 3.6%
Kuether et al, 1998 [34]	Case series	41	Mortality: 5% Morbidity: 7.5%
Cognard et al, 1998 [35]	Case series	71	Mortality: 0% Morbidity: 7%
Eskridge and Song, 1998 [36]	Case series	66	Mortality: 0% Morbidity: 12%
Lot et al, 1999 [37]	Case series	83	Mortality: 0% Morbidity: 4.8%
Murayama et al, 1999 [38]	Case series	109	Mortality: 0% Morbidity: 5.2%
Raftopoulos et al, 2000 [39]	Case series	21	Mortality: 0% Morbidity: 4.8%
Qureshi et al, 2001 [40]	Case series	69	Mortality: 0%
Roy et al, 2001 [41]	Case series	109	Mortality: 0% Morbidity: 4.6%
Wanke et al, 2002 [42]	Case series	33	Mortality: 0% Morbidity: 6%
Goddard et al, 2002 [43]	Case series	50	Morbidity and mortality: 0%
Ng et al, 2002 [30]	Case series	58	Mortality: 0%
Hoh et al, 2003 [44]	Retrospective, population-based	421	Mortality: 1.7% Discharge to other than home: 7.6%

Chapter 26

Table 3. Studies reporting outcomes associated with endovascular coiling of UIA. *Continued.*

Reference	Study design	Patients, n	Outcomes
Lanterna *et al*, 2004 [29]	Systematic review	1,379	Mortality: 0.6% Morbidity: 7%
Gonzalez *et al.*, 2004 [45]	Case series	217	Mortality: 0.5% Morbidity: 5.7%
van Rooij and Sluzewski, 2006 [46]	Case series	149	Mortality: 1.3% Morbidity: 2.6%
Standhardt *et al*, 2008 [47]	Case series	173	Mortality: 0.5% Morbidity: 3.5%
Gallas *et al*, 2008 [48]	Case series	321	Mortality: 1.7% Morbidity: 7.7%
Im *et al*, 2009 [49]	Case series	435	Mortality: 0% Morbidity: 0.27%

UIA = unruptured intracranial aneurysm

substantially, with 62% of studies reporting no deaths, while other studies demonstrated death rates as high as 29%. As a general trend, mortality rates were lower in more recent studies and those with a greater proportion of anterior circulation lesions. Giant aneurysm surgery carried a poor prognosis. Specifically, the authors found the following respective mortality and morbidity rates: giant posterior circulation aneurysms, 9.6% and 37.9%; giant anterior circulation aneurysms, 7.4% and 26.9%; non-giant posterior circulation aneurysms, 3% and 12.9%; and non-giant anterior circulation aneurysms, 0.8% and 1.9%.

The combined morbidity and mortality of microsurgery for UIA was one of the main outcomes assessed by the initial ISUIA publication. The cohort comprised 1,172 patients, 211 of whom had a prior history of SAH [1]. Of these, 996 underwent microsurgical clipping as a treatment strategy. The morbidity and mortality rate at 1 year was 6.5% for patients younger than 45 years, 14.4% for those aged 45-64 years, and 32% for those older than 64 years.

Surprisingly, 3.1% of the treated patients without prior aSAH died from operative complications compared with only 0.9% of those with a history of aSAH. Close inspection, however, reveals that the latter group was younger (47 vs. 53 years) and harbored smaller aneurysms (27% vs. 51% of lesions >10mm) located more often in the anterior circulation (83.4% vs. 73.6%) **(IIa/B)**. It is unclear whether these differences are enough to account for this discrepancy in post-surgical outcomes, particularly since the presence of medical comorbidities, a known risk factor, was not recorded in the ISUIA study.

Coil embolization

Endovascular coil embolization has been employed with increasing frequency in the elective treatment of UIAs. A large number of case series have been published since the early 1990s reporting the clinical outcomes of patients in whom endovascular coiling was employed (Table 3) [29-49]. This literature remains fragmentary, however, with most studies reporting only small numbers of patients and a mix of aneurysm locations, with short follow-ups and variable outcome measures. A review of Table 3 reveals that the mortality rate in these series ranges from approximately 0% to 5%, with morbidity ranging from 0% to 20% **(III/B)**. In general, series published in later years have included a larger number of patients and the outcomes have tended to improve. A 2004 systematic review by Lanterna et al presented an overview of 1,379 patients treated with Guglielmi detachable coils (GDCs) [29]. The combined cohort exhibited an overall case fatality rate of 0.6% and permanent morbidity of 7%. As with all systematic reviews, the applicability of these findings is limited by the heterogeneity of the patient populations and the study designs of the individual series.

Comparison of outcomes between microsurgical clipping and coil embolization

Several non-randomized studies have directly compared the outcomes of patients with UIA treated by endovascular and surgical means, demonstrating mixed results (Table 4) [5, 50-57]. In 2000, Johnston et al performed a single-center blinded comparison of patients with UIA who underwent surgical (n=68) or endovascular (n=62) treatment [50]. All aneurysms in this study were deemed amenable to either surgical or endovascular treatment by a panel of surgeons and interventionalists. The authors reported a higher frequency of post-procedural disability in patients who underwent surgery compared with those treated endovascularly (25% vs. 8%) **(III/B)**. In addition, length of stay and hospital costs were greater for surgery. The same group then reviewed 2,069 patients with treated UIA in a statewide database of California hospital discharges [53]. In this analysis, adverse outcomes were more frequent in the 1,699 patients treated with surgery (25%) than in the 370 treated with endovascular techniques (10%) **(III/B)**. In-hospital death was also more frequent (3.5% vs. 0.5%) and length of stay and hospital costs were greater after surgery. Importantly, adverse outcomes declined over time for endovascular therapy (26% in 1991 vs. 4% in 1998), probably due to improved

technology and increasing interventionalist experience, but not for surgery (26% in 1991 vs. 21% in 1998). A similar retrospective study using a national database was published by Higashida et al in 2007 [55]. A total of 2,535 cases were analyzed, of which 1,881 underwent surgery. Once again, endovascular treatment was associated with lower mortality (0.9% vs. 2.5%), fewer adverse outcomes (6.6% vs. 13.2%), shorter length of stay (4.5 vs. 7.4 days), and lower hospital charges ($42,044 vs. $47,567) than microsurgery **(III/B)**.

These data contrast with those from similar work by Hoh et al, which compared aneurysm coiling with clipping in 565 patients treated at a single institution over 2.5 years [58]. They demonstrated a shorter length of stay in patients undergoing coiling; however, coiling was associated with higher hospital costs, reflecting the increasing costs of endovascular technology over time **(III/B)**. A 2003 observational study from Raftopoulos et al analyzed the experiences of 72 consecutive patients harboring 101 unruptured aneurysms. The interventional neuroradiologists involved in the study decided whether they felt the aneurysm geometry would allow for effective coil embolization and, if so, aneurysms were treated endovascularly. The first-line technique was coil embolization in 41 patients and surgical clipping in 53 patients. Surgery was also offered to 11 patients in whom coil embolization failed, with six patients thus electing to have their aneurysms clipped [51]. Although this study was heavily biased in its patient selection, the surgical clipping group demonstrated higher rates of total aneurysm obliteration (93% vs. 56%), as well as lower rates of permanent complications (1.7% vs. 7.5%) **(III/B)**.

The follow-up ISUIA study, with its large size, prospective design, and multicenter nature, is important to consider for its assessment of outcomes of both surgical and endovascular treatment of UIA. The surgical arm evaluated 1,917 patients at 7 days, discharge, 30 days, and yearly [5]. Findings included a mortality rate of 1.5% and an overall morbidity and mortality rate of 13.2% at 30 days, and rates of 2.3% and 12.2%, respectively, at 1 year. In the microsurgical cohort, asymptomatic patients younger than 50 years of age with UIA of less than 24mm in diameter located in the anterior

Table 4. Studies presenting outcomes of both clipping and coiling of UIA.

Reference	Study design	Patients clip/coil, n	Outcomes, clip vs. coil
Johnston *et al*, 1999 [52]	Retrospective, population-based cohort	2,357/255	Mortality: 2.3% vs. 0.4% (p=0.07) Adverse outcome: 18.5% vs. 10.6% (p=0.002)
Johnston *et al*, 2000 [50]	Retrospective, single-center cohort	68/62	Mortality: 1% vs. 2% Good recovery: 62% vs. 87% Moderate disability: 26% vs. 5% Severe disability: 10% vs. 6%
Johnston *et al*, 2001 [53]	Retrospective, population-based cohort	1,699/370	Mortality: 3.5% vs. 0.5% (p=0.003) Adverse outcome: 25% vs. 10% (p<0.001)
ISUIA Investigators, 2003 [5]	Prospective, multicenter, observational	1,917/451	No previous aSAH: Mortality: 1.8% (30 days), 2.7% (1 year) vs. 2.0% (30 days), 3.4% (1 year) Morbidity or mortality: 13.7% (30 days), 12.6% (1 year) vs. 9.3% (30 days), 9.8% (1 year) Previous aSAH: Mortality: 0.3% (30 days), 0.6% (1 year) vs. 0% (30 days), 0% (1 year) Morbidity or mortality: 11% (30 days), 10.1% (1 year) vs. 7.1% (30 days), 7.1% (1 year)
Raftopoulos *et al*, 2003 [51]	Prospective, single-center, observational	59/41	Morbidity: 1.7% vs. 7.5%
Barker *et al*, 2004 [54]	Retrospective, population-based cohort	3,498/421	Mortality: 2.1% vs. 1.7% (p=0.6) Discharge to other than home: 16.3% vs. 7.4% (p<0.001)
Higashida *et al*, 2007 [55]	Retrospective, population-based cohort	1,881/654	Mortality: 2.5% vs. 0.9% Adverse outcome: 13.2% vs. 6.6% (p<0.05)
Gerlach *et al*, 2007 [56]	Prospective, single-center, observational	81/37	Mortality: 0% vs. 0% Unfavorable outcome (mRS >2): 2.1% vs. 2.6% (p=0.3)
Seifert *et al*, 2008 [57]	Prospective, single-center, observational	126/74	Mortality: 0% vs. 0% Unfavorable outcome (mRS >2): 1.2% vs. 1.3%

M/M = morbidity and mortality; mRS = modified Rankin Scale; UIA = unruptured intracranial aneurysm circulation had the lowest rates of poor outcomes, defined by death, Rankin score 3-5, or impaired cognitive status (5-6% at 1 year) **(IIa/B)**. For comparison, the authors also presented outcome data following endovascular treatment. A total of 451 patients who underwent coiling of a UIA were assessed. Findings included 1.8% and 9.1% mortality and overall morbidity and mortality, respectively, at 30 days, and 3.1% and 9.5% mortality and morbidity, respectively, at 1 year. Once again, rates of poor outcomes were higher in older patients (>50 years) with posterior circulation aneurysms larger than 25mm **(IIa/B)**. When comparing these results with those of other studies, it is important to recognize that both ISUIA studies incorporated cognitive impairment in their analysis, which was not considered in earlier papers.

Conservative therapy

Conservative therapy for UIA encompasses two different paradigms:

◆ The first relates to UIAs where the risks of treatment are thought to outweigh the risk of hemorrhage, given the natural history of these aneurysms.
◆ The second involves incidentally found small aneurysms.

Despite improvements in microsurgical clipping and rapidly developing advances in endovascular therapies, certain aneurysms are better managed conservatively. The size (usually giant), character (calcified), and anatomic configuration (encompassing critical perforators from the dome of the aneurysm, and patients who would not be able to tolerate a bypass) can mean the risks of even the safest treatment outweigh those of the natural history for these few lesions **(IV/C)**. A second class of lesion is the asymptomatic small (<5mm) aneurysm, discovered incidentally. These aneurysms are best followed serially for expansion prior to definitive treatment, given their low rate of rupture in published studies **(IIa/B)**. Despite these recommendations, it must be noted that in practice many ruptured aneurysms are found to be less than 5mm in size, and

further study is necessary to better define which aneurysms are at high risk for rupture.

Recurrence following treatment of UIA

Extensive discussion has centered on the rates of recurrence of treated UIAs as well as the need for repeated procedures for surveillance of recurrent lesions. Microsurgical clipping has repeatedly been demonstrated to provide definitive long-term treatment of cerebral aneurysms **(III/B)**. David et al reviewed 160 surgically managed aneurysms that underwent late angiographic follow-up (mean 4.4 years), of which only 1.5% of initially obliterated lesions exhibited recurrence [59]. In incompletely clipped aneurysms, 25% were enlarged on follow-up imaging, while eight new lesions developed in six patients. These data translated into a 0.52% annual rupture rate for completely clipped aneurysms and a 1.8% annual rate of de novo formation. Tsutsumi et al have also investigated this topic. In 1999, they published data after following 115 patients with surgically treated UIA for an average of 8.8 years [60]. Although four patients suffered aSAH, only one patient bled from a successfully clipped aneurysm, giving a 0.10% annual regrowth rate for completely clipped aneurysms and a 0.20% annual rate of de novo formation. In 2001, the same authors published data after following 140 patients with surgically treated aneurysms for an average of 9.3 years, and found a 0.26% annual regrowth rate for completely clipped aneurysms and a 0.89% annual rate of de novo aneurysm formation [61]. In 2004, Akyuz et al reviewed 166 open surgical clipping cases with late angiography (mean 47 months postoperative) [62]. The authors demonstrated a 99.4% aneurysm cure rate; of the 159 aneurysms confirmed to be occluded on immediate postoperative angiogram, 158 remained obliterated on follow-up.

By contrast, the recurrence rate of coiled aneurysms has been reported to be much higher **(III/B)**. In 2002, Ng et al quoted a 23% recanalization rate in 30 coiled aneurysms with 1-year angiographic follow-up [30]. In the same year, Thornton et al obtained angiographic 1-year follow-up on 143 coiled aneurysms and documented a 1.8% recanalization rate for completely occluded aneurysms and a 28% recanalization rate for those that were incompletely occluded [63]. In 2003, Raymond et al cited a 33.6% recanalization rate in 383 coiled aneurysms with 12.3-month angiographic follow-up [64].

More recently, Murayama et al reported their 11-year experience with embolization of cerebral aneurysms using GDC technology [65]. After analyzing 6- and 12-month angiographic follow-up images for 916 coiled aneurysms, the authors demonstrated a 20.9% overall recanalization rate. The patients were divided into two groups: group A included their initial 5 years' experience with 230 patients (251 aneurysms), and group B included the later 6 years' experience with 588 patients (665 aneurysms). For the combined cohort, complete occlusion was obtained in only 55% of aneurysms, with neck remnants present in 35.4%. The results revealed both a higher complete embolization rate and lower recanalization rate in group B than in group A (56.8% and 17.2% vs. 50.2% and 26.1%, respectively), probably reflecting improved technique, greater experience, and more advanced technology. Of note, recanalization was related to the sizes of the dome and neck of the aneurysm. In small aneurysms (4-10mm) with small necks (<4mm), the overall recanalization rate was only 5.1%. In contrast, among large (11-25mm) and giant aneurysms (>25mm), the overall recanalization rate was 35% and 59.1%, respectively. These data strongly suggest that while clinical and post-embolization outcomes in patients treated with coil embolization have improved over time, larger lesions with wider necks continue to carry a high risk for recanalization **(III/B)**.

Conclusions

When determining a management paradigm for an UIA, one must weigh the natural history of the condition against the risks of intervention. In 2000, the Stroke Council of the American Heart Association issued a scientific statement with the following recommendations for the management of UIA: "In consideration of the apparent low risk of hemorrhage from incidental small (<10mm) aneurysms in patients without previous SAH, treatment rather than observation cannot be generally advocated" [11]. Based on the available literature, we believe that this statement must be revised. The literature regarding the treatment of UIA is characterized by the lack of class I data, and further comparison of the efficacy, morbidity, and long-term durability of both clipping and coiling is imperative. The most conclusive data regarding the natural history of UIA derives from the ISUIA [1, 5] and Helsinki experiences [2]. Murayama's report of aneurysm regrowth after coil embolization provides important insight for comparison with the relative permanence of surgical clipping [65]. Raaymakers' meta-analysis of the literature on surgical morbidity for clipping of UIA [12] fits almost exactly with our own published data [9] and ongoing experience. Studies directly comparing outcomes for clipping and coiling are primarily derived from the retrospective review of population-based databases, and their methodologic limitations preclude meaningful assessment.

In all, although the lack of level I evidence on the subject of UIA management precludes the establishment of rigorous treatment standards, the existing literature does provide at least an imperfect framework for the treatment recommendations listed below. Importantly, we strongly believe that any algorithm for the treatment of UIA must be employed by a multidisciplinary cerebrovascular team of highly experienced microsurgeons and endovascular practitioners working in tandem to offer only low-risk treatment options.

Chapter 26

Recommendations	Evidence level
◆ With rare exceptions, all symptomatic unruptured aneurysms should be treated.	IIb/B
◆ Incidental aneurysms of <5mm should be managed conservatively in virtually all cases, given their exceptionally low rate of rupture.	IIa/B
◆ In young patients with small aneurysms (<5mm) who are psychologically crippled by their knowledge of harboring an UIA, definitive treatment may be justified to improve quality of life and prevent future rupture.	III/B
◆ Aneurysms of >7mm in patients <60 years should be considered for treatment unless there are significant contraindications. Although 7mm was the cut-off in the ISUIA data, there are limitations to using such an exact measurement, particularly since this study was influenced by selection bias. Certainly aneurysms <7mm in diameter are known to infrequently rupture. The accuracy of measurement, even with angiographic data, is at least ±2mm. Therefore, if 7mm is used as a cut-off, some aneurysms will not be treated that should be treated. Our personal practice is to use a standard error of measurement below this cut-off and to treat aneurysms of >5mm in size, to ensure that 99% of patients at risk for rupture are offered treatment.	IIa/B
◆ Incidental aneurysms of >10mm are at relatively increased risk of rupture and should be treated, after accounting for the patient's age, medical health, and treatment morbidity.	IIa/B
◆ When managing older patients (>60 years), the decision to treat becomes less clear, as there is increased treatment morbidity. In these situations, lesion location plays a critical role, as anterior communicating artery, posterior communicating artery, and basilar apex aneurysms carry a higher rupture risk than those in other locations. Thus, we recommend treatment of such lesions, even in older healthy individuals, provided there is low associated treatment morbidity.	IIa/B
◆ Microsurgical clipping may be employed as the treatment of first choice in young patients with small anterior circulation aneurysms. In these cases, the risk of open microsurgery and endovascular surgery is about the same in terms of stroke and death, although endovascular coiling is definitely less invasive. On the other hand, surgical clipping provides a repair that is at least an order of magnitude more durable than coiling.	IIa/B
◆ Endovascular coiling represents a reasonable alternative that should be instituted whenever open surgical intervention carries high risk, such as in elderly or medically ill patients, and where the anatomic characteristics are favorable to coiling (posterior circulation, high neck-to-dome ratio).	IIa/B
◆ Very large and giant aneurysms, and those with high neck-to-dome ratios, will generally benefit more from surgical approaches than from endovascular treatment.	III/B
◆ The improvement in stent and coil technology offers an excellent alternative in this group of poor surgical candidates, even for aneurysms with wide necks and unfavorable neck-to-dome ratios.	III/B

References

1. International Study of Unruptured Intracranial Aneurysms Investigators. Unruptured intracranial aneurysms - risk of rupture and risks of surgical intervention. *N Engl J Med* 1998; 339(24): 1725-33.

2. Juvela S, Porras M, Heiskanen O. Natural history of unruptured intracranial aneurysms: a long-term follow-up study. *J Neurosurg* 1993; 79(2): 174-82.

3. Rinkel GJ, Djibuti M, Algra A, van Gijn J. Prevalence and risk of rupture of intracranial aneurysms: a systematic review. *Stroke* 1998; 29(1): 251-6.

4. Wermer MJ, van der Schaaf IC, Algra A, Rinkel GJ. Risk of rupture of unruptured intracranial aneurysms in relation to patient and aneurysm characteristics: an updated meta-analysis. *Stroke* 2007; 38(4): 1404-10.

5. Wiebers DO, Whisnant JP, Huston J 3rd, *et al*; for the International Study of Unruptured Intracranial Aneurysms Investigators. Unruptured intracranial aneurysms: natural history, clinical outcome, and risks of surgical and endovascular treatment. *Lancet* 2003; 362(9378): 103-10.

6. Juvela S, Porras M, Poussa K. Natural history of unruptured intracranial aneurysms: probability of and risk factors for aneurysm rupture. *J Neurosurg* 2000; 93(3): 379-87.

7. Juvela S, Poussa K, Porras M. Factors affecting formation and growth of intracranial aneurysms: a long-term follow-up study. *Stroke* 2001; 32(2): 485-91.

8. Broderick JP, Sauerbeck LR, Foroud T, *et al*. The Familial Intracranial Aneurysm (FIA) study protocol. *BMC Med Genet* 2005; 6: 17.

9. Solomon RA, Fink ME, Pile-Spellman J. Surgical management of unruptured intracranial aneurysms. *J Neurosurg* 1994; 80(3): 440-6.

10. Rice BJ, Peerless SJ, Drake CG. Surgical treatment of unruptured aneurysms of the posterior circulation. *J Neurosurg* 1990; 73(2): 165-73.

11. Bederson JB, Awad IA, Wiebers DO, *et al*. Recommendations for the management of patients with unruptured intracranial aneurysms: a statement for healthcare professionals from the Stroke Council of the American Heart Association. *Stroke* 2000; 31(11): 2742-50.

12. Raaymakers TW, Rinkel GJ, Limburg M, Algra A. Mortality and morbidity of surgery for unruptured intracranial aneurysms: a meta-analysis. *Stroke* 1998; 29(8): 1531-8.

13. Wirth FP, Laws ER Jr, Piepgras D, Scott RM. Surgical treatment of incidental intracranial aneurysms. *Neurosurgery* 1983; 12(5): 507-11.

14. Inagawa T, Hada H, Katoh Y. Unruptured intracranial aneurysms in elderly patients. *Surg Neurol* 1992; 38(5): 364-70.

15. Asari S, Ohmoto T. Natural history and risk factors of unruptured cerebral aneurysms. *Clin Neurol Neurosurg* 1993; 95(3): 205-214.

16. King JT Jr, Berlin JA, Flamm ES. Morbidity and mortality from elective surgery for asymptomatic, unruptured, intracranial aneurysms: a meta-analysis. *J Neurosurg* 1994; 81(6): 837-42.

17. Khanna RK, Malik GM, Qureshi N. Predicting outcome following surgical treatment of unruptured intracranial aneurysms: a proposed grading system. *J Neurosurg* 1996; 84(1): 49-54.

18. Deruty R, Pelissou-Guyotat I, Mottolese C, Amat D. Management of unruptured cerebral aneurysms. *Neurol Res* 1996; 18(1): 39-44.

19. Orz YI, Hongo K, Tanaka Y, *et al*. Risks of surgery for patients with unruptured intracranial aneurysms. *Surg Neurol* 2000; 53(1): 21-7; discussion 27-9.

20. Barker FG, 2nd, Amin-Hanjani S, Butler WE, Ogilvy CS, Carter BS. In-hospital mortality and morbidity after surgical treatment of unruptured intracranial aneurysms in the United States, 1996-2000: the effect of hospital and surgeon volume. *Neurosurgery* 2003; 52(5): 995-1007; discussion 1007-9.

21. Moroi J, Hadeishi H, Suzuki A, Yasui N. Morbidity and mortality from surgical treatment of unruptured cerebral aneurysms at Research Institute for Brain and Blood Vessels-Akita. *Neurosurgery* 2005; 56(2): 224-31.

22. Ogilvy CS, Carter BS. Stratification of outcome for surgically treated unruptured intracranial aneurysms. *Neurosurgery* 2003; 52(1): 82-7; discussion 87-8.

23. Horn M, Morgan MK, Ingebrigtsen T. Surgery for unruptured intracranial aneurysms in a low-volume neurosurgical unit. *Acta Neurol Scand* 2004; 110(3): 170-4.

24. Krisht AF, Gomez J, Partington S. Outcome of surgical clipping of unruptured aneurysms as it compares with a 10-year nonclipping survival period. *Neurosurgery* 2006; 58(2): 207-16.

25. Nussbaum ES, Madison MT, Myers ME, Goddard J. Microsurgical treatment of unruptured intracranial aneurysms. A consecutive surgical experience consisting of 450 aneurysms treated in the endovascular era. *Surg Neurol* 2007; 67(5): 457-64; discussion 464-6.

26. Aghakhani N, Vaz G, David P, *et al*. Surgical management of unruptured intracranial aneurysms that are inappropriate for endovascular treatment: experience based on two academic centers. *Neurosurgery* 2008; 62(6): 1227-34; discussion 1234-25.

27. Yasunaga H, Matsuyama Y, Ohe K. Risk-adjusted analyses of the effects of hospital and surgeon volumes on postoperative complications and the modified Rankin scale after clipping of unruptured intracranial aneurysms in Japan. *Neurol Med Chir (Tokyo)* 2008; 48(12): 531-38; discussion 538.

28. Hadeishi H, Yasui N, Suzuki A. [Risks of surgical treatment for unruptured intracranial aneurysms]. *No Shinkei Geka* 1991; 19(10): 945-9.

29. Lanterna LA, Tredici G, Dimitrov BD, Biroli F. Treatment of unruptured cerebral aneurysms by embolization with Guglielmi detachable coils: case-fatality, morbidity, and effectiveness in preventing bleeding - a systematic review of the literature. *Neurosurgery* 2004; 55(4): 767-75; discussion 775-8.

30. Ng P, Khangure MS, Phatouros CC, Bynevelt M, ApSimon H, McAuliffe W. Endovascular treatment of intracranial aneurysms with Guglielmi detachable coils: analysis of

midterm angiographic and clinical outcomes. *Stroke* 2002; 33(1): 210-7.

31. Malisch TW, Guglielmi G, Vinuela F, *et al*. Intracranial aneurysms treated with the Guglielmi detachable coil: midterm clinical results in a consecutive series of 100 patients. *J Neurosurg* 1997; 87(2): 176-83.

32. Leber KA, Klein GE, Trummer M, Eder HG. Intracranial aneurysms: a review of endovascular and surgical treatment in 248 patients. *Minim Invasive Neurosurg* 1998; 41(2): 81-5.

33. Debrun GM, Aletich VA, Kehrli P, Misra M, Ausman JI, Charbel F. Selection of cerebral aneurysms for treatment using Guglielmi detachable coils: the preliminary University of Illinois at Chicago experience. *Neurosurgery* 1998; 43(6): 1281-95; discussion 1296-7.

34. Kuether TA, Nesbit GM, Barnwell SL. Clinical and angiographic outcomes, with treatment data, for patients with cerebral aneurysms treated with Guglielmi detachable coils: a single-center experience. *Neurosurgery* 1998; 43(5): 1016-25.

35. Cognard C, Weill A, Castaings L, Rey A, Moret J. Intracranial berry aneurysms: angiographic and clinical results after endovascular treatment. *Radiology* 1998; 206(2): 499-10.

36. Eskridge JM, Song JK. Endovascular embolization of 150 basilar tip aneurysms with Guglielmi detachable coils: results of the Food and Drug Administration multicenter clinical trial. *J Neurosurg* 1998; 89(1): 81-6.

37. Lot G, Houdart E, Cophignon J, Casasco A, George B. Combined management of intracranial aneurysms by surgical and endovascular treatment. Modalities and results from a series of 395 cases. *Acta Neurochir* (Wien) 1999; 141(6): 557-62.

38. Murayama Y, Vinuela F, Duckwiler GR, Gobin YP, Guglielmi G. Embolization of incidental cerebral aneurysms by using the Guglielmi detachable coil system. *J Neurosurg* 1999; 90(2): 207-14.

39. Raftopoulos C, Mathurin P, Boscherini D, Billa RF, Van Boven M, Hantson P. Prospective analysis of aneurysm treatment in a series of 103 consecutive patients when endovascular embolization is considered the first option. *J Neurosurg* 2000; 93(2): 175-82.

40. Qureshi AI, Suri MF, Khan J, *et al*. Endovascular treatment of intracranial aneurysms by using Guglielmi detachable coils in awake patients: safety and feasibility. *J Neurosurg* 2001; 94(6): 880-5.

41. Roy D, Milot G, Raymond J. Endovascular treatment of unruptured aneurysms. *Stroke* 2001; 32(9): 1998-2004.

42. Wanke I, Doerfler A, Dietrich U, *et al*. Endovascular treatment of unruptured intracranial aneurysms. *AJNR Am J Neuroradiol* 2002; 23(5): 756-61.

43. Goddard AJ, Annesley-Williams D, Gholkar A. Endovascular management of unruptured intracranial aneurysms: does outcome justify treatment? *J Neurol Neurosurg Psychiatry* 2002; 72(4): 485-90.

44. Hoh BL, Rabinov JD, Pryor JC, Carter BS, Barker FG 2nd. In-hospital morbidity and mortality after endovascular treatment of unruptured intracranial aneurysms in the United States, 1996-2000: effect of hospital and physician volume. *AJNR Am J Neuroradiol* 2003; 24(7): 1409-20.

45. Gonzalez N, Murayama Y, Nien YL, *et al*. Treatment of unruptured aneurysms with GDCs: clinical experience with 247 aneurysms. *AJNR Am J Neuroradiol* 2004; 25(4): 577-83.

46. van Rooij WJ, Sluzewski M. Procedural morbidity and mortality of elective coil treatment of unruptured intracranial aneurysms. *AJNR Am J Neuroradiol* 2006; 27(8): 1678-80.

47. Standhardt H, Boecher-Schwarz H, Gruber A, Benesch T, Knosp E, Bavinzski G. Endovascular treatment of unruptured intracranial aneurysms with Guglielmi detachable coils: short- and long-term results of a single-centre series. *Stroke* 2008; 39(3): 899-904.

48. Gallas S, Drouineau J, Gabrillargues J, *et al*. Feasibility, procedural morbidity and mortality, and long-term follow-up of endovascular treatment of 321 unruptured aneurysms. *AJNR Am J Neuroradiol* 2008; 29(1): 63-8.

49. Im SH, Han MH, Kwon OK, *et al*. Endovascular coil embolization of 435 small asymptomatic unruptured intracranial aneurysms: procedural morbidity and patient outcome. *AJNR Am J Neuroradiol* 2009; 30(1): 79-84.

50. Johnston SC, Wilson CB, Halbach VV, *et al*. Endovascular and surgical treatment of unruptured cerebral aneurysms: comparison of risks. *Ann Neurol* 2000; 48(1): 11-19.

51. Raftopoulos C, Goffette P, Vaz G, *et al*. Surgical clipping may lead to better results than coil embolization: results from a series of 101 consecutive unruptured intracranial aneurysms. *Neurosurgery* 2003; 52(6): 1280-7; discussion 1287-90.

52. Johnston SC, Dudley RA, Gress DR, Ono L. Surgical and endovascular treatment of unruptured cerebral aneurysms at university hospitals. *Neurology* 1999; 52(9): 1799-805.

53. Johnston SC, Zhao S, Dudley RA, Berman MF, Gress DR. Treatment of unruptured cerebral aneurysms in California. *Stroke* 2001; 32(3): 597-605.

54. Barker FG 2nd, Amin-Hanjani S, Butler WE, *et al*. Age-dependent differences in short-term outcome after surgical or endovascular treatment of unruptured intracranial aneurysms in the United States, 1996-2000. *Neurosurgery* 2004; 54(1): 18-28; discussion 28-30.

55. Higashida RT, Lahue BJ, Torbey MT, Hopkins LN, Leip E, Hanley DF. Treatment of unruptured intracranial aneurysms: a nationwide assessment of effectiveness. *AJNR Am J Neuroradiol* 2007; 28(1): 146-51.

56. Gerlach R, Beck J, Setzer M, *et al*. Treatment-related morbidity of unruptured intracranial aneurysms: results of a prospective single-centre series with an interdisciplinary approach over a 6-year period (1999-2005). *J Neurol Neurosurg Psychiatry* 2007; 78(8): 864-71.

57. Seifert V, Gerlach R, Raabe A, *et al*. The interdisciplinary treatment of unruptured intracranial aneurysms. *Dtsch Arztebl Int* 2008; 105(25): 449-56.

58. Hoh BL, Chi YY, Dermott MA, Lipori PJ, Lewis SB. The effect of coiling versus clipping of ruptured and unruptured cerebral aneurysms on length of stay, hospital cost, hospital reimbursement, and surgeon reimbursement at the university of Florida. *Neurosurgery* 2009; 64(4): 614-19; discussion 619-21.

59. David CA, Vishteh AG, Spetzler RF, Lemole M, Lawton MT, Partovi S. Late angiographic follow-up review of surgically treated aneurysms. *J Neurosurg* 1999; 91(3): 396-401.

60. Tsutsumi K, Ueki K, Usui M, Kwak S, Kirino T. Risk of subarachnoid hemorrhage after surgical treatment of unruptured cerebral aneurysms. *Stroke* 1999; 30(6): 1181-4.

61. Tsutsumi K, Ueki K, Morita A, Usui M, Kirino T. Risk of aneurysm recurrence in patients with clipped cerebral aneurysms: results of long-term follow-up angiography. *Stroke* 2001; 32(5): 1191-4.

62. Akyuz M, Tuncer R, Yilmaz S, Sindel T. Angiographic follow-up after surgical treatment of intracranial aneurysms. *Acta Neurochir* (Wien) 2004; 146(3): 245-50.

63. Thornton J, Debrun GM, Aletich VA, Bashir Q, Charbel FT, Ausman J. Follow-up angiography of intracranial aneurysms treated with endovascular placement of Guglielmi detachable coils. *Neurosurgery* 2002; 50(2): 239-49; discussion 249-50.

64. Raymond J, Guilbert F, Weill A, *et al.* Long-term angiographic recurrences after selective endovascular treatment of aneurysms with detachable coils. *Stroke* 2003; 34(6): 1398-403.

65. Murayama Y, Nien YL, Duckwiler G, *et al.* Guglielmi detachable coil embolization of cerebral aneurysms: 11 years' experience. *J Neurosurg* 2003; 98(5): 959-66.

Chapter 26

Unruptured cerebral aneurysms: observe, clip, or coil?

Chapter 27

Ruptured cerebral aneurysms: clip or coil?

Raqeeb Haque MD, Chief Resident 1
Jonathan Yun MD, Resident 1
Celina M Crisman MD, Resident 2
Brian Y Hwang MD, Resident 3
E Sander Connolly MD, Bennett M Stein Professor of Neurological Surgery;
Vice Chairman of Neurosurgery; Director, Cerebrovascular Research Laboratory 1
Robert A Solomon MD, Byron Stookey Professor of Neurosurgery;
Chairman and Director of Service 1

1 DEPARTMENT OF NEUROLOGICAL SURGERY, THE NEUROLOGIC INSTITUTE OF NEW YORK
COLUMBIA UNIVERSITY, NEW YORK, USA
2 DEPARTMENT OF NEUROLOGICAL SURGERY, UNIVERSITY OF MEDICINE AND
DENTISTRY OF NEW JERSEY, NEWARK, NEW JERSEY, USA
3 DEPARTMENT OF NEUROLOGICAL SURGERY, THE JOHNS HOPKINS UNIVERSITY,
BALTIMORE, MARYLAND, USA

Introduction

Clipping versus coiling in the management of ruptured intracranial aneurysms remains one of the most important controversies in the field of vascular neurosurgery. Patients with ruptured intracranial aneurysms are often eligible for both clipping and coiling. Despite numerous clinical studies and randomized trials, there remains no consensus on the ideal management of ruptured aneurysms, and the decision to clip or coil individual patients remains complex.

Surgical clipping excludes aneurysms from the circulation, and thereby reduces the risk of aneurysmal enlargement or rebleed, while maintaining the integrity of parent vessels and minimizing damage to normal brain. Over the past four decades, surgical clipping has become an established treatment for aneurysm rupture and has been consistently associated with superior results to non-surgical treatments. Nevertheless, endovascular coiling has also gained acceptance in recent years as a generally safe and effective therapy for ruptured aneurysms. While the decision to proceed surgically or through endovascular means must always be rendered on a case-by-case basis, clinical characteristics as well as the risks and benefits of each approach affect treatment considerations.

Methodology

A comprehensive literature search was performed using PubMed from 1976 to May 2010, using the

Chapter 27

search terms 'aneurysm,' 'intracranial,' 'clip,' 'coil,' 'endovascular,' 'surgical,' yielding 81 relevant abstracts for review. Within these abstracts, special attention was focused on abstracts comparing clipping to coiling, especially focusing on the results of the International Subarachnoid Aneurysm Trial. The bibliographies of selected papers were reviewed to identify other related publications.

Patient characteristics

In general, both procedures are well accepted. The decision to coil or clip depends on various factors including patient clinical characteristics, location and size of the lesions, and surgeon experience. For instance, patients with coagulopathy, those who require chronic anticoagulation, and those older than 70 years are frequently considered for endovascular rather than conventional surgery [1]. Clinical grade is important to the decision to intervene. Patients with high-grade subarachnoid hemorrhage (SAH) (Hunt and Hess or World Federation of Neurosurgical Societies [WFNS] grades IV and V) present a greater surgical challenge, as does an edematous or ischemic brain. However, endovascular therapies remain feasible in some cases despite such conditions [2]. A study of endovascular treatment in patients with high-grade aneurysmal SAH (aSAH) reported a favorable outcome in 62% of patients with grade IV SAH, 25% of those with grade V SAH, and 52.5% of total included patients [3] **(III/B)**. A study combining endovascular treatment with aggressive medical management (including hypervolemic hemodilution and hypertensive treatment) in patients with WFNS grade V SAH produced encouraging results [4]. Most patients (55%) experienced a favorable outcome, while the mortality rate was 18% **(III/B)**. Thus, there is growing support for endovascular intervention in patients with high-grade SAH, particularly when coupled with aggressive medical management. However, surgical management may provide a more optimal approach in cases where surgery is needed to evacuate a parenchymal hematoma [5].

Timing of intervention

The timing of the intervention is an appropriate factor in the decision to proceed endovascularly or surgically. Intervention in the care of patients with aSAH is primarily undertaken to prevent rebleeding, an event that increases mortality to 70-90% [6, 7]. The risk of rebleed is the greatest in the first 24 hours, reaching 19%, and by 4 weeks the cumulative risk reaches 40% [6, 8]. Notably, the risk of rebleeding is greatest in those with high clinical grades [8]. Surgical series have yielded conflicting data on the timing of aneurysm clipping, with some studies demonstrating higher rates of vasospasm and concordant morbidity in patients receiving early surgery, while others have shown a benefit associated with very early surgery (0-3 days following rupture). Most studies, however, have yielded similar results with regard to the generally poorer outcome associated with surgical intervention when the risk of vasospasm is greatest, generally 6-10 days post-rupture [9] **(III/B)**.

Endovascular treatment itself has not been associated with increased vasospasm, and endovascular treatment of vasospasm can be undertaken at the time of aneurysm treatment if necessary. For these reasons, the timing issues of conventional surgery do not necessarily hold true for endovascular intervention [10]. A retrospective study divided patients into three groups depending on when they underwent endovascular coil embolization following the development of aSAH: within 48 hours, 3-10 days, or 11-30 days. Statistically, there was no difference in the percent of patients experiencing favorable outcomes within each group [11] **(III/B)**.

Complications

Several specific complications may affect the decision to proceed with surgical or endovascular intervention. The development of an intracerebral hematoma (ICH) following aneurysmal rupture is associated with increased morbidity and mortality compared with SAH alone. The condition often mandates surgery, because of the need for hematoma evacuation and decompression. Clipping of the ruptured aneurysm may be undertaken simultaneously. Despite evacuation of the hemorrhage, particularly in WFNS grade IV/V SAH, mortality in ICH patients remains high, ranging from 21% to 85% [12, 13]. For this reason, a sequential approach involving endovascular aneurysm occlusion followed promptly by surgical evacuation of the hematoma was proposed. One series using this approach in patients with WFNS grade IV/V SAH and ICH due to aneurysm rupture demonstrated favorable outcomes in 48% of patients, with death in 21% [14] **(III/B)**. This strategy may be particularly useful when ICH develops opposite to the side of the ruptured aneurysm. Chung *et al* reported a series of ruptured anterior communicating artery aneurysms complicated by significant ICH, making the ICH difficult to evacuate from the site optimal for aneurysm access [15]. These investigators treated anterior communicating artery aneurysms using endovascular coil occlusion, and then evacuated the ICH through a burr-hole craniotomy. They observed no rebleed during follow-up and more than half of the patients experienced moderate to good recovery [15] **(III/B)**. Thus, evidence suggests that the occlusion of ruptured aneurysms associated with ICH via endovascular means followed by surgical evacuation is a safe and effective approach to this common situation that is traditionally associated with very high mortality.

Location and morphology

Finally, the location and morphology of the aneurysm determine suitability for endovascular treatment. Aneurysms occurring in the posterior circulation are typically better candidates for endovascular treatment based on anatomic considerations. The relationship of these aneurysms to important perforator arteries and cranial nerves creates great risk of surgical morbidity. Patients with multiple aneurysms in different vascular distributions and SAH of uncertain origin are also well served by endovascular treatment. However, aneurysms with tortuous proximal vessels, severe vasospasm, vessels affected by atherosclerosis, or those that are very distally located may present challenges to endovascular access and typically make better surgical candidates [16].

It is widely accepted that aneurysms with small necks, or inflow regions, relative to fundus size, are particularly amenable to endovascular therapy, while giant and fusiform aneurysms are not without the use of adjunctive devices. This is largely due to the tendency of endovascularly placed coils to herniate into the parent vessel. Endovascular techniques and instruments are being developed to meet these issues and have made considerable headway; however, surgical intervention is generally a good choice for these patients.

The middle cerebral artery (MCA) represents one of the most common sites of intracranial aneurysms, accounting for roughly 20%. These are often managed surgically, rather than endovascularly, for several reasons. These aneurysms are easily accessible via craniotomy with minimal brain retraction. Furthermore, MCA aneurysms pose challenges to endovascular treatment, given that they often have wide necks and involve branching vessels. When 53 patients with 58 bifurcation or trifurcation aneurysms of the MCA at one institution were evaluated, 88% of aneurysms had a dome-to-neck ratio of less than two and in 40% branch vessels were incorporated into the aneurysm sac [17] **(III/B)**. However, endovascular therapy, while not generally the preferred option, is not precluded in the case of MCA aneurysms. A recent study of 16 patients with wide-necked MCA aneurysms, including 10 acutely ruptured aneurysms, treated with stent-assisted embolization found no recurrence, rebleeding, or neurologic deterioration at an average of 20 months' follow-up [18] **(III/B)**.

Outcomes

While a number of studies attempted to compare endovascular treatment and surgical clipping, as shown in Table 1 [19-23], the effectiveness of the two procedures was most directly compared in the International Subarachnoid Aneurysm Trial (ISAT) [24]. This study randomized 2,143 patients presenting with SAH attributable to aneurysm rupture after neurosurgical and endovascular teams agreed on the suitability of either modality. It was conducted

Table 1. Summary of surgical and endovascular outcomes for ruptured aneurysm in recent trials comparing treatment modalities.

Reference	Study design	Special considerations	Endovascular treatment	Surgical treatment	Difference	Level of evidence
Kato et al, 2005 [20]	Retrospective	Patients with severe SAH assigned to a treatment group based on clinical grade, age, and aneurysm location	Good outcome in 44% of 59 patients	Good outcome in 69% of 120 patients	Statistical analysis not available, although the authors noted that clipping had a better outcome than coiling	III/B
Hoh et al, 2004 [21]	Retrospective	Decisions regarding treatment modality made by the interventional team; non-randomized	Good outcome in 34% of 79 patients treated with coiling; good outcome in 30% of 23 patients undergoing endovascular coiling with craniotomy	Good outcome in 55% of 413 patients	Clipping had a significantly better outcome than coiling (OR 0.50, 95% CI, 0.27-0.95, p=0.0314); craniotomy with endovascular coiling had a better outcome than coiling (OR 0.53, 95% CI, 0.28-0.985, p=0.045)	III/B
Molyneux et al, 2002 [19]	Randomized	-	23.7% of 801 patients were dead or dependent at 1 year	30.6% of 793 patients were dead or dependent at 1 year	The relative risk reduction in those undergoing endovascular treatment was 22.6% (95% CI, 8.9-34.2)	Ib/A
Bairstow et al, 2002 [22]	Randomized	-	Glasgow Outcome Scale median of 1 at 2 months following discharge (10 patients)	Glasgow Outcome Scale median of 2 at 2 months following discharge (12 patients)	Statistical analysis unavailable; the authors concluded that patients treated endovascularly have better outcomes	Ib/A
Gruber et al, 1998 [23]	Retrospective	Decisions regarding treatment modality made by the interventional team; non-randomized	35.5% of 45 patients remained neurologically intact; 38% had ischemic infarcts	47.7% of 111 patients remained neurologically intact; 22% had ischemic infarcts	Statistical analysis unavailable; however, endovascularly treated patients were in a worse condition at baseline	III/B

CI = confidence interval; OR = odds ratio; SAH = subarachnoid hemorrhage largely in the UK, where 82% of patients received treatment. Of the 2,143 patients, 1,070 underwent microsurgery and 1,073 were treated with a Guglielmi detachable coil (GDC). The two groups were then followed with regard to the incidence of rebleeds and clinical outcomes, including death or dependence (defined as a modified Rankin score >2). At 1 year, death or dependence was 23.7% in the endovascular group compared with 30.6% in the surgical group [24] **(Ib/A)**. The difference between these groups was significant, and the absolute risk reduction in dependence or death associated with endovascular treatment was 6.9%. At this point, the incidence of rebleeds was low; two rebleeds occurred in 1,276 patient-years of follow-up in the endovascular group and none in 1,081 patient-years of follow-up among those undergoing microsurgery. At 5-year follow-up, the dependence rates did not vary significantly between groups. Nevertheless, survival in the endovascular group, even after 7 years of follow-up, remained significantly higher.

In addition to lower mortality, endovascular patients also experienced a substantially lower incidence of seizures, despite a slightly greater incidence of repeat aneurysm rupture. After 3,258 patient-years of follow-up, there were 10 repeat hemorrhages in the endovascular group, compared with three rebleeds in 3,107 patient-years in the surgical group. This may be related in part to the durability of aneurysm occlusion:

66% of follow-up angiograms in the endovascular group demonstrated complete aneurysm occlusion, compared with 82% of surgically clipped aneurysms. Meanwhile, 8% of angiograms from endovascularly treated patients demonstrated incomplete occlusion with aneurysm refilling, compared with 6% of clipped aneurysms [19, 25] **(Ib/A)**. Despite lower rates of complete vascular occlusion, endovascular treatment represents a clinically effective treatment for many cases of ruptured aneurysms, and is well supported by clinical outcomes as an acceptable treatment method in appropriately selected patients with SAH.

Although the ISAT results demonstrate that endovascular coiling is associated with improved short- and long-term clinical outcomes and lower risks of epilepsy, follow-up analysis suggests greater benefits following surgical clipping [26]. Elderly patients with MCA aneurysms seemed to respond better to clipping [26, 27] **(Ib/A)**. Further, there is a decreased risk of rebleeding associated with surgical clipping and a decreased need for retreatment (Table 2) [28]. These findings suggest that a longer follow-up period than that explored in ISAT would reveal lasting benefits of clipping over coiling of aneurysms. Indeed, the Kaplan-Meier analysis of survival in ISAT is suggestive of similar survival in patients at 8 years' follow-up [26]. Given that only 5% of patients were followed for more than 11 years, a longer period of observation is required.

Table 2. Advantages of surgical clipping in the long-term analysis of ISAT (evidence level Ib/A).

	Endovascular, n (%)	Surgical, n (%)	p-value
Cumulative mortality (patients followed for ≥6 years) [33]	165/359 (46)	194/359 (54)	0.085
Independent survival at 5 years' follow-up (mRS ≤2) [33]	626/755 (83)	584/713 (82)	0.61
Late rebleed from target aneurysm [33]	10/13 (77)	3/13 (23)	0.02
Retreatment rate [28]	191/1,096 (17)	39/1,012 (4)	<0.006

ISAT = International Subarachnoid Aneurysm Trial; mRS = modified Rankin Scale

The findings of the ISAT trial concerning occlusion and rebleed rates have been explored and echoed in additional studies. Regarding occlusion, a retrospective review of patients undergoing treatment for a ruptured aneurysm, either endovascularly or surgically, at one of nine centers found that a significantly greater proportion of surgical patients had completely occluded aneurysms. Specifically, the rate of total occlusion was 92% (646/706) in surgically treated patients, compared with 39% (114/295) in the notably fewer endovascular patients [29] **(III/B)**. In addition, a very large long-term study followed patients with aneurysms coiled via GDC embolization over an 11-year period and reported complete occlusion in 55% of patients [30] **(III/B)**. Although this study included both ruptured and unruptured aneurysms, it provides data regarding those aneurysms more likely to be incompletely occluded following embolization. Giant aneurysms presented greater challenges, with 63% being incompletely occluded after embolization, while small aneurysms (4-10mm diameter) with small necks were least likely to result in incomplete occlusion (25.5%). Studies investigating surgical clipping have consistently reported higher rates of complete occlusion. In a study reported in 1999, 91.8% of 160 surgically treated aneurysms were completely occluded [31] **(III/B)**. A similar study, conducted between 1970 and 1980, identified incomplete occlusion in 3.8% of patients [32] **(III/B)**.

The prevention of rehemorrhage is an important measure of successful aneurysm treatment, as rebleed is associated with significant mortality. The phenomenon of late rebleeding, defined as rebleeding more than 1 year post-therapy, has caused concern regarding the long-term durability of coil embolization. Although a relatively rare phenomenon, an analysis of the ISAT dataset published in 2008 reported a significant reduction in late rebleeding in younger patients (<40 years) treated with clipping versus coil embolization by intent-to-treat analysis [27] **(Ib/A)**. Further, late rebleeding from targeted aneurysms was significantly reduced in the surgically treated patient cohort [33] **(Ib/A)**. In light of the fact that recanalization has been reported in up to 21% of patients satisfactorily treated by coil embolization [34], long-term studies of late rebleeding may reveal diminished benefits in this patient cohort **(III/B)**.

Conclusions

The endovascular approach to the treatment of ruptured intracranial aneurysms has seen increased utilization in light of technical advancements, surgeon expertise, and better understanding of optimal patient selection. Patients will likely experience the best outcomes when both the surgical and endovascular option are available, with expertise in both techniques. Patient characteristics, clinical presentations, and anatomical considerations may help guide the surgeon in deciding the best intervention for an aneurysm. Additional long-term outcome studies are necessary to further investigate the advantages of either surgical clipping or endovascular coiling.

Recommendations	Evidence level

♦ Surgical and endovascular approaches to ruptured intracranial aneurysms have both gained widespread acceptance; the decision to proceed through surgical or endovascular means is made on a case-by-case basis and is influenced by various factors, including the patient's clinical characteristics, the location and size of the lesion, and the practitioner's experience.   -

♦ Patients with coagulopathies, elderly patients, and those with severe brain swelling are often considered for endovascular intervention over conventional surgery.   -

♦ Patients with aneurysms of the posterior circulation, multiple aneurysms in different vascular distributions, or SAH of unknown origin are often deemed good endovascular candidates.   III/B

♦ Endovascular treatment is additionally best suited to vessels with small necks relative to fundus size, although approaches and instrumentation, such as stenting, are in development to extend the applicability of endovascular treatment.   -

♦ Tortuous proximal vessels, severe vasospasm, atherosclerotic vessels, and distally located aneurysms render endovascular approaches more challenging. Aneurysms with these characteristics are often addressed through surgery.   III/B

♦ Aneurysms of the MCA are typically managed surgically, given that they are easily accessible with minimal retraction, tend to involve branching vessels, and often have wide necks.   -

♦ Intervention should be undertaken as soon as feasible; studies suggest that outcomes following conventional open surgery are poorer when undertaken while the risk of vasospasm is greatest. Studies imply that this association is not as consistent for endovascular procedures.   III/B

♦ According to ISAT, endovascular coiling produced significantly better clinical outcomes over the short term and up to 7 years, compared with surgical clipping. It was also associated with a lower risk of epilepsy.   Ib/A

♦ Follow-up studies of ISAT patients demonstrated a decreased need for retreatment and decreased rates of late rebleeding in patients treated via surgical clipping.   Ib/A

♦ Surgical clipping appears to produce higher rates of complete occlusion than endovascular coiling.   III/B

♦ There is a need for additional long-term studies comparing strategies in the management of ruptured aneurysms.   -

References

1. Bradac GB, Bergui M, Fontanella M. Endovascular treatment of cerebral aneurysms in elderly patients. *Neuroradiology* 2005; 47(12): 938-41.

2. Johnston SC, Higashida RT, Barrow DL, *et al.* Recommendations for the endovascular treatment of intracranial aneurysms: a statement for healthcare professionals from the Committee on Cerebrovascular Imaging of the American Heart Association Council on Cardiovascular Radiology. *Stroke* 2002; 33(10): 2536-44.

3. Bracard S, Lebedinsky A, Anxionnat R, *et al.* Endovascular treatment of Hunt and Hess grade IV and V aneuryms. *AJNR Am J Neuroradiol* 2002; 23(6): 953-7.

4. van Loon J, Waerzeggers Y, Wilms G, Van Calenbergh F, Goffin J, Plets C. Early endovascular treatment of ruptured cerebral aneurysms in patients in very poor neurological condition. *Neurosurgery* 2002; 50(3): 457-64; discussion 464-5.

5. Bederson JB, Connolly ES Jr, Batjer HH, *et al*. Guidelines for the management of aneurysmal subarachnoid hemorrhage: a statement for healthcare professionals from a special writing group of the Stroke Council, American Heart Association. *Stroke* 2009; 40(3): 994-1025.

6. Inagawa T, Kamiya K, Ogasawara H, Yano T. Rebleeding of ruptured intracranial aneurysms in the acute stage. *Surg Neurol* 1987; 28(2): 93-9.

7. van Gijn J, Kerr RS, Rinkel GJ. Subarachnoid haemorrhage. *Lancet* 2007; 369(9558): 306-18.

8. Rosenorn J, Eskesen V, Schmidt K, Ronde F. The risk of rebleeding from ruptured intracranial aneurysms. *J Neurosurg* 1987; 67(3): 329-32.

9. Taylor B, Harries P, Bullock R. Factors affecting outcome after surgery for intracranial aneurysm in Glasgow. *Br J Neurosurg* 1991; 5(6): 591-600.

10. Yalamanchili K, Rosenwasser RH, Thomas JE, Liebman K, McMorrow C, Gannon P. Frequency of cerebral vasospasm in patients treated with endovascular occlusion of intracranial aneurysms. *AJNR Am J Neuroradiol* 1998; 19(3): 553-8.

11. Baltsavias GS, Byrne JV, Halsey J, Coley SC, Sohn MJ, Molyneux AJ. Effects of timing of coil embolization after aneurysmal subarachnoid hemorrhage on procedural morbidity and outcomes. *Neurosurgery* 2000; 47(6): 1320-9; discussion 1329-31.

12. Jeong JH, Koh JS, Kim EJ. A less invasive approach for ruptured aneurysm with intracranial hematoma: coil embolization followed by clot evacuation. *Korean J Radiol* 2007; 8(1): 2-8.

13. Nowak G, Schwachenwald D, Schwachenwald R, Kehler U, Muller H, Arnold H. Intracerebral hematomas caused by aneurysm rupture. Experience with 67 cases. *Neurosurg Rev* 1998; 21(1): 5-9.

14. Niemann DB, Wills AD, Maartens NF, Kerr RS, Byrne JV, Molyneux AJ. Treatment of intracerebral hematomas caused by aneurysm rupture: coil placement followed by clot evacuation. *J Neurosurg* 2003; 99(5): 843-7.

15. Chung J, Kim BM, Shin YS, Lim YC, Park SK. Treatment of ruptured anterior communicating artery aneurysm accompanying intracerebral hematomas: endovascular coiling followed by hematoma evacuation with burr hole trephination and catheterization. *Acta Neurochir* (Wien) 2009; 151(8): 917-23.

16. Jabbour PM, Tjoumakaris SI, Rosenwasser RH. Endovascular management of intracranial aneurysms. *Neurosurg Clin N Am* 2009; 20(4): 383-98.

17. Jayaraman MV, Do HM, Versnick EJ, Steinberg GK, Marks MP. Morphologic assessment of middle cerebral artery aneurysms for endovascular treatment. *J Stroke Cerebrovasc Dis* 2007; 16(2): 52-6.

18. Yang P, Liu J, Huang Q, *et al*. Endovascular treatment of wide-neck middle cerebral artery aneurysms with stents: a review of 16 cases. *AJNR Am J Neuroradiol* 2010; 31(5): 940-6.

19. Molyneux A, Kerr R, Stratton I, *et al*. International Subarachnoid Aneurysm Trial (ISAT) of neurosurgical clipping versus endovascular coiling in 2143 patients with ruptured intracranial aneurysms: a randomised trial. *Lancet* 2002; 360(9342): 1267-74.

20. Kato Y, Sano H, Dong PT, *et al*. The effect of clipping and coiling in acute severe subarachnoid hemorrhage after international subarachnoid aneurysmal trial (ISAT) results. *Minim Invasive Neurosurg* 2005; 48(4): 224-7.

21. Hoh BL, Topcuoglu MA, Singhal AB, *et al*. Effect of clipping, craniotomy, or intravascular coiling on cerebral vasospasm and patient outcome after aneurysmal subarachnoid hemorrhage. *Neurosurgery* 2004; 55(4): 779-86; discussion 786-9.

22. Bairstow P, Dodgson A, Linto J, Khangure M. Comparison of cost and outcome of endovascular and neurosurgical procedures in the treatment of ruptured intracranial aneurysms. *Australas Radiol* 2002; 46(3): 249-51.

23. Gruber A, Ungersbock K, Reinprecht A, *et al*. Evaluation of cerebral vasospasm after early surgical and endovascular treatment of ruptured intracranial aneurysms. *Neurosurgery* 1998; 42(2): 258-67.

24. Molyneux A, Kerr R, Stratton I, *et al*. International Subarachnoid Aneurysm Trial (ISAT) of neurosurgical clipping versus endovascular coiling in 2143 patients with ruptured intracranial aneurysms: a randomized trial. *J Stroke Cerebrovasc Dis* 2002; 11(6): 304-14.

25. Molyneux AJ, Kerr RS, Yu LM, *et al*. International Subarachnoid Aneurysm Trial (ISAT) of neurosurgical clipping versus endovascular coiling in 2143 patients with ruptured intracranial aneurysms: a randomised comparison of effects on survival, dependency, seizures, rebleeding, subgroups, and aneurysm occlusion. *Lancet* 2005; 366(9488): 809-17.

26. Connolly ES Jr, Meyers PM. Cerebral aneurysms: to clip or to coil? That is no longer the question. *Nat Rev Neurol* 2009; 5(8): 412-3.

27. Mitchell P, Kerr R, Mendelow AD, Molyneux A. Could late rebleeding overturn the superiority of cranial aneurysm coil embolization over clip ligation seen in the International Subarachnoid Aneurysm Trial? *J Neurosurg* 2008; 108(3): 437-42.

28. Campi A, Ramzi N, Molyneux AJ, *et al*. Retreatment of ruptured cerebral aneurysms in patients randomized by coiling or clipping in the International Subarachnoid Aneurysm Trial (ISAT). *Stroke* 2007; 38(5): 1538-44.

29. Johnston SC, Dowd CF, Higashida RT, Lawton MT, Duckwiler GR, Gress DR. Predictors of rehemorrhage after treatment of ruptured intracranial aneurysms: the Cerebral Aneurysm Rerupture After Treatment (CARAT) study. *Stroke* 2008; 39(1): 120-5.

30. Murayama Y, Song JK, Uda K, *et al*. Combined endovascular treatment for both intracranial aneurysm and symptomatic vasospasm. *AJNR Am J Neuroradiol* 2003; 24(1): 133-9.

31. David CA, Vishteh AG, Spetzler RF, Lemole M, Lawton MT, Partovi S. Late angiographic follow-up review of surgically treated aneurysms. *J Neurosurg* 1999; 91(3): 396-401.

32. Feuerberg I, Lindquist C, Lindqvist M, Steiner L. Natural history of postoperative aneurysm rests. *J Neurosurg* 1987; 66(1): 30-4.

33. Molyneux AJ, Kerr RS, Birks J, *et al*. Risk of recurrent subarachnoid haemorrhage, death, or dependence and standardised mortality ratios after clipping or coiling of an intracranial aneurysm in the International Subarachnoid Aneurysm Trial (ISAT): long-term follow-up. *Lancet Neurol* 2009; 8(5): 427-33.

34. Murayama Y, Nien YL, Duckwiler G, *et al*. Guglielmi detachable coil embolization of cerebral aneurysms: 11 years' experience. *J Neurosurg* 2003; 98(5): 959-66.

Chapter 28

Intracranial arteriovenous malformations: epidemiology, natural history, and management

Rudy J Rahme MD, Postdoctoral Research Fellow

Salah G Aoun MD, Postdoctoral Research Fellow

Stephen F Shafizadeh MD PhD, Resident Physician, PGY-6 and
Enfolded Cerebrovascular and Skull Base Fellow

Isaac Josh Abecassis BSc, Medical Student

Bernard R Bendok MD FACS FAANS FAHA, Associate Professor

H Hunt Batjer MD FACS FAANS, Michael J Marchese Professor and Chair

DEPARTMENT OF NEUROLOGICAL SURGERY, NORTHWESTERN UNIVERSITY FEINBERG
SCHOOL OF MEDICINE AND MCGAW MEDICAL CENTER, CHICAGO, ILLINOIS, USA

Introduction

Arteriovenous malformations (AVMs) are vascular lesions composed of a tangled network of dilated arteries directly connected to abnormal 'arterialized' veins without an intervening capillary bed (Figure 1). Intracranial AVMs are a relatively uncommon entity. They are thought to be congenital, forming around the third week of gestation [1]. However rare, AVMs pose a significant problem since they most often affect young and otherwise healthy individuals. Advances and innovations in the last few decades have enhanced our comprehension of AVM pathophysiology and hemodynamics, and added various treatment modalities and techniques. Although originally described by Steinheil over a century ago [2], the natural history of these lesions remains enigmatic. Unfortunately, there are no large-scale randomized controlled trials addressing this issue, or any other aspect of AVMs for that matter. This leaves us with lower levels of evidence that have to be interpreted with caution.

Understanding the epidemiology and natural history of AVMs is important, but has proven difficult to study. The reasons for this are myriad and include the low incidence of AVMs and their heterogeneity with respect to anatomic features, location in the brain, and modes of presentation. Many natural history studies on AVMs are flawed because of short follow-up intervals. Improvements in imaging techniques have further complicated our understanding of this issue; asymptomatic AVMs that would have been previously undetectable are now being increasingly diagnosed.

This chapter reviews the existing literature on intracranial AVMs with particular focus on the epidemiology and natural history, and briefly touches on treatment.

Methodology

A review of the literature using the PubMed/Medline database was performed using the

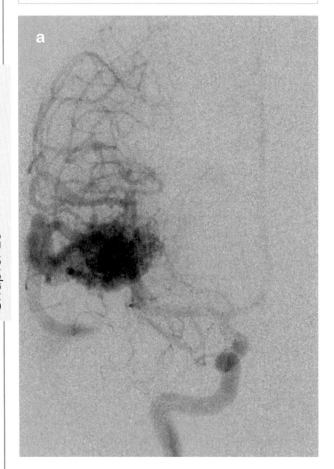

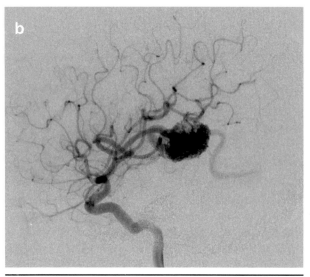

Figure 1. Cerebral angiogram showing a right posterior temporal arteriovenous malformation: a) anteroposterior and b) lateral views.

following key words and combinations of the key words: 'arteriovenous malformation,' 'natural history,' 'epidemiology,' 'hemorrhage,' 'rupture,' and 'seizure.' Our search was limited to papers published in the English language between 1966 and 2010. We then recruited additional studies by reviewing the bibliographies of the papers obtained from our initial search.

Epidemiology

Discerning the incidence and prevalence of AVMs is crucial to understanding their natural history and therefore critical to decision-making. AVMs are mostly congenital lesions and only a certain proportion become symptomatic during a lifetime. The failure of prior studies to completely elucidate the prevalence and incidence of AVMs can be attributed to a number of factors, including retrospective design, the lack of a clear rationale to screen for asymptomatic AVMs, a focus on small, genetically isolated populations, use of non-specific ICD-9 codes, and failure of diagnosis. This in turn partly explains the wide range of quoted prevalence, of 5-613 AVMs per 100,000 persons [3].

What proportion of patients remain asymptomatic with no consequences from their lesions? Can symptomatic patients without prior hemorrhage be managed conservatively? What is the risk of rehemorrhage after a first episode of bleeding? Are certain population subgroups at greater risk of AVM hemorrhage? These questions, among others, remain challenging to answer precisely because of the scant data available.

Before the literature can be discussed, specific epidemiological terms must be defined. Since, at any given time, there may be an uncertain proportion of undiagnosed AVMs, the more semantically correct terms to be used are 'prevalence of detected disease' rather than 'prevalence,' and 'detection rate' rather than 'incidence' [4].

Population-based studies

The most frequently quoted number in terms of AVM prevalence is 0.14% [5-7] **(III/B)**. This number is based on the data from the cooperative study of intracranial aneurysms and subarachnoid hemorrhage, one of the first population-based studies to address the prevalence of AVMs. The cooperative study included 19 centers from the USA and one center located in England [8]. In the final report, out of a total of 6,368 referred patients, Perret and Nishioka analyzed 545 cases of vascular malformations, of which 453 were diagnosed as intracranial AVMs [9]. The overall ratio of AVMs to aneurysms was 1:6.5, with a significant discrepancy between US centers and the center in England. Whereas the ratio was one AVM to 5.3 aneurysms in US centers, it was one AVM to 13.5 aneurysms in the British center. The disparity was thought to be caused by differences in referral patterns. Patients in England were mostly referred to the study center after a bleeding episode. While 36% of AVMs enrolled in US centers had not bled, only 9% of enrolled patients in England had not bled. Overall, the ratio of male to female patients was 1.1:1, with 236 (52%) male and 217 (48%) female patients. Sixty-four percent of AVMs were diagnosed before the age of 40 years.

The prevalence of AVM was then determined based on its relative frequency to that of aneurysms. Using the approximated ratio of 1:7 AVMs to aneurysms from the cooperative study and combining it with an estimated prevalence of 1% for intracranial aneurysm, Michelsen calculated a prevalence of detected AVMs of 0.14% (140 per 100,00 population) [10] **(III/B)**. Unfortunately, Michelsen's calculations were not without a major inaccuracy [4]. Deducing AVM prevalence from aneurysm prevalence rates insinuates that the probability of detecting AVMs – AVMs becoming symptomatic or an incidental finding – is similar to that of aneurysms, an assumption not corroborated by any data in the literature. Berman *et al* argued it would be more accurate to determine the relative detection rate rather than the prevalence. Based on the same data from the cooperative study, they calculated a projected rate of 2.3 detected AVMs per 100,000 person-years in the USA [4] **(III/B)**.

Several other population-based studies have been conducted, arguably the most important of which is the report by Brown *et al* from Olmsted County, Minnesota [11]. The authors used the Mayo Clinic

medical records linkage system to find all cases of intracranial vascular malformations during 1965-1992. A total of 48 cases of intracranial vascular malformations were detected, 26 of which were AVMs, for a detection rate of 1.11 per 100,000 person-years **(III/B)**. Twenty-two of the 26 diagnosed AVMs (85%) were symptomatic. Hemorrhage was the main presenting symptom, comprising 77% of all symptomatic AVMs. Unfortunately, this was not a clean AVM population and no AVM-specific epidemiological data were reported. The prevalence of all vascular malformation was reported to be 19 per 100,000 patient-years. Based on these numbers and using the reported frequency of symptomatic presentation of AVM lesions, Berman *et al* calculated an estimated prevalence of 0.94 per 100,000 person-years [4]. In addition, based on the relative detection rate of AVMs to that of all vascular malformations (1.11 to 2.05 per 100,000 person-years) they calculated an upper limit of prevalence of detected AVMs of 10.3 per 100,000 person-years **(III/B)**.

Population-based longitudinal studies are essential to track trends and determine the natural history of AVM lesions. Their results may not be generalizable, however, since they are performed in specific isolated populations. The variability is reflected in the differences in reported rates between the various population-based studies. Jessurun *et al* reported an annual incidence of 1.1 symptomatic AVMs per 100,000 in the Netherlands Antilles between 1980 and 1990 [12]. This rate should be analyzed carefully, though, as an unusually high proportion of patients had associated hereditary hemorrhagic telangiectasias (six out of 17 patients), suggesting that the rate of AVMs might be higher than in other populations. In addition, five of the 17 patients had multiple AVMs.

Prospective registries

With the growing need for a better understanding of the epidemiological aspects of AVMs coupled with an obvious lack of high-quality data and the shortcomings of retrospective studies, two prospective registries were started in 1999 and 2000 and remain ongoing [3, 13-15]. The Scottish Intracranial Vascular Malformation Study (SIVMS) was a prospective population-based study that collected data on first-time-ever diagnosed intracranial vascular malformations between January 1, 1999 and December 31, 2000 in adults (age ≥16 years) permanently residing in Scotland (estimated adult population of 4,110,956) [14, 15]. The detection rate of brain AVMs was 1.12 (95% confidence interval [CI], 0.90-1.37) per 100,000 adults per year **(IIb/B)**. Out of 92 AVM cases, 19 (21%) were asymptomatic; three of these were discovered on autopsies and the remaining 16 were incidental findings. Interestingly, there were significant differences in the results obtained when various methods of collecting data were analyzed [14]. The SIVMS used ICD-10 coding as well as tertiary-center referrals to collect patients. Only 58 of the 92 AVM cases would have been detected if coding was the only method used. In addition, the population would have been significantly biased toward younger patients with more hemorrhagic presentations, a higher number of angiograms performed, and a higher treatment rate. On the other hand, if patients were exclusively recruited by referrals from collaborators and thus simulating a hospital-based cohort, eight patients would have been missed. Furthermore, those eight patients were statistically different compared with the remaining 84 patients: fewer had had angiograms performed (38% vs. 77%; p=0.014) and fewer had been treated (13% vs. 66%; p=0.003).

The New York Islands AVM study is also an ongoing prospective population-based survey. This study covers Manhattan Island, Staten Island, and Long Island, comprising a population of 9,429,541 inhabitants [3, 13]. The primary objective of the survey is to determine the incidence of AVM-related hemorrhage, as well as subsequent morbidity and mortality. The study was started on March 15, 2000, after which all major New York Islands hospitals and their networks had to prospectively report weekly data on patients with diagnosed AVMs. As of the latest report, published in 2003, 284 patients were enrolled, yielding 21,216,467 person-years of observation [13]. The mean age at diagnosis was 35 years, and women comprised 49% of the population. The average annual detection rate of AVMs was calculated to be 1.34 per 100,000 person-years (95% CI, 1.18-1.49). No differences were detected between men and women **(IIb/B)**.

Autopsy studies

Autopsy studies have contributed some insight into our knowledge of AVM epidemiology. Autopsy data are subject to errors related to a number of factors, including the aggressiveness of the autopsy, the rate of autopsies, the age and cause of death of the patients, and premortem neurologic symptoms or lack thereof [16]. In addition, a center's practice can also potentially influence the results of autopsies, as centers with a specific interest in neurologic diseases will be more inclined to look aggressively for AVM lesions [4].

A series presented by McCormick included 5,754 consecutive autopsies spanning more than 20 years [17]. Thirty AVMs were detected and a calculated prevalence of 521 per 100,000 population (0.52%) was quoted **(III/B)**. Jellinger presented three autopsy series from Austria [18]. Two of these were performed in institutions specializing in neurologic diseases, which could explain the estimated prevalence of 613 AVMs per 100,000 population, one of the highest reported [18] **(III/B)**. On the other hand, the autopsy series performed by Courville, spanning three decades (1918-1948), reported only two AVMs for a prevalence of five per 100,000 population [19] **(III/B)**.

Perhaps the most important conclusion we can draw on this topic is how little we know about the epidemiology of AVMs. Due to the low prevalence of AVMs, the accuracy of estimates will invariably be affected by the small sample size. In fact, to achieve a prevalence with a CI extending less than 10% in either direction, a population of more than 4 million people is needed [4].

Presenting symptoms: hemorrhage

The complexity of the cerebrovascular anatomy of AVMs makes their treatment a challenge with significant inherent risks. Unlike most other diseases where the debate revolves around which type of treatment to administer, in the case of AVMs the debate is more basic: to treat or not to treat. In other words, should we interfere to change the natural course of the disease? While the question is apparently simple, the answer is far from straightforward.

The most common clinical presentation of AVMs is intracranial hemorrhage [5, 20, 21], with reported frequencies ranging from 30% to 82% [22, 23] **(III/B)**. Intraparenchymal hemorrhage is the most common form of AVM-related intracranial hemorrhage [24], although intraventricular and subarachnoid hemorrhages can also occur. The risk of subsequent hemorrhage after initial diagnosis, risk factors for such hemorrhage, and the morbidity and mortality of hemorrhage are important issues to understand and must be measured against the risk of any proposed treatment.

In a prospective observational study, the Northern Manhattan Stroke Study (NOMASS), patients were eligible if they were older than 20 years and had suffered a first-ever stroke between July 1, 1993, and June 30, 1997 [25, 26]. Stapf et al analyzed a specific subset of patients in this study presenting with intracranial hemorrhage, whether intracerebral, intraventricular, or subarachnoid [26]. During 546,492 person-years of observation, 207 patients presented with a first-ever intracranial hemorrhage, three of whom (1.4%) were diagnosed with an underlying brain AVM. All three had been asymptomatic until the bleed. The authors then calculated a first-ever AVM hemorrhage incidence of 0.55 per 100,000 person-years (95% CI, 0.11-1.61).

Hofmeister et al prospectively collected data from three independent brain AVM databases [27]. The largest was a multicenter database comprising 662 patients from centers in Berlin, Paris, the Far East, and the Middle East. The two other databases were from single centers, one in New York (n=337 patients) and the other in Toronto (n=290 patients). Out of a total of 1,289 patients, intracranial hemorrhage was the most common presenting symptom, occurring in 669 patients (53%; 95% CI, 51-56%). After adjusting for AVM size, no difference was detected in hemorrhage rates between the different centers.

The New York Islands AVM study reported an incidence of first-ever hemorrhage of 0.51 per 100,000 person-years (95% CI, 0.41-0.61) [13]. Out of 284 patients, 108 presented with hemorrhage (mean age 31±19 years and 45% women). The estimated prevalence of hemorrhage was 0.68 per 100,000 person-years (95% CI, 0.57-0.79). The major limitation of this study was the short follow-up period of 27 months at the time of reporting.

Most reports in the literature agree that the most common clinical presentation of AVM is hemorrhage, followed by seizures with varying percentages [5, 13, 16, 20, 21, 25, 26, 28-30]. Beyond this, there is very little consensus and even less evidence on the natural history of AVMs.

Natural history

AVM natural history series

In 1990, Ondra et al published what is arguably the most complete and comprehensive AVM natural history series ever written [20]. Based on data from Helsinki University, the authors reported on 160 prospectively followed, untreated, symptomatic AVM patients between 1942 and 1975, with a mean follow-up of 23.7 years. This series is thought to include approximately 90% of AVM lesions in the entire Finnish population for the defined period. The male to female ratio was 3:2, with 99 males and 67 females. The authors did not find any significant difference in the clinical course between men and women. The mean age at presentation was 33.7 years (range 10-70 years), with hemorrhage the most frequent presenting symptom (71% of patients).

During follow-up, 64 patients (40%) suffered at least one major hemorrhagic event for a total of 147 events, with one patient suffering 12 bleeding events. The mean time between initial presentation and hemorrhage was 7.7 years (range 6 weeks-22 years). The calculated rate of yearly hemorrhage risk was 4%. This remained constant over the first 20 years following diagnosis, after which the risk decreased significantly by nearly 50%. The risk of bleeding during follow-up was independent of the initial clinical presentation, whether it was hemorrhage, seizures, headaches, or any other complaints. Eighty-five percent of patients who bled during follow-up suffered major morbidity or mortality, with 23% incurring major morbidity or mortality with their first hemorrhagic event after enrollment.

Mortality rates were also high. Out of 160 patients, 69 (34%) died or experienced major morbidity during the follow-up period. In 37 patients (23%), AVM hemorrhage was the direct cause of death. The mean age at death was 51 years. Patients dying as a direct cause of their AVM had a significantly lower mean age of death than those dying from other causes (44.4 and 59.4 years, respectively). It should be noted that compared with the 73-year life expectancy of the Finnish population at the time, both groups had a lower mean age at death. The calculated yearly rate of death was 1%, and was constant throughout the study period irrespective of the initial clinical presentation. The combined major morbidity and mortality rate was 2.7% per year. This rate was also constant throughout the entire follow-up. This study supported the following:

- The natural history of symptomatic AVMs appeared independent of the initial presentation (III/B).
- The risk of bleeding of an AVM was independent of the initial presentation, and the risk of rebleeding was distant from the initial event (III/B). This emphasizes that clinical AVM series with short-term follow-ups will probably be inadequate to shed light on natural history questions.
- The calculated rates of major morbidity and mortality remained constant during the entire follow-up period. Therefore, it can be deduced that patients are at a risk of hemorrhage and death for their entire lives (III/B).
- Patients with symptomatic AVMs had a lower life expectancy than the general population, regardless of the cause of death (III/B).

This study, however, has limitations. First and foremost, CT imaging was not available at the time of clinical presentation; the diagnosis of hemorrhage was based on clinical history and the presence of fixed neurologic deficits [20]. Therefore, the subgroup of patients with no hemorrhage at presentation might have been overestimated as small hemorrhages might have been missed. Subsequently, any subanalysis based on the division between patients with hemorrhagic presentation and those with non-hemorrhagic presentation could be biased, including evaluation of differences in life expectancy, risk of hemorrhage, and morbidity. Second, the patients were not randomly selected. Patients with inoperable lesions, such as a deep location, or AVMs near eloquent regions were more likely to be referred for enrollment in the study [20]. Third, the statistical methodology was not optimal [29]. The authors did not use Kaplan-Meier life-table analyses to calculate the risk of hemorrhage. Instead, they added the number of bleeds and divided it by the total follow-up time. This will invariably lead to inaccuracies, particularly since the number of hemorrhagic events varied between patients (with one patient having 12 bleeding episodes during follow-up), which could have led to a possible overestimation of the individual risk.

In 2008, Hernesniemi *et al* expanded on the series of Ondra *et al* [20] using the database of the Department of Neurosurgery at Helsinki University Central Hospital. They extended the series to include patients diagnosed between 1942 and 2005 [29]. The study comprised a total of 238 patients. The endpoints were death, AVM rupture, initiation of treatment, or end of 2005. The mean follow-up was 13.5 years (range 1 month-53.1 years). A total of 77 patients suffered an AVM hemorrhage during a total follow-up of 3,222 person-years. Using Kaplan-Meier life-table analyses, the authors calculated an annual rupture rate of 2.4%. The risk of hemorrhage was highest during the first 5 years after diagnosis, with a three-fold higher hemorrhage rate during those first 5 years compared with the remainder of the follow-up (4.6% vs. 1.6%). The lower annual rupture risk compared with the study by Ondra *et al* could be explained by the difference in the statistical methods used, as explained above. Another explanation is that in this study, patients who had a hemorrhage were removed from further follow-up. This was not true for the study by Ondra *et al*, where follow-up was not limited by any clinical event.

Hemorrhage-related mortality

While the study by Ondra *et al* suggested that mortality related to hemorrhage increased with each additional rupture event [20], other studies have suggested otherwise [28, 30]. Fults and Kelly reviewed data from 131 intracranial AVM patients from 1944 to 1982 for a mean follow-up of 7.7 years [28]. The data were based on the North Carolina Baptist Church patient population. Hemorrhage occurred in 61.8% of patients, with a mortality rate of 13.6%. Approximately 67% of survivors suffered a second hemorrhage; the mortality rate in case of a second hemorrhage was 20.7%. A third hemorrhage was fatal in 25% of cases. Although there was a tendency toward increased mortality, it did not reach statistical significance. Unlike in the Helsinki series by Ondra *et al*, the risk of rehemorrhage decreased from 17.9% during the first year to 3% per year after 5 years and to 2% per year after 10 years.

Itoyama *et al* also reported a hospital-based series of 50 AVM patients with an average follow-up of 13.4 years [30]. Twenty-nine patients (58%) presented with hemorrhage. In those patients, 10 suffered a rehemorrhage during follow-up for a total rebleeding rate of 34.5%. The risk of rebleeding decreased with time, from 6.9% in the first year after hemorrhage to 1.91% after 5 years and 0.92% after 15 years. A good clinical outcome was obtained in 19 of the 29 patients (65.5%), with no significant correlation between the number of bleeding episodes and outcome. Among the 21 patients whose initial presenting symptoms were other than hemorrhage, four (19%) experienced a bleeding event during follow-up. The annual hemorrhage rate during the first year after diagnosis was 4.8%. The rate decreased to 1.9% after 5 years and to 1.3% after 10 years. The overall prognosis of the four patients who bled was worse than those who did not bleed. The overall prognosis of patients who presented with hemorrhage was worse than that of patients with non-hemorrhagic presentation.

Currently, an ongoing trial – ARUBA (A Randomized Trial of Unruptured Brain Arteriovenous Malformations) – is comparing prophylactic intervention (endovascular, surgical, and radiotherapy, alone or in combination) to deferral of treatment for unruptured AVMs [31]. The measured outcomes are death, stroke, and functional outcomes, as determined by the modified Rankin Scale. Initially set at 5 years, the follow-up was later extended to 10 years following criticism of what was considered an insufficient follow-up period.

Hemorrhage predictive factors

Ultimately, predicting AVM rupture is the most important aspect of natural history studies. This would allow for a pre-emptive approach to these lesions, potentially significantly decreasing the morbidity and mortality of hemorrhage. In addition, and perhaps just as importantly, it would determine who not to treat, and thereby avoid unnecessary complications and surgical morbidity in patients for whom the natural history would yield better outcomes than intervention.

Kondziolka *et al* presented a hemorrhage risk prediction formula, used to assess the risk of hemorrhage for any particular patient [32]. Based on previous studies quoting a yearly risk of hemorrhage of 2-4%, the authors used an approximate 3% annual rupture rate. Starting with a simple calculation of the yearly rate of hemorrhage-free survival of 1 - 0.03 = 0.97, they applied the multiplicative law of probability and obtained the chance of rupture-free survival after y years = 0.97y. Combining this calculation with the life expectancy of any given patient at any given time, they proposed the following formula:

Risk of bleeding = 1 - 0.97$^{\text{expected years of remaining life}}$ **(III/B)**

In order to apply the formula, two assumptions must be accepted. The first is that the yearly risk of hemorrhage is constant. The second is that the risk of rupture in any year is independent of any event that might have occurred in all other years. Both of these assumptions are probably inaccurate. Even so, this is the only reported method in the literature allowing for the interpretation of statistics on an individual level for AVMs.

According to the data from the Helsinki series by Ondra *et al*, the clinical course, including risk of hemorrhage of AVMs, is constant during a lifetime and is not affected by clinical presentation or previous rupture [20]. These results have been challenged and various factors have been investigated as predictors of AVM rupture, including (but not limited to) history of rupture, location, venous drainage, AVM size, and patient age. Unfortunately, the highest level of evidence we currently have for the role of these factors in AVM rupture is III/B.

Hernesniemi et al performed univariate analyses of risk factors for rupture [29]. Patients who ruptured during follow-up (mean 13.5 years) were significantly younger at admission and were more likely to have a deep lying lesion and a previously ruptured AVM **(III/B)**. A univariate Cox regression analysis revealed a significant two- to 2.5-fold increase in the relative risk of rupture in cases of previous hemorrhage, infratentorial location, and deep location **(III/B)**. This remained true for the entire follow-up. Exclusive deep venous drainage was the highest relative risk factor for hemorrhage, with more than a six-fold increase for the first 5 years, but did not remain as such thereafter **(III/B)**. The highest rupture rate was found with infratentorial AVMs, with a rate of 11.6% during the first 5 years. Age, sex, and AVM size were not correlated with the risk of rupture. Various models of multivariate analyses revealed that previous rupture, large size, and infratentorial and deep locations were independent risk factors. In addition, the interaction between deep location and previous rupture was a significant risk factor, with more than a four-fold relative risk of hemorrhage **(III/B)**.

Laakso et al reported a subanalysis of the same data focusing on Spetzler-Martin (SM) grade IV/V AVMs [33]. A total of 63 patients were identified and the mean follow-up was 11 years. Twenty-three patients (37%) suffered a hemorrhage, for an annual rupture rate of 3.3%. There was a significant difference in the yearly rupture rate between patients presenting with hemorrhage and those with unruptured AVMs (6.0% vs. 1.1%, respectively; p=0.001; hazard ratio 5.09). In addition, the prognosis at 1 year after the first hemorrhage was poor: six patients (26%) died and nine (39%) had a moderate to severe disability.

The Columbia AVM databank is an ongoing prospective study collecting various characteristics of AVM patients, including demographic, clinical, and treatment data. It is based on the patient population admitted to the Columbia-Presbyterian Medical Center since 1989. Multiple analyses have been published based on that database [34-39]. In a report

published in 2006, Stapf et al applied univariate and multivariate logistic regression and Cox proportional hazard models to 622 consecutive patients with a mean follow-up of 829 days, during which 39 patients suffered an AVM-related hemorrhage [39]. The authors analyzed risk factors for hemorrhagic presentation and for hemorrhage during follow-up. A total of 282 had a hemorrhage at presentation. Advanced age (p=0.03), infratentorial and deep location (p<0.0001 and p=0.004, respectively), any or exclusive deep venous drainage (p=0.003 and p<0.0001, respectively), and the presence of an aneurysm (p<0.0001) were risk factors for hemorrhagic presentation in the univariate analyses **(III/B)**, while border-zone location (p<0.0001) and larger AVM size (p<0.0001) were negatively correlated with hemorrhagic presentation. The multivariate analysis model found independent associations between hemorrhagic presentation and larger AVM size (odds ratio [OR] 0.97; 95% CI, 0.96-0.98; p<0.0001), deep location (OR 2.14; 95% CI, 1.09-4.22; p=0.03), border-zone location (OR 0.40; 95% CI, 0.26-0.60; p<0.0001), exclusive deep venous drainage (OR 1.84; 95% CI, 1.11-3.07; p=0.02), and presence of associated aneurysms (OR 2.70; 95% CI, 1.72-4.34; p<0.0001) **(III/B)**. In a separate analysis of the same database, Khaw et al reported that infratentorial AVMs were independently associated with hemorrhagic presentation [37]. The association was also significant for larger AVM size, deep venous drainage, and associated aneurysms in the multivariate logistic regression model [37].

The univariate analysis by Stapf et al revealed that advanced age (p<0.0001), hemorrhagic presentation (p<0.0001), deep location (p=0.001), and exclusive deep venous drainage (p=0.001) were high risk factors for hemorrhage during follow-up [39]. AVM size and the presence of aneurysms did not reach statistical significance **(III/B)**. The multivariate proportional hazard model revealed that increasing age, deep AVM location (attributable risk of 9.4%), exclusive deep venous drainage (13.9%), and hemorrhagic presentation (47.7%) were independent risk factors for hemorrhage during follow-up **(III/B)**. AVM size, sex, and the presence of an associated aneurysm had no significant effect **(III/B)**. The calculated annual hemorrhage rate was 1.3% for unruptured AVM and 5.9% for AVM presenting with a hemorrhage. For patients with none of three risk factors – hemorrhagic presentation, deep location, and deep venous drainage – the yearly hemorrhage rate was 0.9%, compared with 34% for patients who harbored all three risk factors.

Although no high-level evidence exists, deep venous drainage, deep AVM location, and initial hemorrhagic presentation have been consistently associated with an increased risk of hemorrhage in most studies [35, 38-41]. On the other hand, the effect of AVM size on hemorrhage is more controversial. While certain studies did not find any independent correlation between size and hemorrhage [28, 35, 38, 39, 42], others have revealed an increased risk of hemorrhage with either an increase [29, 43, 44] or a decrease [30, 37] in size. The discrepancy, or at least a big part of it, could be clarified by distinguishing between hemorrhagic presentations and hemorrhage during follow-up. Another important nuance is the difference between risk factors and associated factors. Small AVMs with a diameter of less than 3cm (2.5cm in certain studies) [29] are significantly more likely to present with hemorrhage [29, 37, 40, 41] **(III/B)**. This is probably due to the fact that small AVMs are more likely to remain undetected unless they bleed. This, in turn, could lead to a higher rate of hemorrhage during follow-up, not related to lesion size in itself but more probably to previous rupture status, thus potentially confounding the results of risk factor analysis unless multivariate models are used. Of note, none of the studies that used Kaplan-Meier analysis and Cox models found small AVM size to be a risk factor for rupture [29].

Treatment

A comprehensive discussion of the treatment of AVMs is beyond the scope of this chapter. The lack of consensus and the wide variability of treatment options make it impossible to cover all potential scenarios in a single chapter. In addition, treatment varies based on inherent characteristics of the lesion, including location, size, type of venous drainage, associated aneurysms, and so on. Nonetheless, we summarize the literature on microsurgery, embolization, and radiosurgery, focusing on larger and more recent series.

There are three treatment modalities for intracranial AVMs: microsurgery, endovascular embolization, and radiosurgery. These modalities can be used in isolation or combination. There is a paucity of level I evidence supporting any of the treatment modalities. Most of the literature involves retrospective reviews of single-center experiences with varying degrees of methodological rigor.

Microsurgery

Microsurgical resection is touted as a curative option for AVMs, but the results depend on careful patient selection, judicious use of preoperative embolization, and expert planning and execution of the procedure. A review of the literature extending from 2000 to 2011 revealed six studies with a series of at least 20 patients where microsurgery was the primary standalone treatment modality (Table 1) [45-50]. Complete resection rates ranged from 89.7% to 100%. Mortality rates ranged from 0% to 7.5%, but varied significantly depending on lesion characteristics. The highest mortality rate was reported by Zhao et al, in which the series was exclusively comprised of SM grades III-V AVMs [49]. The only two series with no reported mortality included AVMs that were exclusively smaller than 3cm in size [45, 48]. Obviously, all surgical series reflect selection bias (otherwise known as judgment or careful patient selection) [50]. Morbidity rates ranged from 2.7% to 23.3%. The highest morbidity rate was noted in the series by Zhao et al, reflecting, once again, the influence of AVM-specific characteristics and decision-making on outcomes [49].

In our review of the literature, we focused on series reported in the last decade to better analyze current trends in AVM treatment. Interestingly, however, even with all the advances in surgical techniques, the gold standard arguably remains the series reported by Heros et al in 1990 [51]. The authors followed 153 consecutive patients who underwent complete excision of AVM lesions for a mean of 3.8 years. The immediate post-surgical morbidity was 24.2%, dropping to a 7.8% late morbidity rate. The mortality rate was 1.3%. These numbers are even more impressive when we consider that more than 40% of the patients had grade IV/V AVM. The rates reported

Table 1. Major series where microsurgery was used as a standalone treatment for brain AVMs. Series were published between 2000 and 2010, with at least 20 patients included in each study.

Reference	Patients, n	AVM characteristics	Preoperative embolization/ radiosurgery, %	Mortality/ morbidity rates, %	Complete resection rate, %
Pik and Morgan, 2000 [48]	110	<3cm 42% in eloquent regions	8/0	0/2.7	99
Huh et al, 2000 [46]	132	SM grade: I 20.5%, II 50%, III 23.5%, IV 6%, V 0%	0/0	1.5/3.1	89.7
Krivoshapkin and Melidy, 2005 [47]	54	SM grade: I 7%, II 33%, III 28%, IV 17%, V 15%	0/0	1.8/3	100
Akdemir et al, 2007 [45]	25	<3cm	0/0	0/12	96
Zhao et al, 2010 [49]	40	SM grade: III 12.5%, IV 52.5%, V 35%	15/7.5	7.5/23.3	96.5
Davidson and Morgan, 2010 [50]	542 (660 patient series)	SM grade: I/II 56%, III/IV (non-eloquent) 12.3%, III-V (eloquent) 31.6%	NA	9 (overall)	96.9

Cases series were selected after searching the PubMed database and using the following criteria:

- Publication date: 1-1-2000 to 1-1-2011.
- Keywords used in combination: 'brain,' 'AVM,' 'arteriovenous malformations,' 'surgery,' 'microsurgery.'
- Patient load >20 patients.
- Animal and *in vitro* studies were not selected.
- Pediatric studies were not selected.
- Surgery was the primary treatment modality, with no or a minimal percentage of patients undergoing preoperative embolization or radiosurgery.
- The primary endpoint was complete AVM cure.
- Ongoing/unfinished trials were not included.
- Studies where direct preoperative embolization was conducted were not included.
- The publication language was limited to English only.

AVM = arteriovenous malformation; NA = not available; SM = Spetzler-Martin by Heros *et al* are comparable with those obtained from our literature review. No rehemorrhages were noted during follow-up, and over half of the patients who had seizures preoperatively were cured or at least greatly improved. Although the follow-up period was short, the authors stated that most recoveries occurred within the first 6 months, thereby decreasing the significance of this limitation [51]. This paper provides compelling evidence for the following:

♦ The risk of hemorrhage following complete AVM resection is close to non-existent **(III/B)**.
♦ There is a potential for gradual improvement from postoperative deficits **(III/B)**.
♦ Surgical resection has an overall positive outcome on seizure control **(III/B)**.

These concepts have stood the test of time. In addition, the authors retrospectively applied the SM grading system to their patients and concluded that because of the high morbidity and mortality rates of grade V AVMs, these lesions may be best treated conservatively. Although the SM grading system has proven to be a neurosurgeon's ally in determining surgical risk, it has its limitations. Although it is reliable for low grades (I and II), it becomes less accurate with higher grades because of inter-individual and -lesional variability [50]. Certain characteristics that were historically considered good outcome predictors might actually increase surgical risk. An example is the case of a superficial draining vein draped over the lesion. Although system superficial venous drainage is a marker of low surgical risk according to the SM grading, the vein's localization over the lesion renders nidal dissection more complex and delicate.

Hemorrhagic presentation is another outcome predictor absent from the SM grading system that poses a dilemma for treating physicians. Lawton *et al* reported a series of 224 consecutive patients treated microsurgically [52]. Overall, patients presenting with hemorrhage tended to have a neurologic deficit at presentation but improved after surgery. Conversely, patients with non-hemorrhagic presentation were generally neurologically intact preoperatively but had a slight worsening of neurologic status postoperatively. The difference is probably due to 'masking' of the surgical risk by hemorrhagic morbidity. Patients who present with a ruptured AVM will have a neurologic

deficit reflecting the brain injury caused by the hemorrhage. Surgical stress to an already injured area will probably not add to the morbidity. Therefore, these patients are less likely to worsen after surgery and have a wider margin for postoperative clinical improvement. In addition, hemorrhage might present certain advantages to the neurosurgeon, such as a non-anatomical access route, easier dissection plane through the hematoma cavity, gliosis, and so on [52]. Would it therefore be wise to defer surgical treatment until rupture? Or should a patient be treated to avoid hemorrhage-related injury? The answer does not lie in the analysis of a single factor, but rather in an individualized multifactorial assessment of patient- and lesion-specific characteristics.

Embolization

Embolization has been used for palliation, preoperative embolization, and occasionally angiographic cure. Table 2 outlines the outcomes from series in which AVMs were treated with embolization and microsurgery [53-56]. The results reveal wide variability in cure rates and in morbidity and mortality rates. While Hartmann *et al* concluded that combined embolization and surgical therapy for AVMs increases treatment risk [53], Weber *et al* found that preoperative targeted embolization allows safe resection of the lesion [56]. Reported morbidity rates ranged from 3.6% to a staggering 42% [53-56]. The reasons for the discrepancies are not fully clear. These reports are mostly based on single-center experiences and therefore operator experience might partly explain the variability. In addition, AVM angioarchitecture, including the number of feeders, venous drainage, and location, certainly plays a role. The effect of the type of liquid embolic used is less certain.

Table 3 outlines the results of recent series in which embolization was used for a potential cure [57-72]. It is clear that even in highly selected series, cure rates remain low and the morbidity of cure may not compete with that of microsurgery. Morbidity rates ranged from 2% to 14.2%, and mortality rates from 0% to 3.8%. The heterogeneity of AVMs makes definitive statements difficult. This is reflected in the wide range of complete obliteration rates reported in the

Table 2. Major series where embolization was used as an adjuvant treatment aiming to facilitate subsequent surgery. Series were published between 2000 and 2010, with at least 20 patients included in each.

Reference	Patients treated with embolization followed by microsurgery, n	AVM characteristics	Embolic agent used	Overall mortality/ morbidity, %	Cure rate after combined therapy, %	Authors' subjective conclusions
Hartmann et al, 2005 [53]	119	SM grade: I 18%, II 27%, III 40%, IV 22%, V 3%	NBCA	Disabling (mRS ≥3): 0/5 Non-disabling: -/42	96	Increases treatment risk
Weber et al, 2007 [56]	47	SM grade: I-II 53%, III 21%, IV-V 26%	EVOH + DMSO	0/6 (mRS ≥3)	98	Allows targeted embolization and safe resection
Natarajan et al, 2008 [54]	28	SM grade: average 2.75	EVOH + DMSO	3/3.6	96.4	Reduces AVM size and allows surgery
Starke et al, 2009 [55]	175 (202 total series)	SM grade: I 24%, II 29%, III 33%, IV 4%, V 0%	NBCA	NA (for the embolization procedure: 0/2.5 per patient or 1.3 per procedure)	NA	Low incidence of permanent deficits

Cases series were selected after searching the PubMed database and using the following criteria:

- Publication date: 1-1-2000 to 1-1-2011.
- Keywords used in combination: 'brain,' 'AVM,' 'arteriovenous malformation,' 'embolization,' 'surgical,' 'pre-surgical,' 'adjuvant,' 'surgery,' 'microsurgery,' 'preoperative.'
- Patient load: >20 patients.
- Animal and *in vitro* studies were not selected.
- Pediatric studies were not selected.
- Liquid embolics were the principal agent used (>95%); no particulate material or coil studies were included.
- Ongoing/unfinished trials were not included.
- Studies where direct preoperative embolization was conducted were not included.
- The publication language was limited to English only.

AVM = arteriovenous malformation; EVOH = ethylene vinyl alcohol; DMSO = dimethyl sulfoxide; mRS = modified Rankin Scale; NA = not available; NBCA = N-butyl-2-cyano-acrylate; SM = Spetzler-Martin

Table 3. Major series where embolization was used as a standalone treatment for brain AVMs. Series were published between 2000 and 2010, with at least 20 patients included in each study. *Continued overleaf.*

Reference	Patients treated, n	AVM characteristics	Embolic agent used	Mortality/ morbidity rate, %[a]	Complete obliteration rate, %
Liu *et al*, 2000 [62]	103	SM grade: I 2%, II 22.3%, III 30%, IV 36%, V 9.7%	NBCA	2/2 with severe complications	10.7
Yu *et al*, 2004 [72]	27	SM grade: I 11%, II 41%, III 15%, IV 22%, V 11%	Histoacryl	3.8/3.8	22.2
Picard *et al*, 2005 [67]	Total: 728 Cortical: 517 CC: 42	NA	NBCA, EVOH + DMSO	0.96/2.33 (total)	Cortical: 64.99 CC: 73.8
Cronqvist *et al*, 2006 [58]	21	SM grade: II-IV	NBCA, EVOH + DMSO	0/14.2	38
Leonardi *et al*, 2005 [61]	34	SM grade: III-IV	EVOH + DMSO	Severe disability on discharge: 3 Fatal rebleeding: 3	5.9
Haw *et al*, 2006 [59]	306	NA	IBCA, NBCA	3.9 (combined rate)	9.1
Mounayer *et al*, 2007 [65]	94 (53 completed treatment)	SM grade: I 4.5%, II 37%, III 40.5%, IV 17%, V 1%	NBCA, EVOH + DMSO	3.2/8.5	49
van Rooij *et al*, 2007 [69]	44	SM grade: I 9%, II 25%, III 39%, IV 23%, V 4%	EVOH + DMSO	2.3/4.6	16
Weber *et al*, 2007 [70]	93 (94 lesions)	SM grade: I/II 51%, III 26%, IV/V 23%	EVOH + DMSO	0/5.3	20
Andreou *et al*, 2008 [57]	25 (26 lesions)	Nidus <1cm	NBCA	0/4	84.6
Katsaridis *et al*, 2008 [60]	101 (52 completed treatment)	SM grade: I 6.9%, II 17.8%, III 38.6%, IV 32.7%, V 4%	EVOH + DMSO	3/8	53.9

Table 3. Major series where embolization was used as a standalone treatment for brain AVMs. Series were published between 2000 and 2010, with at least 20 patients included in each study. *Continued*

Reference	Patients treated, n	AVM characteristics	Embolic agent used	Mortality/ morbidity rate, %[a]	Complete obliteration rate, %
Panagiotopoulos et al, 2009 [66]	82	SM grade: I-II 72%, III 19.5%, IV/V 8.5%	EVOH + DMSO	2.4/3.8	24.4
Reig et al, 2010 [68]	122	NA	NBCA, EVOH + DMSO	0/5.6	15
Xu et al, 2011 [71]	86	SM grade: I 3.5%, II 15.1%, III 52.3%, IV 22.1%, V 7%	EVOH + DMSO	1.2/3.5	18.6
Lv et al, 2011 [63]	147	SM grade: I 3.4%, II 13.6%, III 36.7%, IV 30%, V 16.3%	NBCA, EVOH + DMSO	0/4.8	19.7
Maimon et al, 2010 [64]	43 (29 completed treatment)	SM grade: I-III 40%, IV/V 60%	EVOH + DMSO	0/6.9	55

Cases series were selected after searching the PubMed database and using the following criteria:

- Publication date: 1-1-2000 to 1-1-2011.
- Keywords used in combination: 'brain,' 'AVM,' 'arteriovenous malformation,' 'embolization'.
- Patient load >20 patients.
- Animal and *in vitro* studies were not selected.
- Pediatric studies were not selected.
- Liquid embolics were the principal agent used (>95%); no particulate material or coil studies were included.
- Cure rate after embolization must be reported.
- AVM cure must be listed as one of the endpoints of the study (no comparative studies between different embolization products were included – the goal of embolization was neither adjuvant to microsurgery or radiosurgery nor palliative).
- Ongoing/unfinished trials were not included.
- The publication language was limited to English only.

[a] = morbidity relates to permanent post-intervention neurologic deficits and not to transient symptoms; AVM = arteriovenous malformation; CC = corpus callosum; EVOH = ethylene vinyl alcohol; DMSO = dimethyl sulfoxide; IBCA = isobutyl-2-cyano-acrylate; NBCA = N-butyl-2-cyano-acrylate; NA = not available; SM = Spetzler-Martin

Table 4. Major series where radiosurgery/Gamma Knife was used to treat brain AVMs. Series were published between 2000 and 2011, with at least 100 patients included in each study. *Continued overleaf.*

Reference	Patients treated, n	Prior surgery/ embolization, %	AVM characteristics	Repeat radiosurgery, %	Mortality/ morbidity, %	Follow-up	Obliteration rates (initial/ repeat), %
Schlienger *et al*, 2000 [79]	169	Combined: 45	Supratentorial: 94% 8-51mm	No	Recurrent hemorrhage: 0/4.7	48-96 months	64/-
Pollock *et al*, 2003 [78]	144	Combined: 16	SM grade: 78% ≥III	One repeat: 18 Two repeats: 1.4	Combined major deficits and deaths: 14	Dead/operated: 3-47 months Others: 23-169 months	76 (total)
Shin *et al*, 2004 [80]	400	Combined: 28.2	SM grade: I 8.25%, II 31.5%, III 40.5%, IV 6.25%, V 0%, VI 3.5	5.5	NA Annual bleeding rate evaluated: 1.9	1-135 months (mean 63 months, median 65 months)	87.3 (total)
Zipfel *et al*, 2004 [81]	268	0/0 Prior radiosurgery: 15	SM grade: I 4%, II 36%, III 41%, IV 19%	No	NA Post-treatment hemorrhage: 9.7	Mean 33 months	44/-
Izawa *et al*, 2005 [75]	237	0/0	SM grade: I 13.9%, II 29.1%, III 43.9%, IV 13.1%, V 0%	No	1.3/9.3	2-12.5 years (mean 6.8±1.1 years)	54.9/-
Inoue, 2006 [74]	114	12.3/18.4	Deep-seated: 42.1%	9.6	3.86/- Annual bleeding rate: 0.7	10-15 years	85.5/55
Liscak *et al*, 2007 [77]	330	19.4/17.6 Prior radiosurgery: 1.8	SM grade: I 11.8%, II 47.3%, III 30.3%, IV 10.6%, V 0%	No	1/3.4	1-118 months (median 38 months)	74/-
Back *et al*, 2008 [73]	150	0/ 3.3 Prior radiosurgery: 20	SM grade: average 2.75	No	NA	≥3 years	72.3/-
Kiran *et al*, 2009 [76]	53 central AVMs	0/9	SM grade: I 0%, II 0%, III 75%, IV 21%, V 4%	No	Rehemorrhage: 0/9.4 Symptomatic radiation change: 15	12-96 months (mean 28 months)	74/-
	255 AVMs at other location	0/18	SM grade: I-II 63%, III 32%, IV 5%, V 0%	No	Rehemorrhage: 0/3 Symptomatic radiation change: 5	-	93/-

Table 4. **Major series where radiosurgery/Gamma Knife was used to treat brain AVMs. Series were published between 2000 and 2011, with at least 100 patients included in each study.** *Continued.*

Cases series were selected after searching the PubMed database and using the following criteria:

♦ Publication date: 1-1-2000 to 1-1-2011.

♦ Keywords used in combination: 'brain,' 'AVM,' 'arteriovenous malformations,' 'radiosurgery,' 'gamma knife.'

♦ Patient load >100 patients.

♦ Animal and *in vitro* studies were not selected.

♦ Pediatric studies were not selected.

♦ The primary endpoint was complete AVM cure.

♦ Ongoing/unfinished trials were not included.

♦ The publication language was limited to English only.

AVM = arteriovenous malformation; NA = not available; SM = Spetzler-Martin

---

literature, from 5.9% to 84.6% [57, 61]. The literature suggests that embolization prior to radiosurgery may not enhance cure rates and may in fact decrease obliteration rates [73]. Again, due to the obvious lack of high-level evidence, no definite conclusions can be drawn on this issue.

Radiosurgery

Radiosurgery has emerged as a viable alternative treatment for select AVMs, particularly surgically 'inaccessible lesions'. The advantage of radiosurgery is its minimally invasive nature. The liability of this approach relates to the latency period for cure and the potential for radiation-related morbidity. Table 4 summarizes radiosurgery series published between 2000 and 2011 that included more than 100 patients [73-81]. Obliteration rates ranged from 44% to 93%. Repeat radiosurgery was performed in three series [74, 78, 80]. Kiran *et al* analyzed their results by separating their patients into two groups based on AVM location: central AVMs and other locations [76]. While central AVMs had a complete obliteration rate of 74%, AVMs at other locations had a cure rate of 93%. Although physician experience is important, this study shows that even within the same center the results can vary significantly depending on AVM characteristics. Although not generalizable, these results emphasize once more the heterogeneity

of AVMs and the importance of a multimodal assessment of all patient- and lesion-specific variables before deciding on a treatment modality.

Morbidity rates in these series ranged from 3.4% to approximately 24%, while mortality rates varied from 0% to 3.86%. Shin *et al* calculated an annual bleeding rate of 1.9% during the latency period in their series of 400 patients [80]. The cumulative risk of rupture during the latency period was 4.6% at 3 years, 10.2% at 5 years, and 14.6% at 10 years. Inoue, on the other hand, found the yearly risk of bleeding during the latency period to be 0.7% [74]. Various potential hemorrhage and other morbidity risk factors during the latency period have been studied, including AVM volume, diffuse nidus, and periventricular and deep locations [75-77, 81]. However, most reports have been based on single-center experiences and no high-level evidence has been produced.

Conclusions

The scarcity of AVMs and their heterogeneity has hindered the production of high-level evidence regarding their natural history and treatment. Nonetheless, our knowledge and ability to treat these fascinating lesions, which can pose a significant risk to those who harbor them, have advanced dramatically over the past three decades. The need for well-designed trials and registries has never been more important, given the expansion of techniques and increase in the diagnosis of asymptomatic lesions. Current treatment depends on a careful and thoughtful synthesis of currently available data, and a thoughtful appraisal of treatment options that takes into account patient wishes, life expectancy, and operator experience.

Recommendations	Evidence level
◆ No level I evidence yet exists to guide AVM treatment.	-
◆ AVMs are thought to be congenital lesions.	-
◆ The most common presenting symptom is hemorrhage followed by seizures.	III/B
◆ The risk of hemorrhage is greatest during the first few years after diagnosis.	III/B
◆ Certain hemorrhage risk factors have been identified: hemorrhagic presentation, deep AVM location, and deep venous drainage.	III/B
◆ Selection of the treatment modality must take into account lesion- and patient-specific factors, including AVM size, angioarchitecture, morphology, location, associated aneurysms, and venous drainage, and patient life expectancy.	-

References

1. Stein BM, Wolpert SM. Arteriovenous malformations of the brain. I: Current concepts and treatment. *Arch Neurol* 1980; 37(1): 1-5.

2. Kombos T, Pietila T, Kern BC, Kopetsch O, Brock M. Demonstration of cerebral plasticity by intra-operative neurophysiological monitoring: report of an uncommon case. *Acta Neurochir* (Wien) 1999; 141(8): 885-9.

3. Stapf C, Mohr JP, Pile-Spellman J, Solomon RA, Sacco RL, Connolly ES Jr. Epidemiology and natural history of arteriovenous malformations. *Neurosurg Focus* 2001; 11(5): e1.

4. Berman MF, Sciacca RR, Pile-Spellman J, *et al*. The epidemiology of brain arteriovenous malformations. *Neurosurgery* 2000; 47(2): 389-96; discussion 397.

5. Arteriovenous malformations of the brain in adults. *N Engl J Med* 1999; 340(23): 1812-8.

6. Graves VB, Duff TA. Intracranial arteriovenous malformations. Current imaging and treatment. *Invest Radiol* 1990; 25(8): 952-60.

7. Mahalick DM, Ruff RM, U HS. Neuropsychological sequelae of arteriovenous malformations. *Neurosurgery* 1991; 29(3): 351-7.

8. Locksley HB, Sahs AL, Knowler L. Report on the cooperative study of intracranial aneurysms and subarachnoid hemorrhage. Section II. General survey of cases in the central registry and characteristics of the sample population. *J Neurosurg* 1966; 24(5): 922-32.

9. Perret G, Nishioka H. Report on the cooperative study of intracranial aneurysms and subarachnoid hemorrhage. Section VI. Arteriovenous malformations. An analysis of 545 cases of cranio-cerebral arteriovenous malformations and fistulae reported to the cooperative study. *J Neurosurg* 1966; 25(4): 467-90.

10. Michelsen WJ. Natural history and pathophysiology of arteriovenous malformations. *Clin Neurosurg* 1979; 26: 307-13.

11. Brown RD Jr, Wiebers DO, Torner JC, O'Fallon WM. Incidence and prevalence of intracranial vascular malformations in Olmsted County, Minnesota, 1965 to 1992. *Neurology* 1996; 46(4): 949-52.

12. Jessurun GA, Kamphuis DJ, van der Zande FH, Nossent JC. Cerebral arteriovenous malformations in The Netherlands Antilles. High prevalence of hereditary hemorrhagic telangiectasia-related single and multiple cerebral arteriovenous malformations. *Clin Neurol Neurosurg* 1993; 95(3): 193-8.

13. Stapf C, Mast H, Sciacca RR, *et al*. The New York Islands AVM Study: design, study progress, and initial results. *Stroke* 2003; 34(5): e29-33.

14. Al-Shahi R, Bhattacharya JJ, Currie DG, *et al*. Scottish Intracranial Vascular Malformation Study (SIVMS): evaluation of methods, ICD-10 coding, and potential sources of bias in a prospective, population-based cohort. *Stroke* 2003; 34(5): 1156-62.

15. Al-Shahi R, Bhattacharya JJ, Currie DG, *et al*. Prospective, population-based detection of intracranial vascular malformations in adults: the Scottish Intracranial Vascular Malformation Study (SIVMS). *Stroke* 2003; 34(5): 1163-9.

16. Ogilvy CS, Stieg PE, Awad I, et al. AHA Scientific Statement: recommendations for the management of intracranial arteriovenous malformations: a statement for healthcare professionals from a special writing group of the Stroke Council, American Stroke Association. Stroke 2001; 32(6): 1458-71.

17. McCormick WF. Pathology of vascular malformations of the brain. In: Intracranial Arteriovenous Malformations. Wilson CB, Stein BM, Eds. Baltimore: Williams & Wilkins, 1984; 44-63.

18. Jellinger K. Vascular malformations of the central nervous system: a morphological overview Neurosurgical Review 1986; 9: 177-216.

19. Courville C. Pathology of the Central Nervous System: A Study Based Upon a Survey of Lesions Found in a Series of Forty Thousand Autopsies. Pacific Press Publishing Association, 1950.

20. Ondra SL, Troupp H, George ED, Schwab K. The natural history of symptomatic arteriovenous malformations of the brain: a 24-year follow-up assessment. J Neurosurg 1990; 73(3): 387-91.

21. Drake CG. Cerebral arteriovenous malformations: considerations for and experience with surgical treatment in 166 cases. Clin Neurosurg 1979; 26: 145-208.

22. Brown RD Jr, Wiebers DO, Torner JC, O'Fallon WM. Frequency of intracranial hemorrhage as a presenting symptom and subtype analysis: a population-based study of intracranial vascular malformations in Olmsted Country, Minnesota. J Neurosurg 1996; 85(1): 29-32.

23. Mast H, Mohr JP, Osipov A, et al. 'Steal' is an unestablished mechanism for the clinical presentation of cerebral arteriovenous malformations. Stroke 1995; 26(7): 1215-20.

24. Morgan M, Sekhon L, Rahman Z, Dandie G. Morbidity of intracranial hemorrhage in patients with cerebral arteriovenous malformation. Stroke 1998; 29(9): 2001-2.

25. Sacco RL, Boden-Albala B, Gan R, et al. Stroke incidence among white, black, and Hispanic residents of an urban community: the Northern Manhattan Stroke Study. Am J Epidemiol 1998; 147(3): 259-68.

26. Stapf C, Labovitz DL, Sciacca RR, Mast H, Mohr JP, Sacco RL. Incidence of adult brain arteriovenous malformation hemorrhage in a prospective population-based stroke survey. Cerebrovasc Dis 2002; 13(1): 43-6.

27. Hofmeister C, Stapf C, Hartmann A, et al. Demographic, morphological, and clinical characteristics of 1289 patients with brain arteriovenous malformation. Stroke 2000; 31(6): 1307-10.

28. Fults D, Kelly DL Jr. Natural history of arteriovenous malformations of the brain: a clinical study. Neurosurgery 1984; 15(5): 658-62.

29. Hernesniemi JA, Dashti R, Juvela S, Vaart K, Niemela M, Laakso A. Natural history of brain arteriovenous malformations: a long-term follow-up study of risk of hemorrhage in 238 patients. Neurosurgery 2008; 63(5): 823-9; discussion 829-31.

30. Itoyama Y, Uemura S, Ushio Y, et al. Natural course of unoperated intracranial arteriovenous malformations: study of 50 cases. J Neurosurg 1989; 71(6): 805-9.

31. Mohr JP, Moskowitz AJ, Stapf C, et al. The ARUBA trial: current status, future hopes. Stroke 2010; 41(8): e537-40.

32. Kondziolka D, McLaughlin MR, Kestle JR. Simple risk predictions for arteriovenous malformation hemorrhage. Neurosurgery 1995; 37(5): 851-5.

33. Laakso A, Dashti R, Juvela S, Isarakul P, Niemela M, Hernesniemi J. Risk of hemorrhage in patients with untreated Spetzler-Martin grade IV and V arteriovenous malformations: a long-term follow-up study in 63 patients. Neurosurgery 2011; 68: 372-8.

34. Choi JH, Mast H, Sciacca RR, et al. Clinical outcome after first and recurrent hemorrhage in patients with untreated brain arteriovenous malformation. Stroke 2006; 37(5): 1243-7.

35. Duong DH, Young WL, Vang MC, et al. Feeding artery pressure and venous drainage pattern are primary determinants of hemorrhage from cerebral arteriovenous malformations. Stroke 1998; 29(6): 1167-76.

36. Hartmann A, Mast H, Mohr JP, et al. Morbidity of intracranial hemorrhage in patients with cerebral malformation. Stroke 1998; 29(5): 931-4.

37. Khaw AV, Mohr JP, Sciacca RR, et al. Association of infratentorial brain arteriovenous malformations with hemorrhage at initial presentation. Stroke 2004; 35(3): 660-3.

38. Mast H, Young WL, Koennecke HC, et al. Risk of spontaneous haemorrhage after diagnosis of cerebral arteriovenous malformation. Lancet 1997; 350(9084): 1065-8.

39. Stapf C, Mast H, Sciacca RR, et al. Predictors of hemorrhage in patients with untreated brain arteriovenous malformation. Neurology 2006; 66(9): 1350-5.

40. Spetzler RF, Hargraves RW, McCormick PW, Zabramski JM, Flom RA, Zimmerman RS. Relationship of perfusion pressure and size to risk of hemorrhage from arteriovenous malformations. J Neurosurg 1992; 76(6): 918-23.

41. Langer DJ, Lasner TM, Hurst RW, Flamm ES, Zager EL, King JT Jr. Hypertension, small size, and deep venous drainage are associated with risk of hemorrhagic presentation of cerebral arteriovenous malformations. Neurosurgery 1998; 42(3): 481-6; discussion 487-9.

42. da Costa L, Wallace MC, Ter Brugge KG, O'Kelly C, Willinsky RA, Tymianski M. The natural history and predictive features of hemorrhage from brain arteriovenous malformations. Stroke 2009; 40(1): 100-5.

43. Mine S, Hirai S, Ono J, Yamaura A. Risk factors for poor outcome of untreated arteriovenous malformation. J Clin Neurosci 2000; 7(6): 503-6.

44. Stefani MA, Porter PJ, terBrugge KG, Montanera W, Willinsky RA, Wallace MC. Large and deep brain arteriovenous malformations are associated with risk of future hemorrhage. Stroke 2002; 33(5): 1220-4.

45. Akdemir H, Oktem S, Menku A, Tucer B, Tugcu B, Gunaldi O. Image-guided microneurosurgical management of small arteriovenous malformation: role of neuronavigation and intraoperative Doppler sonography. Minim Invasive Neurosurg 2007; 50(3): 163-9.

46. Huh SK, Lee KC, Lee KS, Kim DI, Park YG, Chung SS. Selection of treatment modalities for cerebral arteriovenous

malformations: a retrospective analysis of 348 consecutive cases. *J Clin Neurosci* 2000; 7(5): 429-33.

47. Krivoshapkin AL, Melidy EG. Microsurgery for cerebral arteriovenous malformation management: a Siberian experience. *Neurosurg Rev* 2005; 28(2): 124-30.

48. Pik JH, Morgan MK. Microsurgery for small arteriovenous malformations of the brain: results in 110 consecutive patients. *Neurosurgery* 2000; 47(3): 571-5; discussion 575-7.

49. Zhao J, Yu T, Wang S, Zhao Y, Yang WY. Surgical treatment of giant intracranial arteriovenous malformations. *Neurosurgery* 2010; 67(5): 1359-70.

50. Davidson AS, Morgan MK. How safe is arteriovenous malformation surgery? A prospective, observational study of surgery as first-line treatment for brain arteriovenous malformations. *Neurosurgery* 2010; 66(3): 498-504; discussion 504-5.

51. Heros RC, Korosue K, Diebold PM. Surgical excision of cerebral arteriovenous malformations: late results. *Neurosurgery* 1990; 26(4): 570-7; discussion 577-8.

52. Lawton MT, Du R, Tran MN, *et al*. Effect of presenting hemorrhage on outcome after microsurgical resection of brain arteriovenous malformations. *Neurosurgery* 2005; 56(3): 485-93.

53. Hartmann A, Mast H, Mohr JP, *et al*. Determinants of staged endovascular and surgical treatment outcome of brain arteriovenous malformations. *Stroke* 2005; 36(11): 2431-5.

54. Natarajan SK, Ghodke B, Britz GW, Born DE, Sekhar LN. Multimodality treatment of brain arteriovenous malformations with microsurgery after embolization with Onyx: single-center experience and technical nuances. *Neurosurgery* 2008; 62(6): 1213-25; discussion 1225-6.

55. Starke RM, Komotar RJ, Otten ML, *et al*. Adjuvant embolization with N-butyl cyanoacrylate in the treatment of cerebral arteriovenous malformations: outcomes, complications, and predictors of neurologic deficits. *Stroke* 2009; 40(8): 2783-90.

56. Weber W, Kis B, Siekmann R, Jans P, Laumer R, Kuhne D. Preoperative embolization of intracranial arteriovenous malformations with Onyx. *Neurosurgery* 2007; 61(2): 244-52; discussion 252-4.

57. Andreou A, Ioannidis I, Lalloo S, Nickolaos N, Byrne JV. Endovascular treatment of intracranial microarteriovenous malformations. *J Neurosurg* 2008; 109(6): 1091-7.

58. Cronqvist M, Wirestam R, Ramgren B, *et al*. Endovascular treatment of intracerebral arteriovenous malformations: procedural safety, complications, and results evaluated by MR imaging, including diffusion and perfusion imaging. *AJNR Am J Neuroradiol* 2006; 27(1): 162-76.

59. Haw CS, terBrugge K, Willinsky R, Tomlinson G. Complications of embolization of arteriovenous malformations of the brain. *J Neurosurg* 2006; 104(2): 226-32.

60. Katsaridis V, Papagiannaki C, Aimar E. Curative embolization of cerebral arteriovenous malformations (AVMs) with Onyx in 101 patients. *Neuroradiology* 2008; 50(7): 589-97.

61. Leonardi M, Simonetti L, Cenni P, Raffi L. Brain AVM embolization with Onyx®: analysis of treatment in 34 patients. *Interv Neuroradiol* 2005; 11 (Suppl. 1): 185-204.

62. Liu HM, Huang YC, Wang YH. Embolization of cerebral arteriovenous malformations with n-butyl-2-cyanoacrylate. *J Formos Med Assoc* 2000; 99(12): 906-13.

63. Lv X, Wu Z, Jiang C, *et al*. Complication risk of endovascular embolization for cerebral arteriovenous malformation. *Eur J Radiol* 2011; 80(3): 776-9.

64. Maimon S, Strauss I, Frolov V, Margalit N, Ram Z. Brain arteriovenous malformation treatment using a combination of Onyx and a new detachable tip microcatheter, SONIC: short-term results. *AJNR Am J Neuroradiol* 2010; 31(5): 947-54.

65. Mounayer C, Hammami N, Piotin M, *et al*. Nidal embolization of brain arteriovenous malformations using Onyx in 94 patients. *AJNR Am J Neuroradiol* 2007; 28(3): 518-23.

66. Panagiotopoulos V, Gizewski E, Asgari S, Regel J, Forsting M, Wanke I. Embolization of intracranial arteriovenous malformations with ethylene-vinyl alcohol copolymer (Onyx). *AJNR Am J Neuroradiol* 2009; 30(1): 99-106.

67. Picard L, Bracard S, Anxionnat R, Lebedinsky A, Finitsis S. Brain AVM embolization. Retrospective study concerning 728 patients followed between 1984 and 2004. *Interv Neuroradiol* 2005; 11 (Suppl. 1): 45-50.

68. Reig AS, Rajaram R, Simon S, Mercile RA. Complete angiographic obliteration of intracranial AVMs with endovascular embolization: incomplete embolic nidal opacification is associated with AVM recurrence. *J NeuroInterventional Surgery* 2010(2): 202-7.

69. van Rooij WJ, Sluzewski M, Beute GN. Brain AVM embolization with Onyx. *AJNR Am J Neuroradiol* 2007; 28(1): 172-7; discussion 178.

70. Weber W, Kis B, Siekmann R, Kuehne D. Endovascular treatment of intracranial arteriovenous malformations with Onyx: technical aspects. *AJNR Am J Neuroradiol* 2007; 28(2): 371-7.

71. Xu F, Ni W, Liao Y, *et al*. Onyx embolization for the treatment of brain arteriovenous malformations. *Acta Neurochir* (Wien) 2011; 153(4): 869-78.

72. Yu SC, Chan MS, Lam JM, Tam PH, Poon WS. Complete obliteration of intracranial arteriovenous malformation with endovascular cyanoacrylate embolization: initial success and rate of permanent cure. *AJNR Am J Neuroradiol* 2004; 25(7): 1139-43.

73. Back AG, Vollmer D, Zeck O, Shkedy C, Shedden PM. Retrospective analysis of unstaged and staged Gamma Knife surgery with and without preceding embolization for the treatment of arteriovenous malformations. *J Neurosurg* 2008; 109 (Suppl.): 57-64.

74. Inoue HK. Long-term results of Gamma Knife surgery for arteriovenous malformations: 10- to 15-year follow-up in patients treated with lower doses. *J Neurosurg* 2006; 105(Suppl.): 64-8.

75. Izawa M, Hayashi M, Chernov M, *et al*. Long-term complications after Gamma Knife surgery for arteriovenous malformations. *J Neurosurg* 2005; 102(Suppl.): 34-7.

76. Kiran NA, Kale SS, Kasliwal MK, *et al*. Gamma Knife radiosurgery for arteriovenous malformations of basal ganglia, thalamus and brainstem - a retrospective study comparing the results with that for AVMs at other intracranial locations. *Acta Neurochir* (Wien) 2009; 151(12): 1575-82.

77. Liscak R, Vladyka V, Simonova G, *et al.* Arteriovenous malformations after Leksell Gamma Knife radiosurgery: rate of obliteration and complications. *Neurosurgery* 2007; 60(6): 1005-14; discussion 1015-6.

78. Pollock BE, Gorman DA, Coffey RJ. Patient outcomes after arteriovenous malformation radiosurgical management: results based on a 5- to 14-year follow-up study. *Neurosurgery* 2003; 52(6): 1291-6; discussion 1296-7.

79. Schlienger M, Atlan D, Lefkopoulos D, *et al.* Linac radiosurgery for cerebral arteriovenous malformations: results in 169 patients. *Int J Radiat Oncol Biol Phys* 2000; 46(5): 1135-42.

80. Shin M, Maruyama K, Kurita H, *et al.* Analysis of nidus obliteration rates after Gamma Knife surgery for arteriovenous malformations based on long-term follow-up data: the University of Tokyo experience. *J Neurosurg* 2004; 101(1): 18-24.

81. Zipfel GJ, Bradshaw P, Bova FJ, Friedman WA. Do the morphological characteristics of arteriovenous malformations affect the results of radiosurgery? *J Neurosurg* 2004; 101(3): 393-401.

Chapter 29

Extracranial carotid artery stenosis

Rudy J Rahme MD, Postdoctoral Research Fellow

Salah G Aoun MD, Postdoctoral Research Fellow

H Hunt Batjer MD FACS FAANS, Michael J Marchese Professor and Chair

Bernard R Bendok MD FACS FAANS FAHA, Associate Professor

DEPARTMENT OF NEUROLOGICAL SURGERY, NORTHWESTERN UNIVERSITY FEINBERG SCHOOL OF MEDICINE AND McGAW MEDICAL CENTER, CHICAGO, ILLINOIS, USA

Introduction

Stroke is the third leading cause of mortality in the USA [1]. It is also a major source of morbidity and disability, leading to a significant socioeconomic burden on patients, their families, and the health care system as a whole. Atherosclerotic carotid artery disease is thought to be responsible for up to 20% of ischemic strokes [2], making it one of the major preventable causes of cerebral ischemic events.

The first documented surgical carotid artery reconstruction for the prevention of stroke was performed in 1954 [3]. More than a decade later, in 1970, the first randomized trial on carotid endarterectomy (CEA) versus medical treatment for the management of carotid artery stenosis was published [4]. Although the initial results revealed the superiority of surgical over non-surgical management, further analysis failed to confirm this finding. There was no significant difference in the morbidity and mortality rates between the two groups at 42 months' follow-up [5]. Nonetheless, CEA was being performed with increasing frequency. Reports of high rates of complications in addition to the lack of a high level of evidence raised concerns about the safety and efficacy of CEA and led to multiple randomized controlled trials in the early 1990s [6-8].

Methodology

A review of the literature using the PubMed/Medline database was performed using the following key words and combinations of the key words: 'carotid stenosis,' 'angioplasty,' 'stenting,' and 'endarterectomy'. The Cochrane Library database was also reviewed for meta-analyses. The review was limited to papers published in the English language between 1954 and 2010. We then selected the papers with the highest level of evidence.

Carotid endarterectomy

In light of growing criticism of CEA, several trials were designed to answer key questions:

- How does CEA compare with optimal medical treatment?
- Which patients will benefit from CEA?
- What is the long-term benefit of CEA?

Symptomatic patients

The North American Symptomatic Carotid Endarterectomy Trial (NASCET) was the first study to establish the validity of CEA and its superiority over medical management in a specific subset of patients [5]. Symptomatic patients were enrolled and randomized into two groups: medical and surgical. Patients were further subdivided based on the degree of carotid stenosis into severe (70-99%) and moderate (30-69%) [5]. This trial excluded high-surgical-risk patients. In 1991, the first phase of the study revealed an unequivocal benefit of CEA in symptomatic severe stenosis patients, with a 17% absolute reduction in ipsilateral stroke risk [5, 9-11] **(Ib/A)**. Therefore, the monitoring committee recommended that the trial be stopped for patients with a 70% or greater degree of stenosis [5, 9]. The final results revealed a moderate albeit statistically significant decrease in the risk of ipsilateral stroke in symptomatic patients with a 50-69% degree of stenosis. However, no benefits were found for patients with less than 50% stenosis [10] **(Ib/A)**. Male sex, recent hemispheric symptoms, recent stroke, and aspirin at a dose of 650mg or greater per day were associated with greater long-term benefits of CEA [10] **(Ib/A)**. The benefit in women was much lower. For a degree of stenosis of 50-69%, the number needed to treat to prevent any stroke was 12 for men and 67 for women [10]. These results were thought to reflect the initial preintervention lower risk of stroke in women.

The European Carotid Surgery Trial (ECST) also targeted symptomatic patients. This trial reported a clear benefit of CEA for patients with stenosis of 80% and above, with a trend toward diminishing benefit with a decrease in the degree of stenosis **(Ib/A)**. The cut-off point was thought to be somewhere between 70% and 79% [12, 13]. Surgery was harmful in patients with less than 70% stenosis [12-14] **(Ib/A)**.

A meta-analysis combining the two trials (NASCET and ECST) included data from 5,950 symptomatic patients [15]. Patients with ECST-defined stenosis greater than 70% and/or NASCET-defined stenosis greater than 50% (considered as a moderate to high degree of stenosis) had a clear benefit from surgery **(Ia/A)**. The remaining patients (<70% ECST and <50% NASCET stenosis) were actually harmed by CEA, with an increased risk of cerebral ischemic events **(Ia/A)**.

Asymptomatic patients

While NASCET and ECST provided level I evidence for CEA in symptomatic patients, both trials failed to address asymptomatic patients. The Asymptomatic Carotid Atherosclerosis Study (ACAS) provided the first insight into the management of asymptomatic carotid artery stenosis [16]. Asymptomatic patients who were good candidates for surgery and had at least 60% stenosis experienced a 53% reduction in the 5-year aggregate risk of an ipsilateral ischemic event and/or death when CEA was performed in addition to optimal medical therapy [16] **(Ib/A)**. A subanalysis revealed a discrepancy in CEA benefit between men and women. While there was an unquestionable benefit for men, with a 66% 5-year reduction in the rate of stroke or death, the benefit was less certain for women, with only a 17% 5-year reduction in the primary event rate (95% confidence interval [CI], 0.96% to 0.65) [16]. The lower benefit was thought to be due mainly to a high rate of periprocedural events, as revealed by the fact that the 5-year reduction in the rate of stroke or death excluding perioperative complications was 79% for men and 56% for women. Interestingly, however, the overall difference between men and women was not statistically significant (p=0.10) [16].

The Asymptomatic Carotid Surgery Trial (ACST) Collaborative Group reached similar overall conclusions [17]. A total of 3,120 asymptomatic patients with at least 60% reduction in the carotid lumen were randomized to immediate CEA or indefinite deferral of any CEA. The 5-year stroke risk was significantly lower in the CEA group (6.4% vs. 11.8% with deferral; p<0.0001) [17] **(Ib/A)**. The difference remained significant when the endpoint was limited to fatal or disabling stroke (3.5% vs. 6.1%; p=0.004) and to just fatal stroke (2.1% vs. 4.2%; p=0.006). The 5-year benefits of CEA were seen for low-surgical-risk patients younger than 75 years with carotid stenosis of at least 70% and were independent of sex [17]. The 10-year follow-up

Table 1. Landmark carotid endarterectomy trials.

	Stenosis severity, %	Treatment modality, n		Stroke rate, %		p-value
		Medical therapy	CEA	Medical therapy	CEA	
NASCET	≥70	328	331	26	9	<0.001
	50-69	428	430	32.3	23.9	0.026
	≤50	690	678	26.2	25.7	NS
ECST	≥70	389	586	25.9	15.8	<0.001
	50-69	377	582	15.6	17.9	NS
ACAS	≥60	834	825	11	5.1	0.004
ACST[a]	≥60	1,560	1560	17.9	13.4	0.009

[a] = 10-year follow-up; ACAS = Asymptomatic Carotid Atherosclerosis Study; ACST = Asymptomatic Carotid Surgery Trial; CEA = carotid endarterectomy; ECST = European Carotid Surgery Trial; NASCET = North American Symptomatic Carotid Endarterectomy Trial; NS = non-significant

confirmed these findings [18] **(Ib/A)**. At the 10-year mark, 92.5% of patients in the CEA group had actually undergone surgery, compared with 26% of those who were initially allocated to deferral. The rate of all strokes, including any perioperative events, was 13.4% in the CEA group versus 17.9% in the deferral group, resulting in a net reduction of 4.6% with surgery (p=0.009). The reduction in stroke remained significant when only non-perioperative strokes were considered (p<0.0001). Of note, the risk of contralateral strokes was also separately significantly decreased (p=0.01) [18]. The benefits of CEA were independent of sex, cholesterol levels, blood pressure, and ultrasound characteristics of the plaque for patients younger than 75 years of age with stenosis of 60% or greater **(Ib/A)**. Outside these two cut-off points (age and degree of stenosis), the gain from CEA did not differ between age groups or severities of stenosis [18].

The results of these landmark CEA trials are summarized in Table 1.

Carotid endarterectomy versus modern medical management

The data from the various CEA trials [10, 13, 16, 18] and the meta-analysis [15] revealed the unequivocal superiority of CEA over medical management in specific subsets of symptomatic and asymptomatic low-surgical-risk patients. However, patients in the medical management arm were mostly on an aspirin regimen, in addition to statins in more recent years. Antiplatelet therapy has evolved and newer, possibly more efficacious drugs exist today.

Ticlopidine was shown to be slightly better than aspirin in the prevention of cerebral ischemic events in the Ticlopidine Aspirin Stroke Study (TASS) [19]. The Clopidogrel Versus Aspirin in Patients at Risk of Ischaemic Events (CAPRIE) study also revealed the superiority of clopidogrel over aspirin in reducing the risk of ischemic stroke [20]. These facts have raised questions regarding the durability and validity of the above-mentioned trials. However, although these drugs have shown a relative benefit compared with aspirin, the absolute stroke risk reduction was small. A Cochrane review, published in 2009, combined 10 trials comparing aspirin with either clopidogrel or

Chapter 29

Table 2. Summary and level of evidence for carotid endarterectomy

	Evidence level/ recommendation
◆ Symptomatic patients with moderate to severe carotid stenosis (≥50%) should undergo CEA in addition to optimal medical therapy (Ia/A), as long as the surgical risk is ≤6% (IV/C).	Ia/A & IV/C
◆ Symptomatic patients with <50% stenosis should be treated medically.	Ia/A
◆ Asymptomatic patients with moderate to severe carotid stenosis (≥60%) should undergo CEA as long as the operative risk is low.	Ib/A
◆ Asymptomatic patients with low-grade stenosis or who are not candidates for surgery should be treated medically.	Ib/A
◆ The issue of benefit or lack thereof of CEA in women remains controversial.	-

ticlopidine [21]. Although clopidogrel and ticlopidine were somewhat better than aspirin in preventing serious vascular events, the additional benefits were deemed uncertain and possibly negligible. Therefore, the likelihood of clopidogrel or ticlopidine reversing the very significant advantage of CEA over medical management is practically non-existent.

Risks of carotid endarterectomy

CEA is first and foremost performed to reduce the potential risk of subsequent stroke. Although its benefits have been proven, the added surgical complications should be taken into consideration. The cornerstone of medical practice being *primum non nocere* (first, do no harm), the question then becomes, what should be considered as an acceptable surgical risk for a prophylactic intervention mainly performed not for an immediate curative purpose, but for a benefit accumulated over time? According to guidelines from the American Heart Association (AHA), the upper acceptable level of procedural risk for symptomatic and asymptomatic stenosis is 6% and 3%, respectively [22] **(IV/C)**. It should be noted that risk assessment of a surgical

intervention should theoretically take into account the surgeon's expertise as well as the hospital's level of care, in addition to inherent risk factors related to the disease and the surgery itself. Since expertise and level of care cannot be brought down to scientific categorical numbers, however, the level of evidence for the limits set by the AHA is low at best **(IV/C)**.

A summary of recommendations for CEA is shown in Table 2.

Carotid angioplasty and stenting

Advances in endovascular techniques have added yet another treatment modality for carotid artery stenosis. This approach brought forth the promise of a minimally invasive alternative to CEA.

The first angioplasty for carotid stenosis was reported by Mathias *et al* in 1980 [23]. However, the initial experience with this technique revealed a significant increase in neurologic adverse events and high morbidity rates [24, 25]. Questions regarding its validity, efficacy, and safety profile came to prominence.

Endovascular management

The Carotid and Vertebral Artery Transluminal Angioplasty Study (CAVATAS) was the first randomized controlled trial to address endovascular management of carotid artery stenosis [26]. CAVATAS, a multicenter clinical trial, enrolled and randomized 504 patients with carotid stenosis to either CEA (n=253) or endovascular treatment (n=251). Patients in the endovascular arm were treated with angioplasty alone (74%) or with stents (26%). There was no difference in the composite endpoint of major stroke or death between the two trial arms in the short term (periprocedural and within 30 days) or up to a median of 5 years' follow-up [26, 27] **(Ib/A)**. There was, however, a higher risk of minor strokes lasting less than 7 days in the endovascular group, in addition to a significantly higher risk of severe restenosis (defined as >70% stenosis), reaching approximately three times the rate of restenosis in the surgical group (hazard ratio [HR] 3.17; $p<0.0001$) [27-29] **(Ib/A)**. This was partly attributed to the low rate of stent use, which contradicted current practice guidelines. Of note, patients treated with stents had a significantly lower rate of restenosis than those treated with standalone angioplasty ($p=0.04$ for ≥50% stenosis and 0.0003 for ≥70% stenosis) [28]. In addition, no embolic protection devices (EPDs) were used in this trial, which might explain the higher rate of minor periprocedural strokes. On the other hand, the CEA group exhibited significantly higher rates of cranial neuropathy ($p<0.0001$) and combined major groin and neck hematomas ($p<0.0015$) [26].

Carotid artery stenting

The WALLSTENT multicenter trial was designed to determine the equivalence of carotid artery stenting (CAS) to CEA in the treatment of carotid stenosis [30]. The study enrolled and randomized 219 patients with symptomatic carotid artery stenosis of 60-99% to either treatment arm. The primary endpoint was ipsilateral stroke, procedure-related death, or vascular death within 1 year. The stent group included 107 patients and the CEA group 112 patients. The rate of the primary endpoint was 12.1% in the stent group, significantly higher than the 3.6% in the CEA group ($p=0.022$). In addition, significantly higher rates of 30-day periprocedural complications were seen with stenting ($p=0.049$). As a result, the trial was terminated before it reached its recruitment goal. Again, the trial was criticized for the lack of EPD utilization.

The first trial to use EPDs was the Carotid Revascularization Using Endarterectomy or Stenting Systems (CaRESS) trial, which was a multicenter, prospective, non-randomized equivalence study [31-33]. A major advantage of CaRESS was that it closely imitated the clinical setting, in the sense that unlike in other trials, high-risk patients were not excluded. A total of 397 patients were enrolled (254 CEA and 143 stenting). Patients were enrolled if they had symptomatic stenosis of at least 50% and asymptomatic stenosis of at least 75%. Two-thirds of the patients (68%) were asymptomatic. There were no differences in the baseline characteristics of the groups, except that patients in the carotid stenting (CAS) group had more often undergone a carotid intervention prior to enrollment. The groups were similar in the combined death or stroke rates at 30 days (CEA 3.6% vs. CAS 2.1%), 1 year (13.6% vs. 10.0%), and 4 years (26.5% vs. 21.8%) **(IIa/B)**. There was also no difference in residual stenosis, restenosis, repeat angiography, carotid revascularization, and change in quality of life at 30 days and 1 year **(IIa/B)**. There was, however, a higher rate of restenosis ($p=0.014$) in the CAS group at 4 years **(IIa/B)**. Of note, the 4-year incidence of the composite outcome, death and non-fatal stroke, was higher in the CEA group than in the CAS group in patients younger than 80 years ($p=0.049$). This difference was even more pronounced if myocardial infarction (MI) was included ($p=0.030$) **(IIa/B)**, but was not seen in the octogenarian subgroup (80-84 years) [33]. Prior carotid intervention was independently associated with a worse outcome in both groups [31] **(IIa/B)**.

What was considered a strong point for this study could also potentially be considered a source of bias. To achieve the real-world setting professed in the study design, physicians were allowed to examine patients and assess patient-specific factors before assigning them to either treatment arm. This could be part of the reason behind the low periprocedural morbidity and mortality rates achieved in this study.

Although commendable, this real-world setting is a major source of selection bias, which thereby decreases the validity of the study.

CEA versus CAS in high-risk patients

The Stenting and Angioplasty with Protection in Patients at High Risk for Endarterectomy (SAPPHIRE) study was the first randomized trial to compare CEA and CAS in high-risk patients [34]. Unlike in previous trials, where having a severe comorbidity was an exclusion criterion, patients enrolled in SAPPHIRE had to have at least one high-risk factor. Inclusion criteria also included at least 50% stenosis in symptomatic patients and 80% in asymptomatic patients. SAPPHIRE was also the first trial to introduce distal EPDs as mandatory. The study was designed to prove the non-inferiority of CAS to CEA. A total of 334 patients were randomized.

The composite endpoint of death, stroke, or MI occurred in 4.4% of the CAS group and 9.9% of the CEA group in the periprocedural period (p=0.06), and in 12.2% and 20.1%, respectively, at 1 year (p=0.004 for non-inferiority) **(Ib/A)**. There was also significantly less repeat carotid revascularization at 1 year in the CAS arm than in the CEA arm (p=0.04) **(Ib/A)**. When distinguishing between symptomatic and asymptomatic stenosis, the cumulative incidence of the primary endpoint was 16.8% in the CAS group versus 16.5% in the CEA group in symptomatic patients (p=0.95), and 9.9% and 21.5%, respectively, in asymptomatic patients (p=0.02) [34]. Three-year follow-up was available for 260 patients (77.8%). At that point, the incidence of the composite outcome of death, stroke, or MI did not differ between the CEA and CAS groups (26.9% vs. 24.6%, respectively) [35] **(Ib/A)**. Although SAPPHIRE revealed the non-inferiority of CAS to CEA, it was faced with much skepticism and criticism as concerns were raised regarding a potential conflict of interest between the authors and the protection device manufacturer [36].

Non-inferiority trials

The Endarterectomy versus Angioplasty in Patients with Severe Symptomatic Carotid Stenosis (EVA-3S)

and the Stent-Supported Percutaneous Angioplasty of the Carotid Artery versus Endarterectomy (SPACE) studies were two European trials designed to prove the non-inferiority of CAS compared with CEA [37, 38].

EVA-3S randomized symptomatic patients with at least 60% stenosis [37]. It was conducted in 30 centers in France and enrolled 527 patients, with 257 undergoing endarterectomy and 247 being treated endovascularly. The primary and secondary endpoints were any stroke or death at 30 days' and 4 years' follow-up, respectively. The incidence of the primary endpoint was significantly higher in the CAS group (CEA 3.9% vs. CAS 9.6%; relative risk [RR] 2.5). The number needed to harm was 17 [37]. Based on this initial interim analysis, the study was stopped for reasons of safety and futility [37]. At 4 years' follow-up, the incidence of stroke and death was still significantly higher in the CAS group than in the CEA group (11.1% vs. 6.2%; p=0.03) **(Ib/A)**. After accounting for the initial 30-day difference, the 4-year non-procedural risk of stroke was similar in both groups (CAS 4.49% vs. CEA 4.94%; HR 1.02) [39].

The flaws in the trial design significantly reduced its validity. First the use of EPDs was not mandatory until an interim analysis of the first 80 patients randomized in the CAS arm revealed a risk of periprocedural stroke 3.9 times higher in patients treated without an EPD [40]. It was only at that time that the safety committee recommended stopping unprotected CAS [40]. Second, the expertise required for physicians to enroll patients significantly differed between treatment arms. Whereas surgeons had to have performed at least 25 endarterectomy procedures in the year prior to enrollment, interventionalists had to have performed less than half that number (12 carotid-stenting procedures) [37]. In addition, interventionalists were allowed to enroll patients while completing their training. The high number of periprocedural strokes could be explained at least in part by the lack of experience and the lack of EPDs specifically, since after the first 30-day period the incidence of stroke and death was equal between the groups. This trial showcased the utmost importance of EPDs and operator experience.

The second European trial (SPACE) also failed to prove the non-inferiority of CAS to CEA [38] **(Ib/A)**. A total of 1,183 symptomatic patients with stenosis of at least 50% based on the NASCET trial criteria were randomized. The primary endpoint was death or ipsilateral stroke at 30 days post-procedure. The difference between the CAS and CEA arms was non-significant (CAS 6.84% vs. CEA 6.34%; p=0.09 for non-inferiority). Although the criteria for expertise were stricter than in the EVA-3S trial, the use of EPDs was left to the discretion of the physician and EPDs were used in only 27% of cases. It should be noted, however, that a subanalysis of the unprotected and protected CAS subgroups showed no significant difference between the two. The study was stopped early after the second interim analysis for futility and financial reasons after it was revealed that in order to prove the endpoint with good statistical power, 2,500 patients were needed [38]. In another subanalysis, age was associated with worse outcomes in the CAS group but not in the CEA group (CAS p=0.001, CEA p=0.534). The cut-off point was 68 years [41]. A statistical analysis using Kaplan-Meier estimates of ipsilateral stroke up to 2 years' follow-up revealed no difference between the treatment arms. However, the rate of restenosis was significantly higher in the CAS group [42].

Ongoing trials

The International Carotid Stenting Study (ICSS) is an ongoing multicenter, international, randomized controlled trial. It has enrolled 1,713 patients randomized in a 1:1 ratio to stenting (n=855) or endarterectomy (n=858) [43]. The use of EPDs was recommended when considered safe by an interventionalist; EPDs were used in 72% of cases. With a follow-up of 120 days post-procedure, there was a significantly higher rate of stroke, death, or procedural MI in the stenting group (CAS 8.5% vs. CEA 5.2%; HR 1.69, p=0.006). There was also a higher rate of all-cause mortality and of stroke taken separately (HR 2.76 and 1.92, respectively). The rate of disabling stroke or death did not differ significantly between the groups. On the other hand, there were significantly more cranial nerve injuries and hematomas of all severity in the CEA group (p<0.0001 and p=0.0197, respectively). The trial has completed enrollment, but the primary outcome of 3-year follow-up has yet to be reached. Long-term

follow-up will give a clearer picture of the efficacy and safety of CAS.

In a substudy of ICSS, 231 patients (CAS n=124 and CEA n=107) underwent MRI before and after treatment in a bid to determine the incidence of new ischemic brain lesions on diffusion-weighted imaging (DWI) [44]. Significantly more patients in the CAS group had at least one new DWI lesion on day 1 post-treatment (CAS 50% vs. CEA 17%; odds ratio [OR] 5.21; p<0.0001). The use of EPDs did not affect this trend. In a center where EPDs were used with 92% of patients undergoing CAS, the incidence of new DWI lesions on day 1 post-procedure was 73% (37/51), compared with only 17% of patients (8/46) in the CEA group (OR 12.2). This was also true for a center that used EPDs with only 12% of its CAS patients (OR 2.7; p=0.019) [44]. The lack of experience of interventionalists in ICSS was again pinpointed as the main criticism of the trial. Interventionalists were required to have performed only 10 CAS procedures before enrollment, whereas surgeons had to have performed at least 50 CEAs. This asymmetry in credentialing was thought to be partly to blame for the higher incidence of strokes and mortality in the CAS group.

CREST

The Carotid Revascularization Endarterectomy versus Stenting Trial (CREST) [45] was designed with rigorous trial methods including stringent criteria for operator experience. A total of 2,502 symptomatic and asymptomatic patients were enrolled and randomized to either endovascular or surgical treatment in a controlled, blinded fashion. Symptomatic patients were included if they had stenosis of at least 50% on angiography or 70% on ultrasound. In addition, patients with 50-69% stenosis on ultrasound were included if CT angiography or MR angiography showed more than 70% stenosis. Asymptomatic patients were included if they had a stenosis of at least 60% on angiography, at least 70% on ultrasound, or at least 80% on CT or MR angiography with 50-69% stenosis on ultrasound. Particular emphasis was placed on validating the qualifications of the institutional treatment teams. Randomization did not begin until both the interventionalist and the surgeon had been certified. The primary outcomes of the study were stroke, MI, and death in the periprocedural period, and post-procedural ipsilateral stroke within 4 years after treatment. EPDs were used with 96.1% of patients undergoing CAS.

The final analysis showed no significant difference in primary endpoints between CAS and CEA (CAS 7.2% vs. CEA 6.8%; HR 1.11; p=0.51) **(Ib/A)**. There was no difference in the combined incidence of stroke, MI, and death during the periprocedural period (CAS 5.2% vs. CEA 4.5%; HR 1.18; p=0.38). A subanalysis of each separate endpoint revealed that stroke occurred more frequently with CAS than with CEA (4.1% and 2.3%, respectively; p=0.01), while perioperative MI was more prevalent in the CEA group (CAS 1.1% vs. CEA 2.3%; p=0.03). No difference was observed between periprocedural death rates (CAS 0.7% vs. CEA 0.3%; p=0.18), nor between the incidences of stroke in the 4-year follow-up (CAS 2.0% vs. CEA 2.4%; p=0.85). While outcome was not affected by sex, age-curve analysis revealed a slight superiority of CAS in individuals younger than 70 years, while CEA was more suitable for patients older than 70 years **(Ib/A)**. CREST revealed the statistical equivalence of CAS and CEA in a specific population, but a nuanced analysis showed that quality of life, as measured by the Short Form-36 physical and mental component scales, was more affected by stroke than by MI, knowing that stroke was more prevalent in the CAS group and MI more frequent in the CEA group.

It should be noted that although the investigators tried to avoid the mistakes of earlier trials, CREST has its drawbacks. The inclusion of both symptomatic and asymptomatic patients increased the heterogeneity of an already diverse and varied population, which may have confounded the results. For example, a subanalysis of symptomatic patients revealed a significantly higher rate of periprocedural stroke or death in the CAS arm (CEA 3.2% vs. CAS 6.0%; p=0.02) [46]. In addition, the very high standard of credentialing of interventionalists participating in CREST [47], although commendable, contradicts the reality of practice. In fact, only 52% of interventionalists who applied for credentialing were approved [47]. Therefore, the results obtained in CREST might not be generalizable.

The results of these CAS trials are shown in Table 3.

Meta-analyses

The high number of randomized controlled trials still failed to answer the questions of the safety and efficacy of CAS, and a number of meta-analyses were drawn up to try and fill in the blanks [48-52]. Bangalore *et al* combined data from 13 trials, including but not limited to CREST, ICSS, SAPPHIRE, CAVATAS, EVA-3S, and SPACE, for a total of 7,477 patients [50]. CAS was associated with an increased risk of the periprocedural composite outcome of death, MI, or stroke compared with CEA (OR 1.31), but with a decreased risk of cranial nerve injury and MI **(Ia/A)**. In addition, there was a 38% increase in the intermediate- to long-term outcome of death or any stroke with CAS.

A preplanned meta-analysis focusing on short-term outcomes combined data from the EVA-3S, SPACE, and ICSS trials for a total of 3,433 patients [51]. The outcome of stroke or death in the first 120 days after randomization occurred significantly more often in the CAS group (CAS 8.9% vs. CEA 5.8%; RR 1.53; p=0.0006). A subanalysis of different variables revealed that age was the only factor that had a significant effect on treatment **(Ia/A)**. For patients younger than 70 years, there was no difference between CAS and CEA, with a risk of stroke or death of 5.8% and 5.7%, respectively. In those 70 years or older group, however, the risk with CAS was twice that with CEA (12% vs. 5.9%; p=0.0014 for trend) [51].

Another meta-analysis comparing the short- and intermediate-term outcome of CAS and CEA combined 11 trials, including the WALLSTENT, CAVATAS, SAPPHIRE, EVA-3S, SPACE, and ICSS trials, among others, for a total of 4,796 patients [52]. Although the risk of periprocedural stroke or death was lower in the CEA group (CEA 5.4% vs. CAS 7.3%; OR 0.67; p=0.025), there was no difference in the composite outcome of death or disabling stroke (CEA 2.9% vs. CAS 3.8%; p=0.088) **(Ia/A)**. The difference was thought to be due to non-disabling stroke, especially since the mortality rate did not differ significantly between CEA and CAS (p=0.727) [52]. Cranial nerve injuries (CEA 7.5% vs. CAS 0.45%; p<0.001) and MI (CEA 2.6% vs. CAS 0.9%;

Table 3. Landmark carotid artery stenting trials.

Trial (long-term follow-up)	Year of publication	Neurologic status		Treatment modality, n		Rate of 30-day stroke or death, %			Rate of long-term stroke or death, %		
		Symptomatic	Asymptomatic	CEA	CAS	CEA	CAS	p-value	CEA	CAS	p-value
CAVATAS (5 years)	2001	X	X	253	251	9.9	10	NS	23.5	29.7	NS
WALLSTENT	2001	X	X	112	107	4.5	12.1	0.049	NA	NA	NA
CaRESS (4 years)	2003	X	X	254	143	3.6	2.1	NS	26.5	21.8	0.361
SAPPHIRE[a] (3 years)	2004	X	X	167	167	9.8	4.8	0.09	26.9	24.6	0.71
EVA-3S (4 years)	2006	X		257	247	3.9	9.6	0.01	21.6	26.9	0.08
SPACE (2 years)	2006	X		584	599	6.34	6.84	NS	15.1	17.2	NS
ICSS[b]	2010	X		858	855	5.2[b]	8.5[b]	0.006	NA	NA	NA
CREST[c]	2010	X	X	1,240	1,262	4.5	5.2	0.38	6.8	7.2	0.51

[a] = rates in SAPPHIRE include myocardial infarction in addition to stroke and death. The percentages reflect the intent-to-treat analysis; [b] = intent-to-treat analysis outcome at 120 days and not 30 days. Also includes myocardial infarction; [c] = rates include myocardial infarction; CaRESS = Carotid Revascularization Using Endarterectomy or Stenting Systems; CAS = carotid artery stenting; CAVATAS = Carotid and Vertebral Artery Transluminal Angioplasty Study; CEA = carotid endarterectomy; CREST = Carotid Revascularization Endarterectomy versus Stenting Trial; EVA-3S = Endarterectomy versus Angioplasty in Patients with Severe Symptomatic Carotid Stenosis; ICSS = International Carotid Stenting Study; MI = myocardial infarction; NA = not applicable; NS = non-significant; SAPPHIRE = Stenting and Angioplasty with Protection in Patients at High Risk for Endarterectomy; SPACE = Stent-Supported Percutaneous Angioplasty of the Carotid Artery versus Endarterectomy

Chapter 29

p=0.036) were significantly more prevalent in the CEA group. However, there was also no significant difference in intermediate-term outcomes for mortality or stroke. (HR 0.78 and p=0.151 for stroke; HR 1.04 and p=0.779 for mortality) [52].

A Cochrane review of 12 trials, including CAVATAS, EVA-3S, SPACE, SAPPHIRE, WALLSTENT, ACST-2, CREST, and ICSS, collected data from a total of 3,227 patients [48]. Various endpoints were analyzed. There was a significant increase in death or any stroke within 30 days of the procedure with CAS compared with CEA (OR 1.39; p=0.02). Although there was no difference between the two treatment arms in the composite outcome of death or disabling stroke (OR 1.22; p=0.31), or in the incidence of death taken separately within 30 days **(Ia/A)**, there was a significant increase in the incidence of stroke with CAS within 30 days (OR 1.40; p=0.04). On the other hand, there was a significantly higher rate of cranial neuropathy and of death or neurologic complications within 30 days of the procedure in CEA patients. Finally, the composite outcome of death or stroke at any time during follow-up, including and excluding the initial 30-day post-treatment phase, did not differ between endovascular treatment and surgery **(Ia/A)**. This was also the case for stroke at any time during follow-up when the initial 30-day post-procedure events were excluded.

Table 4. Summary and level of evidence for carotid artery stenting.

	Evidence level/ recommendation
◆ CAS is a valid alternative to CEA in high-surgical-risk patients with moderate to severe stenosis.	Ib/A
◆ CAS is associated with a higher risk of stroke in octogenarians.	Ib/A
◆ The periprocedural risk of non-disabling stroke is higher with CAS than with CEA.	Ia/A
◆ Mid- and long-term follow-up, excluding the initial periprocedural complications, revealed equality of CAS and CEA.	Ia/A
◆ Operator experience is the cornerstone of success and safety of the stenting procedure.	-

Summary

The role of CAS in carotid stenosis management is still somewhat unclear. While some studies, such as CREST, have revealed CAS to be a valid alternative to CEA with some limitations, other studies have pointed to significant inferiority of CAS to CEA. Although one comprehensive conclusion is not yet possible, multiple key points can still be drawn up. A summary of recommendations for CAS is shown in Table 4.

Embolic protection devices

Use of EPDs during CAS has been touted as essential for the safety of the procedure. Periprocedural debris released during endovascular manipulation of the stenotic plaque is thought to be a risk factor for micro- as well as macroemboli leading to neurologic deficits, ranging from minor transient symptoms to major disabling stroke or even death [53, 54]. However, there is a glaring lack of evidence supporting this hypothesis.

Kastrup et al conducted a review of the literature between 1990 and 2002, which included 2,537 CAS procedures performed without and 896 procedures with protection devices [55]. The baseline characteristics of both groups were similar. The rate of stroke or death within 30 days post-procedure was significantly higher

in the unprotected group (5.5% without EPDs vs. 1.8% with EPDs; p<0.001) **(III/B)**. The difference was mainly accounted for by strokes, both minor (3.7% without EPDs vs. 0.5% with EPDs; p<0.001) and major (1.1% without EPDs vs. 0.3% with EPDs; p<0.05).

A review by Garg et al yielded essentially the same results [56]. Data from 12,263 protected and 11,198 unprotected CAS patients were compared. Patients who underwent CAS with EPDs had a RR for stroke of 0.62 (95% CI, 0.54-0.72) compared with those who underwent the procedure unprotected **(III/B)**. The difference persisted when patients were divided into symptomatic (RR 0.67; 95% CI, 0.52-0.56) and asymptomatic (RR 0.61; 95% CI, 0.41-0.90) groups (p<0.05) **(III/B)**.

Three non-randomized, prospective, one-sided trials – EPIC, ARMOUR, and EMPiRE – evaluated the effect of specific protection devices on periprocedural stroke rates mainly, but also on mortality and MI rates [57-59]. The EPIC trial evaluated the FiberNet Embolic Protection System (Lumen Biomedical, Inc., Plymouth, MN, USA) [59]. The trial enrolled 237 high-surgical-risk patients. The 30-day rate of stroke, MI, or death was 3% **(IIb/B)**. The ARMOUR pivotal prospective trial enrolled 262 subjects. The EPD used was the Mo.Ma Proximal Cerebral Protection Device (Invatec, Roncadelle, Italy) [57]. The 30-day rate of major adverse cardiac and cerebrovascular events was 2.7% **(IIb/B)**. Finally, the GORE Flow Reversal System (WL Gore and Associates, Flagstaff, AZ, USA) was evaluated in the EMPiRE trial. Here, the 30-day rate of major adverse events, defined as stroke, transient ischemic attack, MI, or death, was 4.5% in 245 enrolled patients [58] **(IIb/B)**. A major disadvantage of these studies is that patients were not randomized.

An ongoing randomized controlled trial – Carotid Stenting versus Surgery of Severe Carotid Artery Disease and Stroke Prevention in Asymptomatic Patients (ACT I) (clinicaltrials.gov study NCT00106938) – might yield better answers. ACT I is a Phase III non-inferiority trial comparing CAS using the Xact stent and Emboshield filter cerebral protection device (Abbott Vascular, Abbott Park, IL, USA) with CEA in asymptomatic patients with severe carotid stenosis. The primary outcome measures are the occurrence of major adverse events 30-day post-procedure and the occurrence of ipsilateral stroke at 1 year.

Summary

The level of evidence conferred by these trials is at most level III. Thousands of patients are needed to conduct randomized controlled trials of CAS with versus without EPDs with enough statistical power to prove superiority [53]. Nonetheless, EPDs continue to be employed as there seems to be a general consensus on their usefulness, fueled mostly by leading authorities in the field, expert opinions, and practice experience. The question then becomes, is it feasible or even ethical to conduct a randomized controlled trial with half of its population treated against what the overwhelming majority of interventionalists perceive as fundamental to the safety of their patients?

Patient selection

When considering treatment modalities for patients with extracranial carotid artery stenosis, five patient- and disease-specific criteria should be considered:

* Symptomatology.
* Degree of stenosis.
* Medical comorbidities and surgical risk.
* Patient age.
* Vascular and local anatomical features.

The evidence available for the combination of symptomatology, degree of stenosis, and surgical risk is shown in Table 5.

Table 5. Evidence for the combination of symptomatology, degree of stenosis, and surgical risk.

Patient	Evidence level/recommendation		
	CEA	**CAS**	**Medical therapy alone**
Symptomatic patient with <50% stenosis	-	-	Ia/A
Symptomatic patient with ≥50% stenosis	Ia/A	-	-
Symptomatic high-surgical-risk patient with moderate to severe stenosis	-	Ib/A	-
Asymptomatic patient with <60% stenosis	-	-	Ia/A
Asymptomatic patient with ≥60% stenosis	Ia/A	-	-
Asymptomatic high-surgical-risk patient with ≥80% stenosis	-	IV/C [60]	-
Asymptomatic high-surgical-risk patient with <80% stenosis	-	-	IV/C [60]
CAS = carotid artery stenting; CEA = carotid endarterectomy			

Cognitive outcome

The pathophysiology of carotid artery stenosis has historically been viewed as embolic rather than hemodynamic. The effects, if any, of increased cerebral perfusion after carotid revascularization have not yet been examined. Previous trials have mainly focused on stroke, MI, and mortality, thus failing to address functional outcomes. Does either CAS or CEA have an effect on quality of life and cognitive and functional outcome? Is there a difference between the treatment modalities in short- and long-term functional outcomes? What are the long-term effects of minor periprocedural transient ischemic strokes? Future trials will have to go a step beyond the current standard clinical endpoints to include cognitive outcomes and quality of life in their analyses.

Conclusions

Much has been said and written about the management of carotid artery stenosis. Even with a large number of randomized controlled trials, the dust is yet to settle on the debate. In addition to often conflicting results, the meta-analyses are hard to interpret. The patient population is widely heterogeneous. Risk factors, various treatment modalities, and techniques, including use of EPDs or lack thereof, and physician expertise can all potentially confound the results of trials and hence the meta-analyses based on those trials. Multiple studies have been stopped early, which may have led to an overestimation of the risk of the endovascular approach. The evolving technology behind EPDs is not yet optimal and could still prove to be the defining factor. Endovascular techniques are fast improving and so is the expertise; medical management is in constant refinement. When all these factors are considered, it becomes clear that the last lines have not yet been written, and the debate is set to continue.

Recommendations	Evidence level
◆ Medical therapy alone is the treatment of choice for symptomatic patients with <50% stenosis and asymptomatic patients with <60% stenosis.	Ia/A
◆ Symptomatic patients at average or low surgical risk with ≥50% stenosis should undergo CEA.	Ia/A
◆ CAS is a valid alternative to CEA in symptomatic high-surgical-risk patients with moderate to severe stenosis.	Ib/A
◆ Asymptomatic low-surgical-risk patients with ≥60% stenosis should undergo CEA.	Ia/A
◆ CAS is a valid alternative in high-surgical-risk patients with >80% stenosis.	IV/C
◆ CEA is superior to CAS in octogenarians.	Ib/A
◆ Operator experience is essential for the success of CAS.	IV/C
◆ The use of EPDs is highly recommended.	III/B

References

1. Lloyd-Jones D, Adams RJ, Brown TM, *et al*. Heart disease and stroke statistics - 2010 update: a report from the American Heart Association. *Circulation* 2010; 121(7): e46-215.

2. Liapis CD, Bell PR, Mikhailidis D, *et al*. ESVS guidelines. Invasive treatment for carotid stenosis: indications, techniques. *Eur J Vasc Endovasc Surg* 2009; 37 (4 Suppl.): 1-19.

3. Eastcott HH, Pickering GW, Rob CG. Reconstruction of internal carotid artery in a patient with intermittent attacks of hemiplegia. *Lancet* 1954; 267(6846): 994-6.

4. Fields WS, Maslenikov V, Meyer JS, Hass WK, Remington RD, Macdonald M. Joint study of extracranial arterial occlusion. V. Progress report of prognosis following surgery or nonsurgical treatment for transient cerebral ischemic attacks and cervical carotid artery lesions. *JAMA* 1970; 211(12): 1993-2003.

5. North American Symptomatic Carotid Endarterectomy Trial. Methods, patient characteristics, and progress. *Stroke* 1991; 22(6): 711-20.

6. Easton JD, Sherman DG. Stroke and mortality rate in carotid endarterectomy: 228 consecutive operations. *Stroke* 1977; 8(5): 565-8.

7. Barnett HJ, Plum F, Walton JN. Carotid endarterectomy - an expression of concern. *Stroke* 1984; 15(6): 941-3.

8. Warlow C. Carotid endarterectomy: does it work? *Stroke* 1984; 15(6): 1068-76.

9. North American Symptomatic Carotid Endarterectomy Trial (NASCET) investigators. Clinical alert: benefit of carotid endarterectomy for patients with high-grade stenosis of the internal carotid artery. National Institute of Neurological Disorders and Stroke Stroke and Trauma Division. *Stroke* 1991; 22(6): 816-7.

10. Barnett HJ, Taylor DW, Eliasziw M, *et al*. Benefit of carotid endarterectomy in patients with symptomatic moderate or severe stenosis. North American Symptomatic Carotid Endarterectomy Trial Collaborators. *N Engl J Med* 1998; 339(20): 1415-25.

11. North American Symptomatic Carotid Endarterectomy Trial Collaborators. Beneficial effect of carotid endarterectomy in symptomatic patients with high-grade carotid stenosis. *N Engl J Med* 1991; 325(7): 445-53.

12. European Carotid Surgery Trialists' Collaborative Group. MRC European Carotid Surgery Trial: interim results for symptomatic patients with severe (70-99%) or with mild (0-29%) carotid stenosis. *Lancet* 1991; 337(8752): 1235-43.

13. European Carotid Surgery Trial. Randomised trial of endarterectomy for recently symptomatic carotid stenosis: final results of the MRC European Carotid Surgery Trial (ECST). *Lancet* 1998; 351(9113): 1379-87.

14. European Carotid Surgery Trial. Endarterectomy for moderate symptomatic carotid stenosis: interim results from the MRC European Carotid Surgery Trial. *Lancet* 1996; 347(9015): 1591-3.

15. Cina CS, Clase CM, Haynes RB. Carotid endarterectomy for symptomatic carotid stenosis. *Cochrane Database Syst Rev* 2000; 2: CD001081.

16. Executive Committee for the Asymptomatic Carotid Atherosclerosis Study. Endarterectomy for asymptomatic carotid artery stenosis. *JAMA* 1995; 273(18): 1421-8.

17. Halliday A, Mansfield A, Marro J, *et al*. Prevention of disabling and fatal strokes by successful carotid endarterectomy in patients without recent neurological symptoms: randomised controlled trial. *Lancet* 2004; 363(9420): 1491-502.

18. Halliday A, Harrison M, Hayter E, *et al*. 10-year stroke prevention after successful carotid endarterectomy for asymptomatic stenosis (ACST-1): a multicentre randomised trial. *Lancet* 2010; 376(9746): 1074-84.

19. Hass WK, Easton JD, Adams HP Jr, *et al*. A randomized trial comparing ticlopidine hydrochloride with aspirin for the prevention of stroke in high-risk patients. Ticlopidine Aspirin Stroke Study Group. *N Engl J Med* 1989; 321(8): 501-7.

20. CAPRIE Steering Committee. A randomised, blinded, trial of Clopidogrel versus Aspirin in Patients at Risk of Ischaemic Events (CAPRIE). *Lancet* 1996; 348(9038): 1329-39.

21. Sudlow CL, Mason G, Maurice JB, Wedderburn CJ, Hankey GJ. Thienopyridine derivatives versus aspirin for preventing stroke and other serious vascular events in high vascular risk patients. *Cochrane Database Syst Rev* 2009; 4: CD001246.

22. Moore WS, Barnett HJ, Beebe HG, *et al*. Guidelines for carotid endarterectomy. A multidisciplinary consensus statement from the Ad Hoc Committee, American Heart Association. *Circulation* 1995; 91(2): 566-79.

23. Mathias K, Gospos C, Thron A, Ahmadi A, Mittermayer C. Percutaneous transluminal treatment of supraaortic artery obstruction. *Ann Radiol* (Paris) 1980; 23(4): 281-2.

24. Jordan WD Jr, Voellinger DC, Fisher WS, Redden D, McDowell HA. A comparison of carotid angioplasty with stenting versus endarterectomy with regional anesthesia. *J Vasc Surg* 1998; 28(3): 397-402; discussion 402-3.

25. Diethrich EB, Ndiaye M, Reid DB. Stenting in the carotid artery: initial experience in 110 patients. *J Endovasc Surg* 1996; 3(1): 42-62.

26. Endovascular versus surgical treatment in patients with carotid stenosis in the Carotid and Vertebral Artery Transluminal Angioplasty Study (CAVATAS): a randomised trial. *Lancet* 2001; 357(9270): 1729-37.

27. Ederle J, Bonati LH, Dobson J, *et al*. Endovascular treatment with angioplasty or stenting versus endarterectomy in patients with carotid artery stenosis in the Carotid and Vertebral Artery Transluminal Angioplasty Study (CAVATAS): long-term follow-up of a randomised trial. *Lancet Neurol* 2009; 8(10): 898-907.

28. Bonati LH, Ederle J, McCabe DJ, *et al*. Long-term risk of carotid restenosis in patients randomly assigned to endovascular treatment or endarterectomy in the Carotid and Vertebral Artery Transluminal Angioplasty Study (CAVATAS): long-term follow-up of a randomised trial. *Lancet Neurol* 2009; 8(10): 908-17.

Chapter 29

29. McCabe DJ, Pereira AC, Clifton A, Bland JM, Brown MM. Restenosis after carotid angioplasty, stenting, or endarterectomy in the Carotid and Vertebral Artery Transluminal Angioplasty Study (CAVATAS). *Stroke* 2005; 36(2): 281-6.

30. Alberts MJ. Results of a multicenter prospective randomized trial of carotid artery stenting vs. carotid endarterectomy (Abstract 53). *Stroke* 2001; 32: 325.

31. Carotid Revascularization Using Endarterectomy or Stenting Systems (CaRESS) Phase I clinical trial: 1-year results. *J Vasc Surg* 2005; 42(2): 213-9.

32. Diethrich E, Fogarty TJ, Zarins CK, et al. CaRESS: carotid revascularization using endarterectomy or stenting systems. *Tech Vasc Interv Radiol* 2004; 7(4): 194-5.

33. Zarins CK, White RA, Diethrich EB, Shackelton RJ, Siami FS. Carotid revascularization using endarterectomy or stenting systems (CaRESS): 4-year outcomes. *J Endovasc Ther* 2009; 16(4): 397-409.

34. Yadav JS, Wholey MH, Kuntz RE, et al. Protected carotid-artery stenting versus endarterectomy in high-risk patients. *N Engl J Med* 2004; 351(15): 1493-501.

35. Gurm HS, Yadav JS, Fayad P, et al. Long-term results of carotid stenting versus endarterectomy in high-risk patients. *N Engl J Med* 2008; 358(15): 1572-9.

36. Thomas DJ. Protected carotid artery stenting versus endarterectomy in high-risk patients reflections from SAPPHIRE. *Stroke* 2005; 36(4): 912-3.

37. Mas JL, Chatellier G, Beyssen B, et al. Endarterectomy versus stenting in patients with symptomatic severe carotid stenosis. *N Engl J Med* 2006; 355(16): 1660-71.

38. Ringleb PA, Allenberg J, Bruckmann H, et al. 30-day results from the SPACE trial of stent-protected angioplasty versus carotid endarterectomy in symptomatic patients: a randomised non-inferiority trial. *Lancet* 2006; 368(9543): 1239-47.

39. Mas JL, Trinquart L, Leys D, et al. Endarterectomy Versus Angioplasty in Patients with Symptomatic Severe Carotid Stenosis (EVA-3S) trial: results up to 4 years from a randomised, multicentre trial. *Lancet Neurol* 2008; 7(10): 885-92.

40. Mas JL, Chatellier G, Beyssen B. Carotid angioplasty and stenting with and without cerebral protection: clinical alert from the Endarterectomy Versus Angioplasty in Patients With Symptomatic Severe Carotid Stenosis (EVA-3S) trial. *Stroke* 2004; 35(1): e18-20.

41. Stingele R, Berger J, Alfke K, et al. Clinical and angiographic risk factors for stroke and death within 30 days after carotid endarterectomy and stent-protected angioplasty: a subanalysis of the SPACE study. *Lancet Neurol* 2008; 7(3): 216-22.

42. Eckstein HH, Ringleb P, Allenberg JR, et al. Results of the Stent-Protected Angioplasty versus Carotid Endarterectomy (SPACE) study to treat symptomatic stenoses at 2 years: a multinational, prospective, randomised trial. *Lancet Neurol* 2008; 7(10): 893-902.

43. Ederle J, Dobson J, Featherstone RL, et al. Carotid artery stenting compared with endarterectomy in patients with symptomatic carotid stenosis (International Carotid Stenting Study): an interim analysis of a randomised controlled trial. *Lancet* 2010; 375(9719): 985-97.

44. Bonati LH, Jongen LM, Haller S, et al. New ischaemic brain lesions on MRI after stenting or endarterectomy for symptomatic carotid stenosis: a substudy of the International Carotid Stenting Study (ICSS). *Lancet Neurol* 2010; 9(4): 353-62.

45. Brott TG, Hobson RW 2nd, Howard G, et al. Stenting versus endarterectomy for treatment of carotid-artery stenosis. *N Engl J Med* 2010; 363(1): 11-23.

46. Berkefeld J, Chaturvedi S. The International Carotid Stenting Study and the North American carotid revascularization endarterectomy versus stenting trial: fueling the debate about carotid artery stenting. *Stroke* 2010; 41(11): 2714-5.

47. Hopkins LN, Roubin GS, Chakhtoura EY, et al. The Carotid Revascularization Endarterectomy versus Stenting Trial: credentialing of interventionalists and final results of lead-in phase. *J Stroke Cerebrovasc Dis* 2010; 19(2): 153-62.

48. Ederle J, Featherstone RL, Brown MM. Percutaneous transluminal angioplasty and stenting for carotid artery stenosis. *Cochrane Database Syst Rev* 2007; 4: CD000515.

49. Murad MH, Flynn DN, Elamin MB, et al. Endarterectomy vs. stenting for carotid artery stenosis: a systematic review and meta-analysis. *J Vasc Surg* 2008; 48(2): 487-93.

50. Bangalore S, Kumar S, Wetterslev J, et al. Carotid artery stenting vs. carotid endarterectomy: meta-analysis and diversity-adjusted trial sequential analysis of randomized trials. *Arch Neurol* 2011; 68(2): 172-84.

51. Bonati LH, Dobson J, Algra A, et al. Short-term outcome after stenting versus endarterectomy for symptomatic carotid stenosis: a preplanned meta-analysis of individual patient data. *Lancet* 2010; 376(9746): 1062-73.

52. Meier P, Knapp G, Tamhane U, Chaturvedi S, Gurm HS. Short term and intermediate term comparison of endarterectomy versus stenting for carotid artery stenosis: systematic review and meta-analysis of randomised controlled clinical trials. *BMJ* 2010; 340: c467.

53. Macdonald S. The evidence for cerebral protection: an analysis and summary of the literature. *Eur J Radiol* 2006; 60(1): 20-5.

54. Cremonesi A, Manetti R, Setacci F, Setacci C, Castriota F. Protected carotid stenting: clinical advantages and complications of embolic protection devices in 442 consecutive patients. *Stroke* 2003; 34(8): 1936-41.

55. Kastrup A, Groschel K, Krapf H, Brehm BR, Dichgans J, Schulz JB. Early outcome of carotid angioplasty and stenting with and without cerebral protection devices: a systematic review of the literature. *Stroke* 2003; 34(3): 813-9.

56. Garg N, Karagiorgos N, Pisimisis GT, et al. Cerebral protection devices reduce periprocedural strokes during carotid angioplasty and stenting: a systematic review of the current literature. *J Endovasc Ther* 2009; 16(4): 412-27.

57. Ansel GM, Hopkins LN, Jaff MR, et al. Safety and effectiveness of the INVATEC MO.MA proximal cerebral protection device during carotid artery stenting: results from

the ARMOUR pivotal trial. *Catheter Cardiovasc Interv* 2010; 76(1): 1-8.

58. Clair DG, Hopkins LN, Mehta M, *et al*. Neuroprotection during carotid artery stenting using the GORE flow reversal system: 30-day outcomes in the EMPiRE Clinical Study. *Catheter Cardiovasc Interv* 2011; 77(3): 420-9.

59. Myla S, Bacharach JM, Ansel GM, Dippel EJ, McCormick DJ, Popma JJ. Carotid artery stenting in high surgical risk patients

using the FiberNet embolic protection system: the EPIC trial results. *Catheter Cardiovasc Interv* 2010; 75(6): 817-22.

60. Hobson RW 2nd, Mackey WC, Ascher E, *et al*. Management of atherosclerotic carotid artery disease: clinical practice guidelines of the Society for Vascular Surgery. *J Vasc Surg* 2008; 48(2): 480-6.

Chapter 29

Extracranial carotid artery stenosis

Chapter 30

Symptomatic intracranial arterial disease: medical therapy, stent, or bypass?

Andria L Ford MD, Assistant Professor of Neurology 1

Jin-Moo Lee MD PhD, Associate Professor of Neurology, Radiology, and Biomedical Engineering; Director, Cerebrovascular Disease Section 2

Colin P Derdeyn MD, Professor of Radiology, Neurology and Neurological Surgery; Director, Stroke and Cerebrovascular Center 3

Gregory J Zipfel MD, Associate Professor of Neurological Surgery and Neurology; Co-Director, Stroke and Cerebrovascular Center 4

WASHINGTON UNIVERSITY DEPARTMENTS OF 1 NEUROLOGY,
2 NEUROLOGY AND RADIOLOGY, 3 RADIOLOGY, NEUROLOGY, AND NEUROSURGERY,
AND 4 NEUROLOGY AND NEUROSURGERY, ST LOUIS, MISSOURI, USA

Introduction

Symptomatic intracranial arterial disease (sICD) is defined as a stroke or transient ischemic attack (TIA) involving the vascular territory distal to a stenotic intracranial artery. It is responsible for nearly 10% of all ischemic strokes in the USA, and is associated with a high risk of recurrent events. Options for treatment include medical therapy, endovascular angioplasty (with or without stenting), and surgical intervention with direct or indirect bypass to revascularize the affected hemisphere. This chapter provides a systematic review of the evidence supporting or refuting the use of these treatment modalities in patients with sICD. Special emphasis is placed on several randomized controlled trials upon which management recommendations can be based.

Methodology

A National Library of Medicine computerized literature search was performed of publications from 1966 to 2011 using each of the following headings separately to build a wide database of articles: 'intracranial atherosclerosis,' 'intracranial arterial disease,' 'symptomatic intracranial atherosclerosis,' 'symptomatic intracranial arterial disease,' 'intracranial angioplasty,' 'intracranial stenting,' 'extracranial-intracranial bypass,' and 'superficial temporal artery-middle cerebral artery bypass.' These headings were then combined with the heading 'evidence-based' to select articles of that nature. The bibliographies of these articles were reviewed for other possible inclusions.

The natural history of symptomatic intracranial arterial disease

Epidemiology and natural history

sICD is responsible for 8-9% of all ischemic strokes in the USA [1, 2], accounting for approximately 65,000 strokes per year [3]. In East Asia, up to one-third of ischemic strokes are secondary to sICD [4, 5].

In the Northern Manhattan Stroke Study, the proportion of patients experiencing the extracranial atherosclerotic stroke subtype was similar among whites, blacks, and Hispanics, while the intracranial atherosclerotic stroke subtype was more prevalent in blacks and Hispanics, having an odds ratio of 5.2 compared with whites [1].

The natural history of sICD portends a high risk of recurrent strokes, which are often moderate in size and disabling. Two large prospective trials have reported recurrent stroke rates of 14% and 19% over 2 years, with most strokes occurring in the first year [6, 7] **(Ib/A)**. In the Warfarin-Aspirin in sICD (WASID) study, 73% of patients with recurrent strokes had strokes in the territory of the symptomatic stenotic artery [6] **(Ib/A)**. Of these strokes, 91% were non-lacunar and 44% were disabling [8]. Of the 27% of patients with strokes in other territories, 48% of strokes were attributed to a previously asymptomatic intracranial arterial stenosis.

Etiologies and risk factors

The vast majority of sICD is caused by atherosclerosis in association with traditional stroke risk factors [9-11]. However, sICD has several less common etiologies, including Moyamoya disease [12], sickle-cell disease [13, 14], infectious meningitis [15, 16], vasculitis [17], dissection [18], and radiation therapy [19]. The common non-modifiable risk factors for sICD include older age, male sex, and African-American, Hispanic, or Asian race [1, 9-11]. Modifiable risk factors include hypertension, hyperlipidemia, ischemic heart disease, and diabetes mellitus [9-11, 20].

Optimal diagnostic imaging

While digital subtraction angiography (DSA) is the gold standard for diagnosing intracranial stenosis, the method requires arterial puncture and contrast to delineate the vasculature and also carries a small risk of procedural stroke. Less invasive diagnostic tests include transcranial Doppler ultrasound (TCD), MR angiography (MRA), and CT angiography (CTA). Until recently, the accuracy of these tests had not been rigorously tested. The Stroke Outcomes and Neuroimaging of Intracranial Atherosclerosis (SONIA) trial was a prospective, multicenter study comparing the diagnostic accuracy of TCD and MRA with that of catheter angiography [21]. The SONIA study reported that both TCD and MRA had high negative predictive values (86% and 91%, respectively), but low positive predictive values (36% and 59%, respectively) **(IIa/B)**. The authors concluded that both TCD and MRA could reliably exclude intracranial stenosis, but that a finding of intracranial stenosis would need confirmation with catheter angiography. A study that compared CTA with DSA measured 475 short segments of intracranial arteries in 41 patients [22]. For detection of at least 50% stenosis, CTA had 97.1% sensitivity and 99.5% specificity. This suggests CTA is an accurate diagnostic tool for detecting sICD, when the technology and experienced neuroradiologists, trained in reading CTAs, are available **(III/B)**.

Medical treatment: antiplatelet therapy, anticoagulation, and risk factor modification

Antiplatelet therapy or anticoagulation?

The belief that anticoagulation is superior to antiplatelet therapy for preventing recurrent stroke in patients with sICD influenced patient management as early as the 1970s [23]. The question was initially addressed in a retrospective trial of 151 patients with stroke or TIA in the distribution of a stenotic intracranial artery who were treated with aspirin or warfarin [24]. Rates of recurrent vascular events, including stroke, myocardial infarction, or sudden death, were significantly lower in patients treated with warfarin compared with aspirin. Aiming to confirm these findings, this retrospective study was followed by WASID, a large, prospective, double-blinded, multicenter trial [6]. More than 500 patients with TIA or non-disabling stroke in the distribution of a stenotic intracranial artery (50-99% by catheter angiography) were randomized to aspirin 650mg twice daily or warfarin 5mg daily (target International Normalized Ratio 2.0-3.0) and followed for a mean of 1.8 years. The combined primary endpoint, which included ischemic stroke, hemorrhagic stroke, or any vascular death, was not significantly different between the two groups, occurring in 22.1% and 21.8% of the aspirin and warfarin treatment groups, respectively **(Ib/A)**. Enrolment into this trial was stopped prematurely because of excessive adverse events (death and major hemorrhage) in the warfarin group compared with the aspirin group. The authors concluded that warfarin offered no benefit over aspirin in patients with sICD. Moreover, warfarin appeared significantly less safe.

Shortly after completion of the WASID trial, a multicenter Asian study tested a low-molecular-weight heparin, nadroparin calcium, within 48 hours of symptom onset in patients with ischemic stroke [25]. Of 603 patients recruited, 353 had at least a moderate degree of intracranial large artery stenosis and were randomly assigned to nadroparin calcium 3800IU subcutaneously twice daily or aspirin 160mg daily for 10 days, followed by aspirin 80-300mg daily (for all enrolled patients) for 6 months. The primary endpoint, good outcome at 6 months (defined as Barthel Index ≥85), did not differ between the two groups **(Ib/A)**.

While guidelines from the American Heart Association and American Stroke Association recommend single-antiplatelet therapy for all patients with acute ischemic stroke [26] **(Ib/A)**, no studies have specifically compared a single antiplatelet agent with placebo in an sICD population. Dual-antiplatelet therapy with the combination of cilostazol (a phosphodiesterase-3 inhibitor) and aspirin was evaluated in a multicenter, double-blind, placebo-controlled trial in 135 patients with sICD [27]. The primary outcome was progression of M1 or basilar stenosis, as measured by MRA. The cilostazol treatment group showed less progression of stenosis, with 24.4% and 15.4% of patients showing regression and 6.7% and 28.8% showing progression of stenosis in the cilostazol plus aspirin and placebo plus aspirin groups, respectively **(Ib/A)**. No recurrent strokes occurred in either group, but the drop-out rate was high at 30% for the cilostazol group and 20% for the placebo group.

More recently, a randomized controlled trial of intracranial stenting versus medical therapy for the prevention of vascular events in patients with sICD (≥70% stenosis randomized within 30 days of stroke or TIA) was stopped prematurely because of an unexpectedly low 30-day event rate in the medical group (4.2% compared with much higher rates in historical controls) and an unexpectedly high event rate in the stenting group (14%) (Stenting vs. Aggressive Medical Management for Preventing Recurrent Stroke in Intracranial Stenosis [SAMMPRIS] trial, see also the endovascular therapy section, below; clinicaltrials.gov NCT00576693) [28]. Both treatment groups received aggressive medical therapy including dual-antiplatelet therapy with aspirin 325mg and clopidogrel 75mg daily for the first 90 days, as well as aggressive lipid and blood-pressure lowering. It is possible that the low event rate in the medical arm was due to very early dual-antiplatelet therapy, which has been shown to be more beneficial than single-antiplatelet therapy in patients with acute coronary syndromes [29]. However, given the potential bleeding risks with dual-antiplatelet therapy, this regimen requires further study in a randomized trial.

Factors influencing recurrent stroke

A prespecified aim of the WASID study was to identify patients with sICD who were at particularly high risk of recurrent stroke in the territory of the stenotic artery. A univariate analysis of more than 20 baseline characteristics identified five factors significantly associated with recurrent stroke [30]:

* Female sex.
* History of diabetes.
* Score of more than 1 for the qualifying event on the National Institutes of Health Stroke Scale (NIHSS).
* Enrollment within 17 days or less of the qualifying event.
* Stenosis of 70% or more.

A multivariate model included variables hypothesized to increase the risk of recurrent stroke in the territory of the symptomatic stenotic artery and any remaining significant variables from the univariate analysis. Female sex (p=0.054), NIHSS score above 1 (p=0.005), enrollment within 17 days or less

Chapter 30

(p=0.026), and 70% or more stenosis (p=0.004) continued to be associated with recurrent stroke, while history of diabetes did not (p=0.49) **(IIa/B)**. Factors initially hypothesized to be associated with an increased risk of recurrent stroke, but were not, included: the qualifying event being stroke versus TIA, the qualifying event being anterior versus posterior circulation, being on antithrombotic therapy at the time of the qualifying event, age at least 64 years or younger than 64 years, and race. While black race was not independently associated with a higher risk for the primary endpoint in WASID, blacks were significantly more likely than whites to have risk factors for stroke, such as hypertension, diabetes, and high total cholesterol/low-density lipoprotein (LDL) [31]. In addition, the rate of the primary endpoint (28% vs. 20%) and of ischemic stroke alone (25% vs. 16%) was higher in blacks than whites. A similar differentiation was seen by sex, with 2-year rates of the primary endpoint of 28% for women and 17% for men [32]. Women were less likely to drink alcohol or use tobacco, but were more likely to have a sedentary lifestyle and higher total cholesterol/LDL. Sociodemographic comparisons demonstrated that women with recurrent stroke were more likely than men to be black, unmarried, unemployed, and living alone.

Risk factor modification and recurrent stroke risk in WASID

The WASID study monitored vascular and lifestyle risk factors at baseline and throughout the 2-year follow-up. Overall, 61% of participants were taking statin medications at baseline, increasing to 82% during follow-up [33]. Of patients with a history of hypertension and diabetes, 96% and 91% were prescribed antihypertensive agents and diabetes medications, respectively. While total cholesterol, LDL, and glycated hemoglobin levels significantly decreased over the study period, blood pressure did not change. Multivariate analysis showed that mean systolic blood pressure (SBP) 140mmHg or more (p=0.0009), no alcohol consumption (p=0.002), and total cholesterol 200mg/dL or more (p=0.048) were associated with an increased risk of stroke, myocardial infarction, or vascular death **(Ib/A)**. These same

factors were significantly associated with ischemic stroke alone. A closer look at the relationship between blood pressure and recurrent stroke risk demonstrated a continuous escalation of risk with increasing SBP and diastolic blood pressure [34]. The significance for SBP was largely driven by the highest blood pressure group (SBP ≥160mm Hg). A common clinical practice regarding blood pressure management following sICD is to withhold antihypertensive therapy, allowing permissive hypertension and prevention of hemodynamic ischemic events in the territory of the stenotic artery. The above relationship between higher blood pressure and increased recurrent stroke risk suggests this practice is not beneficial and may be harmful.

Based on the subgroup analyses of the WASID population, the SAMMPRIS trial (see the endovascular therapy section below for details), was designed to include 'aggressive medical therapy' in both treatment arms. This included dual-antiplatelet therapy, lipid lowering (LDL target of <70mg/dL), and blood-pressure lowering (SBP target of <130mmHg in those with diabetes and <140mmHg in those without). Given the lower than anticipated event rate in the medical arm relative to historical controls, it is likely that one or more aspects of the aggressive medical management regimen conferred the benefits in the medical therapy arm.

The question of 'failed' medical therapy

Given the lack of rigorous studies testing neurointerventional versus medical therapies for sICD, referrals for intervention are commonly made in the setting of 'failed' medical therapy. An early retrospective analysis of sICD patients on antithrombotic therapy found high rates of recurrence, near 55% [35]. The conclusion was that patients in whom thrombotic therapy 'fails' may be at higher risk of recurrent stroke and may benefit from more aggressive interventions such as angioplasty and stenting. The WASID investigators compared rates of stroke and vascular death in patients on (n=299) versus off (n=269) antithrombotics at the time of their qualifying event [36]. Neither univariate nor multivariate analyses showed a difference in events between the two groups. The authors concluded that both groups of patients were at high risk of recurrence and, therefore, interventional trials for sICD should not be limited to patients in whom antithrombotic therapy fails **(IIa/B)**.

Summary

sICD is responsible for up to 10% of all ischemic strokes and is associated with a risk of recurrent stroke as high as 10% per year. Digital subtraction angiography remains the gold standard for diagnosis, although CTA and MRA may be useful as screening examinations. Current evidence supports single-antiplatelet therapy over anticoagulation for the prevention of recurrent strokes in sICD. Factors such as female sex, recent stroke, more than 70% stenosis, elevated SBP, and elevated total cholesterol are likely to increase the risk of recurrent stroke related to sICD.

Endovascular treatment

With continued improvements in angiographic imaging equipment, as well as angioplasty balloon and stent technology, the endovascular treatment of intracranial stenosis has become feasible and even routine at some institutions (Figure 1). Most of the published experience is with presumed sICD, with several small case series for intracranial dissections. Endovascular options for either vasculopathy include the following:

◆ Angioplasty alone.
◆ Angioplasty followed by placement of balloon-expandable stents.

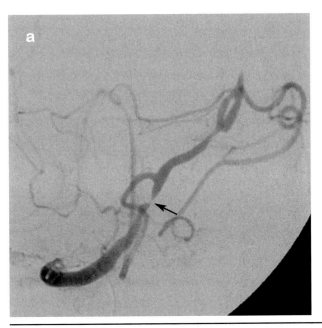 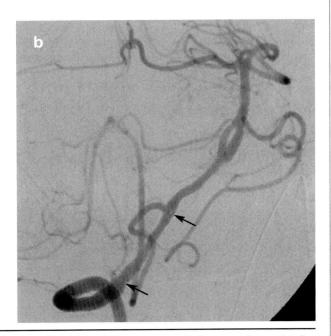

Figure 1. An endovascular stent in a 59-year-old with recurrent posterior circulation strokes. a) The oblique view after right vertebral artery injection demonstrates high-grade stenosis (black arrow) just proximal to the posterior inferior cerebellar artery. Note the distal fenestration and lack of antegrade flow beyond the midbasilar. The left vertebral artery was occluded. The posterior communicating arteries were not patent and the distal basilar territory was supplied from pial collaterals from the middle cerebral artery. b) Repeat angiogram after angioplasty and stenting with the Wingspan device shows good restoration of luminal diameter and distal flow. Black arrows indicate the proximal and distal markers of the stent.

* Angioplasty followed by placement of self-expanding stents.

This is an area of rapid evolution and ongoing clinical trials. Interest has been driven in part by the WASID trial, which documented a very high risk for recurrent stroke in patients with sICD [6].

Until very recently, the only balloons and stents small and flexible enough to be navigated into the cerebral circulation were coronary devices. In many patients, however, the acute angles and bony confines of the skull base do not allow passage of these relatively stiff devices. Newer devices designed for intracranial use have made these procedures much safer and easier. A second limitation of coronary devices is the relatively high pressures used for angioplasty. The cerebral vessels have no supporting soft tissue and are free in the subarachnoid space. Vessel rupture is a generally fatal complication of intracranial angioplasty, and may be more common with coronary balloons than with lower-pressure balloons designed for neurologic applications.

To date, most published studies have been case series. Few have reported long-term outcome and restenosis rates. The early (30-day) outcomes of one randomized trial of angioplasty versus medical therapy have been published. This study (SAMMPRIS) [28] and one other are ongoing. This section reviews the published literature describing angioplasty and stenting for sICD.

Angioplasty alone

The first endovascular procedures for coronary, carotid, and intracranial atherosclerotic stenosis involved angioplasty alone, as this was the only technology available at the time. The first reported cases of balloon angioplasty for intracranial stenoses were from Sundt et al in 1980 [37].

With modern balloons and imaging equipment, technical success (defined as reduction of stenosis to <50%) can be achieved in more than 80% of patients, and the rate of stroke or death within 30 days of angioplasty has varied between 4% and 40% in several retrospective angioplasty studies [38-47]. Two possible reasons for the wide range of complication rates are variability in the time from the presenting ischemic event to treatment and the heterogeneity of lesions being treated. Largely elective procedures have been associated with lower complication rates (4-6%) [42, 43, 45]. Restenosis rates following angioplasty alone range from 24% to 40% [42, 43]. There are limited data on the long-term outcomes after intracranial angioplasty alone. In 2006, Marks et al eported an annual stroke rate of 4.4% (3.2% in the territory of stenosis) in a retrospective review of 120 patients who underwent intracranial angioplasty at four sites [42]. The actual stroke rate is uncertain, given the retrospective nature of the study and the lack of adjudication of events by neurologists.

Stenting

Stents were developed to address the limitations of bare angioplasty: vessel recoil and dissection. Stents prop the diameter of the vessel open and resist recoil, and also tack down any intimal flaps caused by stretching the plaque with balloons. In general and in most circulations, stents are preferred over angioplasty alone. A meta-analysis from Siddiq et al published in 2009 concluded that 1-year stroke and death rates were lower with angioplasty and stenting than with angioplasty alone [48] **(III/B)**. Technical success and symptomatic restenosis rates (11-14%) were similar between the techniques. Complication rates appeared similar with moderate (50-69%) and severe (70-99%) stenosis [49].

Until recently, most data on the safety and efficacy of intracranial stenting have been limited to single-center series [50-60]. These data suggest that intracranial stenting can be performed relatively safely and with high technical success. Larger, more recent studies suggest that the rate of stroke in patients with 70-99% stenosis may be substantially lower after stenting than was reported with medical therapy alone in the WASID study. Data exist for two categories of stents: balloon-expandable and self-expanding stents.

Balloon-expandable stents

A balloon-expandable stent is a relatively rigid stainless-steel stent mounted on a non-compliant angioplasty balloon. The device is placed across the stenosis and deployed in a single inflation. The advantage of this approach, similar to angioplasty alone, is the simplicity of the procedure. The disadvantage is that the combination of the stent and the balloon creates a very inflexible segment, and it is sometimes not possible to navigate it into the cerebral circulation. These devices are generally designed and approved for coronary use. Some balloon-mounted stents are drug-eluting, and the safety and efficacy of these agents in the cerebral circulation remains unknown. Overall, modern case series of intracranial angioplasty and stenting with balloon-mounted stents have reported high rates of technical success (91-98%) [61] **(III/B)**.

An industry-sponsored multicenter Phase I trial of a balloon-expandable bare-metal stent for intracranial stenosis (Neurolink, Guidant Corporation) provided encouraging data on the safety and potential efficacy of stenting for this indication. The Stenting of Symptomatic Atherosclerotic Lesions in the Vertebral or Intracranial Arteries (SSYLVIA) trial was a non-randomized, multicenter study that evaluated the safety and performance of primary stenting in 61 patients with intracranial arterial stenosis (n=43), vertebral pre-posterior inferior communicating artery (PICA) stenosis (n=12), or vertebral ostium stenosis (n=6) of 50% or more [62]. Deployment of the stent was successful in 58 of 61 patients (95%). In the first 30 days after stenting, four of 55 patients with intracranial or pre-PICA stenosis (defined as intracranial in WASID) experienced a stroke (30-day rate 7.2%; 95% confidence interval [CI], 2.0-17.6%) and there were no deaths. The frequency of stroke within 1 year (including the 30-day rate) was 10.9% (6/55 patients; 95% CI, 4.1-22.3%). All strokes were in the territory of the treated artery. Recurrent stenosis (≥50%) at 6 months was documented by angiography in 18 of 51 patients (35%; 95% CI, 22.2-48.4%). Factors significantly associated with restenosis were diabetes, post-procedure stenosis of more than 30%, and small vessel diameter. These features have also been associated with higher restenosis rates after

coronary stenting. This device was never taken to market.

A more recent study published by Jiang et al in 2007 reported a 7.2% rate of stroke or symptomatic brain hemorrhage at 1 year after stenting in patients with intracranial stenosis of 70% or more [49]. This study used a balloon-expandable stent that is not available in the USA. Coronary drug-eluting stents have been used in the cerebral circulation, with the aim of reducing in-stent stenosis [63, 64]. However, the stiffness of the currently available stents makes them difficult to consistently deliver in the tortuous cerebral circulation.

In 2007 and 2008, data were reported on two new balloon-mounted stents designed to treat intracranial stenosis. The Apollo stent (MicroPort Medical) was studied in a small single-center series of 46 patients [65]. It had a technical success rate of 91.7%, but delivery of the stent was limited by vessel tortuosity and the restenosis rate was 28%. In another study, the Pharos intracranial stent (Micrus Endovascular) was used to treat 21 patients with acute or chronic intracranial stenoses [66]. Among the 14 patients treated non-emergently, the technical success was 85.7% and the procedure-related complication rate was 28.5%.

Self-expanding stents

Self-expanding stents are nitinol devices that apply some degree of outward radial force to the vessel. They are the preferred device in some circulations, such as the extracranial carotid artery. Placement involves an initial angioplasty, followed by removal of the balloon over an exchange wire. The stent deployment catheter is then placed over the exchange wire and deployed. The advantage of this system in the intracranial circulation is its flexibility. The disadvantage is the extra step relative to balloon-mounted stents.

The bare-metal self-expanding Wingspan stent (Boston Scientific), designed specifically to treat intracranial stenosis, was approved by the US Food and Drug Administration on August 3, 2005, for use under a humanitarian device exemption (HDE) for

Chapter 30

patients with intracranial stenosis "who are refractory to medical therapy." This approval was based on a European/Asian study of 45 patients with symptomatic 50-99% stenosis who had recurrent stroke while on antithrombotic therapy. The main findings of the study were that the stent was successfully deployed in 44 of 45 patients (98%; 95% CI, 88.2-99.9%), the 30-day rate of stroke or death was 4.4% (95% CI, 0.5-15.2%), and the 12-month rate of ipsilateral stroke or death was 9.3% (4/43 patients; 95% CI, 2.6-22.1%). Only three of 40 patients (7.5%; 95% CI, 1.6-20.4%) had restenosis at 6 months and none was symptomatic [67]. Of the 45 patients, 29 entered the study with 70-99% stenosis. Of these 29 patients, three (10.3%) had a stroke in the territory or died within 1 year (95% CI, 2.2-27.4%).

Since the initial Wingspan HDE study, additional data on the safety and success of Wingspan have been reported from two multicenter registries. The first report included data from five centers on 78 patients with 82 symptomatic intracranial stenoses (50-99%), and demonstrated a technical success rate of 98.8% and a periprocedural rate of major neurologic complications of 6.1% [68]. The second registry, the National Institutes of Health multicenter Wingspan registry, focused on 129 patients with 70-99% symptomatic intracranial stenosis at 16 centers [69]. The rationale for this registry was based on the WASID findings of higher risk in this population. The technical success rate was 96.7% and the frequency of any stroke, intracerebral hemorrhage, or death within 30 days or ipsilateral stroke beyond 30 days was 14% at 6 months **(III/B)**. These data compared favorably with the outcomes of WASID and formed the basis for the SAMMPRIS trial that examined angioplasty and stenting versus best medical management (aspirin 325mg and clopidogrel 75mg daily for the first 90 days, plus aggressive lipid and blood-pressure lowering) for sICD patients.

Enrollment in the SAMMPRIS study was halted in April 2011 on the recommendation of the Data and Safety Monitoring Board, owing to higher than expected 30-day morbidity and mortality in the stenting group and a lower than expected stroke rate in the medical group [28]. Follow-up and medical treatment are continuing and the trial will be completed in 2014. A total of 451 of the planned 764 patients (59%) were enrolled at 50 participating sites in the USA. Overall, 14% of the patients randomized to stenting had a stroke or died within 30 days of enrollment, compared with an estimated figure of 5.2-9.6% from the registries. The 30-day risk of stroke or death in the medically treated patients was 5.8%, compared with a 30-day risk of 10.7% in WASID. There were five stroke-related deaths within 30 days in the stent group as compared with one in the medical arm. The risks of recurrent stroke beyond 30 days were similar between the two groups, but less than half of the patients had reached 1-year follow-up at the time of this analysis. The authors considered the data sufficient to conclude that medical management (as per the SAMMPRIS protocol) was superior to angioplasty and stenting in this patient population.

Since the initial reports of the Wingspan registries, additional follow-up data have become available. Restenosis rates (≥50% on follow-up angiogram) of 25-32% have been reported [69, 70] and appear to be higher in younger patients, especially those with supraclinoid carotid stenosis [71]. However, the restenosis is usually asymptomatic [69, 72]. This phenomenon raises the question as to the underlying occlusive vasculopathy in this population. The location of stenosis and the demographics of this patient group are similar to those of North American patients with Moyamoya phenomenon [73]. These patients may have a similar underlying occlusive vasculopathy, but lack the proliferative signals that result in Moyamoya collateral formation.

Summary

Angioplasty with stenting has the potential to benefit patients with symptomatic intracranial atherosclerotic disease, but the failure of the SAMMPRIS trial suggests that the identification of high-risk patient subgroups and further advances in technology may be required. Two randomized trials are underway. The results of these trials and developments in devices and medical regimens will lead to further improvements in the endovascular treatment of these patients. At present, it is reasonable to consider angioplasty and stenting in patients with unstable symptoms or a chronic fixed lesion with recurrent symptoms despite aggressive medical management.

Extracranial-intracranial bypass

Surgical revascularization for sICD was initially explored soon after the superficial temporal artery-middle cerebral artery (STA-MCA) bypass was developed by Yasargil and Donaghy in the late 1960s (Figure 2) [74, 75]. Several subsequent retrospective

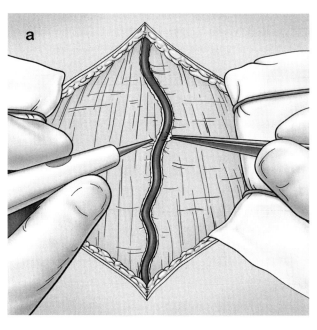

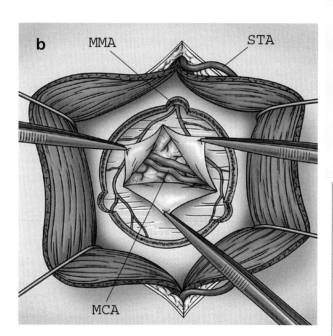

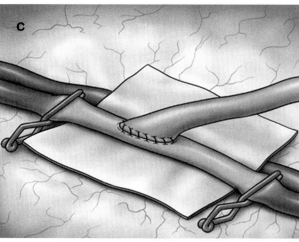

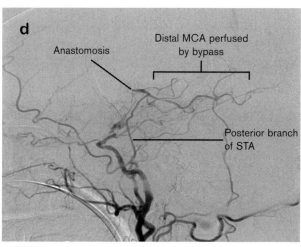

Chapter 30

Figure 2. Superficial temporal artery (STA)-middle cerebral artery (MCA) bypass. a) The posterior branch of the STA is dissected free from the scalp. b) The STA is then mobilized out of the field, the temporal muscle is divided, and a temporal craniotomy is performed over the sylvian fissure to expose a cortical MCA branch. c) An end-to-side anastomosis between the STA and the cortical MCA branch is performed under EEG-burst suppression for neuroprotection. d) Lateral view of the common carotid artery injection, demonstrating patency of an STA-MCA bypass performed for the treatment of symptomatic Moyamoya disease. *Figures a) b) and c) reproduced with permission from: Zipfel GJ, Fox DJ Jnr, Rivet DJ. Moyamoya disease in adults: the role of cerebral revascularization. Skull Base 2005; 15: 27-41.*

case series published in the 1970s and 1980s documented high bypass patency rates and relatively low perioperative complication rates in patients undergoing STA-MCA bypass for ischemic cerebrovascular disease [76-79]. These early positive results established STA-MCA bypass as a common therapeutic approach for sICD patients in whom medical therapy had failed. However, this early enthusiasm was tempered by discouraging results from the International Cooperative Study of Extracranial/Intracranial Arterial Anastomosis (EC-IC Bypass Study), published in 1985 [80]. Since then, STA-MCA bypass and other less common techniques for establishing a direct EC-IC bypass (e.g., radial artery or saphenous vein high-flow bypass) have been infrequently used for treating patients with sICD. Some have suggested that assessing cerebral hemodynamic impairment with sophisticated imaging techniques may identify a subgroup of sICD patients who would benefit from surgical revascularization [81-83]. Others have begun to explore potentially less morbid indirect revascularization techniques to treat patients with sICD [84]. This section reviews the published literature describing both direct and indirect bypass procedures for sICD, with an emphasis on the EC-IC Bypass Study – the only available large-scale randomized controlled trial evaluating surgical revascularization for this patient population [80].

Direct bypass

Several single-institution retrospective case series have examined the technical success and perioperative safety of direct EC-IC bypass for ischemic cerebrovascular disease. Most of these studies have evaluated patients with a variety of cerebrovascular conditions including sICD (but also extracranial carotid occlusion, Moyamoya disease, and/or carotid dissection), while a minority have specifically examined patients with sICD. All were retrospective studies, and none included adjudication of cerebrovascular events by neurologists.

Gratzl et al reported data from a series of 65 patients who underwent STA-MCA bypass for primarily ischemic cerebrovascular disease [76]. Forty-five patients had sICD. The authors documented 95% bypass patency, 3.1% perioperative morbidity, and 7.7% perioperative mortality for the entire series. Yasargil and Yonekawa reported on a series of 84 patients who underwent 82 STA-MCA and four occipital-MCA bypass procedures for ischemic cerebrovascular disease [77]. Fifty-one patients had sICD. They documented 87% bypass patency, 5.8% perioperative morbidity (from stroke or subdural hematoma), and 3.5% perioperative mortality for the entire series **(III/B)**. Sundt et al reported on a series of 403 patients who underwent 415 STA-MCA bypass procedures for predominantly ischemic cerebrovascular disease [78]. A total of 115 patients had sICD. They documented 99% bypass patency, 4% perioperative morbidity, and 1% perioperative mortality for the entire series. Perioperative mortality for sICD patients alone was 2.8% **(III/B)**. Tummala et al reported on a series of 65 patients who underwent 71 STA-MCA bypass procedures for predominantly ischemic cerebrovascular disease [85]. Sixteen patients had sICD. They reported 0% morbidity and 0% mortality for the entire series. Bypass patency was not assessed with vascular imaging **(III/B)**.

Very few studies have exclusively examined patients with sICD. The report of Weinstein et al was the first such study [79]. They reported on a series of 105 patients who underwent STA-MCA bypass procedures for sICD. They documented 97% bypass patency, 2.8% perioperative morbidity (from stroke), and 1% perioperative mortality. They also examined long-term outcomes after surgery, reporting a late stroke rate of 1.5% per year – a rate that compared favorably to the natural history of medically treated patients with sICD **(III/B)**. Most recently, Tsai et al reported on a series of 11 patients who underwent STA-MCA bypass for sICD (all MCA stenosis or occlusion) [86]. They documented 100% bypass patency, 0% perioperative morbidity, and 0% perioperative mortality. The late stroke rate in long-term follow-up was not reported **(III/B)**.

In 1985, the landmark EC-IC Bypass Trial was published [80]. It remains the largest prospective, third-party adjudicated study examining the safety and efficacy of STA-MCA bypass for patients with ischemic cerebrovascular disease, including those with sICD. Patients were eligible for the trial if they suffered one or more TIAs or minor ischemic strokes within 3 months of enrollment and had angiographic evidence of: stenosis or occlusion of the major trunk or branches of the MCA; stenosis of the internal carotid artery (ICA) at or above the C2 vertebral body (i.e., at a place inaccessible to carotid endarterectomy); or occlusion of the ICA. Therefore, many (about a third) but not all patients included in this study had sICD. Patients were randomized to STA-MCA bypass or non-surgical management. All patients received aspirin (325mg four time daily) throughout the trial, unless contraindicated or not tolerated. The primary study endpoints were post-randomization fatal or non-fatal stroke. These endpoints were adjudicated by a non-participating neurologist and a neurosurgeon blinded to the patients' treatment category.

The results for patients undergoing STA-MCA bypass were as follows **(Ib/A)**:

* Bypass patency rate: 96%.
* Perioperative cerebral and retinal ischemic event rate: 12.2%.
* Perioperative major stroke rate: 4.5%.
* Perioperative mortality rate: 1.1%.

The incidence of fatal and non-fatal strokes was higher in patients randomized to STA-MCA bypass than in those randomized to medical therapy alone. When considering only patients with sICD, a similar negative result for surgery was noted: the incidence of fatal and non-fatal stroke was 32.4% in the surgical group and 27.6% in the medical group. An even greater difference in outcome was noted for sICD patients with intracranial stenosis rather than occlusion: the incidence of fatal and non-fatal stroke for patients with severe ICA or MCA stenosis was 40.2% in the surgical group and 30.5% in the medical group. Many have attributed this finding to post-bypass stasis at the stenotic arterial segment

(probably the result of competing antegrade flow from the native artery vs. retrograde flow from the arterial bypass), which would promote thromboembolic complications. These overwhelmingly negative results led to a dramatic reduction in the use of STA-MCA bypass for the management of sICD patients in whom medical therapy had failed.

Several commentators have suggested that one of the key reasons for failure of the EC-IC Bypass Trial was lack of assessment of cerebral hemodynamics to identify a subgroup of patients with reduced cerebral perfusion pressure, in whom STA-MCA bypass may be more beneficial [81-83]. Several methods have now been developed to quantitatively examine cerebral hemodynamic impairment in patients with ischemic cerebrovascular disease. These include cerebral blood-flow measurements before and after a vasodilatory stimulus; cerebral blood volume and/or mean transit time measurements via single positron emission CT (SPECT), positron emission tomography (PET), or MR/CT perfusion; and oxygen extraction fraction (OEF) measurement with PET (for review, see Grubb et al [87]).

Of these, PET-based assessment of hemodynamic impairment has been the most rigorously studied, with two prospective observational studies showing that patients with recently symptomatic ischemic cerebrovascular disease and increased OEF have a markedly elevated risk of subsequent ipsilateral ischemic stroke (as compared with those with normal OEF) [88, 89]. However, only 10 of the 121 patients included in these two studies had sICD (the remainder had ICA occlusion), making conclusions regarding the value of hemodynamic assessment in patients with sICD difficult. Given the paucity of cerebral hemodynamic data for sICD patients, along with the aforementioned increased risk of STA-MCA bypass for patients with severe ICA or MCA stenosis [80] and the premature stoppage of the Carotid Occlusion Surgery Study (a randomized controlled trial comparing STA-MCA bypass vs. best medical therapy for patients with recently symptomatic ICA occlusion and increased OEF [87]), it is unlikely that direct EC-IC bypass for sICD patients – even for those in whom medical therapy has failed and who have documented impaired cerebral hemodynamics – will be proven effective.

Indirect bypass

One recent alternative approach to surgical revascularization for sICD patients is an indirect bypass, with the aim of promoting angiogenesis and improving cerebral blood flow over time. Komotar *et al* have reported a case series of 12 patients with sICD and impaired cerebral hemodynamics (assessed by SPECT measurement of cerebral blood flow before and after acetazolamide challenge) who were treated with indirect bypass: 11 underwent encephaloduroarteriosynangiosis (EDAS) and one received burr holes with dural and arachnoid incisions [84]. Perioperative morbidity was 27% (two patients developed minor neurologic deficits and one developed temporary hemisensory loss and weakness that returned to baseline 2 months later). Perioperative mortality was 0% **(III/B)**. On late follow-up, only two patients demonstrated increased perfusion in previously hypoperfused areas by SPECT, while five patients suffered repeat ischemic infarction. When compared with a meta-analysis evaluating four studies of medically treated patients with symptomatic ICA occlusion and severe hemodynamic failure, the authors found that indirect surgical revascularization provided no protection against subsequent ischemic stroke **(III/B)**. Based on this small retrospective case series, indirect surgical revascularization for patients with sICD is not indicated and does not appear to hold much promise **(III/B)**.

Summary

Direct and indirect surgical revascularization for the treatment of sICD is not supported by the available literature. In particular, STA-MCA bypass for patients with symptomatic severe ICA or MCA stenosis appears not only ineffective, but probably harmful. Further studies examining the utility of PET and other techniques for assessing cerebral hemodynamic impairment in sICD patients appear warranted.

Conclusions

sICD remains a significant contributor to the large societal health burden of stroke, both as a primary cause of ischemic stroke and as a secondary source of recurrent ischemic events. Current minimally invasive imaging techniques allow identification of sICD, creating an opportunity for both accurate diagnosis and investigation into effective treatments for stroke prevention. The current evidence supports antiplatelet therapy over anticoagulation for the prevention of recurrent strokes in sICD. Failure of the SAMMPRIS trial suggests that angioplasty and stenting should not be recommended before treating with aggressive medical therapy. Moreover, neither direct and indirect bypass for patients with symptomatic stenosis or occlusion of the ICA or MCA is supported by clinical trials to date. As technology and interventional and surgical techniques advance, select patient subgroups may be identified that will benefit from endovascular or surgical intervention; however, these interventions will need to be tested in randomized controlled trials.

Recommendations	Evidence level
◆ Patients with sICD experience a high rate of recurrent strokes (14-19% over 2 years).	Ib/A
◆ TCD and MRA have high sensitivity but low specificity for detecting intracranial stenosis compared with DSA (the gold standard). These are reasonable screening tools for ICAD.	IIa/B
◆ CTA appears to have both high sensitivity and specificity compared with DSA.	III/B
◆ Antiplatelet therapy with aspirin (50-325mg daily), aspirin plus extended-release dipyridamole, or clopidogrel are recommended for all patients with non-cardioembolic ischemic stroke or TIA to reduce the risk of recurrent stroke.	Ib/A
◆ Anticoagulation with warfarin offers no benefit over aspirin for preventing recurrent strokes in patients with sICD and is associated with a higher rate of adverse events.	Ib/A
◆ Low-molecular-weight heparin is not superior to aspirin for preventing recurrent strokes in patients with sICD <48 hours from stroke onset.	Ib/A
◆ Compared with aspirin alone, dual-antiplatelet therapy with cilostazol and aspirin may slow the progression of stenosis in patients with sICD, but has unknown effects on clinical outcomes.	Ib/A
◆ Female sex, NIHSS score >1, recent symptom onset (≤17 days), and ≥70% stenosis are associated with a high risk of recurrent stroke in patients with sICD.	IIa/B
◆ sICD patients with SBP ≥140mmHg, no alcohol consumption, and cholesterol ≥200mg/dL are at increased risk of recurrent stroke.	Ib/A
◆ One-year stroke and death rates are lower for sICD patients treated with angioplasty and stenting vs. angioplasty alone.	III/B
◆ Rates of technical success for angioplasty and stenting (self-expanding stents) for sICD are high (>95%).	III/B
◆ The frequency of perioperative stroke or death plus ipsilateral stroke at >30 days for sICD patients treated with angioplasty and stenting (self-expanding stents) compares favorably with the outcomes for those treated with medical therapy alone.	III/B
◆ Direct EC-IC bypass for patients with sICD does not reduce the incidence of fatal and non-fatal strokes as compared with medical therapy alone.	Ib/A
◆ Indirect EC-IC bypass for patients with sICD does not reduce the incidence of subsequent ischemic stroke as compared with medical therapy alone.	III/B

Chapter 30

References

1. Sacco RL, Kargman DE, Gu Q, Zamanillo MC. Race-ethnicity and determinants of intracranial atherosclerotic cerebral infarction. The Northern Manhattan Stroke Study. *Stroke* 1995; 26: 14-20.

2. Wityk RJ, Lehman D, Klag M, Coresh J, Ahn H, Litt B. Race and sex differences in the distribution of cerebral atherosclerosis. *Stroke* 1996; 27: 1974-80.

3. Lloyd-Jones D, Adams RJ, Brown TM, *et al*. Executive summary: heart disease and stroke statistics - 2010 update: a report from the American Heart Association. *Circulation* 2010; 121: 948-54.

Chapter 30

4. Wong KS, Huang YN, Gao S, Lam WW, Chan YL, Kay R. Intracranial stenosis in Chinese patients with acute stroke. *Neurology* 1998; 50: 812-3.

5. Wong KS, Li H, Chan YL, *et al.* Use of transcranial Doppler ultrasound to predict outcome in patients with intracranial large-artery occlusive disease. *Stroke* 2000; 31: 2641-7.

6. Chimowitz MI, Lynn MJ, Howlett-Smith H, *et al.* Comparison of warfarin and aspirin for symptomatic intracranial arterial stenosis. *N Engl J Med* 2005; 352: 1305-16.

7. Mazighi M, Tanasescu R, Ducrocq X, *et al.* Prospective study of symptomatic atherothrombotic intracranial stenoses: the GESICA study. *Neurology* 2006; 66: 1187-91.

8. Famakin BM, Chimowitz MI, Lynn MJ, Stern BJ, George MG. Causes and severity of ischemic stroke in patients with symptomatic intracranial arterial stenosis. *Stroke* 2009; 40: 1999-2003.

9. Bae HJ, Lee J, Park JM, *et al.* Risk factors of intracranial cerebral atherosclerosis among asymptomatics. *Cerebrovasc Dis* 2007; 24: 355-60.

10. Huang HW, Guo MH, Lin RJ, *et al.* Prevalence and risk factors of middle cerebral artery stenosis in asymptomatic residents in Rongqi County, Guangdong. *Cerebrovasc Dis* 2007; 24: 111-5.

11. Uehara T, Tabuchi M, Mori E. Risk factors for occlusive lesions of intracranial arteries in stroke-free Japanese. *Eur J Neurol* 2005; 12: 218-22.

12. Scott RM, Smith ER. Moyamoya disease and Moyamoya syndrome. *N Engl J Med* 2009; 360: 1226-37.

13. Adams RJ, Nichols FT, McKie V, McKie K, Milner P, Gammal TE. Cerebral infarction in sickle cell anemia: mechanism based on CT and MRI. *Neurology* 1988; 38: 1012-7.

14. Pavlakis SG, Bello J, Prohovnik I, *et al.* Brain infarction in sickle cell anemia: magnetic resonance imaging correlates. *Ann Neurol* 1988; 23: 125-30.

15. Palacio S, Hart RG, Vollmer DG, Kagan-Hallet K. Late-developing cerebral arteropathy after pyogenic meningitis. *Arch Neurol* 2003; 60: 431-3.

16. Lu CH, Chang WN, Chang HW, *et al.* Clinical relevance of intracranial arterial stenoses in tuberculous and cryptococcal meningitis. *Infection* 2007; 35: 359-63.

17. Cantu C, Pineda C, Barinagarrementeria F, *et al.* Noninvasive cerebrovascular assessment of Takayasu arteritis. *Stroke* 2000; 31: 2197-202.

18. Chaves C, Estol C, Esnaola MM, *et al.* Spontaneous intracranial internal carotid artery dissection: report of 10 patients. *Arch Neurol* 2002; 59: 977-81.

19. Rogers LR. Cerebrovascular complications in cancer patients. *Neurol Clin* 2003; 21: 167-92.

20. Suwanwela NC, Chutinet A, Phanthumchinda K. Inflammatory markers and conventional atherosclerotic risk factors in acute ischemic stroke: comparative study between vascular disease subtypes. *J Med Assoc Thai* 2006; 89: 2021-7.

21. Feldmann E, Wilterdink JL, Kosinski A, *et al.* The Stroke Outcomes and Neuroimaging of Intracranial Atherosclerosis (SONIA) trial. *Neurology* 2007; 68: 2099-106.

22. Nguyen-Huynh MN, Wintermark M, English J, *et al.* How accurate is CT angiography in evaluating intracranial atherosclerotic disease? *Stroke* 2008; 39: 1184-8.

23. Feldmeyer JJ, Merendaz C, Regli F. [Symptomatic stenoses of the middle cerebral artery.] *Rev Neurol* (Paris) 1983; 139: 725-36.

24. Chimowitz MI, Kokkinos J, Strong J, *et al.* The Warfarin-Aspirin Symptomatic Intracranial Disease Study. *Neurology* 1995; 45: 1488-93.

25. Wong KS, Chen C, Ng PW, *et al.* Low-molecular-weight heparin compared with aspirin for the treatment of acute ischaemic stroke in Asian patients with large artery occlusive disease: a randomised study. *Lancet Neurol* 2007; 6: 407-13.

26. Adams RJ, Albers G, Alberts MJ, *et al.* Update to the AHA/ASA recommendations for the prevention of stroke in patients with stroke and transient ischemic attack. *Stroke* 2008; 39: 1647-52.

27. Kwon SU, Cho YJ, Koo JS, *et al.* Cilostazol prevents the progression of the symptomatic intracranial arterial stenosis: the multicenter double-blind placebo-controlled trial of cilostazol in symptomatic intracranial arterial stenosis. *Stroke* 2005; 36: 782-6.

28. Chimowitz MI, Lynn MJ, Derdeyn CP, *et al.*; SAMMPRIS Trial Investigators. Stenting versus aggressive medical therapy for intracranial arterial stenosis. *N Engl J Med* 2011; 365: 993-1003.

29. Yusuf S, Zhao F, Mehta SR, Chrolavicius S, Tognoni G, Fox KK; Clopidogrel in Unstable Angina to Prevent Recurrent Events Trial Investigators. Effects of clopidogrel in addition to aspirin in patients with acute coronary syndromes without ST-segment elevation. *N Engl J Med* 2001; 345: 494-502.

30. Kasner SE, Chimowitz MI, Lynn MJ, *et al.* Predictors of ischemic stroke in the territory of a symptomatic intracranial arterial stenosis. *Circulation* 2006; 113: 555-63.

31. Waddy SP, Cotsonis G, Lynn MJ, *et al.* Racial differences in vascular risk factors and outcomes of patients with intracranial atherosclerotic arterial stenosis. *Stroke* 2009; 40: 719-25.

32. Williams JE, Chimowitz MI, Cotsonis GA, Lynn MJ, Waddy SP. Gender differences in outcomes among patients with symptomatic intracranial arterial stenosis. *Stroke* 2007; 38: 2055-62.

33. Chaturvedi S, Turan TN, Lynn MJ, *et al.* Risk factor status and vascular events in patients with symptomatic intracranial stenosis. *Neurology* 2007; 69: 2063-8.

34. Turan TN, Cotsonis G, Lynn MJ, Chaturvedi S, Chimowitz M. Relationship between blood pressure and stroke recurrence in patients with intracranial arterial stenosis. *Circulation* 2007; 115: 2969-75.

35. Thijs VN, Albers GW. Symptomatic intracranial atherosclerosis: outcome of patients who fail antithrombotic therapy. *Neurology* 2000; 55: 490-7.

36. Turan TN, Maidan L, Cotsonis G, *et al.* Failure of antithrombotic therapy and risk of stroke in patients with symptomatic intracranial stenosis. *Stroke* 2009; 40: 505-9.

37. Sundt TM Jr, Smith HC, Campbell JK, Vlietstra RE, Cucchiara RF, Stanson AW. Transluminal angioplasty for basilar artery stenosis. *Mayo Clin Proc* 1980; 55: 673-80.

38. Higashida RT, Tsai FY, Halbach VV, *et al*. Transluminal angioplasty for atherosclerotic disease of the vertebral and basilar arteries. *J Neurosurg* 1993; 78: 192-8.

39. Clark WM, Barnwell SL, Nesbit G, O'Neill OR, Wynn ML, Coull BM. Safety and efficacy of percutaneous transluminal angioplasty for intracranial atherosclerotic stenosis. *Stroke* 1995; 26: 1200-4.

40. Takis C, Kwan ES, Pessin MS, Jacobs DH, Caplan LR. Intracranial angioplasty: experience and complications. *AJNR Am J Neuroradiol* 1997; 18: 1661-8.

41. Marks MP, Marcellus M, Norbash AM, Steinberg GK, Tong D, Albers GW. Outcome of angioplasty for atherosclerotic intracranial stenosis. *Stroke* 1999; 30: 1065-9.

42. Marks MP, Wojak JC, Al-Ali F, *et al*. Angioplasty for symptomatic intracranial stenosis: clinical outcome. *Stroke* 2006; 37: 1016-20.

43. Connors JJ 3rd, Wojak JC. Percutaneous transluminal angioplasty for intracranial atherosclerotic lesions: evolution of technique and short-term results. *J Neurosurg* 1999; 91: 415-23.

44. Alazzaz A, Thornton J, Aletich VA, Debrun GM, Ausman JI, Charbel F. Intracranial percutaneous transluminal angioplasty for arteriosclerotic stenosis. *Arch Neurol* 2000; 57: 1625-30.

45. Nahser HC, Henkes H, Weber W, Berg-Dammer E, Yousry TA, Kuhne D. Intracranial vertebrobasilar stenosis: angioplasty and follow-up. *AJNR Am J Neuroradiol* 2000; 21: 1293-301.

46. Gress DR, Smith WS, Dowd CF, Van Halbach V, Finley RJ, Higashida RT. Angioplasty for intracranial symptomatic vertebrobasilar ischemia. *Neurosurgery* 2002; 51: 23-7; discussion 27-9.

47. Gupta R, Schumacher HC, Mangla S, *et al*. Urgent endovascular revascularization for symptomatic intracranial atherosclerotic stenosis. *Neurology* 2003; 61: 1729-35.

48. Siddiq F, Memon MZ, Vazquez G, Safdar A, Qureshi AI. Comparison between primary angioplasty and stent placement for symptomatic intracranial atherosclerotic disease: meta-analysis of case series. *Neurosurgery* 2009; 65: 1024-33; discussion 33-4.

49. Jiang WJ, Xu XT, Du B, *et al*. Long-term outcome of elective stenting for symptomatic intracranial vertebrobasilar stenosis. *Neurology* 2007; 68: 856-8.

50. Gomez CR, Misra VK, Campbell MS, Soto RD. Elective stenting of symptomatic middle cerebral artery stenosis. *AJNR Am J Neuroradiol* 2000; 21: 971-3.

51. Gomez CR, Misra VK, Liu MW, *et al*. Elective stenting of symptomatic basilar artery stenosis. *Stroke* 2000; 31: 95-9.

52. Rasmussen PA, Perl J, 2nd, Barr JD, *et al*. Stent-assisted angioplasty of intracranial vertebrobasilar atherosclerosis: an initial experience. *J Neurosurg* 2000; 92: 771-8.

53. Levy EI, Hanel RA, Boulos AS, *et al*. Comparison of periprocedure complications resulting from direct stent placement compared with those due to conventional and staged stent placement in the basilar artery. *J Neurosurg* 2003; 99: 653-60.

54. Kim DJ, Lee BH, Kim DI, Shim WH, Jeon P, Lee TH. Stent-assisted angioplasty of symptomatic intracranial

vertebrobasilar artery stenosis: feasibility and follow-up results. *AJNR Am J Neuroradiol* 2005; 26: 1381-8.

55. de Rochemont Rdu M, Turowski B, Buchkremer M, Sitzer M, Zanella FE, Berkefeld J. Recurrent symptomatic high-grade intracranial stenoses: safety and efficacy of undersized stents - initial experience. *Radiology* 2004; 231: 45-9.

56. Liu JM, Hong B, Huang QH, *et al*. [Safety and short-term results of stent-assisted angioplasty for the treatment of intracranial arterial stenosis.] *Zhonghua Wai Ke Za Zhi* 2004; 42: 169-72.

57. Zhang QZ, Miao ZR, Li SM, *et al*. [Complications of stent-assistant angioplasty of symptomatic intracranial artery stenosis.] *Zhonghua Yi Xue Za Zhi* 2003; 83: 1402-5.

58. Jiang WJ, Du B, Wang YJ, Wang SX, Wang GH, Jin M. [Symptomatic intracranial artery stenosis: angiographic classifications and stent-assisted angioplasty.] *Zhonghua Nei Ke Za Zhi* 2003; 42: 545-9.

59. Jiang WJ, Wang YJ, Du B, *et al*. Stenting of symptomatic M1 stenosis of middle cerebral artery: an initial experience of 40 patients. *Stroke* 2004; 35: 1375-80.

60. Lylyk P, Vila JF, Miranda C, *et al*. Endovascular reconstruction by means of stent placement in symptomatic intracranial atherosclerotic stenosis. *Neurol Res* 2005; 27(Suppl. 1): S84-8.

61. Leung TW, Kwon SU, Wong KS. Management of patients with symptomatic intracranial atherosclerosis. *Int J Stroke* 2006; 1: 20-5.

62. SSYLVIA Study Investigators. Stenting of Symptomatic Atherosclerotic Lesions in the Vertebral or Intracranial Arteries (SSYLVIA): study results. *Stroke* 2004; 35: 1388-92.

63. Gupta R, Al-Ali F, Thomas AJ, *et al*. Safety, feasibility, and short-term follow-up of drug-eluting stent placement in the intracranial and extracranial circulation. *Stroke* 2006; 37: 2562-6.

64. Abou-Chebl A, Bashir Q, Yadav JS. Drug-eluting stents for the treatment of intracranial atherosclerosis: initial experience and midterm angiographic follow-up. *Stroke* 2005; 36: e165-8.

65. Jiang WJ, Xu XT, Jin M, Du B, Dong KH, Dai JP. Apollo stent for symptomatic atherosclerotic intracranial stenosis: study results. *AJNR Am J Neuroradiol* 2007; 28: 830-4.

66. Kurre W, Berkefeld J, Sitzer M, Neumann-Haefelin T, du Mesnil de Rochemont R. Treatment of symptomatic high-grade intracranial stenoses with the balloon-expandable Pharos stent: initial experience. *Neuroradiology* 2008; 50: 701-8.

67. Bose A, Hartmann M, Henkes H, *et al*. A novel, self-expanding, nitinol stent in medically refractory intracranial atherosclerotic stenoses: the Wingspan study. *Stroke* 2007; 38: 1531-7.

68. Fiorella D, Levy EI, Turk AS, *et al*. US multicenter experience with the Wingspan stent system for the treatment of intracranial atheromatous disease: periprocedural results. *Stroke* 2007; 38: 881-7.

69. Zaidat OO, Klucznik R, Alexander MJ, *et al*. The NIH registry on use of the Wingspan stent for symptomatic 70-99% intracranial arterial stenosis. *Neurology* 2008; 70: 1518-24.

70. Albuquerque FC, Levy EI, Turk AS, *et al*. Angiographic patterns of Wingspan in-stent restenosis. *Neurosurgery* 2008; 63: 23-7; discussion 27-8.

71. Turk AS, Levy EI, Albuquerque FC, *et al*. Influence of patient age and stenosis location on Wingspan in-stent restenosis. *AJNR Am J Neuroradiol* 2008; 29: 23-7.

72. Levy EI, Turk AS, Albuquerque FC, *et al*. Wingspan in-stent restenosis and thrombosis: incidence, clinical presentation, and management. *Neurosurgery* 2007; 61: 644-50; discussion 650-1.

73. Goyal MS, Hallemeier CL, Zipfel GJ, *et al*. Clinical features and outcome in North American adults with idiopathic basal arterial occlusive disease without Moyamoya collaterals. *Neurosurgery* 2010; 67: 278-85.

74. Yasargil MG. *Microsurgery, Applied to Neurosurgery*. Stuttgart: Georg Thieme, 1969.

75. Donaghy RMP. What's new in surgery: neurological surgery. *Surg Gynecol Obstet* 1972; 134: 269-71.

76. Gratzl O, Schmiedek P, Spetzler R, Steinhoff H, Marguth F. Clinical experience with extra-intracranial arterial anastomosis in 65 cases. *J Neurosurg* 1976; 44: 313-24.

77. Yasargil MG, Yonekawa Y. Results of microsurgical extra-intracranial arterial bypass in the treatment of cerebral ischemia. *Neurosurgery* 1977; 1: 22-4.

78. Sundt TM Jr, Whisnant JP, Fode NC, Piepgras DG, Houser OW. Results, complications, and follow-up of 415 bypass operations for occlusive disease of the carotid system. *Mayo Clin Proc* 1985; 60: 230-40.

79. Weinstein PR, Rodriguez y Baena R, Chater NL. Results of extracranial-intracranial arterial bypass for intracranial internal carotid artery stenosis: review of 105 cases. *Neurosurgery* 1984; 15: 787-94.

80. The EC/IC Bypass Study Group. Failure of extracranial-intracranial arterial bypass to reduce the risk of ischemic stroke. Results of an international randomized trial. *N Engl J Med* 1985; 313: 1191-200.

81. Day AL, Rhoton AL Jr, Little JR. The extracranial-intracranial bypass study. *Surg Neurol* 1986; 26: 222-6.

82. Schmiedek P, Piepgras A, Leinsinger G, Kirsch CM, Einhupl K. Improvement of cerebrovascular reserve capacity by EC-IC arterial bypass surgery in patients with ICA occlusion and hemodynamic cerebral ischemia. *J Neurosurg* 1994; 81: 236-44.

83. Yonas H, Gur D, Good BC, *et al*. Stable xenon CT blood flow mapping for evaluation of patients with extracranial-intracranial bypass surgery. *J Neurosurg* 1985; 62: 324-33.

84. Komotar RJ, Starke RM, Otten ML, *et al*. The role of indirect extracranial-intracranial bypass in the treatment of symptomatic intracranial atheroocclusive disease. *J Neurosurg* 2009; 110: 896-904.

85. Tummala RP, Chu RM, Nussbaum ES. Extracranial-intracranial bypass for symptomatic occlusive cerebrovascular disease not amenable to carotid endarterectomy. *Neurosurg Focus* 2003; 14: e8.

86. Tsai ST, Yen PS, Wang YJ, Chiu TL. Superficial temporal artery-middle cerebral artery bypass for ischemic atherosclerotic middle cerebral artery disease. *J Clin Neurosci* 2009; 16: 1013-7.

87. Grubb RL Jr, Powers WJ, Derdeyn CP, Adams HP Jr, Clarke WR. The Carotid Occlusion Surgery Study. *Neurosurg Focus* 2003; 14: e9.

88. Grubb RL Jr, Derdeyn CP, Fritsch SM, *et al*. Importance of hemodynamic factors in the prognosis of symptomatic carotid occlusion. *JAMA* 1998; 280: 1055-60.

89. Yamauchi H, Fukuyama H, Nagahama Y, *et al*. Significance of increased oxygen extraction fraction in five-year prognosis of major cerebral arterial occlusive diseases. *J Nucl Med* 1999; 40: 1992-8.

Chapter 30

Chapter 31

Cerebral vasospasm following aneurysmal subarachnoid hemorrhage

Gregory J Velat MD, Clinical Lecturer

Matthew Kimball MD, Resident Physician

Brian L Hoh MD, Associate Professor

University of Florida, Department of Neurological Surgery, Gainesville, Florida, USA

Introduction

Aneurysmal subarachnoid hemorrhage (aSAH) accounts for approximately 5% of all strokes, affecting some 30,000 Americans annually [1]. The incidence of aSAH varies internationally, ranging from two to 23 cases per 100,000 population [2, 3]. Case-fatality rates range from 32% to 67% [4], although recent evidence suggests slightly declining mortality rates worldwide [5]. Cerebral vasospasm accounts for the majority of morbidity and mortality for patients who survive to undergo treatment following aSAH. Angiographic vasospasm is observed in 30-70% of patients, occurring between days 5 and 14 following the ictus [6, 7]. Approximately 50% of patients with angiographic vasospasm will develop delayed ischemic neurologic deficit (DIND), with 15-20% of these patients suffering stroke or death despite maximal therapy [8, 9].

Methodology

In January 2010, we conducted a literature search of Medline, the Cochrane Controlled Trials Registry, and the National Institutes of Health/National Library of Medicine clinical trials registry. The following search terms were used: 'cerebral vasospasm,' or 'delayed cerebral ischemia,' or 'DIND,' with 'aneurysm' and 'SAH.' No limitation was applied to the publication date. Only articles written in English and enrolling at least 10 patients were included in the analysis. All articles were reviewed and classified into five categories:

- Meta-analysis.
- Randomized controlled trial (RCT).
- Randomized case series.
- Non-randomized case-control trial.
- Case series.

A detailed analysis of all meta-analyses and RCTs was performed. Studies examining different endpoints on the same patient cohort were excluded. Significant findings were defined as alpha values ≤0.05.

Triple-H therapy

Hypertension, hypervolemia, and hemodilution, also known as triple-H therapy, has been used since the early 1970s to prevent vasospasm and DIND following aSAH. The overall benefit of triple-H therapy is not clear, and this treatment may in fact pose

Table 1. Randomized controlled trials using triple-H therapy for vasospasm treatment.

Reference	n	Major findings
Rosenwasser et al, 1983 [13]	30	Reduced preoperative vasospasm in hypertensive patients treated with vasodilatory drugs compared with diuretics and volume restriction [a]
Lennihan et al, 2000 [12]	82	No reduction in vasospasm incidence with hypervolemic therapy vs. euvolemia
Egge et al, 2001 [11]	32	No reduction in vasospasm incidence for patients who received prophylactic triple-H therapy vs. normovolemic therapy

[a] = statistically significant

significant physiologic risks including myocardial infarction, pulmonary edema, cerebral edema, renal failure, and even potential rupture of additional intracranial aneurysms. The goal of triple-H therapy is to augment cerebral blood flow by expanding intravascular volume to increase leptomeningeal collateral perfusion, decreasing the viscosity of blood to improve hemodynamic flow, and counteracting elevated cerebrovascular resistance by increasing in-flow pressure. Triple-H therapy is not standardized, and varying parameters for goal blood pressures and hematocrit levels are found throughout the literature.

Sixteen studies of triple-H therapy following aSAH for the treatment or prevention of vasospasm were identified. These included one meta-analysis [10], three RCTs [11-13], one non-randomized case-control study [14], and 11 case series [15-25], for a total of 1,506 patients. Most case series reported improvement in either neurologic status or cerebral blood-flow measurements in patients undergoing triple-H therapy [15-17, 19-21, 23-25]. Significant complications directly attributable to aggressive triple-H therapy were cited in two case series, including pulmonary edema [18] and worsening intracranial edema with hemorrhagic transformation [22] **(III/B)**.

A retrospective, non-randomized case-control trial with 348 patients published by Vermeij et al in 1998 found significantly improved 3-month clinical outcomes for patients who received triple-H therapy (p=0.006) [14] **(III/B)**. Aneurysm rebleeding was more

likely to contribute to mortality in patients who received triple-H treatment relative to controls. The results of this study are difficult to interpret as many additional factors varied between the two cohorts, including use of tranexamic acid, management of hydrocephalus, and definitive aneurysm treatment.

Three RCTs were identified (Table 1). Rosenwasser et al reported a significant reduction in the incidence of preoperative vasospasm in 15 patients who were treated for hypertension using centrally acting drugs or vasodilators compared with 15 control patients who were managed using diuretics and volume restriction [13] **(Ib/A)**. Lennihan et al failed to observe a significant reduction in the incidence of symptomatic vasospasm among 82 patients who were randomized to receive hypervolemic therapy compared with euvolemia [12] **(Ib/A)**. Hypervolemic therapy increased cardiac filling pressures and fluid intake, but did not improve cerebral blood flow or blood volume. Glasgow Outcome Scale (GOS) scores were similar between the groups at 14 days and at 3-, 6-, and 12-month follow-up. Egge et al randomized 16 patients to prophylactic triple-H therapy and another 16 subjects to normovolemic therapy [11]. Triple-H therapy did not result in a significant difference in vasospasm rate, clinical outcomes, transcranial Doppler (TCD) velocities or single positron emission CT (SPECT) scanning compared with controls **(Ib/A)**. Triple-H therapy incurred increased costs and was associated with more frequent complications.

Table 2. Randomized controlled trials of calcium-channel blockers for vasospasm treatment.

Reference	n	Major findings
Nimodipine		
Allen *et al*, 1983 [30]	125	Reduced incidence of vasospasm in nimodipine-treated patients [a]
Neil-Dwyer *et al*, 1987 [34]	75	Reduced mortality at 3-month follow-up in nimodipine-treated patients [a]
Messeter *et al*, 1987 [33]	20	Improved carbon dioxide vessel reactivity and reduced DCI in nimodipine-treated patients
Jan *et al*, 1988 [31]	127	Reduced mortality from severe vasospasm in nimodipine-treated patients [a]
Petruk *et al*, 1988 [36]	154	Reduced incidence of delayed ischemic neurological deficit and improved clinical outcomes in nimodipine-treated patients [a]
Philippon *et al*, 1986 [37]	70	Reduced incidence of vasospasm-related neurologic deficits with a trend toward improved clinical outcomes in nimodipine-treated patients
Pickard *et al*, 1989 [38]	554	Reduced incidence of DCI in nimodipine-treated patients [a]
Ohman *et al*, 1991 [35]	213	Reduced incidence of DCI and vasospasm-related mortality in nimodipine-treated patients [a]
Karinen *et al*, 1999 [32]	127	Increased life expectancy with reduced 3-month mortality in nimodipine-treated patients [a]
Nicardipine		
Haley *et al*, 1993 [51]	906	Reduced vasospasm incidence, without improved clinical outcomes, for patients treated with IV nicardipine [a]
Barth *et al*, 2007 [50]	32	Reduced incidence of angiographic vasospasm, with improved 1-year clinical outcomes, in proximal intracranial arteries treated with nicardipine prolonged-release implants [a]

[a] = statistically significant; DCI = delayed cerebral infarction

One meta-analysis by Treggiari *et al* reviewed four prospective papers (two RCTs, one non-randomized case-control trial, and one case series) on triple-H therapy to prevent clinical vasospasm and DIND in 488 patients [10]. Compared with no preventative measures, triple-H therapy was associated with a significantly reduced risk of symptomatic vasospasm (relative risk [RR] 0.45; 95% confidence interval [CI], 0.32-0.65), but not DIND (RR 0.54; 95% CI, 0.2- 1.49) **(Ia/A)**. The mortality rate was significantly higher (RR 0.68; 95% CI, 0.53-0.87) for patients not receiving triple-H therapy.

Calcium-channel blockers

Calcium-channel blockers (CCB) decrease the influx of calcium into vascular smooth muscle cells, thereby reducing vasospasm. They may also possess neuroprotective properties. Numerous studies have analyzed the effects of various CCBs in the prevention and treatment of cerebral vasospasm. Four main CCBs have been identified:

- Nimodipine.
- Nicardipine.
- Nitroprusside.
- Verapamil.

Four meta-analyses have been performed [26-29], the most recent of which was published by Dorhout Mees *et al* in 2007 [27]. This study analyzed data from 16 RCTs involving 3,361 patients. Overall, CCBs reduced the risk of a poor outcome (RR 0.81; 95% CI, 0.72-0.92), with oral nimodipine being associated with the most significant reductions (RR 0.67; 95% CI, 0.55-0.82) **(Ia/A)**. A non-significant trend toward reduced secondary ischemia and fatality were also observed. The trials are reviewed by CCB below, with the results of influential RCTs highlighted and summarized in Table 2.

Nimodipine

Nimodipine is a dihydropyridine calcium antagonist that in 1989 gained US Food and Drug Administration approval for the treatment and prevention of vasospasm in patients with aSAH admitted in good neurologic condition (Hunt and Hess grades 1-3). We reviewed 19 studies that investigated the use of nimodipine: nine RCTs [30-38], two randomized case series [39, 40], one non-randomized case-control study [41], and seven case series [42-48], enrolling a total of 2,335 patients.

The results of the case series were varied and based largely on oral nimodipine dosing, although both intravenous (IV) [44, 47] and intra-arterial (IA) [49] administration were also used. Seiler *et al* observed a significant reduction in the severity of vasospasm on TCD studies without a reduction in vasospasm incidence [41] **(IIa/B)**. Gilsbach *et al* failed to find a difference in the incidence of DIND using two different IV nimodipine dosages [39] **(IIb/B)**. Kronvall *et al* observed no difference in the incidence of vasospasm, associated DIND, or clinical outcomes in a randomized non-controlled trial using both IV and oral nimodipine [40] **(IIb/B)**.

Oral nimodipine was administered in the majority of RCTs [30, 34, 36-38], while IV nimodipine was used in four trials [31-33, 35]. Allen *et al* illustrated a significant reduction in the incidence of symptomatic vasospasm for patients who received oral nimodipine compared with placebo [30] **(Ib/A)**. In the largest RCT, Pickard *et al* observed significant reductions in the incidence of cerebral infarction and poor clinical outcome in patients treated with oral nimodipine [38] **(Ib/A)**. IV nimodipine was found to be cost-effective by Karinen *et al*; patients who received the drug lived 3.46 years longer than controls, saving $223 (US$1996) per life-year gained [32] **(Ib/A)**.

Nicardipine

Nicardipine is a dihydropyridine calcium antagonist that possesses virtually equivalent pharmacologic activity to nimodipine. It is widely available in an IV formulation, which allows for drug titration in the event of iatrogenic hypotension or the need for induced hypertension. A total of 13 studies were included for analysis: two RCTs [50, 51], one randomized case series [52], two non-randomized case-control studies [53, 54], and eight case series [55-62], enrolling a total of 1,998 patients. One additional RCT was not included in our review because it analyzed different outcomes for patients included in another study [63].

Early case series used IV nicardipine with a relatively low incidence of symptomatic vasospasm and delayed cerebral infarction (DCI) [56, 57] **(III/B)**. Nicardipine prolonged-release implants (NPRI) placed at the time of aneurysm clipping to deliver low doses of nicardipine postoperatively showed promise in preventing vasospasm in more proximal rather than distal intracranial arteries [58, 59] **(III/B)**. Kasuya *et al* observed a non-significant reduction in the incidence of DIND for patients treated with NPRI (6%) compared with placebo (11%) in a non-randomized case-control trial [53] **(IIa/B)**. More recently, IA nicardipine was shown to dilate vessels in vasospasm and transiently improve neurologic deficits in several small case series [55, 60, 62] **(III/B)**. Haley *et al* failed to observe a difference in the incidence of symptomatic vasospasm and 3-month clinical outcomes for patients randomized to receive high- or low-dose IV nicardipine [52] **(IIb/B)**. Prophylactic intrathecal nicardipine infusion successfully reduced the incidence of symptomatic vasospasm by 26% and improved 30-day clinical outcomes by 15% in a non-randomized case-control trial, with two cases of meningitis reported in 50 treated patients [54] **(IIa/B)**.

The largest RCT using nicardipine to date was published by Haley *et al* in 1993 [51]. In this study, 449 patients treated with IV nicardipine had a significantly reduced incidence of vasospasm compared with 457 placebo-treated patients (32% vs. 46%; p<0.001), but clinical outcomes were similar among the cohorts at 3-month follow-up **(Ib/A)**. More recently, Barth *et al* showed benefit for 16 patients randomized to receive NPRI compared with 16 control patients [50] **(Ib/A)**. The treated patients had a significant reduction in angiographic vasospasm (p<0.05) as well as improved modified Rankin Scale scores at 1-year follow-up (p=0.0001).

Nitroprusside

Sodium nitroprusside is an inorganic compound that dissociates to form nitric oxide, thereby relaxing vascular smooth muscle cells and affecting vasodilation. Because of its relatively short half-life in the bloodstream, it has been used intrathecally in three studies, totaling 58 patients, for the prevention and treatment of vasospasm [64-66]. In a prospective, non-randomized case-control trial published in 2009, Agrawal *et al* administered sodium nitroprusside intrathecally to 10 patients and placebo to 10 controls [64]. TCD velocities and Glasgow Coma Scale scores improved for the treated patients during the trial period **(IIa/B)**. Intrathecal sodium nitroprusside has also shown anecdotal improvement in vasospasm and neurologic condition in two case series [65, 66] **(III/B)**.

Verapamil

Verapamil is an L-type CCB that has recently been used for the prevention and treatment of cerebral vasospasm. Four case series were identified [67-70], studying 66 patients. Because of the potential systemic effects of verapamil, IA administration was used in all of the studies. Two studies observed improvements in arterial diameter without significant side effects [68, 69], while one trial failed to show arterial diameter improvement following IA verapamil treatment [70] **(III/B)**. In the most recent study, continuous high-dose verapamil was administered to 12 patients with medically refractory vasospasm through indwelling microcatheters [67]. The treatment was effective, and only four vessels required balloon angioplasty **(III/B)**. No adverse complications occurred.

Fasudil

Fasudil, developed and studied in Japan as AT877, inhibits Rho kinase activity with the functional effect of a CCB. It antagonizes the vasoconstrictive effects of endothelin by dilating cerebral arteries in animal vasospasm models [71]. Fasudil has been studied in two RCTs [71, 72], one non-randomized case-control series [73], and six case series [74-79], for a total of 6,292 patients. Several studies have demonstrated prevention of cerebral vasospasm using IV fasudil [71-73, 75-77] or selective IA administration [74, 78, 79]. Nakashima *et al* observed a reduced incidence of cerebral vasospasm and DCI in patients who received combination IV fasudil and ozagrel (a thromboxane synthetase inhibitor) compared with IV ozagrel alone [73] **(IIa/B)**. In a large case series, patients who received IV fasudil alone (n=3,690), compared with those who received combination IV fasudil and ozagrel (n=1,138), had a significantly reduced incidence of symptomatic vasospasm and corresponding low-density areas on head CT (p<0.001) without a significant difference in clinical outcome [77] **(III/B)**.

Two RCTs have investigated fasudil for the treatment of vasospasm (Table 3). Shibuya *et al* reported an RCT of 267 patients [72]. IV fasudil was administered three times daily to 131 patients for 14 days following aSAH. Significant reductions in angiographic vasospasm (p=0.002), symptomatic vasospasm (p=0.025), and low-density areas on head CT (p=0.001) were observed for patients treated with fasudil compared with placebo **(Ib/A)**, and 1-month GOS scores were significantly improved (p=0.015).

Table 3. Randomized controlled trials using fasudil for vasospasm treatment.

Reference	n	Major findings
Shibuya *et al*, 1992 [72]	267	Reduced incidence of angiographic and symptomatic vasospasm, with improved 1-month clinical outcomes, for patients treated with fasudil [a]
Zhao *et al*, 2006 [71]	72	Reduced incidence of symptomatic vasospasm for patients treated with IV fasudil compared with IV nimodipine

[a] = statistically significant; IV = intravenous

Zhao *et al* compared fasudil with nimodipine for the prevention of vasospasm following aSAH [71]. Patients were randomized to receive IV fasudil three times daily (n=37) or continuous IV nimodipine infusion (n=35) for 14 days following aSAH. A non-significant reduction in symptomatic vasospasm was observed for patients who received fasudil compared with nimodipine (15.6% vs. 28.1%; p=0.125) **(Ib/A)**. No significant differences were observed in the incidence of DCI, angiographic vasospasm, or clinical outcome between the groups.

Papaverine

Papaverine is an alkaloid substance that induces vasodilation of the cerebral and coronary arteries through direct interactions on smooth muscle cells. Mechanistically, papaverine acts by inhibiting cyclic adenosine monophosphate and cyclic guanosine 3,5-monophosphate phosphodiesterase activity [80]. Fourteen publications studying 468 patients from 1986 to 2004 were identified: three non-randomized case-control studies [81-83] and 11 case series [84-94]. No RCT or meta-analyses were found.

Segawa *et al* used intracisternal papaverine twice daily to treat 15 patients with symptomatic vasospasm following aSAH, with good angiographic results [93] **(III/B)**. Clinical improvement occurred in seven patients, with one iatrogenic intracerebral hemorrhage. Kaku *et al* used combination balloon angioplasty and IA papaverine to successfully dilate vasospastic arteries in eight of 10 patients (80%), with corresponding neurologic improvement observed in four subjects [87]

(III/B). The first use of IA papaverine alone for the treatment of cerebral vasospasm was described by Kassell *et al* in 1992 [88]. Two-thirds of affected patients showed marked angiographic improvement following treatment, with clinical improvement occurring in four of 12 patients (33.3%) **(III/B)**. Multiple publications have described successful treatment of cerebral vasospasm using IA papaverine with good angiographic and clinical results [81, 82, 84-91, 93, 94]. Two studies, however, did not find clinical benefit following IA papaverine therapy [83, 92].

In a non-randomized case-control study, Dalbasti *et al* reported a significantly reduced incidence of symptomatic vasospasm and improved GOS scores in patients treated with papaverine controlled-release pellets implanted at the time of aneurysm clipping compared with controls (2.3% vs. 46.6%; p<0.001) [81] **(IIa/B)**.

Transluminal balloon angioplasty

Transluminal balloon angioplasty (TBA) for vasospasm has been reported in 26 publications from 1984 to 2008, enrolling 1,028 patients. Most of these (92%) are retrospective case series. Improvements in vessel diameters and neurologic deficits have been observed in most studies following TBA [95-117]. Successful treatment of vessels with TBA translated into a reduced incidence of DCI on radiographic imaging in several trials [97, 108, 110, 111, 115].

The temporal relationship between the onset of symptomatic vasospasm and TBA has been examined

Table 4. Randomized controlled trials using transluminal balloon angioplasty for vasospasm treatment.

Reference	n	Major findings
Zwienenberg-Lee *et al*, 2008 [117]	170	Patients treated with prophylactic TBA experienced a lower incidence of DIND (NS) and reduced need for therapeutic angioplasty [a]

[a] = statistically significant; NS = non-significant

by Rosenwasser *et al*, who observed a significant improvement in clinical outcome for patients who underwent TBA less than 2 hours from the time of symptomatic decline [113] **(III/B)**. Bejjani *et al* reported similar results for patients treated with TBA within 24 hours of neurologic decline [98] **(III/B)**. Several studies have compared TBA to IA papaverine or combination therapy. Lewis *et al* observed a significant improvement in TCD velocities and cerebral perfusion analyzed using SPECT imaging for vessels treated with TBA compared with IA papaverine [118] **(III/B)**. Three other trials failed to show any significant clinical benefit for patients managed with TBA compared with IA papaverine or combination therapy [109, 119, 120]. Complications of TBA, including vessel perforation [107, 110, 111, 117], hematoma formation [98], and death [110, 111, 117], have been described.

A multicenter RCT studying prophylactic TBA in the setting of aSAH was published by Zwienenberg-Lee in 2008 (Table 4) [117]. Eighty-five patients with Fisher grade III aSAH underwent prophylactic TBA within 96 hours of rupture. Target vessels were the bilateral A1, M1, P1, and the basilar artery, and the intradural segment of the dominant vertebral artery. Patients who underwent TBA had a lower incidence of DIND (p=0.30) **(Ib/A)**. A statistically significant reduction in the number of TBA-treated patients requiring therapeutic angioplasty was observed compared with controls (p=0.03), and a trend toward favorable 3-month clinical outcomes was observed for TBA-treated patients. Four patients suffered vessel perforations during TBA, resulting in three deaths. Before completion of the study, the treatment protocol was revised to exclude angioplasty of the bilateral A1 and P1 segments because of complications related to TBA in these vessels.

Thrombolytics

Intracisternal thrombolytic therapy to expedite the lysis and clearance of subarachnoid blood following aSAH has been used in the prevention and treatment of vasospasm. Both urokinase and tissue plasminogen activator (tPA) have been studied, often in combination with cerebrospinal fluid (CSF) drainage. Eighteen studies were identified enrolling a total of 1,201 patients: two RCTs [121, 122], six non-randomized case-control trials [123-128], and 10 case series [129-138]. One meta-analysis studying 652 patients was found [139], but included only one RCT. Twelve studies used tPA [121, 123-126, 129, 130, 132, 134, 136-138], while urokinase was used in five [122, 128, 131, 133, 135]. One non-randomized case-control trial studied both tPA and urokinase [127]. The majority of case series and non-randomized trials observed a low incidence of, or relative reduction in, vasospasm and DCI.

Two RCTs have been published using thrombolytics for the treatment of vasospasm (Table 5). Findlay *et al* randomized 100 patients to receive either 10mg intracisternal tPA (n=51) or placebo (n=49) at the time of surgical clipping [121]. A trend toward reduced vasospasm severity was observed in the tPA-treated patients. A 56% RR reduction of severe vasospasm was observed for patients with thick subarachnoid clot on admission head CT scanning who received tPA compared with placebo (p=0.02) **(Ib/A)**. Hamada *et al* reported a benefit of intrathecal urokinase infusion following coil embolization of ruptured intracranial aneurysms [122]. A total of 110 patients were randomized to receive intrathecal urokinase (60,000 IU over 20 minutes, n=53) or no adjuvant thrombolytic therapy (n=57) following aneurysm coiling. A significant reduction in

Table 5. Randomized controlled trials using thrombolytics for vasospasm treatment.

Reference	n	Major findings
Findlay et al, 1995 [121]	100	Reduced vasospasm severity in patients who received intracisternal tissue plasminogen activator (NS), with a significant reduction for patients with thick subarachnoid blood [a]
Hamada et al, 2003 [122]	110	Decreased vasospasm incidence and improved clinical outcomes in patients who received intrathecal urokinase [a]

[a] = statistically significant; NS = non-significant

the primary endpoint, symptomatic vasospasm, was observed in patients who received intrathecal urokinase therapy compared with controls (8.8% vs. 30.2%; p=0.012) **(Ib/A)**. The mortality rate was similar in each group, but a significant improvement in 6-month GOS scores was observed in urokinase-treated patients (p=0.036).

Cisternal drainage

CSF diversion has been analyzed in eight clinical studies enrolling 942 patients: five non-randomized case-control trials [140-144] and three case series [145-147]. Preliminary case series described an anecdotal reduction in vasospasm incidence when subarachnoid clot was evacuated acutely following aneurysm rupture [146, 147] **(III/B)**. Fenestration of the lamina terminalis and Liliequist membrane to achieve enhanced intraoperative CSF drainage showed benefit in a non-randomized case-control trial [141] **(IIa/B)**. Inagawa et al found a non-significant decrease in symptomatic vasospasm and associated DCI for patients treated with increased CSF drainage [145] **(III/B)**. Klimo et al observed a significant reduction in clinical vasospasm, need for balloon angioplasty, and DCI in 81 patients who received prolonged lumbar cisternal drainage compared with controls who had either no CSF diversion or CSF drainage using an external ventricular catheter [143] **(IIa/B)**. Head-shaking maneuvers have been combined with cisternal drainage in several studies, with significant reductions in symptomatic vasospasm and DCI [142] and improved long-term clinical outcomes [140] **(IIa/B)**.

Endothelin receptor antagonists

Endothelin 1 is a peptide that is believed to be the most potent and persistent vasoconstrictive agent discovered to date. Its activity is primarily mediated through selective endothelin A receptors found on vascular smooth muscle cells. Clazosentan, a non-peptide endothelin receptor A antagonist, and bosentan, which competitively inhibits both endothelin A and B receptors, have been investigated in several human trials. Five studies published from 2000 to 2008 were reviewed that used endothelin receptor antagonists in the treatment and prevention of cerebral vasospasm. Three RCTs (Table 6) [148-150] and one case series [151] were identified, studying 875 patients. One RCT [152] was excluded because it analyzed different outcomes in patients from a previously published trial.

Shaw et al published a large RCT that enrolled 420 patients [149]. A total of 207 patients were randomized to receive a 10-day course of an IV endothelin antagonist (TAK-044) while 213 patients received placebo. Although there was a trend toward decreased DIND at 3 months in TAK-044-treated patients (29.5% vs. 36.6%; RR 0.8; 95% CI, 0.61-1.06), no differences were seen in GOS scores **(Ib/A)**. Another RCT initially randomized 32 patients to receive a continuous IV clazosentan infusion (n=15) or placebo [150]. Six patients (40%) randomized to clazosentan and 15 patients (88%) in the placebo group suffered angiographic vasospasm during the study (p=0.008) **(Ib/A)**. The second part of the study allowed for cross-over between the placebo and study

Table 6. Randomized controlled trials using endothelin receptor antagonists for vasospasm treatment.

Reference	n	Major findings
Shaw et al, 2000 [149]	420	Decreased incidence of delayed ischemic events in patients treated with an endothelin receptor antagonist compared with placebo, with no improvement in clinical outcome
Vajkoczy et al, 2005 [150]	32	Reduced vasospasm incidence and severity in patients treated with an endothelin receptor antagonist [a]
Macdonald et al, 2008 [148]	413	Dose-dependent reduction in the incidence of moderate and severe angiographic vasospasm in patients treated with an endothelin receptor antagonist [a]

[a] = statistically significant

drug groups for patients with angiographically confirmed vasospasm. A total of 19 patients entered this part of the study (seven initially treated with clazosentan and 12 with placebo). Fifty percent of patients who crossed into the treatment arm experienced a reversal of vasospasm following treatment with the study drug. A trend toward a decreased rate of DCI was observed for patients initially randomized to receive clazosentan (15% vs. 44%; p=0.13). Macdonald et al published their results from the Clazosentan to Overcome Neurological Ischemia and Infarction Occurring after Subarachnoid Hemorrhage (CONSCIOUS-1) trial in 2008 [148]. This study randomized 413 patients to receive either dose-escalated clazosentan (n=313; 1, 5, or 15mg/hour dosing) or placebo (n=96). A statistically significant reduction in moderate and severe vasospasm was observed in patients who received high-dose clazosentan (15mg/hour) compared with placebo (RR 0.65; 95% CI, 0.47-0.78; p<0.0001) **(Ib/A)**. A non-significant reduction in the incidence of DIND and DCI was observed for patients who received the study drug compared with placebo. Clazosentan was associated with increased rates of pulmonary complications, hypotension, and anemia.

Magnesium

Magnesium, which has demonstrated success in the management of pre-eclampsia and eclampsia in obstetric patients, has been studied as a treatment for cerebral vasospasm. Magnesium is believed to act through multimodal mechanisms. Chemically functioning as a divalent cation, magnesium directly antagonizes voltage-dependent calcium channels, thereby preventing smooth muscle contraction. It also provides a neuroprotective benefit by inhibiting the release of glutamate and blocking N-methyl-D-aspartate receptors. Magnesium increases cardiac contractility, which may improve cerebral perfusion in the setting of cerebral dysautoregulation following aSAH.

A review of the literature yielded 13 studies published between 2000 and 2009 in which magnesium was used in the management of cerebral vasospasm following aSAH: one meta-analysis [153], five RCTs [154-158], two non-randomized case-control series [159, 160], and five case series [161-165], totaling 1,187 patients. Magnesium was typically administered IV [153-162, 165], although IA [164] and intracisternal [163] dosing were also utilized.

The results of the five small case series and two non-randomized case-control trials varied, but generally showed favorable radiographic and/or clinical responses to magnesium [159-165]. One randomized trial failed to show a benefit for IV magnesium over IV nimodipine in preventing vasospasm-induced DCI or improving clinical outcome [158] **(Ib/A)**. Four placebo-controlled RCTs were identified (Table 7). Veyna *et al* observed a non-significant trend toward reduced mean middle cerebral artery TCD velocities and improved GOS scores in patients treated with IV magnesium (n=20) compared with placebo (n=20) [156] **(Ib/A)**. The results from the Magnesium in Aneurysmal Subarachnoid Hemorrhage (MASH) trial, which enrolled 283 patients, were published in 2005 [155]. Patients who received continuous IV magnesium infusion had non-significant reductions of 34% for DCI (hazard ratio 0.66; 95% CI, 0.38-1.14) and 23% for poor clinical outcomes at 3 months (RR 0.77; 95% CI, 0.54-1.09) **(Ib/A)**. Wong *et al* reported a decreased incidence of symptomatic vasospasm in patients who received continuous IV magnesium infusion (n=30) compared with placebo (n=30) (43% vs. 23%; p=0.06), without an improvement in clinical outcome [157] **(Ib/A)**. A significant reduction in the duration of elevated TCD velocities was observed for the magnesium-treated patients (p<0.01). Muroi *et al* demonstrated improved clinical outcomes at 3 months based on actual treatment in patients who received IV magnesium infusion compared with control patients (p=0.17) [154] **(Ib/A)**. The incidences of iatrogenic hypocalcemia

(p=0.005) and hypotension (p=0.04) were significantly increased in patients who received magnesium.

A 2009 meta-analysis by Zhao *et al* revealed a statistically significant reduction in poor outcomes, including vegetative state and dependency (OR 0.54; 95% CI, 0.36-0.81), for patients who received magnesium therapy following aSAH, without a difference in mortality [153] **(Ia/A)**. The Phase III MASH II trial is currently underway, with a goal of randomizing 1,200 patients to receive either IV magnesium or placebo.

Statins

Hydroxymethylglutaryl coenzyme A reductase inhibitors, also known as statins, have been the focus of many recent research efforts for the prevention of vasospasm. Although initially developed as cholesterol-lowering agents, statins have been shown to reduce inflammation and cell proliferation, upregulate the production of

Table 7. Randomized controlled trials using magnesium for vasospasm treatment.

Reference	n	Major findings
Veyna *et al*, 2002 [156]	40	Magnesium-treated patients had improved middle cerebral artery transcranial Doppler velocities without a reduced incidence of symptomatic vasospasm
van den Bergh *et al*, 2005 [155]	283	IV magnesium reduced the risk of delayed cerebral ischemia and the 3-month risk of poor clinical outcome
Wong *et al*, 2006 [157]	60	Symptomatic vasospasm rates were reduced in patients who received IV magnesium compared with placebo
Schmid-Elsaesser *et al*, 2006 [158]	104	Similar cerebral infarction rates were observed for patients who received magnesium and those who received nimodipine, with no difference in clinical outcomes
Muroi *et al*, 2008 [154]	58	IV magnesium improved 3-month clinical outcomes based on actual treatment analysis compared with placebo, with higher incidences of hypotension and hypocalcemia in magnesium-treated patients [a]

[a] = statistically significant; IV = intravenous

Table 8. Randomized controlled trials using statins for vasospasm treatment.

Reference	n	Major findings
Tseng et al, 2005 [172]	80	Reduced incidence of vasospasm, delayed ischemic neurological deficit, and mortality in patients treated with statins compared with placebo [a]
Lynch et al, 2005 [170]	39	Reduced vasospasm incidence and highest middle cerebral artery TCD velocities in patients treated with statins [a]
McGirt et al, 2005 [171]	17	Reduced incidence of TCD-defined vasospasm in patients who received statins compared with placebo
Chou et al, 2008 [169]	39	No differences in vasospasm or cerebral infarction rates or clinical outcomes in patients treated with statins vs. placebo
Vergouwen et al, 2009 [173]	32	No differences in TCD velocities, clinical signs of delayed cerebral ischemia, or outcome in patients who received statins vs. placebo

[a] = statistically significant; NS = non-significant; TCD = transcranial Doppler

endothelial nitric oxide synthase, and inhibit thrombogenesis [166, 167].

A total of 13 clinical studies from 2005 to 2009 were identified, enrolling 2,040 patients. One meta-analysis [168], five RCTs (Table 8) [169-173], and seven case series [174-180] were analyzed. Tseng et al first described the beneficial effects of statin therapy in a Phase II RCT in 2005 [172]. Eighty patients with aSAH were randomized to receive 40mg oral pravastatin daily or placebo. Vasospasm incidence, measured by TCD, was reduced by 32% in patients who received statin therapy (p=0.006) **(Ib/A)**. The incidences of vasospasm-related DIND (p<0.001) and mortality (p=0.037) were also significantly reduced in the treatment group. Similar results were obtained by Lynch et al in a smaller RCT [170]. Only five of 19 patients (26.3%) who received high-dose oral simvastatin (80mg/day) compared with 12 of 20 placebo-treated patients (60%) developed vasospasm based on TCD velocities or cerebral angiography (p<0.05) **(Ib/A)**. McGirt et al observed a non-significant decreased incidence of TCD-defined vasospasm among nine patients who received statin therapy compared with eight placebo-treated patients [171] **(Ib/A)**. Serum surrogate markers of vascular and cerebral injury were significantly reduced in the statin

patients. Tseng et al further analyzed the effects of statin therapy on cerebral autoregulation [181], long-term patient outcomes [182], and biological markers [183] following aSAH in three additional publications, which detailed different outcome measures for the patients enrolled in the initial 2005 report. The 2007 report by Tseng et al provides the most extensive long-term clinical follow-up for patients treated with statins [182]. In this study, patients given statins were found to have non-significantly improved 6-month modified Rankin Scale and Short Form-36 scores compared with placebo-treated patients **(Ib/A)**.

Chou et al randomized 39 adult patients with Fisher grade 3 aSAH to receive 80mg of oral daily simvastatin or placebo [169]. Angiographically confirmed vasospasm occurred in five of 19 simvastatin-treated patients (26.3%) and eight of 20 patients (40%) who received placebo. Vasospasm-induced DCI developed in two of 19 study patients (10.5%) and five of 20 controls (25%). A trend toward decreased vasospasm incidence and DIND was observed **(Ib/A)**. In the study by Vergouwen et al, 32 patients were randomized to receive either 80mg of oral daily simvastatin or placebo for 14 days following aSAH. This study failed to find a significant reduction in vasospasm incidence, DCI, or poor

Chapter 31

clinical outcomes for patients who received statin therapy [173] **(Ib/A)**. Twelve of 16 active-treatment patients (75%) and 11 of 16 control patients (68.8%) developed vasospasm during the trial, defined using TCD parameters. No significant clinical differences in GOS scores were observed between the groups at 3 and 6 months' follow-up.

A 2008 meta-analysis of three RCTs enrolling a total of 158 patients described a statistically significant reduction in vasospasm incidence (RR 0.73; 95% CI, 0.54-0.99), DIND (RR 0.38; 95% CI, 0.17-0.83), and mortality (RR 0.22; 95% CI, 0.06-0.82) for patients treated with statins following aSAH [168] **(Ia/A)**. The results of this meta-analysis may be biased by potential variability among the included trials regarding the definition of TCD-diagnosed vasospasm.

Tirilazad

Tirilazad mesylate is a non-glucocorticoid aminosteroid that inhibits lipid peroxidation,

functioning as a free-radical scavenger. It has been shown to have neuroprotective effects in experimental stroke and aSAH models.

Five RCTs enrolling a total of 3,799 patients (Table 9) [184-188] and one meta-analysis [189] were identified in the literature. Haley *et al* published an initial Phase II dose-escalation study on 245 patients in 1995 [184]. A trend toward improved 3-month clinical outcomes was observed in patients who received 2mg/kg/day tirilazad compared with controls **(Ib/A)**, but there was no significant difference in symptomatic vasospasm incidence between the two groups. Results from the cooperative tirilazad trial in Europe, Australia, and New Zealand, which enrolled 1,023 patients, were first detailed in 1996 [186]. Patients who were randomized to receive high-dose tirilazad (6mg/kg/day) had significantly reduced overall mortality and improved 3-month clinical outcomes compared with those randomized to placebo (p=0.01) **(Ib/A)**. The improved outcomes, however, were probably not secondary to prevention of vasospasm as a non-statistically significant reduction in symptomatic vasospasm was observed in the high-

Table 9. Randomized controlled trials using tirilazad for vasospasm treatment.

Reference	n	Major findings
Haley *et al*, 1995 [184]	245	Improved 3-month outcomes for patients treated with tirilazad compared with placebo
Kassell *et al*, 1996 [186]	1,023	Moderate reduction in vasospasm incidence for patients treated with tirilazad compared with placebo (NS); decreased mortality rates for patients treated with high-dose tirilazad, with improved 3-month clinical outcomes [a]
Haley *et al*, 1997 [185]	897	No improvement in mortality rates, 3-month clinical outcome, or employment status in patients treated with tirilazad vs. placebo
Lanzino *et al*, 1999 [188]	819	Reduced rates of symptomatic vasospasm, cerebral infarction, and need for triple-H therapy in patients treated with tirilazad vs. placebo[a]; no differences in 3-month mortality rate or clinical outcome were observed
Lanzino *et al*, 1999 [187]	823	Reduced mortality rates in patients who presented in poor clinical status treated with high-dose tirilazad vs. placebo[a]; no differences in symptomatic vasospasm incidence or severity were observed

[a] = statistically significant; NS = non-significant

dose tirilazad patients. Male patients seemed to derive more benefit from the study drug than females. In the North American multicenter cooperative tirilazad trial, 897 patients were randomized to receive low- (2mg/kg/day) or high-dose (6mg/kg/day) tirilazad or placebo [185]. Symptomatic vasospasm occurred in 88 of 298 patients (29.5%) in the low-dose group, 98 of 299 patients (32.8%) in the high-dose group, and 100 of 300 controls (33%) **(Ib/A)**. The incidence of DCI and neurologic decline was actually lower in the placebo arm, and no significant difference in 3-month GOS scores was observed between the groups.

The last two RCTs using tirilazad studied female subjects only using a higher dosage of the medication (15mg/kg/day) to potentially counteract any physiologic differences in drug metabolism. A cooperative study published in 1999 randomized 819 women patients to tirilazad (n=405) or placebo (n=414) at 56 centers in Europe, Australia, New Zealand, and South Africa [188]. A significant reduction in symptomatic vasospasm was observed in tirilazad-compared with placebo-treated patients (33.7% vs. 24.8%; p=0.005) **(Ib/A)**. The incidence of DCI was also significantly reduced in patients who received tirilazad compared with placebo (8% vs. 13%; p<0.04). However, no significant difference was observed for the 3-month mortality rate, the primary endpoint of the trial. A similar study was conducted with 823 women with aSAH in North America [187]. No significant differences in symptomatic vasospasm, vasospasm severity, or clinical outcome were observed between the study groups **(Ib/A)**, although mortality rates were significantly reduced in patients with poor admission World Federation of Neurological Surgeons (WFNS) grades (IV/V) who received tirilazad compared with placebo (p=0.016). Patients with good admission WFNS grades (I, II, or III) who received placebo actually had significantly better 3-month clinical outcomes than those who received tirilazad (p=0.04).

A 2009 meta-analysis by Jang et al analyzed all five RCTs using tirilazad [189]. This study found a significant reduction in symptomatic vasospasm for patients treated with tirilazad compared with placebo (OR 0.80; 95% CI, 0.69-0.93), although a significant reduction in unfavorable clinical outcomes was not observed **(Ia/A)**. On subset analyses, no significant benefit was conferred to patients based on sex or admission WFNS grade.

Miscellaneous

Multiple additional therapies outside the scope of this review have been studied for the prevention and treatment of cerebral vasospasm. Nine RCTs were identified. Suzuki et al observed a significant reduction in vasospasm incidence for patients treated with a thromboxane synthetase inhibitor compared with placebo [190] **(Ib/A)**. Tsementzis et al found increased mortality and reduced cerebral blood flow for patients treated with tranexamic acid, an antifibrinolytic agent, compared with control patients [191] **(Ib/A)**. Free-radical scavenger and antioxidant agents have been demonstrated to improve clinical outcome while reducing vasospasm incidence and severity in several RCTs [192-194] **(Ib/A)**. Wurm et al observed a significant reduction in vasospasm-induced DCI with associated improved 1-month clinical outcomes for patients treated with low-molecular-weight enoxaparin compared with placebo [195] **(Ib/A)**. These results were not supported by a study by Siironen et al, which failed to demonstrate clinical benefit for patients treated with enoxaparin [196] **(Ib/A)**. In 2009, IV erythropoietin was reported to significantly reduce vasospasm severity and associated DCI with improved neurologic outcomes at the time of discharge compared with placebo [197] **(Ib/A)**. However, a previous study by Springborg et al failed to find a clinical benefit for patients who received erythropoietin compared with placebo [198] **(Ib/A)**.

Conclusions

The evidence suggests that cerebral vasospasm following aSAH can be prevented or treated with the routine use of oral nimodipine. Other CCBs, triple-H therapy, fasudil, thrombolytics, cisternal drainage, endothelin receptor antagonists, magnesium, and statins may provide benefit but require additional study. Rescue therapy using TBA and IA vasodilatory agents should be considered in cases of refractory symptomatic vasospasm, but limited information is

Table 10. Evidence-based recommendations for vasospasm treatment.

Treatment	Recommendation	Evidence level/ recommendation
Triple-H	Triple-H therapy should be used judiciously in patients with symptomatic vasospasm. Its effectiveness has not been demonstrated in any single large RCT, but it was found to reduce the incidence of symptomatic vasospasm and mortality in one meta-analysis. Prophylactic triple-H therapy is not recommended.	Ia/A
CCBs	Oral nimodipine effectively improves clinical outcomes by reducing the incidence of secondary cerebral ischemia and should be routinely used in the treatment and prevention of vasospasm. Other CCBs, including nicardipine, may also provide benefit.	Ia/A
Fasudil	Fasudil may reduce the incidence of vasospasm and improves clinical outcomes following aneurysmal SAH, but is not superior to CCBs.	Ib/A
Papaverine	Papaverine may be considered for the treatment of symptomatic vasospasm as it has been shown to dilate vessels in vasospasm. It is unclear whether papaverine improves clinical outcomes, as it has never been studied in an RCT.	IIa/B
TBA	TBA may provide more durable treatment of symptomatic vasospasm than intra-arterial medications, but should be used cautiously because of potential risks of arterial rupture and dissection. Prophylactic TBA is not recommended, although it has been shown to reduce the need for therapeutic angioplasty in one RCT.	Ib/A
Thrombolytics	Intrathecal thrombolytics can be considered for the prevention of cerebral vasospasm. Thrombolytics have been shown to reduce the incidence of vasospasm and improve clinical outcomes in two small RCTs.	Ib/A
Cisternal drainage	Cisternal drainage can be considered to treat associated hydrocephalus following aneurysmal SAH. No recommendations can be made regarding cisternal drainage and cerebral vasospasm, as this question has not been analyzed in any RCT.	IIa/B
Endothelin receptor antagonists	Endothelin receptor antagonists have been shown to reduce vasospasm severity, but not to improve clinical outcomes.	Ib/A
Magnesium	The routine use of magnesium can be considered, as it appears to have a neuroprotective benefit that may confer improved clinical outcomes.	Ia/A
Statins	Statins can be considered as they appear to reduce the incidence of symptomatic vasospasm and delayed ischemic neurologic deficit. Statins may improve clinical outcomes, although several RCTs have failed to identify a long-term benefit compared with placebo.	Ia/A
Tirilazad	The routine use of tirilazad is not recommended for the treatment of cerebral vasospasm as it has not been shown to improve clinical outcomes in several large RCTs.	Ia/A

CCB = calcium-channel blocker; RCT = randomized controlled trial; SAH = subarachnoid hemorrhage; TBA = transluminal balloon angioplasty

available from prospective RCTs. There is not enough evidence to support the use of tirilazad for the prevention or treatment of cerebral vasospasm. Table 10 summarizes the various treatment modalities for cerebral vasospasm.

Recommendations	Evidence level

♦ Triple-H therapy should be initiated in patients with symptomatic vasospasm, although its effectiveness has not been shown in a large RCT. — Ia/A

♦ Nimodipine is the only CCB demonstrated to improve clinical outcomes in the treatment of cerebral vasospasm. — Ia/A

♦ Fasudil may reduce vasospasm and improves clinic outcomes following vasospasm. — Ib/A

♦ Papaverine has not been shown to improve clinical outcomes in the treatment of symptomatic vasospasm in randomized trials. Conflicting evidence regarding its clinical utility exists in the literature. Papaverine has been shown to effectively dilate vessels in vasospasm. — IIa/B

♦ Prophylactic TBA reduced the need for therapeutic angioplasty for vasospasm in one RCT, but carries significant iatrogenic risk. — Ib/A

♦ Thrombolytics may reduce vasospasm incidence and improve clinical outcomes following aSAH. — Ib/A

♦ Cisternal drainage has unclear effects on cerebral vasospasm following aSAH. — IIa/B

♦ Endothelin receptor antagonists reduce vasospasm severity, but do not improve overall clinical outcomes. — Ib/A

♦ Magnesium may improve clinical outcomes following aSAH. — Ia/A

♦ The effect of statins on the incidence of symptomatic vasospasm and DIND is unclear due to mixed clinical outcomes in studies. — Ia/A

♦ Tirilazad should not be used as prophylaxis for vasospasm as it has failed to demonstrate improved clinical outcomes in several large RCTs. — Ia/A

References

1. King JT Jr. Epidemiology of aneurysmal subarachnoid hemorrhage. *Neuroimaging Clin N Am* 1997; 7(4): 659-68.

2. Inagawa T, Takechi A, Yahara K, *et al*. Primary intracerebral and aneurysmal subarachnoid hemorrhage in Izumo City, Japan. Part I: incidence and seasonal and diurnal variations. *J Neurosurg* 2000; 93(6): 958-66.

3. Ingall T, Asplund K, Mahonen M, Bonita R. A multinational comparison of subarachnoid hemorrhage epidemiology in the WHO MONICA stroke study. *Stroke* 2000; 31(5): 1054-61.

4. Hop JW, Rinkel GJ, Algra A, van Gijn J. Case-fatality rates and functional outcome after subarachnoid hemorrhage: a systematic review. *Stroke* 1997; 28(3): 660-4.

5. Stegmayr B, Eriksson M, Asplund K. Declining mortality from subarachnoid hemorrhage: changes in incidence and case fatality from 1985 through 2000. *Stroke* 2004; 35(9): 2059-63.

6. Fisher CM, Roberson GH, Ojemann RG. Cerebral vasospasm with ruptured saccular aneurysm - the clinical manifestations. *Neurosurgery* 1977; 1(3): 245-8.

7. Heros RC, Zervas NT, Varsos V. Cerebral vasospasm after subarachnoid hemorrhage: an update. *Ann Neurol* 1983; 14(6): 599-608.

8. Haley EC Jr, Kassell NF, Torner JC. The International Cooperative Study on the Timing of Aneurysm Surgery. The North American experience. *Stroke* 1992; 23(2): 205-14.

9. Longstreth WT Jr, Nelson LM, Koepsell TD, van Belle G. Clinical course of spontaneous subarachnoid hemorrhage: a population-based study in King County, Washington. *Neurology* 1993; 43(4): 712-8.

10. Treggiari MM, Walder B, Suter PM, Romand JA. Systematic review of the prevention of delayed ischemic neurological deficits with hypertension, hypervolemia, and hemodilution therapy following subarachnoid hemorrhage. *J Neurosurg* 2003; 98(5): 978-84.

11. Egge A, Waterloo K, Sjoholm H, Solberg T, Ingebrigtsen T, Romner B. Prophylactic hyperdynamic postoperative fluid therapy after aneurysmal subarachnoid hemorrhage: a clinical, prospective, randomized, controlled study. *Neurosurgery* 2001; 49(3): 593-605; discussion 605-6.

12. Lennihan L, Mayer SA, Fink ME, *et al*. Effect of hypervolemic therapy on cerebral blood flow after subarachnoid

hemorrhage: a randomized controlled trial. *Stroke* 2000;
31(2): 383-91.

13. Rosenwasser RH, Delgado TE, Buchheit WA, Freed MH.
Control of hypertension and prophylaxis against vasospasm in
cases of subarachnoid hemorrhage: a preliminary report.
Neurosurgery 1983; 12(6): 658-61.

14. Vermeij FH, Hasan D, Bijvoet HW, Avezaat CJ. Impact of
medical treatment on the outcome of patients after
aneurysmal subarachnoid hemorrhage. *Stroke* 1998; 29(5):
924-30.

15. Awad IA, Carter LP, Spetzler RF, Medina M, Williams FC Jr.
Clinical vasospasm after subarachnoid hemorrhage:
response to hypervolemic hemodilution and arterial
hypertension. *Stroke* 1987; 18(2): 365-72.

16. Darby JM, Yonas H, Marks EC, Durham S, Snyder RW,
Nemoto EM. Acute cerebral blood flow response to
dopamine-induced hypertension after subarachnoid
hemorrhage. *J Neurosurg* 1994; 80(5): 857-64.

17. Hadeishi H, Mizuno M, Suzuki A, Yasui N. Hyperdynamic
therapy for cerebral vasospasm. *Neurol Med Chir* (Tokyo)
1990; 30(5): 317-23.

18. Medlock MD, Dulebohn SC, Elwood PW. Prophylactic
hypervolemia without calcium channel blockers in early
aneurysm surgery. *Neurosurgery* 1992; 30(1): 12-6.

19. Origitano TC, Wascher TM, Reichman OH, Anderson DE.
Sustained increased cerebral blood flow with prophylactic
hypertensive hypervolemic hemodilution ('triple-H' therapy)
after subarachnoid hemorrhage. *Neurosurgery* 1990; 27(5):
729-39; discussion 739-40.

20. Otsubo H, Takemae T, Inoue T, Kobayashi S, Sugita K.
Normovolaemic induced hypertension therapy for cerebral
vasospasm after subarachnoid haemorrhage. *Acta Neurochir*
(Wien) 1990; 103(1-2): 18-26.

21. Raabe A, Beck J, Keller M, Vatter H, Zimmermann M, Seifert
V. Relative importance of hypertension compared with
hypervolemia for increasing cerebral oxygenation in patients
with cerebral vasospasm after subarachnoid hemorrhage. *J
Neurosurg* 2005; 103(6): 974-81.

22. Shimoda M, Oda S, Tsugane R, Sato O. Intracranial
complications of hypervolemic therapy in patients with a
delayed ischemic deficit attributed to vasospasm. *J
Neurosurg* 1993; 78(3): 423-9.

23. Solomon RA, Fink ME, Lennihan L. Early aneurysm surgery
and prophylactic hypervolemic hypertensive therapy for the
treatment of aneurysmal subarachnoid hemorrhage.
Neurosurgery 1988; 23(6): 699-704.

24. Tanabe T, Saitoh T, Tachibana S, Takagi H, Yada K. Effect of
hyperdynamic therapy on cerebral ischaemia caused by
vasospasm associated with subarachnoid haemorrhage. *Acta
Neurochir* (Wien) 1982; 63(1-4): 291-6.

25. Yano K, Kuroda T, Tanabe Y, Yamada H. Preventive therapy
against delayed cerebral ischaemia after aneurysmal
subarachnoid haemorrhage: trials of thromboxane A2
synthetase inhibitor and hyperdynamic therapy. *Acta
Neurochir* (Wien) 1993; 125(1-4): 15-9.

26. Barker FG, 2nd, Ogilvy CS. Efficacy of prophylactic
nimodipine for delayed ischemic deficit after subarachnoid

hemorrhage: a meta-analysis. *J Neurosurg* 1996; 84(3): 405-
14.

27. Dorhout Mees SM, Rinkel GJ, Feigin VL, *et al.* Calcium
antagonists for aneurysmal subarachnoid haemorrhage.
Cochrane Database Syst Rev 2007; 3: CD000277.

28. Feigin VL, Rinkel GJ, Algra A, Vermeulen M, van Gijn J.
Calcium antagonists in patients with aneurysmal
subarachnoid hemorrhage: a systematic review. *Neurology*
1998; 50(4): 876-83.

29. Rinkel GJ, Feigin VL, Algra A, van den Bergh WM, Vermeulen
M, van Gijn J. Calcium antagonists for aneurysmal
subarachnoid haemorrhage. *Cochrane Database Syst Rev*
2005; 1: CD000277.

30. Allen GS, Ahn HS, Preziosi TJ, *et al.* Cerebral arterial spasm
- a controlled trial of nimodipine in patients with subarachnoid
hemorrhage. *N Engl J Med* 1983; 308(11): 619-24.

31. Jan M, Buchheit F, Tremoulet M. Therapeutic trial of
intravenous nimodipine in patients with established cerebral
vasospasm after rupture of intracranial aneurysms.
Neurosurgery 1988; 23(2): 154-7.

32. Karinen P, Koivukangas P, Ohinmaa A, Koivukangas J,
Ohman J. Cost-effectiveness analysis of nimodipine treatment
after aneurysmal subarachnoid hemorrhage and surgery.
Neurosurgery 1999; 45(4): 780-4; discussion 784-5.

33. Messeter K, Brandt L, Ljunggren B, *et al.* Prediction and
prevention of delayed ischemic dysfunction after aneurysmal
subarachnoid hemorrhage and early operation. *Neurosurgery*
1987; 20(4): 548-53.

34. Neil-Dwyer G, Mee E, Dorrance D, Lowe D. Early intervention
with nimodipine in subarachnoid haemorrhage. *Eur Heart J*
1987; 8 (Suppl. K): 41-7.

35. Ohman J, Servo A, Heiskanen O. Long-term effects of
nimodipine on cerebral infarcts and outcome after aneurysmal
subarachnoid hemorrhage and surgery. *J Neurosurg* 1991;
74(1): 8-13.

36. Petruk KC, West M, Mohr G, *et al.* Nimodipine treatment in
poor-grade aneurysm patients. Results of a multicenter
double-blind placebo-controlled trial. *J Neurosurg* 1988;
68(4): 505-17.

37. Philippon J, Grob R, Dagreou F, Guggiari M, Rivierez M, Viars
P. Prevention of vasospasm in subarachnoid haemorrhage. A
controlled study with nimodipine. *Acta Neurochir* (Wien)
1986; 82(3-4): 110-4.

38. Pickard JD, Murray GD, Illingworth R, *et al.* Effect of oral
nimodipine on cerebral infarction and outcome after
subarachnoid haemorrhage: British aneurysm nimodipine
trial. *BMJ* 1989; 298(6674): 636-42.

39. Gilsbach JM, Reulen HJ, Ljunggren B, *et al.* Early aneurysm
surgery and preventive therapy with intravenously
administered nimodipine: a multicenter, double-blind, dose-
comparison study. *Neurosurgery* 1990; 26(3): 458-64.

40. Kronvall E, Undren P, Romner B, Saveland H, Cronqvist M,
Nilsson OG. Nimodipine in aneurysmal subarachnoid
hemorrhage: a randomized study of intravenous or peroral
administration. *J Neurosurg* 2009; 110(1): 58-63.

41. Seiler RW, Grolimund P, Zurbruegg HR. Evaluation of the
calcium-antagonist nimodipine for the prevention of

Chapter 31

vasospasm after aneurysmal subarachnoid haemorrhage. A prospective transcranial Doppler ultrasound study. *Acta Neurochir* (Wien) 1987; 85(1-2): 7-16.

42. Auer LM. Acute operation and preventive nimodipine improve outcome in patients with ruptured cerebral aneurysms. *Neurosurgery* 1984; 15(1): 57-66.

43. Biondi A, Ricciardi GK, Puybasset L, *et al.* Intra-arterial nimodipine for the treatment of symptomatic cerebral vasospasm after aneurysmal subarachnoid hemorrhage: preliminary results. *AJNR Am J Neuroradiol* 2004; 25(6): 1067-76.

44. Grotenhuis JA, Bettag W. Prevention of symptomatic vasospasm after SAH by constant venous infusion of nimodipine. *Neurol Res* 1986; 8(4): 243-9.

45. Hanggi D, Beseoglu K, Turowski B, Steiger HJ. Feasibility and safety of intrathecal nimodipine on posthaemorrhagic cerebral vasospasm refractory to medical and endovascular therapy. *Clin Neurol Neurosurg* 2008; 110(8): 784-90.

46. Kazner E, Sprung C, Adelt D, *et al.* Clinical experience with nimodipine in the prophylaxis of neurological deficits after subarachnoid hemorrhage. *Neurochirurgia* (Stuttg) 1985; 28 (Suppl. 1): 110-3.

47. Koos WT, Perneczky A, Auer LM, *et al.* Nimodipine treatment of ischemic neurological deficits due to cerebral vasospasm after subarachnoid hemorrhage. Clinical results of a multicenter study. *Neurochirurgia* (Stuttg) 1985; 28 (Suppl. 1): 114-7.

48. Saveland H, Ljunggren B, Brandt L, Messeter K. Delayed ischemic deterioration in patients with early aneurysm operation and intravenous nimodipine. *Neurosurgery* 1986; 18(2): 146-50.

49. Hanggi D, Turowski B, Beseoglu K, Yong M, Steiger HJ. Intra-arterial nimodipine for severe cerebral vasospasm after aneurysmal subarachnoid hemorrhage: influence on clinical course and cerebral perfusion. *AJNR Am J Neuroradiol* 2008; 29(6): 1053-60.

50. Barth M, Capelle HH, Weidauer S, *et al.* Effect of nicardipine prolonged-release implants on cerebral vasospasm and clinical outcome after severe aneurysmal subarachnoid hemorrhage: a prospective, randomized, double-blind Phase IIa study. *Stroke* 2007; 38(2): 330-6.

51. Haley EC Jr, Kassell NF, Torner JC. A randomized controlled trial of high-dose intravenous nicardipine in aneurysmal subarachnoid hemorrhage. A report of the Cooperative Aneurysm Study. *J Neurosurg* 1993; 78(4): 537-47.

52. Haley EC Jr, Kassell NF, Torner JC, Truskowski LL, Germanson TP. A randomized trial of two doses of nicardipine in aneurysmal subarachnoid hemorrhage. A report of the Cooperative Aneurysm Study. *J Neurosurg* 1994; 80(5): 788-96.

53. Kasuya H, Onda H, Sasahara A, Takeshita M, Hori T. Application of nicardipine prolonged-release implants: analysis of 97 consecutive patients with acute subarachnoid hemorrhage. *Neurosurgery* 2005; 56(5): 895-902.

54. Shibuya M, Suzuki Y, Enomoto H, Okada T, Ogura K, Sugita K. Effects of prophylactic intrathecal administrations of nicardipine on vasospasm in patients with severe aneurysmal

subarachnoid haemorrhage. *Acta Neurochir* (Wien) 1994; 131(1-2): 19-25.

55. Badjatia N, Topcuoglu MA, Pryor JC, *et al.* Preliminary experience with intra-arterial nicardipine as a treatment for cerebral vasospasm. *AJNR Am J Neuroradiol* 2004; 25(5): 819-26.

56. Beck DW, Adams HP, Flamm ES, Godersky JC, Loftus CM. Combination of aminocaproic acid and nicardipine in treatment of aneurysmal subarachnoid hemorrhage. *Stroke* 1988; 19(1): 63-7.

57. Flamm ES, Adams HP Jr, Beck DW, *et al.* Dose-escalation study of intravenous nicardipine in patients with aneurysmal subarachnoid hemorrhage. *J Neurosurg* 1988; 68(3): 393-400.

58. Kasuya H, Onda H, Takeshita M, Okada Y, Hori T. Efficacy and safety of nicardipine prolonged-release implants for preventing vasospasm in humans. *Stroke* 2002; 33(4): 1011-5.

59. Krischek B, Kasuya H, Onda H, Hori T. Nicardipine prolonged-release implants for preventing cerebral vasospasm after subarachnoid hemorrhage: effect and outcome in the first 100 patients. *Neurol Med Chir* (Tokyo) 2007; 47(9): 389-94; discussion 394-6.

60. Linfante I, Delgado-Mederos R, Andreone V, Gounis M, Hendricks L, Wakhloo AK. Angiographic and hemodynamic effect of high concentration of intra-arterial nicardipine in cerebral vasospasm. *Neurosurgery* 2008; 63(6): 1080-6; discussion 1086-7.

61. Suzuki M, Doi M, Otawara Y, Ogasawara K, Ogawa A. Intrathecal administration of nicardipine hydrochloride to prevent vasospasm in patients with subarachnoid hemorrhage. *Neurosurg Rev* 2001; 24(4): 180-4.

62. Tejada JG, Taylor RA, Ugurel MS, Hayakawa M, Lee SK, Chaloupka JC. Safety and feasibility of intra-arterial nicardipine for the treatment of subarachnoid hemorrhage-associated vasospasm: initial clinical experience with high-dose infusions. *AJNR Am J Neuroradiol* 2007; 28(5): 844-8.

63. Haley EC Jr, Kassell NF, Torner JC. A randomized trial of nicardipine in subarachnoid hemorrhage: angiographic and transcranial Doppler ultrasound results. A report of the Cooperative Aneurysm Study. *J Neurosurg* 1993; 78(4): 548-53.

64. Agrawal A, Patir R, Kato Y, Chopra S, Sano H, Kanno T. Role of intraventricular sodium nitroprusside in vasospasm secondary to aneurysmal subarachnoid haemorrhage: a 5-year prospective study with review of the literature. *Minim Invasive Neurosurg* 2009; 52(1): 5-8.

65. Pachl J, Haninec P, Tencer T, *et al.* The effect of subarachnoid sodium nitroprusside on the prevention of vasospasm in subarachnoid haemorrhage. *Acta Neurochir* Suppl 2005; 95: 141-5.

66. Thomas JE, Rosenwasser RH, Armonda RA, Harrop J, Mitchell W, Galaria I. Safety of intrathecal sodium nitroprusside for the treatment and prevention of refractory cerebral vasospasm and ischemia in humans. *Stroke* 1999; 30(7): 1409-16.

67. Albanese E, Russo A, Quiroga M, Willis RN, Mericle RA, Ulm AJ. Ultrahigh-dose intraarterial infusion of verapamil through

an indwelling microcatheter for medically refractory severe vasospasm: initial experience. *J Neurosurg* 2010; 113(4): 913-22.

68. Feng L, Fitzsimmons BF, Young WL, *et al*. Intraarterially administered verapamil as adjunct therapy for cerebral vasospasm: safety and 2-year experience. *AJNR Am J Neuroradiol* 2002; 23(8): 1284-90.

69. Keuskamp J, Murali R, Chao KH. High-dose intraarterial verapamil in the treatment of cerebral vasospasm after aneurysmal subarachnoid hemorrhage. *J Neurosurg* 2008; 108(3): 458-63.

70. Mazumdar A, Rivet DJ, Derdeyn CP, Cross DT, 3rd, Moran CJ. Effect of intraarterial verapamil on the diameter of vasospastic intracranial arteries in patients with cerebral vasospasm. *Neurosurg Focus* 2006; 21(3): E15.

71. Zhao J, Zhou D, Guo J, *et al*. Effect of fasudil hydrochloride, a protein kinase inhibitor, on cerebral vasospasm and delayed cerebral ischemic symptoms after aneurysmal subarachnoid hemorrhage. *Neurol Med Chir* (Tokyo) 2006; 46(9): 421-8.

72. Shibuya M, Suzuki Y, Sugita K, *et al*. Effect of AT877 on cerebral vasospasm after aneurysmal subarachnoid hemorrhage. Results of a prospective placebo-controlled double-blind trial. *J Neurosurg* 1992; 76(4): 571-7.

73. Nakashima S, Tabuchi K, Shimokawa S, Fukuyama K, Mineta T, Abe M. Combination therapy of fasudil hydrochloride and ozagrel sodium for cerebral vasospasm following aneurysmal subarachnoid hemorrhage. *Neurol Med Chir* (Tokyo) 1998; 38(12): 805-10; discussion 810-1.

74. Iwabuchi S, Yokouchi T, Hayashi M, Uehara H, Ueda M, Samejima H. Intra-arterial administration of fasudil hydrochloride for vasospasm following subarachnoid hemorrhage - analysis of time-density curve with digital subtraction angiography. *Neurol Med Chir* (Tokyo) 2006; 46(11): 535-9; discussion 540.

75. Shibuya M, Suzuki Y, Sugita K, *et al*. Dose escalation trial of a novel calcium antagonist, AT877, in patients with aneurysmal subarachnoid haemorrhage. *Acta Neurochir* (Wien) 1990; 107(1-2): 11-5.

76. Suzuki Y, Shibuya M, Satoh S, Sugimoto Y, Takakura K. A postmarketing surveillance study of fasudil treatment after aneurysmal subarachnoid hemorrhage. *Surg Neurol* 2007; 68(2): 126-31; discussion 131-2.

77. Suzuki Y, Shibuya M, Satoh S, Sugiyama H, Seto M, Takakura K. Safety and efficacy of fasudil monotherapy and fasudil-ozagrel combination therapy in patients with subarachnoid hemorrhage: sub-analysis of the post-marketing surveillance study. *Neurol Med Chir* (Tokyo) 2008; 48(6): 241-7; discussion 247-8.

78. Tachibana E, Harada T, Shibuya M, *et al*. Intra-arterial infusion of fasudil hydrochloride for treating vasospasm following subarachnoid haemorrhage. *Acta Neurochir* (Wien) 1999; 141(1): 13-9.

79. Tanaka K, Minami H, Kota M, Kuwamura K, Kohmura E. Treatment of cerebral vasospasm with intra-arterial fasudil hydrochloride. *Neurosurgery* 2005; 56(2): 214-23.

80. Bolton TB. Mechanisms of action of transmitters and other substances on smooth muscle. *Physiol Rev* 1979; 59(3): 606-718.

81. Dalbasti T, Karabiyikoglu M, Ozdamar N, Oktar N, Cagli S. Efficacy of controlled-release papaverine pellets in preventing symptomatic cerebral vasospasm. *J Neurosurg* 2001; 95(1): 44-50.

82. Liu JK, Tenner MS, Gottfried ON, *et al*. Efficacy of multiple intraarterial papaverine infusions for improvement in cerebral circulation time in patients with recurrent cerebral vasospasm. *J Neurosurg* 2004; 100(3): 414-21.

83. Polin RS, Hansen CA, German P, Chadduck JB, Kassell NF. Intra-arterially administered papaverine for the treatment of symptomatic cerebral vasospasm. *Neurosurgery* 1998; 42(6): 1256-64; discussion 1264-57.

84. Clouston JE, Numaguchi Y, Zoarski GH, Aldrich EF, Simard JM, Zitnay KM. Intraarterial papaverine infusion for cerebral vasospasm after subarachnoid hemorrhage. *AJNR Am J Neuroradiol* 1995; 16(1): 27-38.

85. Fandino J, Kaku Y, Schuknecht B, Valavanis A, Yonekawa Y. Improvement of cerebral oxygenation patterns and metabolic validation of superselective intraarterial infusion of papaverine for the treatment of cerebral vasospasm. *J Neurosurg* 1998; 89(1): 93-100.

86. Firlik KS, Kaufmann AM, Firlik AD, Jungreis CA, Yonas H. Intra-arterial papaverine for the treatment of cerebral vasospasm following aneurysmal subarachnoid hemorrhage. *Surg Neurol* 1999; 51(1): 66-74.

87. Kaku Y, Yonekawa Y, Tsukahara T, Kazekawa K. Superselective intra-arterial infusion of papaverine for the treatment of cerebral vasospasm after subarachnoid hemorrhage. *J Neurosurg* 1992; 77(6): 842-7.

88. Kassell NF, Helm G, Simmons N, Phillips CD, Cail WS. Treatment of cerebral vasospasm with intra-arterial papaverine. *J Neurosurg* 1992; 77(6): 848-52.

89. Little N, Morgan MK, Grinnell V, Sorby W. Intra-arterial papaverine in the management of cerebral vasospasm following subarachnoid haemorrhage. *J Clin Neurosci* 1994; 1(1): 42-6.

90. Morgan MK, Jonker B, Finfer S, Harrington T, Dorsch NW. Aggressive management of aneurysmal subarachnoid haemorrhage based on a papaverine angioplasty protocol. *J Clin Neurosci* 2000; 7(4): 305-8.

91. Numaguchi Y, Zoarski GH. Intra-arterial papaverine treatment for cerebral vasospasm: our experience and review of the literature. *Neurol Med Chir* (Tokyo) 1998; 38(4): 189-95.

92. Sawada M, Hashimoto N, Tsukahara T, Nishi S, Kaku Y, Yoshimura S. Effectiveness of intra-arterially infused papaverine solutions of various concentrations for the treatment of cerebral vasospasm. *Acta Neurochir* (Wien) 1997; 139(8): 706-71.

93. Segawa H, Saito I, Okada T, *et al*. [Efficacy of intracisternal papaverine on symptomatic vasospasm.] *No Shinkei Geka* 1986; 14(7): 847-54.

94. Yoshimura S, Tsukahara T, Hashimoto N, Kazekawa K, Kobayashi A. Intra-arterial infusion of papaverine combined with intravenous administration of high-dose nicardipine for cerebral vasospasm. *Acta Neurochir* (Wien) 1995; 135(3-4): 186-90.

95. Andaluz N, Tomsick TA, Tew JM Jr, van Loveren HR, Yeh HS, Zuccarello M. Indications for endovascular therapy for

Chapter 31

refractory vasospasm after aneurysmal subarachnoid hemorrhage: experience at the University of Cincinnati. *Surg Neurol* 2002; 58(2): 131-8.

96. Armonda RA, Thomas JE, Rosenwasser RH. Early and aggressive treatment of medically intractable cerebral vasospasm with pentobarbital coma, cerebral angioplasty and ICP reduction. *Neurosurg Focus* 1998; 5(4): e7.

97. Beck J, Raabe A, Lanfermann H, *et al*. Effects of balloon angioplasty on perfusion- and diffusion-weighted magnetic resonance imaging results and outcome in patients with cerebral vasospasm. *J Neurosurg* 2006; 105(2): 220-7.

98. Bejjani GK, Bank WO, Olan WJ, Sekhar LN. The efficacy and safety of angioplasty for cerebral vasospasm after subarachnoid hemorrhage. *Neurosurgery* 1998; 42(5): 979-86; discussion 986-7.

99. Coyne TJ, Montanera WJ, Macdonald RL, Wallace MC. Percutaneous transluminal angioplasty for cerebral vasospasm after subarachnoid hemorrhage. *Can J Surg* 1994; 37(5): 391-6.

100. Elliott JP, Newell DW, Lam DJ, *et al*. Comparison of balloon angioplasty and papaverine infusion for the treatment of vasospasm following aneurysmal subarachnoid hemorrhage. *J Neurosurg* 1998; 88(2): 277-84.

101. Eskridge JM, McAuliffe W, Song JK, *et al*. Balloon angioplasty for the treatment of vasospasm: results of first 50 cases. *Neurosurgery* 1998; 42(3): 510-6; discussion 516-7.

102. Eskridge JM, Newell DW, Pendleton GA. Transluminal angioplasty for treatment of vasospasm. *Neurosurg Clin N Am* 1990; 1(2): 387-99.

103. Firlik AD, Kaufmann AM, Jungreis CA, Yonas H. Effect of transluminal angioplasty on cerebral blood flow in the management of symptomatic vasospasm following aneurysmal subarachnoid hemorrhage. *J Neurosurg* 1997; 86(5): 830-9.

104. Fujii Y, Takahashi A, Yoshimoto T. Effect of balloon angioplasty on high grade symptomatic vasospasm after subarachnoid hemorrhage. *Neurosurg Rev* 1995; 18(1): 7-13.

105. Higashida RT, Halbach VV, Cahan LD, *et al*. Transluminal angioplasty for treatment of intracranial arterial vasospasm. *J Neurosurg* 1989; 71(5 Pt 1): 648-53.

106. Higashida RT, Halbach VV, Dormandy B, Bell J, Brant-Zawadzki M, Hieshima GB. New microballoon device for transluminal angioplasty of intracranial arterial vasospasm. *AJNR Am J Neuroradiol* 1990; 11(2): 233-8.

107. Higashida RT, Halbach VV, Dowd CF, Dormandy B, Bell J, Hieshima GB. Intravascular balloon dilatation therapy for intracranial arterial vasospasm: patient selection, technique, and clinical results. *Neurosurg Rev* 1992; 15(2): 89-95.

108. Jestaedt L, Pham M, Bartsch AJ, *et al*. The impact of balloon angioplasty on the evolution of vasospasm-related infarction after aneurysmal subarachnoid hemorrhage. *Neurosurgery* 2008; 62(3): 610-7.

109. Katoh H, Shima K, Shimizu A, *et al*. Clinical evaluation of the effect of percutaneous transluminal angioplasty and intra-arterial papaverine infusion for the treatment of vasospasm following aneurysmal subarachnoid hemorrhage. *Neurol Res* 1999; 21(2): 195-203.

110. Muizelaar JP, Zwienenberg M, Mini NA, Hecht ST. Safety and efficacy of transluminal balloon angioplasty in the prevention of vasospasm in patients with Fisher Grade 3 subarachnoid hemorrhage: a pilot study. *Neurosurg Focus* 15 1998; 5(4): e5.

111. Muizelaar JP, Zwienenberg M, Rudisill NA, Hecht ST. The prophylactic use of transluminal balloon angioplasty in patients with Fisher Grade 3 subarachnoid hemorrhage: a pilot study. *J Neurosurg* 1999; 91(1): 51-8.

112. Newell DW, Eskridge JM, Mayberg MR, Grady MS, Winn HR. Angioplasty for the treatment of symptomatic vasospasm following subarachnoid hemorrhage. *J Neurosurg* 1989; 71(5 Pt 1): 654-60.

113. Rosenwasser RH, Armonda RA, Thomas JE, Benitez RP, Gannon PM, Harrop J. Therapeutic modalities for the management of cerebral vasospasm: timing of endovascular options. *Neurosurgery* 1999; 44(5): 975-79; discussion 979-80.

114. Terry A, Zipfel G, Milner E, *et al*. Safety and technical efficacy of over-the-wire balloons for the treatment of subarachnoid hemorrhage-induced cerebral vasospasm. *Neurosurg Focus* 2006; 21(3): E14.

115. Turowski B, du Mesnil de Rochemont R, Beck J, Berkefeld J, Zanella FE. Assessment of changes in cerebral circulation time due to vasospasm in a specific arterial territory: effect of angioplasty. *Neuroradiology* 2005; 47(2): 134-43.

116. Zubkov YN, Nikiforov BM, Shustin VA. Balloon catheter technique for dilatation of constricted cerebral arteries after aneurysmal SAH. *Acta Neurochir* (Wien) 1984; 70(1-2): 65-79.

117. Zwienenberg-Lee M, Hartman J, Rudisill N, *et al*. Effect of prophylactic transluminal balloon angioplasty on cerebral vasospasm and outcome in patients with Fisher grade III subarachnoid hemorrhage: results of a Phase II multicenter, randomized, clinical trial. *Stroke* 2008; 39(6): 1759-65.

118. Lewis DH, Paul Elliott J, Newell DW, Eskridge JM, Richard Winn H. Interventional endovascular therapy: SPECT cerebral blood flow imaging compared with transcranial Doppler monitoring of balloon angioplasty and intraarterial papaverine for cerebral vasospasm. *J Stroke Cerebrovasc Dis* 1999; 8(2): 71-5.

119. Coenen VA, Hansen CA, Kassell NF, Polin RS. Endovascular treatment for symptomatic cerebral vasospasm after subarachnoid hemorrhage: transluminal balloon angioplasty compared with intraarterial papaverine. *Neurosurg Focus* 1998; 5(4): e6.

120. Polin RS, Coenen VA, Hansen CA, *et al*. Efficacy of transluminal angioplasty for the management of symptomatic cerebral vasospasm following aneurysmal subarachnoid hemorrhage. *J Neurosurg* 2000; 92(2): 284-90.

121. Findlay JM, Kassell NF, Weir BK, *et al*. A randomized trial of intraoperative, intracisternal tissue plasminogen activator for the prevention of vasospasm. *Neurosurgery* 1995; 37(1): 168-76; discussion 177-8.

122. Hamada J, Kai Y, Morioka M, *et al*. Effect on cerebral vasospasm of coil embolization followed by microcatheter intrathecal urokinase infusion into the cisterna magna: a

Chapter 31

prospective randomized study. *Stroke* 2003; 34(11): 2549-54.

123. Gorski R, Zabek M, Jarmuzek P. Influence of intraoperative using of recombinant tissue plasminogen activator on the development of cerebral angiospasm after subarachnoid haemorrhage in patients with ruptured intracranial aneurysms. *Neurol Neurochir Pol* 2000; 34(6 Suppl.): 41-7.

124. Majchrzak H, Lech A, Kopera M, Gajos L, Dragan T, Ladzinski P. [Application of alteplase in prevention of cerebral vasospasm and its sequelae in patients after aneurysmal subarachnoid hemorrhage from ruptured cerebral aneurysm.] *Neurol Neurochir Pol* 1995; 29(3): 379-87.

125. Mizoi K, Yoshimoto T, Takahashi A, Fujiwara S, Koshu K, Sugawara T. Prospective study on the prevention of cerebral vasospasm by intrathecal fibrinolytic therapy with tissue-type plasminogen activator. *J Neurosurg* 1993; 78(3): 430-7.

126. Seifert V, Stolke D, Zimmermann M, Feldges A. Prevention of delayed ischaemic deficits after aneurysmal subarachnoid haemorrhage by intrathecal bolus injection of tissue plasminogen activator (rTPA). A prospective study. *Acta Neurochir* (Wien) 1994; 128(1-4): 137-43.

127. Usui M, Saito N, Hoya K, Todo T. Vasospasm prevention with postoperative intrathecal thrombolytic therapy: a retrospective comparison of urokinase, tissue plasminogen activator, and cisternal drainage alone. *Neurosurgery* 1994; 34(2): 235-44; discussion 244-5.

128. Yamada K, Yoshimura S, Enomoto Y, Yamakawa H, Iwama T. Effectiveness of combining continuous cerebrospinal drainage and intermittent intrathecal urokinase injection therapy in preventing symptomatic vasospasm following aneurysmal subarachnoid haemorrhage. *Br J Neurosurg* 2008; 22(5): 649-53.

129. Findlay JM, Weir BK, Kassell NF, Disney LB, Grace MG. Intracisternal recombinant tissue plasminogen activator after aneurysmal subarachnoid hemorrhage. *J Neurosurg* 1991; 75(2): 181-8.

130. Kinouchi H, Ogasawara K, Shimizu H, Mizoi K, Yoshimoto T. Prevention of symptomatic vasospasm after aneurysmal subarachnoid hemorrhage by intraoperative cisternal fibrinolysis using tissue-type plasminogen activator combined with continuous cisternal drainage. *Neurol Med Chir* (Tokyo) 2004; 44(11): 569-75; discussion 576-7.

131. Kodama N, Sasaki T, Kawakami M, Sato M, Asari J. Cisternal irrigation therapy with urokinase and ascorbic acid for prevention of vasospasm after aneurysmal subarachnoid hemorrhage. Outcome in 217 patients. *Surg Neurol* 2000; 53(2): 110-7; discussion 117-8.

132. Mizoi K, Yoshimoto T, Fujiwara S, Sugawara T, Takahashi A, Koshu K. Prevention of vasospasm by clot removal and intrathecal bolus injection of tissue-type plasminogen activator: preliminary report. *Neurosurgery* 1991; 28(6): 807-12; discussion 812-3.

133. Moriyama E, Matsumoto Y, Meguro T, *et al.* Combined cisternal drainage and intrathecal urokinase injection therapy for prevention of vasospasm in patients with aneurysmal subarachnoid hemorrhage. *Neurol Med Chir* (Tokyo) 1995; 35(10): 732-6.

134. Ohman J, Servo A, Heiskanen O. Effect of intrathecal fibrinolytic therapy on clot lysis and vasospasm in patients with aneurysmal subarachnoid hemorrhage. *J Neurosurg* 1991; 75(2): 197-201.

135. Sasaki T, Kodama N, Kawakami M, *et al.* Urokinase cisternal irrigation therapy for prevention of symptomatic vasospasm after aneurysmal subarachnoid hemorrhage: a study of urokinase concentration and the fibrinolytic system. *Stroke* 2000; 31(6): 1256-62.

136. Sasaki T, Ohta T, Kikuchi H, *et al.* A Phase II clinical trial of recombinant human tissue-type plasminogen activator against cerebral vasospasm after aneurysmal subarachnoid hemorrhage. *Neurosurgery* 1994; 35(4): 597-604; discussion 604-5.

137. Stolke D, Seifert V. Single intracisternal bolus of recombinant tissue plasminogen activator in patients with aneurysmal subarachnoid hemorrhage: preliminary assessment of efficacy and safety in an open clinical study. *Neurosurgery* 1992; 30(6): 877-81.

138. Zabramski JM, Spetzler RF, Lee KS, *et al.* Phase I trial of tissue plasminogen activator for the prevention of vasospasm in patients with aneurysmal subarachnoid hemorrhage. *J Neurosurg* 1991; 75(2): 189-96.

139. Amin-Hanjani S, Ogilvy CS, Barker FG 2nd. Does intracisternal thrombolysis prevent vasospasm after aneurysmal subarachnoid hemorrhage? A meta-analysis. *Neurosurgery* 2004; 54(2): 326-34; discussion 334-5.

140. Hanggi D, Liersch J, Turowski B, Yong M, Steiger HJ. The effect of lumboventricular lavage and simultaneous low-frequency head-motion therapy after severe subarachnoid hemorrhage: results of a single center prospective Phase II trial. *J Neurosurg* 2008; 108(6): 1192-9.

141. Ito U, Tomita H, Yamazaki S, Takada Y, Inaba Y. Enhanced cisternal drainage and cerebral vasospasm in early aneurysm surgery. *Acta Neurochir* (Wien) 1986; 80(1-2): 18-23.

142. Kawamoto S, Tsutsumi K, Yoshikawa G, *et al.* Effectiveness of the head-shaking method combined with cisternal irrigation with urokinase in preventing cerebral vasospasm after subarachnoid hemorrhage. *J Neurosurg* 2004; 100(2): 236-43.

143. Klimo P Jr, Kestle JR, MacDonald JD, Schmidt RH. Marked reduction of cerebral vasospasm with lumbar drainage of cerebrospinal fluid after subarachnoid hemorrhage. *J Neurosurg* 2004; 100(2): 215-24.

144. Yamamoto I, Shimoda M, Yamada S, *et al.* Indications for cisternal drainage in conjunction with early surgery in ruptured aneurysms and timing of its discontinuation. *Neurol Med Chir* (Tokyo) 1989; 29(5): 407-13.

145. Inagawa T, Kamiya K, Matsuda Y. Effect of continuous cisternal drainage on cerebral vasospasm. *Acta Neurochir* (Wien) 1991; 112(1-2): 28-36.

146. Mizukami M, Kawase T, Usami T, Tazawa T. Prevention of vasospasm by early operation with removal of subarachnoid blood. *Neurosurgery* 1982; 10(3): 301-7.

147. Ohta H, Ito Z, Yasui N, Suzuki A. Extensive evacuation of subarachnoid clot for prevention of vasospasm - effective or not? *Acta Neurochir* (Wien) 1982; 63(1-4): 111-6.

148. Macdonald RL, Kassell NF, Mayer S, et al. Clazosentan to overcome neurological ischemia and infarction occurring after subarachnoid hemorrhage (CONSCIOUS-1): randomized, double-blind, placebo-controlled Phase 2 dose-finding trial. Stroke 2008; 39(11): 3015-21.

149. Shaw MD, Vermeulen M, Murray GD, Pickard JD, Bell BA, Teasdale GM. Efficacy and safety of the endothelin, receptor antagonist TAK-044 in treating subarachnoid hemorrhage: a report by the Steering Committee on behalf of the UK/Netherlands/Eire TAK-044 Subarachnoid Haemorrhage Study Group. J Neurosurg 2000; 93(6): 992-7.

150. Vajkoczy P, Meyer B, Weidauer S, et al. Clazosentan (AXV-034343), a selective endothelin A receptor antagonist, in the prevention of cerebral vasospasm following severe aneurysmal subarachnoid hemorrhage: results of a randomized, double-blind, placebo-controlled, multicenter Phase IIa study. J Neurosurg 2005; 103(1): 9-17.

151. Nogueira RG, Bodock MJ, Koroshetz WJ, et al. High-dose bosentan in the prevention and treatment of subarachnoid hemorrhage-induced cerebral vasospasm: an open-label feasibility study. Neurocrit Care 2007; 7(3): 194-202.

152. Barth M, Capelle HH, Munch E, et al. Effects of the selective endothelin A (ET(A)) receptor antagonist clazosentan on cerebral perfusion and cerebral oxygenation following severe subarachnoid hemorrhage - preliminary results from a randomized clinical series. Acta Neurochir (Wien) 2007; 149(9): 911-8.

153. Zhao XD, Zhou YT, Zhang X, Zhuang Z, Shi JX. A meta analysis of treating subarachnoid hemorrhage with magnesium sulfate. J Clin Neurosci 2009; 16(11): 1394-7.

154. Muroi C, Terzic A, Fortunati M, Yonekawa Y, Keller E. Magnesium sulfate in the management of patients with aneurysmal subarachnoid hemorrhage: a randomized, placebo-controlled, dose-adapted trial. Surg Neurol 2008; 69(1): 33-9.

155. van den Bergh WM, Algra A, van Kooten F, et al. Magnesium sulfate in aneurysmal subarachnoid hemorrhage: a randomized controlled trial. Stroke 2005; 36(5): 1011-5.

156. Veyna RS, Seyfried D, Burke DG, et al. Magnesium sulfate therapy after aneurysmal subarachnoid hemorrhage. J Neurosurg 2002; 96(3): 510-4.

157. Wong GK, Chan MT, Boet R, Poon WS, Gin T. Intravenous magnesium sulfate after aneurysmal subarachnoid hemorrhage: a prospective randomized pilot study. J Neurosurg Anesthesiol 2006; 18(2): 142-8.

158. Schmid-Elsaesser R, Kunz M, Zausinger S, Prueckner S, Briegel J, Steiger HJ. Intravenous magnesium versus nimodipine in the treatment of patients with aneurysmal subarachnoid hemorrhage: a randomized study. Neurosurgery 2006; 58(6): 1054-65.

159. Chia RY, Hughes RS, Morgan MK. Magnesium: a useful adjunct in the prevention of cerebral vasospasm following aneurysmal subarachnoid haemorrhage. J Clin Neurosci 2002; 9(3): 279-81.

160. Stippler M, Crago E, Levy EI, et al. Magnesium infusion for vasospasm prophylaxis after subarachnoid hemorrhage. J Neurosurg 2006; 105(5): 723-9.

161. Boet R, Mee E. Magnesium sulfate in the management of patients with Fisher grade 3 subarachnoid hemorrhage: a pilot study. Neurosurgery 2000; 47(3): 602-6; discussion 606-7.

162. Brewer RP, Parra A, Lynch J, Chilukuri V, Borel CO. Cerebral blood flow velocity response to magnesium sulfate in patients after subarachnoid hemorrhage. J Neurosurg Anesthesiol 2001; 13(3): 202-6.

163. Mori K, Yamamoto T, Nakao Y, et al. Initial clinical experience of vasodilatory effect of intra-cisternal infusion of magnesium sulfate for the treatment of cerebral vasospasm after aneurysmal subarachnoid hemorrhage. Neurol Med Chir (Tokyo) 2009; 49(4): 139-44; discussion 144-5.

164. Shah QA, Memon MZ, Suri MF, et al. Super-selective intra-arterial magnesium sulfate in combination with nicardipine for the treatment of cerebral vasospasm in patients with subarachnoid hemorrhage. Neurocrit Care 2009; 11(2): 190-8.

165. Yahia AM, Kirmani JF, Qureshi AI, Guterman LR, Hopkins LN. The safety and feasibility of continuous intravenous magnesium sulfate for prevention of cerebral vasospasm in aneurysmal subarachnoid hemorrhage. Neurocrit Care 2005; 3(1): 16-23.

166. Liao JK, Laufs U. Pleiotropic effects of statins. Annu Rev Pharmacol Toxicol 2005; 45: 89-118.

167. Miida T, Takahashi A, Ikeuchi T. Prevention of stroke and dementia by statin therapy: experimental and clinical evidence of their pleiotropic effects. Pharmacol Ther 2007; 113(2): 378-93.

168. Sillberg VA, Wells GA, Perry JJ. Do statins improve outcomes and reduce the incidence of vasospasm after aneurysmal subarachnoid hemorrhage: a meta-analysis. Stroke 2008; 39(9): 2622-6.

169. Chou SH, Smith EE, Badjatia N, et al. A randomized, double-blind, placebo-controlled pilot study of simvastatin in aneurysmal subarachnoid hemorrhage. Stroke 2008; 39(10): 2891-3.

170. Lynch JR, Wang H, McGirt MJ, et al. Simvastatin reduces vasospasm after aneurysmal subarachnoid hemorrhage: results of a pilot randomized clinical trial. Stroke 2005; 36(9): 2024-6.

171. McGirt MJ, Woodworth GF, Pradilla G, et al. Galbraith Award: simvastatin attenuates experimental cerebral vasospasm and ameliorates serum markers of neuronal and endothelial injury in patients after subarachnoid hemorrhage: a dose-response effect dependent on endothelial nitric oxide synthase. Clin Neurosurg 2005; 52: 371-8.

172. Tseng MY, Czosnyka M, Richards H, Pickard JD, Kirkpatrick PJ. Effects of acute treatment with pravastatin on cerebral vasospasm, autoregulation, and delayed ischemic deficits after aneurysmal subarachnoid hemorrhage: a Phase II randomized placebo-controlled trial. Stroke 2005; 36(8): 1627-32.

173. Vergouwen MD, Meijers JC, Geskus RB, et al. Biologic effects of simvastatin in patients with aneurysmal subarachnoid hemorrhage: a double-blind, placebo-controlled randomized trial. J Cereb Blood Flow Metab 2009; 29(8): 1444-53.

174. Kern M, Lam MM, Knuckey NW, Lind CR. Statins may not protect against vasospasm in subarachnoid haemorrhage. *J Clin Neurosci* 2009; 16(4): 527-30.

175. Kramer AH, Gurka MJ, Nathan B, Dumont AS, Kassell NF, Bleck TP. Statin use was not associated with less vasospasm or improved outcome after subarachnoid hemorrhage. *Neurosurgery* 2008; 62(2): 422-7; discussion 427-30.

176. McGirt MJ, Blessing R, Alexander MJ, *et al*. Risk of cerebral vasospasm after subarachnoid hemorrhage reduced by statin therapy: a multivariate analysis of an institutional experience. *J Neurosurg* 2006; 105(5): 671-4.

177. McGirt MJ, Garces Ambrossi GL, Huang J, Tamargo RJ. Simvastatin for the prevention of symptomatic cerebral vasospasm following aneurysmal subarachnoid hemorrhage: a single-institution prospective cohort study. *J Neurosurg* 2009; 110(5): 968-74.

178. Moskowitz SI, Ahrens C, Provencio JJ, Chow M, Rasmussen PA. Prehemorrhage statin use and the risk of vasospasm after aneurysmal subarachnoid hemorrhage. *Surg Neurol* 2009; 71(3): 311-7, discussion 317-8.

179. Parra A, Kreiter KT, Williams S, *et al*. Effect of prior statin use on functional outcome and delayed vasospasm after acute aneurysmal subarachnoid hemorrhage: a matched controlled cohort study. *Neurosurgery* 2005; 56(3): 476-84; discussion 476-84.

180. Singhal AB, Topcuoglu MA, Dorer DJ, Ogilvy CS, Carter BS, Koroshetz WJ. SSRI and statin use increases the risk for vasospasm after subarachnoid hemorrhage. *Neurology* 2005; 64(6): 1008-13.

181. Tseng MY, Czosnyka M, Richards H, Pickard JD, Kirkpatrick PJ. Effects of acute treatment with statins on cerebral autoregulation in patients after aneurysmal subarachnoid hemorrhage. *Neurosurg Focus* 2006; 21(3): E10.

182. Tseng MY, Hutchinson PJ, Czosnyka M, Richards H, Pickard JD, Kirkpatrick PJ. Effects of acute pravastatin treatment on intensity of rescue therapy, length of inpatient stay, and 6-month outcome in patients after aneurysmal subarachnoid hemorrhage. *Stroke* 2007; 38(5): 1545-50.

183. Tseng MY, Hutchinson PJ, Turner CL, *et al*. Biological effects of acute pravastatin treatment in patients after aneurysmal subarachnoid hemorrhage: a double-blind, placebo-controlled trial. *J Neurosurg* 2007; 107(6): 1092-100.

184. Haley EC Jr, Kassell NF, Alves WM, Weir BK, Hansen CA. Phase II trial of tirilazad in aneurysmal subarachnoid hemorrhage. A report of the Cooperative Aneurysm Study. *J Neurosurg* 1995; 82(5): 786-90.

185. Haley EC Jr, Kassell NF, Apperson-Hansen C, Maile MH, Alves WM. A randomized, double-blind, vehicle-controlled trial of tirilazad mesylate in patients with aneurysmal subarachnoid hemorrhage: a cooperative study in North America. *J Neurosurg* 1997; 86(3): 467-74.

186. Kassell NF, Haley EC Jr, Apperson-Hansen C, Alves WM. Randomized, double-blind, vehicle-controlled trial of tirilazad mesylate in patients with aneurysmal subarachnoid hemorrhage: a cooperative study in Europe, Australia, and New Zealand. *J Neurosurg* 1996; 84(2): 221-8.

187. Lanzino G, Kassell NF. Double-blind, randomized, vehicle-controlled study of high-dose tirilazad mesylate in women with aneurysmal subarachnoid hemorrhage. Part II. A cooperative study in North America. *J Neurosurg* 1999; 90(6): 1018-24.

188. Lanzino G, Kassell NF, Dorsch NW, *et al*. Double-blind, randomized, vehicle-controlled study of high-dose tirilazad mesylate in women with aneurysmal subarachnoid hemorrhage. Part I. A cooperative study in Europe, Australia, New Zealand, and South Africa. *J Neurosurg* 1999; 90(6): 1011-7.

189. Jang YG, Ilodigwe D, Macdonald RL. Meta-analysis of tirilazad mesylate in patients with aneurysmal subarachnoid hemorrhage. *Neurocrit Care* 2009; 10(1): 141-7.

190. Suzuki S, Sano K, Handa H, *et al*. Clinical study of OKY-046, a thromboxane synthetase inhibitor, in prevention of cerebral vasospasms and delayed cerebral ischaemic symptoms after subarachnoid haemorrhage due to aneurysmal rupture: a randomized double-blind study. *Neurol Res* 1989; 11(2): 79-88.

191. Tsementzis SA, Hitchcock ER, Meyer CH. Benefits and risks of antifibrinolytic therapy in the management of ruptured intracranial aneurysms. A double-blind placebo-controlled study. *Acta Neurochir* (Wien) 1990; 102(1-2): 1-10.

192. Asano T, Takakura K, Sano K, *et al*. Effects of a hydroxyl radical scavenger on delayed ischemic neurological deficits following aneurysmal subarachnoid hemorrhage: results of a multicenter, placebo-controlled double-blind trial. *J Neurosurg* 1996; 84(5): 792-803.

193. Munakata A, Ohkuma H, Nakano T, Shimamura N, Asano K, Naraoka M. Effect of a free radical scavenger, edaravone, in the treatment of patients with aneurysmal subarachnoid hemorrhage. *Neurosurgery* 2009; 64(3): 423-8; discussion 428-9.

194. Saito I, Asano T, Sano K, *et al*. Neuroprotective effect of an antioxidant, ebselen, in patients with delayed neurological deficits after aneurysmal subarachnoid hemorrhage. *Neurosurgery* 1998; 42(2): 269-77; discussion 277-8.

195. Wurm G, Tomancok B, Nussbaumer K, Adelwohrer C, Holl K. Reduction of ischemic sequelae following spontaneous subarachnoid hemorrhage: a double-blind, randomized comparison of enoxaparin versus placebo. *Clin Neurol Neurosurg* 2004; 106(2): 97-103.

196. Siironen J, Juvela S, Varis J, *et al*. No effect of enoxaparin on outcome of aneurysmal subarachnoid hemorrhage: a randomized, double-blind, placebo-controlled clinical trial. *J Neurosurg* 2003; 99(6): 953-9.

197. Tseng MY, Hutchinson PJ, Richards HK, *et al*. Acute systemic erythropoietin therapy to reduce delayed ischemic deficits following aneurysmal subarachnoid hemorrhage: a Phase II randomized, double-blind, placebo-controlled trial. Clinical article. *J Neurosurg* 2009; 111(1): 171-80.

198. Springborg JB, Moller C, Gideon P, Jorgensen OS, Juhler M, Olsen NV. Erythropoietin in patients with aneurysmal subarachnoid haemorrhage: a double blind randomised clinical trial. *Acta Neurochir* (Wien) 2007; 149(11): 1089-101.

Chapter 32

Deep intracranial hemorrhage

Hamad Farhat MD, Clinical Assistant Professor 1
Jacques J Morcos MD FRCS(Eng) FRCS(Ed)
Professor of Clinical Neurosurgery and Otolaryngology 2

1 DEPARTMENT OF NEUROLOGICAL SURGERY, NORTHSHORE UNIVERSITY HEALTHSYSTEM, EVANSTON, ILLINOIS, USA
2 DEPARTMENT OF NEUROLOGICAL SURGERY, UNIVERSITY OF MIAMI, MIAMI, FLORIDA, USA

Introduction

Since McKissock, Richardson, and Taylor reported on their evaluation of surgical and conservative treatment in 180 unselected cases of 'primary intracerebral haemorhage' in 1961, operative approaches for intracerebral hemorrhage (ICH) have been heavily debated [1]. This chapter defines deep intracranial hemorrhage as hemorrhage into the brain parenchyma in the absence of causal trauma or a structural disease process on a macroscopic level, such as a tumor, aneurysm, vascular malformation, or arteriovenous fistula (primary ICH). In this chapter, we first review the different clinical characteristics of primary ICH and then critically review current management strategies.

Methodology

A computerized literature search using PubMed from 1960 through 2010 was performed with the subject headings 'intracranial hemorrhage,' 'hypertensive brain hemorrhage,' and 'hemorrhagic stroke' used separately. The abstracts were carefully reviewed, and those relevant to deep intracranial hemorrhage were selected. Articles covering medical management were reviewed, as were articles describing various surgical techniques in the management of deep hemorrhages. In addition, the references of selected papers were carefully reviewed to identify other related articles. Several reviews and book chapters were also selected and used in the writing of this chapter.

Historical review

As discussed by Donley, in 1658 John James Wepfer first described the relationship between circulating blood and cerebral function, and the consequences of effusion of blood in the head, in *De Apoplexia* [2]. In their historical reviews, Clarke and Fazio *et al* note that Hoffman (1660-1742) first introduced the concept of ICH [3, 4]. They also say that Morgagni (1682-1771) described the difference between apoplexy associated with hemorrhage into the cerebral parenchyma and the ventricular system in *De Sedibus*.

In 1888, MacEwen described the first successful operation for spontaneous ICH [5]. In 1903, Cushing reported the first surgical evacuation of a cerebral hematoma and attributed increased intracranial pressure (ICP) to the mass effect caused by the hematoma [6]. During the next three decades, the surgical treatment of ICH was occasionally reported. Bagley first described surgical indications based on the location of the hematoma [7]. He suggested that surgical treatment was ineffective for hemorrhages in the basal ganglia and best reserved for subcortical hematomas associated with increased ICP. He also hypothesized that a ruptured aneurysm or rupture of an atherosclerotic or congenitally weak blood-vessel wall without an aneurysm often caused spontaneous ICH. In 1932, Robinson suggested the possibility of spontaneous recovery in patients with small hemorrhages [8].

The advent of cerebral angiography in 1929 provided an impetus for the surgical treatment of hematomas and resulted in multiple publications in the French literature in the 1940s and 1950s [9, 10]. In 1959, Lazorthes reported the results of 52 cases, sparking a resurgence of interest in the surgical management of ICH [10]. In 1961, McKissock et al reported no difference in outcomes between surgical and medical management, and cast serious doubt on the benefit of surgical treatment [1]. The advent of CT in 1973 and MRI in 1982 allowed a much better recognition and understanding of the occurrence, evolution, and precise localization of ICH.

Epidemiology and relevance

ICH causes 10-15% of first-ever strokes. In 2002, an estimated 67,000 patients in the USA experienced an ICH; of these, only 20% were expected to be functionally independent at 6 months [11]. ICH carries an exceedingly high 30-day mortality rate of 35-52%; half of the deaths occur in the first 2 days [11, 12].

ICH is more common in men than women, and is particularly seen in those older than 55 years. There is a high incidence of ICH among Japanese and Afro-American populations at 55 per 100,000 population [13, 14], roughly twice the incidence in white Western populations. ICH is rare before the age of 45 years and becomes increasingly more frequent with

advancing age. Among those 80 years and older, the incidence is 25 times that of the total population [15]. Because of the increasing age of the Western population, it is predicted that ICH rates will steadily rise despite more accurate blood pressure (BP) control [16, 17]. Primary ICH is believed to account for 78-88% of cases [13, 18].

Causes

Trauma is the most common cause of ICH. Chronic arterial hypertension is the most common cause in the non-traumatic group, accounting for approximately 50% of cases. High BP has consistently been reported as a major risk factor for ICH [12, 19-22]. A meta-analysis and review by Ariesen et al estimated a crude odds ratio (OR) of 3.68 for hypertension and ICH compared with normotensives [16]. Sturgeon et al studied risk factors for ICH in a pooled cohort of the Atherosclerosis Risk in Communities (ARIC) study and the Cardiovascular Health Study (CHS) [14]. The ARIC cohort was recruited from 1987 to 1989 and involved 15,792 men and women, aged 45-64 years at baseline, sampled from four US communities. The CHS cohort was recruited from 1989 to 1993 and involved 5,888 men and women, aged 65 years or older at baseline, again sampled from four US communities. The follow-up was more than 263,400 person-years. In this prospective study assessing baseline risk factors and the subsequent occurrence of ICH, higher age, Afro-American ethnicity (versus white), and hypertension were positively associated with the incidence of ICH. Participants with a systolic BP (SBP) of 160mmHg or more or a diastolic BP of 110mmHg or more had 5.55 times (95% confidence interval [CI], 3.07-10.0) the rate of ICH as those without hypertension.

The most common locations of spontaneous ICH are the putamen, subcortical white matter, cerebellum, thalamus, and brainstem. Kase and Mohr studied 100 cases of spontaneous ICH and found that 34 patients had putaminal hemorrhage, 24 lobar hemorrhage, 20 thalamic hemorrhage, seven cerebellar hemorrhage, and six pontine hemorrhage [23]. Hemorrhages in the caudate nucleus, putamen, thalamus, brainstem, and cerebellum occur in the distribution of small perforating arteries with a diameter of 50-200μm. These deep penetrating arteries are small non-branching end arteries that arise directly from much larger arteries (e.g., the middle cerebral artery, anterior choroidal artery, anterior cerebral artery, posterior cerebral artery, posterior communicating artery, cerebellar arteries, basilar artery). Their small size and proximal position predispose them to the development of microatheroma and lipohyalinosis. Electron microscope studies suggest that most bleeding occurs at or near the bifurcation of affected arteries, where prominent degeneration of the media and smooth muscles can be seen [24].

In 1868, Charcot and Bouchard introduced the concept of ICH arising from the rupture of miliary microaneurysms [25]. Russell and Cole, and Yates confirmed the presence of microaneurysms in an anatomic distribution closely correlated with that of hypertensive hemorrhages [26, 27]. Russell also found an association between miliary aneurysms of 300-900μm in size and hypertension. A few aneurysms were observed in normotensive controls (diastolic BP <110mmHg), but 84% of those patients were aged 60 years or older. Cole and Yates noted that microaneurysms of 50-2,500μm in diameter were uncommon in those younger than 50 years, even in the setting of hypertension. We can therefore conclude that both hypertension and age appear to be risk factors in the formation of microaneurysms.

Fisher studied the pathological process affecting small cerebral arteries in hypertension and coined the term 'lipohyalinosis' to describe a destructive vascular process that was previously referred to as 'fibrinoid necrosis,' 'angionecrosis,' or 'hyaline arterionecrosis' [28-30]. High arterial pressure alters the walls of small (80-300μm) cerebral arterioles and leads to subintimal fibrinoid deposition and fat-filled macrophages. The integrity of the elastica and media is eventually lost, and the artery dilates locally to form a microaneurysm. Fisher also found that lipohyalinosis, by virtue of occlusion of the vascular lumen, was the cause of many lacunar infarcts. However, he could not confirm that microaneurysms were the source of massive ICH.

Clinical presentation and diagnosis

The symptoms and signs of ICH depend substantially on the location and size of the hematoma. The ictus often occurs during activity and manifests with the sudden onset of a neurologic deficit, which gradually progresses. Important insights with regard to the presentation can be taken from the prospective 1978 Harvard Cooperative Stroke Registry study [31]. Only one-third of patients have maximal deficits from the onset of symptoms. The history and physical examination are distinct from those in patients with subarachnoid hemorrhage. As is often the case, a thorough history and examination can give decisive clues even before the CT scan is obtained. Additional information from witnesses and relatives is very helpful. Although patients may present with sudden-onset headache, with or without vomiting, this is usually not as acute as in patients with subarachnoid hemorrhage. In the above-mentioned registry study, only 36% of awake patients (19/54) presented with headache. Less than half of the patients (44%) presented with vomiting. Clearly the absence of such symptoms does not rule out a severe ICH. Seizures are rare. A history of chronic arterial hypertension should alert physicians to the possibility of hypertensive ICH, which must be differentiated from the acute hypertension present in patients with elevated ICP. Previous strokes, seizures, liver disease, coagulopathy, primary or metastatic brain tumor, or valvular heart disease may suggest an underlying cause for the ICH.

Impaired consciousness is the most relevant neurologic sign. Such a finding was described in 60% of the cases reported in the Harvard Cooperative Stroke Registry study [31]. The degree of impaired consciousness is subject to the location, size, and extension of the hematoma in deep structures or ventricles. A large hematoma results in increased ICP and direct compression or distortion of the thalamic and brainstem reticular activating system [32]. Patients with hematomas in deep locations present with a significant decrease in the level of consciousness and dense, lateralized neurologic deficits. Patients with more peripherally located hematomas are more alert with corresponding focal deficits.

The hallmark of brainstem involvement is a mixture of coma, long tract signs, and cranial nerve deficits. The presentation of cerebellar hemorrhage is unique and so distinct from that of supratentorial ICH that a clinical diagnosis of location can be made after the physical examination and prior to a CT scan. The classic symptoms and typical findings of cerebellar hemorrhage have been summarized by Heros (Table 1) [33].

Table 1. Clinical features of cerebellar hemorrhage.

Symptoms	Signs
Early	
Headache	Truncal or appendicular ataxia
Nausea	Dysarthria
Dizziness	Nystagmus
Lack of balance	Stiff neck
Vomiting	
Intermediate	
Confusion	Abducens palsy
Somnolence, stupor	Gaze paresis
	Peripheral facial palsy
	Depressed corneal reflex
	Horner's syndrome
	Babinski's sign
	Mild hemiparesis
Late	
Stupor	Pinpoint pupils
Coma	Ataxic respirations
	Decerebrate posture

A third to a quarter of initially alert patients experience a deterioration in consciousness within 24 hours [34, 35]. Rather than initial clinical signs, the most accurate predictor is large hematoma volume and ventricular extension [35]. Consequently, these patients need to be very closely monitored during the first 24 hours, especially if they are still awake and alert despite a large hematoma volume. Expansion of the hematoma

is the most common cause of neurologic deterioration and death within the first 3 hours of the ictus [34, 35]. Progression of mass effect due to edema can essentially occur within two distinct time intervals [36]:

- Early, within the first 2 days.
- Late, within the second and third week.

Radiology

The initial radiologic work-up consists of a plain CT scan of the brain. This will be fast and easy to interpret. The location and size of the hematoma and the presence or absence of mass effect, perilesional edema, and ventricular extension can be depicted; all of these image criteria are important in the acute phase to decide on a management plan. Contrast enhancement can offer the possibility of diagnosing associated abnormalities such as arteriovenous malformations, aneurysms, and tumors, but this depends on the size of the masking blood clot. Blood on a CT scan usually presents with a hyperdense signal within 4 hours. In the face of acute blood caused by ICH, MRI will not provide more useful information and is in fact often a source of confusion because of the variable interpretation of blood-clot-producing signal inhomogeneities. After about 7-10 days, the high attenuation values of the hematoma start decreasing peripherally. Depending on its size, the whole hematoma may become isodense in 2-3 weeks and resolve completely to an area of decreased density within 2 months. Occasionally a resolving hematoma may give the appearance of ring enhancement, because of either increased vascularity at the periphery or disruption of the blood-brain barrier.

Clinical profile of patients with deep ICH

Putaminal hemorrhage

Putaminal hemorrhage is the most common form of ICH and can present in different ways, depending on the size and extent of the hematoma. Initially there is acute onset of headaches. However, these are different from the thunderclap-type headaches of subarachnoid hemorrhage. They soon are followed by a gradual progression of focal neurologic signs and, depending on the overall size, with a worsening level of consciousness. A marked deficit from the beginning is unusual. Common neurologic findings are as follows [28, 37]:

- Hemiparesis.
- Hemisensory syndrome.
- Homonymous hemianopsia.
- Horizontal gaze palsy.
- Aphasia (dominant hemisphere) or hemineglect (non-dominant hemisphere).

Pronounced neurologic deficits associated with coma suggest large hematomas and are associated with a poor prognosis. Intraventricular extension of the hemorrhage is a sign of extensive parenchymal dissection or destruction and another bad prognosticator [38, 39]. In contrast, patients who are alert and have only limited motor deficits, normal extraocular movements, a full visual field, and a hematoma that does not extend laterally or upward out of the putaminal region fare better. This has been ascribed to reversible compression of the capsular fibers as opposed to destruction [38].

Thalamic hemorrhage

Thalamic hemorrhages account for 10-15% of all ICHs [28, 40]. The bleeding originates from thalamic perforators of the posterior cerebral arteries and may extend laterally into the internal capsule, medially into the ventricles, superiorly into the corona radiata, and inferiorly into the subthalamus and midbrain [41].

The clinical presentation depends on the size and pattern of extension of the hematoma. In contrast to putaminal hemorrhages, thalamic bleeds instantly result in gross neurologic deficit with sensorimotor loss, a higher likelihood of vomiting, variable presence of headaches, and occasionally coma [4, 40, 42]. The ocular findings in thalamic lesions are pathognomonic [4, 28, 40, 42]:

- Upward gaze palsy.
- Convergence gaze.

- Miotic unreactive pupils because of compression of the midbrain tectum.
- Less commonly, retraction nystagmus on upward gaze and skew deviation (vertical misalignment of the eyes caused by abnormal prenuclear vestibular input to the ocular motor nuclei).

Different characteristics of the so-called 'thalamic syndrome' were described at the beginning of the 19th century by Dejerine and Roussy [43], followed by Lhermitte in 1925 [44] and Baudouin *et al* in 1930 [45]. In 1959, Fisher emphasized language disorders and ocular motility disturbances [46]. In 1995, Kumral *et al* provided an excellent study based on 100 patients, with a very detailed correlation of different symptoms (sensorimotor, oculomotor, and neurobehavioral) to four defined topographic types of thalamic hemorrhage [47]:

- Posterolateral thalamic hemorrhage: severe sensorimotor deficit, frequently transcortical aphasia with left-sided lesions, anosognosia with right-sided lesions, several variants of vertical gaze dysfunction, ocular skew deviation, gaze preference toward the side of the lesion, and miotic pupils (particularly with a large hemorrhage).
- Ventrolateral thalamic hemorrhage: severe sensorimotor deficits, less frequent language and oculomotor deficits compared with posterolateral lesions.
- Medial thalamic hemorrhages: sensorimotor deficits (moderate in small lesions and severe in large lesions) because of involvement of the internal capsule. Language disturbances with large left medial lesions, and neglect in large right medial lesions.
- Dorsal thalamic hemorrhage: usually rare, mild, and transient sensorimotor deficits. Oculomotor and neuropsychologic deficits with large lesions only.

Caudate hemorrhage

Caudate hematomas represent approximately 5-7% of ICH cases [39]. The most common cause of caudate hemorrhage is arterial hypertension [39, 48-52].

The head of the caudate nucleus receives its blood supply from Heubner's artery and the anterior lenticulostriate and lateral lenticulostriate arteries, which also supply the anterior internal capsule and putamen [52]. A rupture in these arteries causes parenchymal hemorrhage.

The presentation is that of abrupt headache and vomiting, followed by a decreased level of consciousness. Patients are usually disoriented and have evidence of neck stiffness [39]. Occasionally patients experience seizures and horizontal gaze paresis. On CT scan, ventricular extension of the hematoma into the frontal horn is common, with secondary hydrocephalus. Occasionally the hemorrhage extends into the anterior portion of the thalamus. Such patients present with transient but significant short-term memory deficits [38]. In a series of eight cases from Stein et al, most patients recovered fully with no significant neurologic deficits [39]. Weisberg also reported a small series of caudate hemorrhages, this time with poor outcomes; stupor and a massive amount of intraventricular hemorrhage (IVH) were associated with poor outcome [48]. More recently, Liliang et al looked at clinical data from 36 consecutive patients with hypertensive caudate hemorrhage [53]. In this relatively large study, multivariate analysis and stepwise logistic regression revealed that hydrocephalus was the only independent prognostic factor for poor outcome (p<0.001).

Cerebellar hemorrhage

The frequency of cerebellar hemorrhage ranges between 5% and 10% [28, 54, 55]. One of the major differences with supratentorial hemorrhages is the entirely different prognosis once coma has occurred. If the diagnosis is made early and surgical intervention is prompt, coma is reversible after a cerebellar hemorrhage [56-59]. A 2008 study by Smajlovic et al on 30-day prognosis and risk factors in 352 treated patients for ICH confirmed, once again, that compared with all other ICHs, cerebellar hematoma is associated with the best outcomes after the first month; brainstem and multilobar ICHs had the worst [60]. The dentate nuclei are the most common substrate. The hematoma extends into the hemispheric white matter and often into

the fourth ventricle, causing either brainstem compression or direct invasion. Rarely, cerebellar hemorrhage involves only the vermis. Hypertension and anticoagulation are the two most important causative factors in cerebellar hemorrhage [56, 61].

As mentioned above, the presentation of cerebellar hemorrhage is unique and a clinical diagnosis of location can be made after the physical examination and before a CT scan (Table 1). Loss of consciousness at onset is rare. On admission to hospital, about one-third of patients are obtunded [56]. The early physical signs are appendicular or truncal ataxia, dysarthria, ipsilateral horizontal gaze palsy, peripheral facial palsy, nystagmus, and sixth nerve palsy. In a review of 56 cases by Ott et al, at least two of the three characteristic clinical signs – appendicular ataxia, ipsilateral gaze palsy, and peripheral facial palsy – were present in 73% of cases [56].

The clinical course of cerebellar hemorrhage is unpredictable. These patients, whether alert or lethargic on admission, can deteriorate quickly to coma and die with no warning [56, 62]. Little et al reported on two groups of patients with cerebellar hemorrhage [63]. The first group, who required surgery, presented with abrupt onset, a progressive course, and low level of consciousness. CT in this group showed cerebellar hematomas 3cm or greater in diameter, obstructive hydrocephalus, and extension of the hemorrhage into the fourth ventricle [64, 65]. The second group of patients were awake and stable and had hematomas smaller than 3cm in diameter. These patients were treated medically, with good outcomes [63].

Brainstem hemorrhage

The pons is the most common location for non-vascular causes of ICH in the brainstem. Spontaneous non-traumatic midbrain and medullary hematomas are comparably rare. The first person to evaluate a large number of pontine hemorrhages was Attwater in 1911 [66]. After performing autopsies on 77 subjects with pontine hemorrhages, Attwater was able to differentiate between primary and secondary brainstem hemorrhages. He attributed some pontine hemorrhages to elevated ICP. Several years later, in a monograph, Duret also described this phenomenon, which now bears his name [67]. 'Duret hemorrhage' describes a characteristic slit-like bleed in the upper brainstem (mesencephalon and pons) [68]. It must be noted, however, that this does not automatically imply spontaneous ICH as a cause. As Parizel *et al* have pointed out, Duret hemorrhage also occurs in victims of craniocerebral trauma [68].

In an autopsy review of 30 cases of pontine hemorrhage among 511 cases of ICH at Boston City Hospital, two-thirds of the patients were comatose on presentation and had massive hemorrhages that extended into the midbrain or fourth ventricle. Within 48 hours, 78% of the patients died. Fisher suggested that primary hemorrhage, by virtue of a pressure effect, caused the surrounding vessels to rupture, initiating a cascade of gradual enlargement of the hematoma [69]. The bleeding in hypertensive patients was attributed to leakage from tiny penetrating vessels damaged by lipohyalinosis and containing small microaneurysms [69, 70].

Pinpoint (miotic) reactive pupils are a hallmark of pontine lesions. Among the possible various ophthalmic findings with pontine hemorrhage are the following:

* Absent horizontal gaze movement, when the paramedian pontine reticular formation is bilaterally damaged.
* One-and-a-half syndrome after a unilateral pontine tegmental or abducent nucleus lesion that results in a horizontal conjugate gaze palsy in one direction, plus an internuclear ophthalmoplegia in the other [71].
* Ocular bobbing – Fisher was the first to describe these brisk, conjugate downward eye movements, followed by a slower 'bobbing' back up to the primary position [72].

Massive pontine hemorrhages are usually fatal, but death may not be instantaneous. Some patients with medium-sized hematomas and most of those with small basal or lateral tegmental hematomas survive, with various degrees of residual neurologic deficits.

Medical management

The clinical course of ICH after medical management can be dismal. Mortality rates range from 27% to 77% [73-76]. However, optimizing medical care with regard to managing BP, controlling ICP, limiting hematoma expansion, and stabilizing the cardiorespiratory system can have important effects on outcome and help prevent deterioration. The American Heart Association guidelines for the management of spontaneous ICH, published in July 2010, attempt to examine the current evidence for and against several diagnostic and therapeutic procedures utilized in the management of ICH [77]. Despite this concerted effort, uncertainty remains in several aspects of treatment.

Steroids

The use of steroids in patients with ICH is controversial. Batjer *et al* used steroids (4mg dexamethasone intravenously every 6 hours) in their protocol [76]. The rationale for using steroids in the treatment of ICH is that they might lessen the damaging effects of cerebral edema, increased ICP, a disrupted blood-brain barrier, and stress [78]. In a well-designed study reported in 1987, Poungvarin *et al* studied 93 patients (aged 40-80 years) using a double-blind randomized design [79]. Patients with documented primary supratentorial ICH were randomly assigned to either dexamethasone (10mg intravenously and then 5mg every 6 hours) or placebo. The mortality rate was identical in both groups at day 21 (dexamethasone 21/46 patients, placebo 21/47 patients; p=0.93). In contrast, the rate of complications (mostly infections and complications of diabetes) was 11 times higher in the dexamethasone group (p<0.001). This led to early termination of the study **(Ib/A)**.

Blood pressure management

The single most important factor in determining rapid expansion of an ICH is BP. In studies of patients with hypertensive ICH, persistently elevated BP has increased the risk of hematoma progression [80-82]. In a retrospective review of 320 patients with hypertensive ICH, 10 patients showed rapid expansion of the hematoma on serial CT scans [82] (III/B) obtained an average of 1.7 and 48.9 hours after hemorrhage. Of the 10 patients with radiographic evidence of expansion, all had persistent hypertension and half deteriorated neurologically. The average BP of this group on admission was 179/110mmHg, and the average BP recorded before deterioration was 190/121mmHg. The first 24 hours seem to be particularly critical. In a more recent retrospective study of 76 consecutive patients with hypertensive ICH, Ohwaki et al observed that maximum SBP was significantly associated with hematoma enlargement (p=0.0074) [83]. Target SBPs of 160mmHg or less were significantly associated with hematoma enlargement compared with those of 150mmHg or less (p=0.025) (III/B).

The degree to which BP should be controlled is controversial. Patients with a history of chronic hypertension have impaired autoregulation and overzealous lowering of the BP can lower cerebral perfusion pressure, producing secondary ischemic damage. This is especially true of patients with a decreased level of consciousness, who may have elevated ICP. Some authors recommend lowering SBP to less than 160mmHg [84]; others recommend lowering it to normotensive levels but not below [85]. In a prospective randomized trial of putaminal ICH that compared craniotomy with medical therapy, patients were initially treated with sodium nitroprusside to decrease SBP by 25% during the first 24 hours [76]. During the next 48-72 hours, BP decreased to normotensive levels. In this study, mean admission SBP was 234mmHg. Despite the tight BP control, the 6-month mortality rate was 77%. Because this study did not report the cause of death or the time of deterioration, it is difficult to determine whether the degree of BP control was adequate.

In theory, there might be at least two conflicting trends in the immediate hours after ICH: the development of a perilesional microcirculatory insufficiency with a propensity to render brain ischemic; and a propensity to rehemorrhage. The former would necessitate increased perfusion, the latter strict BP control. Qureshi et al looked at the rate

of 24-hour BP decline and mortality after spontaneous ICH [86]. A total of 105 patients with ICH were included in this retrospective study. Logistic regression analysis showed that the rate of decline of BP in the first 24 hours was an independent predictor of mortality but did not affect the functional outcome of survivors (III/B). More recently, the Antihypertensive Treatment of Acute Cerebral Hemorrhage (ATACH) trial set out to establish the optimal BP range in the first 24 hours after an ICH [87]. This was a multicenter open-label pilot that aimed to determine the tolerability and safety of three escalating levels of antihypertension treatment goals (110-140, 140-170, and 170-210mmHg) for acute hypertension in 60 subjects with supratentorial ICH. Each subject was followed for 3 months. A total of 18, 20, and 22 patients were enrolled in the respective three tiers of SBP treatment goals. Seven subjects experienced neurologic deterioration: one (6%), two (10%), and four (18%) in tier one, two, and three, respectively. Serious adverse events were observed in one subject (5%) in tier two and in three subjects (14%) in tier three. Three (17%), two (10%), and five (23%) subjects in tiers one, two, and three, respectively, died within 3 months. This trial confirmed the safety and tolerability of antihypertensive treatment in hypertensive patients with ICH. The underlying mechanism of this beneficial effect is presumably through a reduction in the rate and magnitude of hematoma expansion, observed in approximately 70% of these patients. The results favor pharmacologic reduction of SBP in patients with acute ICH (IIb/B).

Experimental rat studies suggest that although transient alterations in blood flow occur within minutes of hemorrhage, the severe alterations in perihematoma microcirculation that cause ischemia are not maximal until 4 hours thereafter [88, 89]. In addition, the formation of edema is not maximal until 6-8 hours [90]. However, the period associated with the maximal risk of hemorrhage progression in the presence of persistent hypertension is 3-6 hours [15, 82, 91, 92]. Therefore, an argument can be made to reduce BP dramatically during the first 4 hours after hemorrhage to decrease the risk of rehemorrhage, and then raise the BP slowly to perfuse ischemic areas.

Intracranial pressure management

Elevated ICP is considered a major contributor to mortality after ICH and should be treated vigorously [93]. ICP can be managed through osmotherapy, controlled hyperventilation, surgery, and other measures. Therapeutic goals are ICP of less than 20mmHg and cerebral perfusion pressure of higher than 70mmHg.

Mannitol effectively and safely decreases ICP and can be used alone or with urea to potentiate its effect. In a study following ICP-monitored patients, aggressive medical treatment with urea, mannitol, or both adequately controlled ICP and was associated with better outcomes and lower mortality rates [94]. The beneficial effect of sustained hyperventilation on ICP is unresolved and has not been systematically examined in this condition. In theory, reduction of ICP by hyperventilation ceases when the pH of the cerebrospinal fluid reaches equilibrium. If hyperventilation is instituted for elevated ICP, PCO_2 should be maintained between 30 and 35mmHg. An induced barbiturate coma or therapeutic hypothermia are considered last-ditch options and are not part of a standardized algorithm for the treatment of elevated ICP in patients with ICH. Short-acting barbiturates such as thiopental have been shown to effectively reduce elevated ICP [95, 96]. The effect is presumably mediated through reduction of cerebral blood flow and volume. In addition to reducing the volume of the normal brain, barbiturates reduce brain swelling and may act as free-radical scavengers [1, 97]. Moderate hypothermia (32-35°C) can be neuroprotective and decreases ICP by lowering the cerebral blood volume (via lowered metabolic demand) [98].

Studies looking specifically at ICP management in ICH are limited, and most current knowledge about the topic is derived from the head trauma literature. ICH patients with a Glasgow Coma Scale (GCS) score of 8 or less, clinical evidence of herniation, or significant IVH or hydrocephalus may be considered for ICP monitoring and treatment, with a reasonable ICP goal of 50-70mmHg [77] (IV/C). The role of hydrocephalus in predicting poor outcome was well substantiated in a secondary analysis of data from the Surgical Trial in ICH (STICH) [99]. The institution of ventricular drainage as treatment for hydrocephalus is therefore reasonable in patients with impaired consciousness (Ib/A).

Seizures after intracerebral hemorrhage

Seizure activity can result in neuronal injury and worsening of an already critically ill patient and must be treated aggressively [100-107] (Ia/A). The incidence of immediate seizures following supratentorial parenchymal ICH in published series ranges from 1.4% to 17% [100-107].

In a prospective observational study of 761 consecutive patients with non-traumatic, non-aneurysmal ICH, Passero et al reported a cumulative actuarial risk of experiencing seizures of 7.2% in the first 5 days and 8.1% within 30 days [107]. Lobar location of a hemorrhage was also found to be an independent predictor of early seizures, as had been previously recognized [100, 102-104]. However, prospective studies have found no impact of clinical seizures on morbidity and mortality [108, 109]. In addition, the use of prophylactic phenytoin appears to worsen outcomes at 3 months [110] (IIa/B).

EEG monitoring also seems to have a role in management. It may unmask subclinical seizures in the patient with a level of coma unexplained by the significance of the IVH [111].

It may be reasonable to conclude the following:

* Prophylactic anticonvulsants should not be used (IIa/B).
* Clinical seizures should be treated with antiepileptics (Ia/A).
* EEG monitoring is probably indicated in select patients (III/B).
* Treatment should be started if electrographic seizures are unmasked (IV/C).

Recombinant activated factor VII

Multiple studies have demonstrated that the volume of the hematoma is a critical determinant of mortality and functional outcome after ICH [92, 112], and early hematoma growth is an important cause of neurologic deterioration [15, 91, 113, 114]. Early hematoma growth occurs in the absence of coagulopathy and appears to result from continued bleeding or rebleeding at multiple sites within the first few hours of onset [113]. Recombinant activated factor VII (rFVIIa) is approved to treat bleeding in patients with hemophilia, and it has also been reported to reduce bleeding in patients without coagulopathy [115]. Furthermore, a dose-escalation safety study found that doses of rFVIIa ranging from 5 to 160µg/kg body weight were not associated with a high frequency of thromboembolic complications in patients with acute ICH [116].

In 2005, Mayer et al published the results of a double-blind, placebo-controlled trial in which 399 patients with ICH were randomly assigned to receive a single intravenous dose of rFVIIa 40, 80, or 160µg/kg or placebo [117]. Treatment was instituted within 4 hours of symptom onset. Mortality at 90 days was 29% for patients who received placebo, as compared with 18% in the three rFVIIa groups combined (p=0.02). Serious thromboembolic adverse events, mainly myocardial or cerebral infarction, occurred in 7% of rFVIIa-treated patients and 2% of those given placebo (p=0.12). From these data, the authors concluded that treatment with rFVIIa within 4 hours of the onset of ICH limits the growth of the hematoma, reduces mortality, and improves functional outcomes at 90 days, despite a small increase in the frequency of thromboembolic adverse events **(Ib/A)**.

To confirm the treatment advantage with respect to outcome, the Phase III Factor Seven for Acute Hemorrhagic Stroke (FAST) trial was conducted by the same group [118]. A total of 841 patients with ICH were randomly assigned to receive placebo (n=268), rFVIIa 20µg/kg (n=276), or rFVIIa 80µg/kg (n=297) within 4 hours of the onset of the ictus. Surprisingly, despite a reconfirmed significant reduction in growth of the hemorrhage volume, rFVIIa therapy did not improve survival or functional outcomes **(Ib/A)**. The proportion of patients with a poor clinical outcome at 90 days did not differ between the groups (placebo 24%, rFVIIa 20µg/kg 26%, rFVIIa 80µg/kg 29%) **(Ib/A)**.

In conclusion, although rFVIIa can limit the extent of hematoma expansion in patients who are not

coagulopathic, it also increases thromboembolic phenomena. As a result, there is no clear clinical benefit to its use in unselected patients **(Ib/A)**.

Intracerebral hemorrhage due to impaired hemostasis

This topic is not discussed in this chapter. However, an extensive literature review prompted the writing group of the American Heart Association/American Stroke Association 2010 guidelines to reach the following conclusions [77]:

- Patients with severe coagulation factor deficiency or severe thrombocytopenia should receive appropriate factor or platelet replacement, respectively **(IV/C)**.
- Patients on anticoagulants with an elevated International Normalized Ratio (INR) should have warfarin withheld, and receive INR-correcting vitamin K-dependent factors and vitamin K **(IV/C)**.
- Prothrombin complex concentrates (containing Factors II, VII, IX, and X) do not achieve better outcomes than fresh frozen plasma, but may have a safer profile and are a reasonable alternative **(Ib/A)**.
- rFVIIa may lower INR, but does not replace all clotting factors. It is not recommended as the sole agent to reverse the effect of anticoagulants **(IV/C)**.

Summary of medical treatment of intracerebral hemorrhage

Randomized medical trials of ICH examining steroids, glycerol, and hemodilution have not shown significant benefits for any of these therapies [78, 119, 120] **(Ib/A)**. General measures to control BP, reduce ICP, prevent seizures, and maintain systemic health are important in preventing the progression of hemorrhage, edema, and brain ischemia. Despite disappointing results thus far, these parameters should be controlled aggressively. The optimal reduction of BP needed to adequately perfuse the brain yet prevent rebleeding or progression is controversial. The patient's state of consciousness is the best guide to prognosis [1, 121] and may help to determine the degree of BP and ICP control that should be instituted. If neurologic deterioration occurs or ICP cannot be controlled, surgical evacuation should be considered.

Surgical management

Supratentorial hematoma

Hematoma volume

In 1977, Hier *et al* reviewed 5,000 CT scans to correlate the volume of putaminal hematomas with presentation and prognosis [38]. The authors defined three groups:

- Patients with small hematomas (<35cm^3) showed mild to moderate hemiparesis or hemisensory loss, preservation of higher cortical function, and a good prognosis, regardless of treatment.
- Patients with moderate hematomas (mean 120cm^3) had classic flaccid hemiplegia, hemisensory defect, lateral gaze preference, homonymous hemianopsia, and either aphasia or apractagnosia.
- Massive hemorrhages (>200cm^3) produced coma, fixed and dilated pupils, papilledema, absent eye movements, bilateral fixed plantar response, and rapid death.

These correlations suggested that patients with moderate hematomas might be candidates for a controlled clinical comparison of surgical and conservative treatments.

In a retrospective review of 188 cases of supratentorial ICH, Broderick *et al* showed that hematoma volume was the strongest predictor of 30-day mortality and functional outcome at all locations (putaminal, thalamic, and subcortical) [92] **(III/B)**. The 30-day mortality rates for deep hemorrhages less than 30cm^3, between 30 and 60cm^3, and greater than 60cm^3 were 23%, 64%, and 93%, respectively. Mortality rates for lobar hemorrhages at these volumes were 7%, 60%, and 71%, respectively. Half

of the patients who died did so within the first 2 days. Of 71 patients surviving with hematoma volumes larger than 30cm^3, only one (1.4%) was independent at 30 days. In contrast, of the 91 patients who survived with hematoma volumes less than 30cm^3, 16 (18%) were independent. Combining hematoma volumes with admission GCS scores proved to be 97% sensitive and 97% specific for 30-day mortality. The probability of death at 30 days was 91% for patients with GCS scores less than 8 and hematoma volumes greater than 60cm^3, compared with 19% for those with GCS scores higher than 9 and hematoma volumes less than 30cm^3. Although this study did not aim to evaluate the effectiveness of treatment, operative removal was associated with a decreased 30-day mortality rate, although overall surgical morbidity and mortality rates were not significantly different from those associated with conservative treatment.

Volpin *et al* retrospectively reviewed outcomes following medical treatment and craniotomy in 132 cases of supratentorial ICH with respect to hematoma volume, regardless of location [122]. Compared with conservative treatment, surgery decreased the mortality rate of comatose patients with hematoma volumes between 26 and 85cm^3, but the probability of discharge with a severe deficit was high. All patients with hematoma volumes greater than 85cm^3 died, irrespective of treatment, and all patients with hematoma volumes less than 26cm^3 survived without surgery.

In contrast, a retrospective comparison of surgery and conservative therapy in 182 patients with putaminal hemorrhage found that the size of the hematoma on CT was a statistically significant predictor of outcome, despite treatment modality [49]. Localized hematomas or those extending into either limb of the internal capsule (groups I-III) were compared with those that extended into both limbs of the internal capsule, the thalamus, or both (groups IV and V). The 30-day mortality rate was significantly lower in groups I-III than in groups IV and V (12% vs. 57%).

A randomized prospective study comparing endoscopic removal of supratentorial ICH with medical management found surgery to be beneficial for hematomas of all volumes, especially subcortical hematomas [123]. Interestingly, patients with hematoma volumes less than 50cm³ had better outcomes after surgery than after conservative treatment (25% vs. 0% with an activities of daily living score of 1), although the mortality rate was the same. For large hematomas (>50cm³), there was no difference in functional outcome between the two groups, but the mortality rate was lower in the surgical group than in the conservative group (48% vs. 90%). This study suggests that surgical evacuation may play a life-saving role in patients with large hematomas by sparing viable local brain function by decreasing mass effect, progressive edema, or impaired cerebral perfusion. The overall lower surgical mortality rate (30%) in this study compared with others may reflect surgical technique and is discussed later in this chapter. However, this study did suffer from certain statistical issues in the analysis of multiple variables and outcomes that weaken its impact.

Large-volume thalamic hematomas are more devastating than similarly sized subcortical or putaminal hematomas. In a study of 29 patients with thalamic hemorrhages, those with volumes greater than 10cm³ or with a maximal diameter greater than 3cm had activity of daily living scores of 4 or 5 [124]. Thalamic hematomas with a long axis greater than 3cm are associated with poor outcomes [40, 42, 48]. In a comparison of 75 patients with thalamic hemorrhages who underwent either stereotactic aspiration or conservative treatment, 31 of 40 surgical patients (78%) with hematoma diameters larger than 3.3cm returned to useful activity in 6 months [125]. This finding suggests that the less invasive nature of stereotactic aspiration may improve therapeutic outcomes, despite the size and location of the hematoma **(III/B)**.

Hematoma volume also seems to be related to the risk of deterioration. In a retrospective study of 182 African-Americans, the presence of an ICH greater than 30cm³ increased the risk of deterioration and death in the first 24 hours by 6.78 and 6.66 times, respectively [35]. Of 46 non-comatose patients, 15 deteriorated during the initial 24 hours. In this study, hematoma volume was a better early predictor of poor outcome than admission GCS score.

Time course

Understanding the natural time course of an acute ICH and its effect on clinical deterioration is critical to therapeutic decision-making. Before CT was available, ICH was considered to be a monophasic event that stopped quickly as a result of clotting and tamponade by the surrounding regions [126]. This impression is incorrect, as demonstrated by CT scans showing that hematomas expand over time [15, 114]. The radiographic progression of a hematoma and its correlation with clinical course have been well studied. Rehemorrhage typically occurs within the first 6 hours of the primary ictus [91, 92]. Most of the extravasation of contrast in the angiograms of patients with ICH is seen within 3-6 hours of onset [127, 128]. If deterioration occurs later than 6 hours after hemorrhage then other factors (e.g., edema, hydrocephalus, new IVH, or a metabolic abnormality) must be contributing.

In a study of 419 patients, Fujii et al obtained the first CT scan within 24 hours of onset and a follow-up scan 24 hours after admission [113]. They found that hematomas had enlarged in 14% of patients. In another study, Kazui et al obtained sequential CT scans from 204 patients with acute ICH [114]. Hematomas enlarged by 40% in 20% of patients. This was seen when the scans were obtained early; none of the patients showed an increase in hematoma size after 24 hours.

To define the progression over time more closely, Brott et al prospectively studied 103 patients with ICH at all locations who underwent CT within 3 hours of onset [15]. The patients were rescanned 1 and 20 hours after the first scan. On the 1-hour follow-up scan, 26% of patients exhibited hematoma growth (>33% enlargement). An additional 12% showed growth between 1 and 20 hours. Therefore, 38% of patients exhibited hematoma progression within 24 hours of hemorrhage. Of these patients, 33% deteriorated within the first hour, and an additional 25% deteriorated within the next 20 hours. Therefore, the clinical condition of more than 50% of all patients showing progression on serial CT deteriorated. This finding implies that early hematoma evacuation may not only reduce perihematoma ischemia [89, 129, 130] and the toxic effects of blood products [89, 131, 132], but also contain potential hemorrhagic progression.

Bae *et al* reported similar results from their retrospective study of 320 patients with ICH who underwent serial CTs [82]. Overall, 3% of patients showed rapid hematoma progression. The mean follow-up scan was obtained at 48.9 hours after hemorrhage (range 10.5-149 hours), and 50% of patients showing progression deteriorated before 24 hours had elapsed. In this study, the most important risk factor for progression was persistent hypertension.

When Qureshi *et al* retrospectively reviewed 182 African-American patients to identify independent predictors of early deterioration and death, 23% of the patients with GCS scores higher than 12 showed early deterioration (mean 7.9 hours) [35]. An ICH volume greater than $30cm^3$ and ventricular extension were independent predictors of early deterioration (OR 6.78 and 4.67, respectively) and death (OR 6.66 and 4.23, respectively) **(III/B)**.

Goals of surgery

The goals of the surgical evacuation of a hematoma are to reduce the mass effect, block the release of neuropathic products from the hematoma, and prevent prolonged interaction between the hematoma and normal tissue, which can initiate pathologic processes [62]. From the data available, it is clear that within the spectrum of ICH there are some patients (with large or space-occupying ICH) who require surgery for neurologic deterioration and others with small hematomas who should be managed conservatively. There is equipoise about the management of patients between these two extremes. Some patients have a penumbra of functionally impaired but potentially viable tissue around the ICH; surgical removal of the clot may improve the function and recovery in this penumbra [133]. As suggested by the aforementioned studies, early surgery may play an important role in preventing secondary deterioration, and the timing of surgery becomes an important question that needs to be elucidated.

Timing of surgery

Credible experimental evidence indicates that early evacuation of hematomas improves cerebral blood flow [88, 89, 130-132], histologic changes [134], brain edema [90], ischemia [89], and outcomes [130]. The natural history of ICH reveals that 50% of related deaths occur within 48 hours of hemorrhage [92], and radiographic expansion or rebleeding occur maximally within 3-4 hours but for as long as 24 hours thereafter [15]. Therefore, early surgery may improve outcomes for many reasons. Extensive clinical evidence also supports early surgery [135-137]. A single lenticulostriate branch rupture that bleeds for a brief time creates a significant hypertensive hematoma [138]. Consequently, direct early vessel coagulation seems advantageous. Exacerbation occurs suddenly and usually within 4-6 hours of bleeding [15]; thus, early surgery might prevent clinical progression. Because secondary changes such as edema occur 7-8 hours after a hemorrhage, evacuation before that time may prevent these changes.

In an important retrospective study of ultra-early surgery, Kaneko *et al* reviewed 100 putaminal hemorrhages, all of which were operated on within 7 hours [136]. All patients were hemiplegic, with GCS scores between 6 and 12 and hematoma volumes greater than $20-30cm^3$. The mortality rate was 7%, and the 6-month rate of 'useful recovery' was 83%. Two patients died from rapid exacerbation before surgery, and two died from reaccumulation of hematoma. These results are favorable when compared with the series of Yukawa and Kanaya, which did not emphasize early surgery and reported a 29% mortality rate and 63% rate of useful recovery [139] **(III/B)**. The patients in the Kaneko *et al* study had better immediate preoperative neurologic grades, implying that earlier surgery limited the time available for further deterioration [136]. However, this study did not address patients with GCS scores of 13 and hematoma volumes between 20 and $30cm^3$.

These results are supported by a retrospective analysis that showed that a subgroup of patients with moderate-sized putaminal hematomas had better outcomes when operated on within 6 hours of hemorrhage [137] **(III/B)**. Furthermore, in a prospective study by Juvela *et al*, 52 patients with GCS scores

Deep intracranial hemorrhage

Table 2. Summary of retrospective trials: surgery versus medical therapy for intracerebal hemorrhage. *Continued overleaf.*

Reference	Total cases, n		Preoperative neurologic grade		Good outcome, n (%)		Fair outcome, n (%)		Poor outcome, n (%)		Group-stratified mortality, n (%)		Outcome	Overall mortality, n (%)
	Surgical	Medical	Surgical	Medical	Surgical	Medical	Surgical	Medical	Surgical	Medical	Surgical	Medical		
Guillaume et al, 1957	128	-	NA	NA	NA	NA	NA	NA	NA	NA	NA	NA	-	41 (32)
McKissock et al, 1961	89	91	NA	NA	10 (11)	12 (13)	8 (9)	21 (23)	13 (15)	15 (17)	58 (65)	46 (51)	-	89 (58)
Cuatico et al, 1965	99	-	2.6	-	35 (35)	NA	23 (23)	NA	33 (33)	NA	-	-	-	8 (8)
Mitsuno et al, 1966	43	-	NA	NA	NA	NA	NA	NA	NA	NA	NA	NA	-	19 (43)
Luessenhop et al, 1967	37	27	NA	NA	NA	NA	NA	NA	NA	NA	12 (32)	12 (44)	-	24 (38)
Scott and Werthan, 1970	17	25	3.2	2.8	3 (18)	4 (16)	3 (18)	2 (8)	0 (0)	3 (12)	11 (65)	15 (60)	-	23 (55)
Mitsuno et al, 1971	514	436	NA	NA	NA	NA	NA	NA	NA	NA	NA	NA	-	180 (35)
Mizukami et al, 1972	72	-	NA	NA	NA	NA	NA	NA	NA	NA	NA	NA	-	19 (26)
Pailas and Alliez, 1973	137	-	NA	NA	NA	NA	NA	NA	NA	NA	NA	NA	-	64 (47)
Kanaya and Handa, 1974	1558	-	NA	NA	NA	NA	NA	NA	NA	NA	NA	NA	-	476 (31)
Tedeschi et al, 1975	57	14	NA	NA	8 (14)	0 (0)	13 (23)	2 (14)	14 (25)	6 (43)	22 (39)	6 (43)	-	28 (39)
Kanaya et al, 1976	174	-	NA	NA	NA	NA	NA	NA	NA	NA	NA	NA	-	59 (33.9)
Kanaya et al, 1978	410	204	1		(89)	(89)	NA	NA	NA	NA	(2.7)	(2.0)	At 6 months	(25.9)
			2		(59)	(59)					(9.3)	(9.3)		
			3		(33)	(5)					(17.8)	(52.7)		
			4A		(47)	(8)					(28.2)	(58.2)		
			4B		(0)	(0)					(57.1)	(100.0)		
			5		(0)	(0)					(87.5)	(100.0)		
Matsumoto et al, 1980	94	-	1		(92)	-	(0)	-	(0)		(8)	-	-	(13)
			2		(50)		(50)		(0)		(0)			
			3		(58)		(38)		(0)		(4)			
			4A		(0)		(25)		(50)		(25)			
			4B		(0)		(0)		(50)		(50)			
			5		(0)		(0)		(0)		(0)			

Table 2. Summary of retrospective trials: surgery versus medical therapy for intracerebal hemorrhage. *Continued.*

Reference	Total cases, n		Preoperative neurologic grade		Good outcome, n (%)		Fair outcome, n (%)		Poor outcome, n (%)		Group-stratified mortality, n (%)		Outcome	Overall mortality, n (%)
	Surgical	Medical	Surgical	Medical	Surgical	Medical	Surgical	Medical	Surgical	Medical	Surgical	Medical		
Kanaya et al, 1981	3216	-	1		(61.6)	-	(34.7)	-	(3.7)	-	(5.3)	-	At 6 months	(20.7)
			2		(55.9)	-	(37.2)	-	(6.9)	-	(9.4)	-		
			3		(38.7)	-	(45.4)	-	(15.9)	-	(16.8)	-		
			4A		(27.2)	-	(44.0)	-	(28.8)	-	(29.3)	-		
			4B		(16.2)	-	(47.6)	-	(36.2)	-	(57.8)	-		
			5		(0)	-	(15.4)	-	(84.6)	-	(75.9)	-		
Kaneko et al, 1983[a]	100	87	1		(0)	(81)	(0)	(19)	(0)	(0)	(0)	(0)	-	Overall: (22)
			2		(70)	(47)	(20)	(33)	(0)	(13)	(10)	(7)		Total surgical: (7)
			3		(53)	(8)	(37)	(39)	(6)	(31)	(4)	(23)		Total medical: (39)
			4A		(39)	(0)	(28)	(0)	(33)	(50)	(0)	(50)		
			4B		(0)	(0)	(25)	(0)	(0)	(0)	(75)	(100)		
			5		(0)	(0)	(0)	(0)	(0)	(4)	(0)	(96)		
Zuccarello et al, 1983	167	139	NA		NA		NA		NA		(52.1)	(21.5)	-	-
Bolander et al, 1983[b]	39	35	NA		(16)	(16)	(19)	(28)	(38)	(25)	(27)	(29)	At 3 months	-
Brambilla et al, 1983	37	49	NA		NA		NA		NA		(52)	(43)	At 30 days	-
Volpin et al, 1984	32	34	1		(100)	(67)	(0)	(33)	(0)	(0)	(0)	(0)	-	(16) (32)
			2		(100)	(71)	(0)	(21)	(0)	(0)	(0)	(7)		
			3		(20)	(16.7)	(60)	(33)	(0)	(0)	(0)	(50)		
			4A, 4B, 5		(18)	(0)	(50)	(0)	(9)	(0)	(23)	(100)		
Kanno et al, 1984[a]	154	305	Mild		(84.4)	(83)	(7.4)	(7.5)	(7.4)	(9.4)	-		-	-
			Moderate		(36.6)	(30)	(30.0)	(5.0)						
			Severe		(41.0)	(45)	(33.0)	(54.0)						
			Fulminant		NA	NA	NA	NA						
			Very severe		(0)	(0)	(0)	(0)						
Coraddu et al, 1990[c]	31	28	NA		NA		NA		NA		(17)	(0)	At 30 days	-

[a] = Putamen; [b] = all locations; [c] = supra- and infratentorial; ADL = activities of daily living; NA = data not available

Outcomes: good = ADL 1-2; fair = ADL 3; poor = ADL 4-5

Neurologic grades: 1 = alert or confused; 2 = somnolent; 3 = stuporous; 4A = semicomatose without herniation signs; 4B = semicomatose with herniation signs; 5 = deep coma

Deep intracranial hemorrhage

Table 3. Summary of prospective randomized controlled trials: surgery (open craniotomy) versus medical therapy in intracerebral hemorrhage. *Continued overleaf.*

Reference	Location	Inclusion criteria	Total cases	Mean hematoma size	Preoperative neurologic status	Independent at 6 months, n (%)	Dependent at 6 months, n (%)	Dead at 6 months, n (%)	Time from onset to surgery, hours (mean)	Odds ratio (95% CI)	Comments
McKissock, 1961	All	Not clear	S: 89 M: 91	NA	Equal groups	S: 18 (20) M: 31 (34)	S: 13 (15) M: 14 (15)	S: 58 (65) M: 46 (51)	72	2.04 (1.04-3.98)	Method of randomization not described Pre-CT era
Juvela et al, 1989	All	'Unconscious and/or severe hemiparesis or dysphasia' Excluded patients 'not responding to pain'	S: 26 M: 26	S: 56.2cc M: 66.7cc	Mean GCS: S: 9 M: 12	S: 1 (4) M: 5 (19)	S: 13 (50) M: 11 (42)	S: 12 (46) M: 10 (39)	48 (14.5)	5.95	Surgical group had overall lower pretreatment GCS score and increased incidence of IVH (p<0.05) Four patients in ICP and medically managed group
Batjer, 1990	Putamen	>3cm diameter ICH, alert and 2/5, lethargic and 2/5, obtunded, or stuporous but purposeful with hemiplegia	S: 8 M: 9	>3cm	No. of patients in grade 3: S: 2 M: 2	S: 2 (25) M: 2 (22)	S: 2 (25) M: 0 (0)	S: 4 (50) M: 7 (78)	24	0.86 (0.09-8.09)	Unclear if assessor blinded Exact time to surgery not mentioned
Morgenstern, 1998	Lobe putamen	GCS 5-15 ICH >9cc Excluded: large IVH, GCS 15 and 10-20cc, and antigravity strength	S: 17 M: 17	S: 49cc M: 43.8cc	Mean GCS: S: 10 M: 11	S: 6 (35) M: 7 (41)	S: 8 (47) M: 6 (35)	S: 3 (18) M: 4 (24)	12 (8.3)	1.28	Single site Small sample size Surgical group mostly had lobar ICH Surgical group had worse pretreatment neurologic grades
Zucarrello, 1999	All	Age >18 years ICH >10cc and focal neurologic deficit GCS >4	S: 9 M: 11	Median: S: 35cc M: 30cc	Mean GCS: S: 12.2 M: 10.2	S: 5 (56) M: 4 (36)	S: 2 (22) M: 4 (36)	S: 2 (22) M: 3 (18)	24 (8.5)	0.45	4/9 cases performed stereotactically
Teernstra (STX), 2001	-	Age >45 years ICH >10cc Treatment within 72 hours	S: 36 M: 34	-	Glasgow eye motor score 2-10	-	-	-	-	0.52 (1.2-2.3) Odds ratio of mortality not statistically significant	Trial prematurely stopped because of slow patient accrual

Table 3. Summary of prospective randomized controlled trials: surgery (open craniotomy) versus medical therapy in intracerebral hemorrhage. *Continued.*

Reference	Location	Inclusion criteria	Total cases	Mean hematoma size	Preoperative neurologic status	Independent at 6 months, n (%)	Dependent at 6 months, n (%)	Dead at 6 months, n (%)	Time from onset to surgery, hours (mean)	Odds ratio (95% CI)	Comments
Mendelow, 2005	All	GCS ≥5 ICH ≥2cm ICH within 72 hours	S: 503 M: 530	S: 40cc M: 37cc	Equal	S: 152 (33) M: 137 (28)	S: 312 (67) M: 351 (72)	S: 173 (36) M: 189 (37)	30	-	Superficial hematomas might benefit from surgery
Subtotal	-	-	S: 688 M: 718	-	-	S: 184 (30) M: 186 (29)	S: 350 (58) M: 386 (61)	S: 252 (40) M: 260 (39)	-	1.71	-
Endoscopic Auer, 1989	All	Age 30-80 years ICH >10cc 'With neurologic deficit and/or disturbance of consciousness'	S: 50 M: 50	>50 cc: S: 44% M: 48%	-	S: 22 (44) M: 13 (26)	S: 7 (14) M: 2 (4)	S: 21 (42) M: 35 (70)	48	0.45 (0.19-1.98)	Did not use a valid statistical subgroup analysis No statistical adjustments made for multiple testing of multiple outcome categories
Stereotactic Hattori, 2004	Putamen	Age 35-85 years Treatment started within <24 hours	S: 121 M: 121	S: 48cc M: 40cc	Equal	S: 61 (50) M: 39 (32)	S: 51 (42) M: 62 (51)	S: 9 (7) M: 20 (17)	-	-	Benefit for stereotactic evacuation with regards to ADL using multiple regression analysis
Total	-	-	**S: 859 M: 893**	-	-	**S: 267 (34) M: 238 (29)**	**S: 408 (53) M: 450 (56)**	**S: 282 (35) M: 315 (38)**	-	1.21	-

ADL = activities of daily living; CI = confidence interval; CT = computed tomography; GCS = Glasgow Coma Scale; ICH = intracerebral hemorrhage; IVH = intraventricular hemorrhage; M = medical group; S = surgical group between 7 and 10 did not benefit from surgery performed after 24 hours, but mortality rates improved when surgery occurred within 13 hours [140].

A prospective randomized controlled trial has evaluated the feasibility of early surgery [141]. The median time from symptom onset to hospitalization was 3.3 hours, and time to surgery was 8.5 hours (beyond the range of <6 hours). There was no difference in outcomes between surgery and medical treatment, but there was a trend toward a lower 3-month morbidity rate with surgery **(Ib/A)**. This study suggests that there are logistic barriers to ultra-early surgery, and this is where the bulk of the 'brain-attack' effort is directed (i.e., educating primary physicians, paramedics, and the public).

The need to gain robust evidence to support clinical decision-making led to the initiation of the Surgical Trial in ICH (STICH), funded by the Medical Research Council and the Stroke Association and activated in 1998 [142]. This was a prospective randomized trial to compare early surgery with initial conservative treatment for patients with spontaneous supratentorial ICH. Early surgery combined hematoma evacuation (within 24 hours of randomization) with best medical treatment. Initial conservative treatment used best medical treatment, although delayed evacuation was allowed if it became necessary. Analysis was on an intention-to-treat basis. At 6 months, of 468 patients randomized to early surgery, 122 (26%) had a favorable outcome compared with 118 of 496 (24%) randomized to initial conservative treatment (OR 0.89; 95% confidence interval [CI], 0.66-1.19; p=0.414). These results suggested no overall benefit from early surgery when compared with initial conservative treatment **(Ib/A)**. Detailed analysis of the CT images from STICH has shown that 42% of patients included in the trial had an associated IVH. The prognosis for patients with IVH with or without hydrocephalus is much worse than that for ICH alone. Removing these patients from the analysis and focusing on superficial hematomas presents a better picture for surgery. Using prognosis-based Rankin score as the outcome variable, a significant benefit was observed for surgical patients in this subgroup (p=0.013) **(IIa/B)**. Further analysis of the subgroups of patients with lobar hematomas from

the trials of Auer *et al* and Teernstra *et al* support the hypothesis that this subgroup might benefit from early surgery [123, 143]. This evidence supports the ongoing STICH-II trial, which aims to evaluate the role of early surgery in patients with superficial supratentorial lobar hematomas without IVH.

Infratentorial hematoma

With cerebellar hemorrhages, identifying the appropriate clinical progression is paramount to guiding surgical evacuation. When hematomas are near the brainstem, however, irreversible deterioration can occur without warning. Many studies recommend surgery for all hematomas greater than 3cm in diameter [37, 56, 144]. Smaller lesions have a more benign course. However, the patient's clinical profile must still be followed carefully because spatial accommodation is, by necessity, more limited here than supratentorially.

Cerebellar hemorrhage tends to progress rapidly and to cause death because of its proximity to the brainstem. It has been recommended that patients with GCS scores of 13 or less or hemorrhages of 4cm or more should undergo surgical evacuation [137] **(III/B)**. Other authors, however, contend that rapid progression of particular cerebellar and cranial nerve syndromes (see earlier) represents a surgical emergency, despite these criteria [33, 145].

Timing of surgery

With cerebellar hemorrhage, ultra-early surgery is vital in patients with signs of brainstem compression. At the earliest sign of clinical change, immediate evacuation without CT can be life- and function-saving. Without brainstem signs, however, the timing of surgery is controversial **(IV/C)**. Ott *et al* studied the natural history of cerebellar hemorrhage [56]. Their review of 56 cases showed that nine of 28 patients treated conservatively died precipitously up to 2 weeks after hemorrhage. Fifty percent deteriorated within 2 days, and an additional 25% deteriorated within 1 week. Only after 8 days did awake or drowsy patients treated conservatively have a lower mortality rate than those undergoing surgery. Therefore, patients presenting in the first week of hemorrhage may still benefit from surgery **(III/B)**.

Research from Yanaka *et al* supports the notion that even deeply comatose patients with cerebellar hemorrhage benefit from surgical evacuation, provided evacuation is immediate, especially if the time between coma onset and surgery can be kept to less than 2 hours [58] **(III/B)**.

Death is usually within the first 2 days, but can occur later. Progressive hematomas produce consistent clinical findings that must be promptly recognized. With the first sign of deterioration, patients must undergo immediate surgical evacuation.

Summary of surgical treatment of intracerebral hemorrhage

Tables 2 and 3 summarize the retrospective and prospective randomized controlled trials, respectively,

of surgery versus medical therapy for intracerebal hemorrhage.

Conclusions

Spontaneous ICH has multiple facets and the best management of these challenging lesions is still somewhat controversial. Immediate and aggressive medical care in an intensive care unit setting, emphasizing the control of BP, offers the best chance of recovery for mildly disabled patients at ictus. Emergent surgical evacuation of a large hematoma offers devastated patients the best chance of survival, but without much recovery of function over and above what medical management might have achieved. The ideal treatment of patients that lie between these two extremes remains unclear. At our institution, we advocate that a hypertensive putaminal, lobar, or subcortical ICH large enough to cause a neurologic deficit is an acute 'brain attack' that needs to be evacuated emergently with standard open microsurgical techniques.

Recommendations	Evidence level
◆ Dexamethasone is not useful, and potentially harmful, in the medical treatment of ICH.	Ib/A
◆ Untreated hypertension in the first few hours after a spontaneous ICH increases the risk of hematoma expansion and mortality.	IIb/B
◆ Aggressive treatment of hypertension to within a range of 110-140mmHg in the first 24 hours after ICH reduces hematoma expansion, mortality, and neurologic deterioration.	IIb/B
◆ ICH patients with a GCS 8, clinical evidence of herniation, or significant IVH or hydrocephalus may be considered for ICP monitoring and treatment, with a reasonable goal of ICP of 50-70mmHg.	IV/C
◆ The institution of ventricular drainage as treatment for hydrocephalus is reasonable in patients with impaired consciousness.	Ib/A
◆ Prophylactic anticonvulsants should not be used.	IIa/B
◆ Clinical seizures should be treated with antiepileptics.	Ia/A
◆ EEG monitoring is probably indicated in select patients.	III/B
◆ Treatment should be started if electrographic seizures are unmasked.	IV/C

Continued

Recommendations *continued* | **Evidence level**

- rFVIIa, when used generally for all patients with ICH, does not improve survival or functional outcome. — Ib/A

- Patients with severe coagulation factor deficiency or severe thrombocytopenia should receive appropriate factor or platelet replacement, respectively. — IV/C

- Patients on anticoagulants with an elevated INR should have warfarin withheld, and receive INR-correcting vitamin K-dependent factors and vitamin K. — IV/C

- Prothrombin complex concentrates (containing Factors II, VII, IX, and X) do not achieve better outcomes than fresh frozen plasma, but may have a safer profile and are a reasonable alternative. — Ib/A

- rFVIIa may lower INR, but does not replace all clotting factors. It is not recommended as the sole agent to reverse the effect of anticoagulants. — IV/C

- For most patients with ICH, the usefulness of surgery is uncertain. — Ib/A

- For patients with large and superficial hematomas, craniotomy for evacuation is an option. — IIa/B

- Early surgical evacuation of intracranial hematomas is beneficial in some subgroups of patients. — III/B

- If median time from onset to surgery is 8.5 hours, the outcomes of surgical evacuation are no better than those of medical treatment. — Ib/A

- If all patients with supratentorial ICH and IVH are considered indiscriminately, early surgery or initial conservative management yield similar 6-month outcomes. — Ib/A

- Subgroup analysis reveals that patients with superficial hematomas achieve better Rankin scores after surgical evacuation, compared with medical therapy. — IIa/B

- Ultra-early surgery for supratentorial ICH has not been shown to improve outcomes in general. — Ib/A

- The use of minimally invasive clot evacuation techniques is considered investigational at this point, in view of inconsistent results. — IIb/B

- Patients with cerebellar hemorrhage and signs of mass effect benefit from early surgery. — III/B

- For those without clinical mass effect, the role of surgery remains controversial. — IV/C

Chapter 32

References

1. McKissock W, Richardson A, Taylor J. Primary intracerebral haemorrhage; a controlled trial of surgical and conservative treatment in 180 unselected cases. *Lancet* 1961; ii: 221-6.

2. Donley J. John James Wepfer: a renaissance student of apoplexy. *Bull Johns Hopkins Hosp* 1990; 20: 1-2.

3. Clarke E. Cerebrovascular system - historical aspects. In: *Radiology of the Skull and Brain*, vol. 2, book 1. Newton T, Potts D, Eds. New York: Mosby, 1974; 875-89.

4. Fazio C, Sacco G, Bugiani O. The thalamic hemorrhage. An anatomo-clinical study. *Eur Neurol* 1973; 9: 30-43.

5. MacEwen W. An address on the surgery of the brain and spinal cord. *BMJ* 1888; 2: 302-9.

6. Cushing H. The blood-pressure reaction of acute cerebral compression, illustrated by cases of intracranial hemorrhage. *Am J Med Sci* 1903; 125: 1017-44.

7. Bagley C. Spontaneous cerebral hemorrhage: discussion of four types, with surgical considerations. *Arch Neurol Psychiatry* 1932; 27: 1113-74.

8.   Robinson G. Encapsulated brain hemorrhages. A study of their frequency and pathology. *Arch Neurol Psychiatry* 1932; 27: 1441-4.

9.   Guillome J, Roger R. Indications chirurgicales dans les hemorragies cerebrales. *Presse Med* 1957; 63: 827-9.

10. Lazorthes G. Surgery of cerebral hemorrhage; report on the results of 52 surgically treated cases. *J Neurosurg* 1959; 16: 355-64.

11. Broderick J, Connolly S, Feldmann E, *et al.* Guidelines for the management of spontaneous intracerebral hemorrhage in adults; 2007 update: a guideline from the American Heart Association/American Stroke Association Stroke Council, High Blood Pressure Research Council, and the Quality of Care and Outcomes in Research Interdisciplinary Working Group. *Stroke* 2007; 38: 2001-23.

12. Foulkes MA, Wolf PA, Price TR, *et al.* The Stroke Data Bank: design, methods, and baseline characteristics. *Stroke* 1988; 19: 547-54.

13. Qureshi AI, Giles WH, Croft JB. Racial differences in the incidence of intracerebral hemorrhage: effects of blood pressure and education. *Neurology* 1999; 52: 1617-21.

14. Sturgeon JD, Folsom AR, Longstreth WT Jr, *et al.* Risk factors for intracerebral hemorrhage in a pooled prospective study. *Stroke* 2007; 38: 2718-25.

15. Brott T, Broderick J, Kothari R, *et al.* Early hemorrhage growth in patients with intracerebral hemorrhage. *Stroke* 1997; 28: 1-5.

16. Ariesen MJ, Claus SP, Rinkel GJ, *et al.* Risk factors for intracerebral hemorrhage in the general population: a systematic review. *Stroke* 2003; 34: 2060-5.

17. Hanggi D, Steiger HJ. Spontaneous intracerebral haemorrhage in adults: a literature overview. *Acta Neurochir* (Wien) 2008; 150: 371-9.

18. Woo D, Sauerbeck LR, Kissela BM, *et al.* Genetic and environmental risk factors for intracerebral hemorrhage: preliminary results of a population-based study. *Stroke* 2002; 33: 1190-5.

19. Woodward M, Huxley H, Lam TH, *et al.* A comparison of the associations between risk factors and cardiovascular disease in Asia and Australasia. *Eur J Cardiovasc Prev Rehabil* 2005; 12: 484-91.

20. Neaton JD, Wentworth DN, Cutler J, *et al.* Risk factors for death from different types of Stroke. Multiple Risk Factor Intervention Trial Research Group. *Ann Epidemiol* 1993; 3: 493-9.

21. Leppälä JM, Virtamo J, Fogelholm R, *et al.* Different risk factors for different stroke subtypes: association of blood pressure, cholesterol, and antioxidants. *Stroke* 1999; 30: 2535-40.

22. Thrift AG, McNeil JJ, Forbes A, *et al.* Risk factors for cerebral hemorrhage in the era of well-controlled hypertension. Melbourne Risk Factor Study (MERFS) Group. *Stroke* 1996; 27: 2020-5.

23. Kase C, Mohr J. Intracerebral hemorrhage. In: S*troke: Pathophysiology, Diagnosis and Management.* Barnett HH, Ed. New York: Churchill Livingstone.

24. Cole FM, Yates PO. Pseudo-aneurysms in relationship to massive cerebral hemorrhage. *J Neurol Neurosurg Psychiatry* 1967; 30: 61-6.

25. Charcot J, Bouchard C. Nouvelles recherches sur la pathogenie de lhemorragie cerebrale. *Arch Physiol Normale Pathol* 1868; 110-27, 643-65, 725-34.

26. Russell R. Observations on intracerebral aneurysms. *Brain* 1963; 86: 425-42.

27. Cole FM, Yates PO. The occurrence and significance of intracerebral micro-aneurysms. *J Pathol Bacteriol* 1967; 93: 393-411.

28. Fisher C. Clinical syndromes in cerebral hemorrhage. In: *Pathogenesis and Treatment of Cerebrovascular Disease.* Fields E, Ed. Springfield, IL: Charles C Thomas, 1961.

29. Fisher C. Cerebral miliary aneurysms in hypertension. *Am J Pathol* 1972; 66: 313-24.

30. Fisher C. The arterial lesions underlying lacunes. *Acta Neuropathol* 1969; 12: 1-15.

31. Mohr JP, Caplan LR, Melski JW, *et al.* The Harvard Cooperative Stroke Registry: a prospective registry. *Neurology* 1978; 28: 754-62.

32. Andrews BT, Chiles BW 3rd, Olsen WL, Pitts LH. The effect of intracerebral hematoma location on the risk of brain-stem compression and on clinical outcome. *J Neurosurg* 1988; 69: 518-22.

33. Heros RC. Cerebellar hemorrhage and infarction. *Stroke* 1982; 13: 106-9.

34. Mayer SA, Sacco RL, Shi T, Mohr JP. Neurologic deterioration in noncomatose patients with supratentorial intracerebral hemorrhage. *Neurology* 1994; 44: 1379-84.

35. Qureshi AI, Safdar K, Weil J, *et al.* Predictors of early deterioration and mortality in black Americans with spontaneous intracerebral hemorrhage. *Stroke* 1995; 26: 1764-7.

36. Zazulia AR, Diringer MN, Derdeyn CP, Powers WJ. Progression of mass effect after intracerebral hemorrhage. *Stroke* 1999; 30: 1167-73.

37. Ojemann, RG, Heros RC. Spontaneous brain hemorrhage. *Stroke* 1983; 14: 468-75.

38. Hier DB, Davis KR, Richardson EP Jr, Mohr JP. Hypertensive putaminal hemorrhage. *Ann Neurol* 1977; 1: 152-9.

39. Stein RW, Kase CS, Hier DB, *et al.* Caudate hemorrhage. *Neurology* 1984; 34: 1549-54.

40. Walshe TM, Davis KR, Fisher CM. Thalamic hemorrhage: a computed tomographic-clinical correlation. *Neurology* 1977; 27: 217-22.

41. Ojemann, RG, Mohr JP. Hypertensive brain hemorrhage. *Clin Neurosurg* 1976; 23: 220-44.

42. Barraquer-Bordas L, Illa I, Escartin A, *et al.* Thalamic hemorrhage. A study of 23 patients with diagnosis by computed tomography. *Stroke* 1981; 12: 524-7.

43. Dejerine J, Roussy G. Le syndrome thalamique. *Rev Neurol* 1906; 14: 521-32.

44. Lhermitte J. Les syndromes thalamiques dissocié: les formes analgique et hémialgique. *Ann Méd* 1925; 17: 488-501.

45. Baudouin A, Lhermitte J, Lerebouillet J. Une observation anatomo-clinique d'hémorragie du thalamus. *Rev Neurol* 1930; 2: 102-9.

46. Fisher C. The pathologic and clinical aspects of thalamic hemorrhage. *Trans Am Neurol Assoc* 1959; 84: 56-9.

47. Kumral E, Kocaer T, Ertübey NO, Kumral K. Thalamic hemorrhage: a prospective study of 100 patients. *Stroke* 1995; 26: 964-70.

48. Weisberg LA. Caudate hemorrhage. *Arch Neurol* 1984; 41: 971-4.

49. Waga S, Miyazaki M, Okada M, *et al.* Hypertensive putaminal hemorrhage: analysis of 182 patients. *Surg Neurol* 1986; 26: 159-66.

50. Asakura K, Mizuno M, Yasui N. [Clinical analysis of 24 cases of caudate hemorrhage.] *Neurol Med Chir* (Tokyo) 1989; 29: 1107-12.

51. Fuh J. Caudate hemorrhage: clinical features, neuropsychological assessments and radiological findings. *Clin Neurol Neurosurg* 1995; 18: 445-50.

52. Kumral E, Evyapan D, Balkir K. Acute caudate vascular lesions. *Stroke* 1999; 30: 1734-5.

53. Liliang P, Liang C, Lu CH, *et al.* Hypertensive caudate hemorrhage prognostic predictor, outcome, and role of external ventricular drainage. *Stroke* 2001; 32: 1195-200.

54. Dinsdale HB. Spontaneous hemorrhage in the posterior fossa. A study of primary cerebellar and pontine hemorrhages with observations on their pathogenesis. *Arch Neurol* 1964; 10: 200-17.

55. Freeman RE, Onofrio BM, Okazaki H, Dinapoli RP. Spontaneous intracerebellar hemorrhage. Diagnosis and surgical treatment. *Neurology* 1973; 23: 84-90.

56. Ott KH, Kase CS, Ojemann RG, Mohr JP. Cerebellar hemorrhage: diagnosis and treatment. A review of 56 cases. *Arch Neurol* 1974; 31: 160-7.

57. Brennan RW, Bergland RM. Acute cerebellar hemorrhage. Analysis of clinical findings and outcome in 12 cases. *Neurology* 1977; 27: 527-32.

58. Yanaka K, Meguro K, Fujita K, Narushima K, Nose T. Immediate surgery reduces mortality in deeply comatose patients with spontaneous cerebellar hemorrhage. *Neurol Med Chir* (Tokyo) 2000; 40: 295-9.

59. Morioka J, Fujii M, Kato S, *et al.* Surgery for spontaneous intracerebral hemorrhage has greater remedial value than conservative therapy. *Surg Neurol* 2006; 65: 67-72; discussion 72-3.

60. Smajlovic D, Salihovic D, Ibrahimagic O, *et al.* Analysis of risk factors, localization and 30-day prognosis of intracerebral hemorrhage. *Bosn J Basic Med Sci* 2008; 8: 121-5.

61. Fisher CM, Picard EH, Polak A, *et al.* Acute hypertensive cerebellar hemorrhage: diagnosis and surgical treatment. *J Nerv Ment Dis* 1965; 140: 38-57.

62. Kaufman, HH. Treatment of deep spontaneous intracerebral hematomas. A review. *Stroke* 1993; 24(12 Suppl.): I101-6; discussion I107-8.

63. Little JR, Tubman DE, Ethier R. Cerebellar hemorrhage in adults. Diagnosis by computerized tomography. *J Neurosurg* 1978; 48: 575-9.

64. Elkind MS, Mohr JP. Cerebellar hemorrhage. *New Horiz* 1997; 5: 352-8.

65. Pollak L, Rabey JM, Gur R, Schiffer J. Indication to surgical management of cerebellar hemorrhage. *Clin Neurol Neurosurg* 1998; 100: 99-103.

66. Attwater H. Pontine hemorrhage. *Guys Hosp Rep* 1911; 65: 339-89.

67. Duret H. Traumatismes Cranio-Cerebraux. Paris: Librairie Felix Alcan, 1919.

68. Parizel PM, Makkat S, Jorens PG, *et al.* Brainstem hemorrhage in descending transtentorial herniation (Duret hemorrhage). *Intensive Care Med* 2002; 28: 85-8.

69. Fisher CM. Pathological observations in hypertensive cerebral hemorrhage. *J Neuropathol Exp Neurol* 1971; 30: 536-50.

70. Cole FM Yates PO. Intracerebral microaneurysms and small cerebrovascular lesions. *Brain* 1967; 90: 759-68.

71. Wall M, Wray SH. The one-and-a-half syndrome - a unilateral disorder of the pontine tegmentum: a study of 20 cases and review of the literature. *Neurology* 1983; 33: 971-80.

72. Fisher C. Ocular bobbing. *Arch Neurol* 1964; 11: 543-6.

73. Helweg-Larsen S, Sommer W, Strange P, *et al.* Prognosis for patients treated conservatively for spontaneous intracerebral hematomas. *Stroke* 1984; 15: 1045-8.

74. Scott M, Werthan M. The fate of hypertensive patients with clinically proven spontaneous intracerebral hematomas treated without intracranial surgery. *Stroke* 1970; 1: 286-300.

75. Kutsuzawa T, Ito K, Kawakami H. [Conserative treatment of hypertensive cerebral hemorrhage: results of 104 patients of acute stage.] *Neurol Med Chir* (Tokyo) 1976; 16(1 Pt 2): 29-36.

76. Batjer HH, J. S. Reisch, Allen BC, *et al.* Failure of surgery to improve outcome in hypertensive putaminal hemorrhage. A prospective randomized trial. *Arch Neurol* 1990; 47: 1103-6.

77. Morgenstern LB, Hemphill JC 3rd, Anderson C, *et al*, on behalf of the American Heart Association Stroke Council and Council on Cardiovascular Nursing. Guidelines for the management of spontaneous intracerebral hemorrhage: a guideline for healthcare professionals from the AHA/ASA. *Stroke* 2010; 41: 2108-29.

78. Tellez H, Bauer RB. Dexamethasone as treatment in cerebrovascular disease. 1. A controlled study in intracerebral hemorrhage. *Stroke* 1973; 4: 541-6.

79. Poungvarin N, Bhoopat W, Viriyavejakul A, *et al.* Effects of dexamethasone in primary supratentorial intracerebral hemorrhage. *N Engl J Med* 1987; 316: 1229-33.

80. Kelley RE, Berger JR, Scheinberg P, Stokes N. Active bleeding in hypertensive intracerebral hemorrhage: computed tomography. *Neurology* 1982; 32: 852-6.

81. Kase C. Pathophysiologie, diagnosis and management. In: *Stroke*, vol 1. Kase C, Ed. New York: Churchill Livingstone, 1986.

82. Bae HG, Lee KS, Yun IG, *et al.* Rapid expansion of hypertensive intracerebral hemorrhage. *Neurosurgery* 1992; 31: 35-41.

83. Ohwaki K, Yano E, Nagashima H, *et al.* Blood pressure management in acute intracerebral hemorrhage. Relationship between elevated blood pressure and hematoma enlargement. *Stroke* 2004; 35: 1364-7.

84. Zabramski J, Hamilton M. Intracerebral hematomas. In: *Neurovascular Surgery*. Spetzler RF, Carter LP, Hamilton MG, Eds. New York: McGraw-Hill, 1995; 477-96.

85. Crowell R, Ojemann R. Cerebellar hemorrhage. In: *Surgery of the Posterior Fossa*. Buchheit W, Truex R, Eds. New York: Raven Presss, 1979; 562-76.

86. Qureshi AI, Bliwise DL, Bliwise NG, *et al*. Rate of 24-hour blood pressure decline and mortality after spontaneous intracerebral hemorrhage: a retrospective analysis with a random effects regression model. *Crit Care Med* 1999; 27: 480-5.

87. Qureshi AI, Tariq N, Divani AA, *et al*. Antihypertensive treatment of acute cerebral hemorrhage. The Antihypertensive Treatment of Acute Cerebral Hemorrhage (ATACH) investigators. *Crit Care Med* 2010; 38(2): 637-48.

88. Nehls DG, Mendelow AD, Graham DI, *et al*. Experimental intracerebral hemorrhage: progression of hemodynamic changes after production of a spontaneous mass lesion. *Neurosurgery* 1988; 23: 439-44.

89. Mendelow AD. Mechanisms of ischemic brain damage with intracerebral hemorrhage. *Stroke* 1993; 24(12 Suppl.): I115-7; discussion I118-9.

90. Wagner KR, Xi G, Hua Y, *et al*. Lobar intracerebral hemorrhage model in pigs: rapid edema development in perihematomal white matter. *Stroke* 1996; 27: 490-7.

91. Fujitsu K, Muramoto M, Ikeda Y, *et al*. Indications for surgical treatment of putaminal hemorrhage. Comparative study based on serial CT and time-course analysis. *J Neurosurg* 1990; 73: 518-25.

92. Broderick JP, Brott TG, Duldner JE, *et al*. Volume of intracerebral hemorrhage. A powerful and easy-to-use predictor of 30-day mortality. *Stroke* 1993; 24: 987-93.

93. Janny P, Papo I, Chazal J, *et al*. Intracranial hypertension and prognosis of spontaneous intracerebral haematomas. A correlative study of 60 patients. *Acta Neurochir* (Wien) 1982; 61: 181-6.

94. Duff TA, Ayeni S, Levin AB, Javid M. Nonsurgical management of spontaneous intracerebral hematoma. *Neurosurgery* 1981; 9: 387-93.

95. Smith DS, Rehncrona S, Siesjö BK. Barbiturates as protective agents in brain ischemia and as free radical scavengers *in vitro*. *Acta Physiol Scand Suppl* 1980; 492: 129-34.

96. Murphy PG, Davies MJ, Columb MO, Stratford N. Effect of propofol and thiopentone on free radical mediated oxidative stress of the erythrocyte. *Br J Anaesth* 1996; 76: 536-43.

97. Magladery J. The natural course of cerebrovascular hemorrhage. *Clin Neurosurg* 1963; 9: 106-13.

98. Shiozaki T, Sugimoto H, Taneda M, *et al*. Effect of mild hypothermia on uncontrollable intracranial hypertension after severe head injury. *J Neurosurg* 1993; 79: 363-8.

99. Bhattathiri PS, Gregson B, Prasad KS, Mendelow AD; STICH Investigators. Intraventricular hemorrhage and hydrocephalus after spontaneous intracerebral hemorrhage: results from the STICH trial. *Acta Neurochir* Suppl 2006; 96: 65.

100. Berger AR, Lipton RB, Lesser ML, *et al*. Early seizures following intracerebral hemorrhage: implications for therapy. *Neurology* 1988; 38: 1363-5.

101. Shinton RA, Gill JS, Melnick SC, *et al*. The frequency, characteristics and prognosis of epileptic seizures at the onset of stroke. *J Neurol Neurosurg Psychiatry* 1988; 51: 273-6.

102. Faught E, Peters D, Bartolucci A, *et al*. Seizures after primary intracerebral hemorrhage. *Neurology* 1989; 39: 1089-93.

103. Sung CY, Chu NS. Epileptic seizures in intracerebral haemorrhage. *J Neurol Neurosurg Psychiatry* 1989; 52: 1273-6.

104. Weisberg LA, Shamsnia M, Elliott D. Seizures caused by nontraumatic parenchymal brain hemorrhages. *Neurology* 1991; 41: 1197-9.

105. Burn J, Dennis M, Bamford J, *et al*. Epileptic seizures after a first stroke: the Oxfordshire Community Stroke Project. *BMJ* 1997; 315: 1582-7.

106. Labovitz DL, Hauser WA. Preventing stroke-related seizures: when should anticonvulsant drugs be started? *Neurology* 2003; 60: 365-6.

107. Passero S, Rocchi R, Rossi S, *et al*. Seizures after spontaneous supratentorial intracerebral hemorrhage. *Epilepsia* 2002; 43: 1175-80.

108. Andaluz N, Zuccarello M. Recent trends in the treatment of spontaneous intracerebral hemorrhage: analysis of a nationwide inpatient database. *J Neurosurg* 2009; 110: 403-10.

109. Szaflarski JP, Rackley AY, Kleindorfer DO, *et al*. Incidence of seizures in the acute phase of stroke: a population-based study. *Epilepsia* 2008; 49: 974-81.

110. Messe SR, Sansing LH, Cucchiara BL, CHANT investigators. Prophylactic antiepileptic drug use is associated with poor outcome following ICH. *Neurocrit Care* 2009; 11: 38-44.

111. Claassen J, Jette N, Chum F, *et al*. Electrographic seizures and periodic discharges after intracerebral hemorrhage. *Neurology* 2007; 69: 1356-65.

112. Hemphill JC 3rd, Bonovich DC, Besmertis L, *et al*. The ICH score: a simple, reliable grading scale for intracerebral hemorrhage. *Stroke* 2001; 32: 891-7.

113. Fujii Y, Tanaka R, Takeuchi S, *et al*. Hematoma enlargement in spontaneous intracerebral hemorrhage. *J Neurosurg* 1994; 80: 51-7.

114. Kazui S, Naritomi H, Yamamoto H, *et al*. Enlargement of spontaneous intracerebral hemorrhage. Incidence and time course. *Stroke* 1996; 27: 1783-7.

115. Friederich PW, Henny CP, Messelink EJ, *et al*. Effect of recombinant activated factor VII on perioperative blood loss in patients undergoing retropubic prostatectomy: a double-blind placebo-controlled randomised trial. *Lancet* 2003; 361: 201-5.

116. Mayer SA, Brun NC, Broderick J, *et al*. Safety and feasibility of recombinant factor VIIa for acute intracerebral hemorrhage. *Stroke* 2005; 36: 74-9.

117. Mayer SA, Brun NC, Begtrup K, *et al*. Recombinant activated factor VII for acute intracerebral hemorrhage. *N Engl J Med* 2005; 352: 777-85.

118. Mayer SA, Brun NC, Begtrup K, *et al*. Efficacy and safety of recombinant activated factor VII for acute intracerebral hemorrhage. *N Engl J Med* 2008; 358: 2127-37.

119. Yu YL, Kumana CR, Lauder IJ, *et al*. Treatment of acute cerebral hemorrhage with intravenous glycerol. A double-blind, placebo-controlled, randomized trial. *Stroke* 1992; 23: 967-71.

120. Italian Acute Stroke Study Group. Haemodilution in acute stroke: results of the Italian haemodilution trial. *Lancet* 1988; 1: 318-21.

121. Benes V, Koukolik F, Obrovska D. Two types of spontaneous intracerebral hemorrhage due to hypertension. *J Neurosurg* 1972; 37: 509-13.

122. Volpin L, Cervellini P, Colombo F, Zanusso M, Benedetti A. Spontaneous intracerebral hematomas: a new proposal about the usefulness and limits of surgical treatment. *Neurosurgery* 1984; 15: 663-6.

123. Auer LM, Deinsberger W, Niederkorn K, *et al*. Endoscopic surgery versus medical treatment for spontaneous intracerebral hematoma: a randomized study. *J Neurosurg* 1989; 70: 530-5.

124. Kwak R, Kadoya S, Suzuki T. Factors affecting the prognosis in thalamic hemorrhage. *Stroke* 1983; 14: 493-500.

125. Niizuma H, Yonemitsu T, Jokura H, *et al*. Stereotactic aspiration of thalamic hematoma. Overall results of 75 aspirated and 70 nonaspirated cases. *Stereotact Funct Neurosurg* 1990; 54-55: 438-44.

126. Herbstein DJ, Schaumberg HH. Hypertensive intracerebral hematoma. An investigation of the initial hemorrhage and rebleeding using chromium Cr 51-labeled erythrocytes. *Arch Neurol* 1974; 30: 412-4.

127. Takada I. [On the phenomena of extravasation of contrast media in cerebral angiogram of the case of hypertensive intracerebral hematoma and their clinical significance-analysis of 14 cases.] *No Shinkei Geka* 1976; 4: 471-8.

128. Ebina K, Okabe S, Manabe H, Iwabuchi T. [Experimental study on liquefaction of intracranial hematoma: usefulness of tissue-plasminogen activator (t-PA), a hematolytic agent, and its combination.] *No Shinkei Geka* 1990; 18: 927-34.

129. Nath FP, Jenkins A, Mendelow AD, *et al*. Early hemodynamic changes in experimental intracerebral hemorrhage. *J Neurosurg* 1986; 65: 697-703.

130. Nehls DG, Mendelow DA, Graham DI, Teasdale GM. Experimental intracerebral hemorrhage: early removal of a spontaneous mass lesion improves late outcome. *Neurosurgery* 1990; 27: 674-82.

131. Ropper AH, Zervas NT. Cerebral blood flow after experimental basal ganglia hemorrhage. *Ann Neurol* 1982; 11: 266-71.

132. Jenkins A, Mendelow AD, Graham DI, *et al*. Experimental intracerebral haematoma: the role of blood constituents in early ischaemia. *Br J Neurosurg* 1990; 4: 45-51.

133. Siddique MS, Fernandes HM, Wooldridge TD, *et al*. Reversible ischemia around intracerebral hemorrhage: a single-photon emission computerized tomography study. *J Neurosurg* 2002; 96: 736-41.

134. Takasugi S, Ueda S, Matsumoto K. Chronological changes in spontaneous intracerebral hematoma - an experimental and clinical study. *Stroke* 1985; 16: 651-8.

135. Mizukami M, Araki G, Mihara H, Tomita T. [Surgical treatment of hypertensive cerebral hemorrhage. 4. The prognosis based on cerebral angiography.] *No To Shinkei* 1972; 24: 579-83.

136. Kaneko M, Tanaka K, Shimada T, *et al*. Long-term evaluation of ultra-early operation for hypertensive intracerebral hemorrhage in 100 cases. *J Neurosurg* 1983; 58: 838-42.

137. Kanno T, Sano H, Shinomiya Y, *et al*. Role of surgery in hypertensive intracerebral hematoma. A comparative study of 305 nonsurgical and 154 surgical cases. *J Neurosurg* 1984; 61: 1091-9.

138. Takebayashi S, Kaneko M. Electron microscopic studies of ruptured arteries in hypertensive intracerebral hemorrhage. *Stroke* 1983; 14: 28-36.

139. Yukawa H, Kanaya H. [Indication for surgery in hypertensive intracerebral hemorrhage - a statistical study.] *Neurol Med Chir* (Tokyo) 1978; 18: 361-5.

140. Juvela S, Heiskanen O, Poranen A, *et al*. The treatment of spontaneous intracerebral hemorrhage. A prospective randomized trial of surgical and conservative treatment. *J Neurosurg* 1989; 70: 755-8.

141. Zuccarello M, Brott T, Derex L, *et al*. Early surgical treatment for supratentorial intracerebral hemorrhage: a randomized feasibility study. *Stroke* 1999; 30: 1833-9.

142. Mendelow AD, Gregson BA, Fernandes HM, *et al*. Early surgery versus initial conservative treatment in patients with spontaneous supratentorial intracerebral haematomas in the International Surgical Trial in Intracerebral Haemorrhage (STICH): a randomised trial. *Lancet* 2005; 365: 387-97.

143. Teernstra OP, Evers SM, Lodder J, *et al*. Stereotactic treatment of intracerebral hematoma by means of a plasminogen activator: a multicenter randomized controlled trial (SICHPA). *Stroke* 2003; 34: 968-74.

144. Almaani WS, Awidi AS. Spontaneous intracranial bleeding in hemorrhagic diathesis. *Surg Neurol* 1982; 17: 137-40.

145. Heros RC. Surgical treatment of cerebellar infarction. *Stroke* 1992; 23: 937-8.

Introduction

Neurotrauma

Alex Valadka MD

Chief Executive Officer

SETON BRAIN AND SPINE INSTITUTE, AUSTIN, TEXAS, USA

Surgeons are not passive people. They often take decisive action to help their patients improve. Indeed, one reason physicians choose surgery as a specialty is the satisfaction of helping others in a very tangible way. But what if uncertainty exists regarding the indication for surgery? And to make things worse, what if a patient is critically ill, and failure to make the right decision could result in serious harm?

Uncertainty about the optimal course of action arises in part from the continuous updating of medical knowledge. What physicians learn in residency will be refined as new data continue to accrue. But such progress is not linear. Often, surgeons begin treating patients in a given manner. This may result in a fad, which is then elevated to dogma – only to be replaced by a better-informed way of doing things. Fortunately, books such as this one help keep physicians up to date regarding current perspectives on the best ways to manage patients.

A core principle of treating patients with severe traumatic brain injury (TBI) is that they require intracranial pressure (ICP) monitoring. Adherence to this principle has been proposed as a quality criterion for trauma centers. But is this dogma really true? After all, ICP monitoring in TBI patients has not been shown to improve outcomes. In Chapter 33, Chesnut reviews this concept as well as several other widely held beliefs about ICP monitoring after TBI. Such questioning of established practices is a healthy undertaking, even if the ultimate result turns out to be a reaffirmation of existing practices.

Decompressive craniectomy for severe TBI has been embraced aggressively at some centers and in some parts of the world. Other neurosurgeons, however, remain troubled about the poor outcomes of many of these patients and the risks and complications of this procedure. Undoubtedly, craniectomy is the ideal treatment for some TBI patients, but identifying the appropriate candidates is often difficult. Chapter 34 synthesizes the published and ongoing work in this area.

Prompt decompression of an acutely traumatized spinal cord would appear reasonable. Yet despite very supportive laboratory evidence, this concept has not translated into clinical practice as smoothly as one might have expected. Indeed, a few older reports suggested that early surgery may actually be deleterious in some patients. However, some surgeons continued to forge ahead, and a growing body of literature now suggests that early decompression may indeed be beneficial. Chapter 35 presents a nice review of this topic.

When to decompress a patient with acute spinal cord injury, whether to perform a decompressive craniectomy, when to monitor ICP – these questions arise on a daily basis. Uncertainty often clashes with a surgeon's instinct to be bold and aggressive. The guidance in these chapters will allow surgeons to provide definitive emergency care while still adhering to the overriding principle to first do no harm.

Chapter 33

Use of intracranial pressure and ventriculostomy in traumatic brain injury

Randall M Chesnut MD FCCM FACS, Integra Endowed Professor of Neurotrauma; Chief of Neurotrauma and Neurosurgical Spine Surgery, Department of Neurological Surgery; Professor, Department of Orthopaedic Surgery; Adjunct Professor, School of Global Health

HARBORVIEW MEDICAL CENTER, UNIVERSITY OF WASHINGTON, SEATTLE, WASHINGTON, USA

Introduction

Monitoring and treating intracranial hypertension is central to the current treatment of severe traumatic brain injury (sTBI), although it is neither universally practiced nor based on such solid scientific evidence as to render its role unassailable. As such, it is important to understand its evidentiary underpinnings in order to take a rational approach to sTBI management and to facilitate proper interpretation of the related literature.

Various topics related to the monitoring of intracranial pressure (ICP) in TBI have been covered as part of a series of evidence reports on the management of sTBI in adults [1-3] and children [4], as well as in penetrating brain injury [5]. These works have been widely received as definitive and are routinely reviewed and updated under the aegis of the Brain Trauma Foundation (www.braintrauma.org). Within these publications, the topics of ICP monitoring technology, indications for ICP monitoring, and ICP treatment thresholds have been specifically addressed, and the role of ICP in other aspects of sTBI management has been included in other sections wherever relevant. As such, the reader is referred to these documents for specific evidence reports on these topics.

Given the availability of the aforementioned referenced works, there is little rationale for performing another evidence review covering the same topics. What is valuable, however, is to address the issue of integrating the current body of evidence into the current practice of sTBI management in a manner that respects the available evidence in accordance with its rigor, while recognizing that many treatment decisions will have to be made without definitive direction from the published literature. This is the thrust of this chapter.

Methodology

A National Library of Medicine computerized literature search from 1966 to 2010 was performed based primarily on the expanded heading 'brain injuries' plus 'trauma,' 'intracranial pressure, intracranial hypertension, or ICP' and 'monitoring or treatment.' As appropriate to subsections of the text, headings of 'threshold,' 'cerebral perfusion pressure or CPP,' 'complications,' 'techniques,' and 'outcomes' were combined to parse these references into relevant subgroups. Pearling included these selected articles, plus a search of the Cochrane database (using similar search terms) and a review of evidence reports on TBI over the same time period.

Intracranial pressure and outcomes

The seminal work of Lundberg [6] and Guillaume and Janny [7] established that ICP elevation is common after sTBI, not consistently reflected in the clinical examination, and associated with less favorable outcomes. Although, as evidenced by patients with pseudotumor (benign intracranial hypertension), markedly elevated ICP does not universally portend severe neurologic dysfunction, numerous studies have established that ICP elevation after sTBI is associated with a higher likelihood of death or unfavorable outcomes, often in a statistically independent fashion [8-15]. As a result, during the 1970s and 1980s, the manipulation of ICP became a central focus of sTBI management [9, 11]. A plethora of articles appeared during this period associating the 'new wave' of aggressive management of sTBI with improved outcomes, of which the publications by Becker *et al* and Marshall *et al* are prime examples [9, 11]. Although such articles are often quoted as strongly supporting the benefits of monitoring and managing ICP, these publications are powerfully confounded by the concomitant development of many other aspects of TBI care. These include the initiation of neurocritical care, marked improvements in prehospital management, and the hugely influential availability of early CT imaging. In essence, the concept that ICP was treatable changed the focus of TBI management from the evacuation of mass lesions to the supportive care of the injured brain. Unfortunately, the role of ICP monitor-based treatment of intracranial hypertension cannot be isolated within these publications.

The virtually universal inclusion of ICP monitoring in current publications on TBI management maintains this confounding. As a result, monitoring ICP as a means of guiding such treatment has become widely (although not universally [16, 17]) adopted. This has obvious research-design implications for the study of ICP monitoring within nations that have ready access to monitoring technology and where ICP monitor-based treatment is considered 'standard of practice.'

Despite the wide acceptance of the association between severe intracranial hypertension and less favorable outcomes following sTBI, and the resultant fervor for ICP management in this setting, the conclusion that sTBI patients will benefit from reversing intracranial hypertension does not directly follow and is less well established. First, it must be established whether intracranial hypertension is a treatable entity or a marker of disease severity. In those patients with extreme intracranial hypertension, the latter is clearly the case. At what point outcome becomes dependent on ICP control is currently unclear. Second, if intracranial hypertension is to be considered a treatable entity, the treatment threshold (the definition of intracranial hypertension) must be empirically established. Finally, it is necessary to determine the relative contribution of ICP *per se* toward determining outcome, versus its acting as a proxy for or a component of other physiological processes that might actually be the critical determinants.

Although there are certainly questions regarding the details of treating intracranial hypertension, it is the role of monitoring in directing such treatment that is of interest here. This can be broken down into several questions:

- Does ICP management improve outcomes following sTBI?
- Who is at risk for intracranial hypertension?
- What is the proper ICP treatment threshold? (Or, is there an actual set treatment threshold?)

Does intracranial pressure management improve outcomes following sTBI?

Central to the discussion of the utility of ICP monitoring is the question of the efficacy of ICP treatment in improving outcome. Although this efficacy is often considered self-evident, and this feeling has prompted almost universal adoption of ICP management schemes into TBI care, the actual evidentiary base remains relatively weak and not entirely consistent.

Intracranial pressure monitoring

In an early publication widely cited in support of ICP monitoring, Becker *et al* reported retrospectively on 160 patients treated with a standardized protocol that included control of ICP in addition to early imaging and surgical management of intracranial mass lesions, widespread mechanical ventilation, and diligent critical care [9]. They felt that the 3-month mortality of 30% with this protocol compared favorably with the 50% mortality in the historical comparison group of 700 patients treated without ICP monitoring published by Jennett et al [18] (III/B). No attempt was made to statistically tease out the independence of ICP monitoring from the other uncontrolled confounders in the analysis.

In a study of 200 consecutive sTBI patients admitted to five hospitals in the San Diego area, Bowers and Marshall reported significantly better outcomes for the group that underwent ICP monitoring and treatment of intracranial hypertension [19] (III/B). They did not test the independence of this factor with respect to outcome, however, and there was no control for variable indications for monitoring or different modes of ICP management.

In an early prospective study of 225 sTBI patients from one institution, Miller et al noted a strong correlation between ICP elevation and its response to therapy in terms of outcome [20] (III/B). Patients whose ICP remained below 20mmHg throughout their course had a mortality rate of 18% and a favorable outcome rate of 74% (Glasgow Outcome Scale [GOS] score 4-5). Patients whose ICP rose above 20mmHg but was reducible with therapy had rates of 26% and 55%, respectively, while patients whose ICP was elevated and refractory to treatment had rates of 92% and 3%, respectively. While the authors admitted to a lack of published data answering the question, 'Can you show that ICP monitoring results in a lower mortality and thereby justifies the risks of intracranial infection which are entailed?', they did conclude that ICP monitoring was an important part of their therapeutic approach to sTBI. In addition, they reported the incidence of intracranial hypertension was only less than 25% in ventilated patients with normal CT imaging, and suggested that detection of ICP elevations required physiological monitoring. It is notable that this trial differed in many ways from prior studies, as well as from present management. It represented an early example of the routine use of

early CT imaging, widespread employment of ICP monitoring in sTBI, and a protocol-based management approach. In contrast to current practice, however, steroids were uniformly used, hyperventilation (to as low a $PaCO_2$ as 20mmHg) was common, and fluid restriction was routine. Nevertheless, the paper supports a strong interaction between 'ICP/ICP responsiveness to therapy' and outcomes following sTBI.

In contrast, a retrospective study by Stuart et al with 100 sTBI patients managed without ICP monitoring in Australia reported 34% mortality, with 49% achieving favorable outcomes [21] (III/B). ICP was not treated outside of baseline steroid administration (thought to be beneficial at that time) and aggressive responses to signs of herniation. The large transport distances, non-inclusion of patients who did not survive transportation, and occasional surgical management at district hospitals before transfer may have influenced the outcomes.

Saul and Ducker reported on consecutive prospective cohorts of patients treated within one institution before and after a change in the ICP treatment threshold [22]. A total of 127 sTBI patients treated between 1977 and 1978 at a threshold of 20-25mmHg had a mortality rate of 46%; 106 patients treated between 1979 and 1980 at a threshold of 15mmHg had a mortality rate of 28%. The authors stated that management was comparable between groups, with the exception of the ICP treatment (patients in the latter group were randomized into a high-dose barbiturate study if their ICP was >25mmHg). All sTBI patients received hyperventilation and steroids. The authors felt their data supported the correlation between early, aggressive ICP management and improved outcomes (and that patients may benefit from a lower ICP treatment threshold) (IIb/B).

Two studies have looked at the efficacy of ICP-based therapy using contemporaneous control groups from centers that differ in their use of ICP monitoring. Colohan et al prospectively compared 822 sTBI patients treated with ICP monitoring in Virginia, USA, with 551 sTBI patients treated without ICP monitoring in New Delhi, India [23]. The overall mortality for all sTBI patients was similar when the groups were compared by motor score. The relative mortalities for the subset of patients who localized to painful stimuli (Glasgow Coma Scale [GCS] motor score of 5) were 4.8% and 12.5%. Although the authors felt that ICP-monitor-based management played a role in the difference in outcomes, they were unable to present data isolating this from the myriad other differences between these centers **(IIb/B)**.

Harris *et al* prospectively studied TBI of any severity at a center in Atlanta, Georgia (n=632), and two hospitals on the island of Jamaica (combined n=610) [24]. ICP monitoring was commonly used for patients with sTBI at the center in Georgia (n=161) but rarely at the other two centers (combined n=108). Although the overall mortality for all grades of TBI did not differ between sites, the mortality rate following sTBI at the center in Georgia was 32% versus 57% and 54% at the two Jamaican centers **(IIb/B)**. As in the Colohan *et al* study, the authors noted prominent differences in operative interventions, intensive care unit (ICU) admissions, and CT imaging, in addition to the different ICP monitoring between centers. Both of these studies were significantly compromised by such confounding differences between centers, and therefore provide only indirect support for a correlation between ICP management and improved outcomes following sTBI.

Bulger *et al* examined prospectively collected data from 34 academic level I and II trauma centers in the USA contained in the University Hospitals Consortium database, evaluating discharge mortality for 182 patients admitted with sTBI plus a long bone fracture [25]. They divided the centers into two groups – aggressive and non-aggressive – based on the criterion of placing ICP monitors in at least 50% of patients with an admission GCS score of 8 or less and an abnormal CT scan (in accordance with the criteria for monitoring from the first edition of the guidelines for the management of severe brain injury from the Brain Trauma Foundation [1]). Eleven of the 34 centers, managing 74 of the 180 study patients (41%), met this criterion. Notably, all centers treated ICP, with or without a monitor. The overall mortality at the aggressive centers was 27% versus 45% at the non-aggressive centers, producing an adjusted

hazard ratio for death of 0.43 for aggressive compared with non-aggressive centers **(IIb/B)**. Other significant management differences, such as the frequency of CT imaging, were also seen between aggressive and non-aggressive centers.

Ghajar *et al* prospectively studied discharge outcomes in a cohort of sTBI patients treated at a single center with a monitor-based ICP management protocol (n=34) versus no monitoring or treatment (n=15) for intracranial hypertension [26]. Mortality was lower (12% vs. 53%) and the proportion living independently was higher (59% vs. 20%) for the monitored patients versus those not treated for ICP **(IIb/B)**. The overall incidence of intracranial hypertension (ICP >20mmHg) within the monitored group was rather low (10%), however, and there were significant differences in demographic variables such as age and admission GCS between the small study groups.

Smith *et al* examined the need for ICP monitoring in guiding ICP treatment in a prospective randomized trial of sTBI patients [27]. Both groups were monitored and underwent similar CT imaging schedules. All patients were mechanically ventilated and hyperventilated to 25-30mmHg. One group (n=37) was treated for ICP higher than 25mmHg with doses of mannitol. Refractory intracranial hypertension was treated with high-dose pentobarbital, and treatment was weaned based on ICP. The other group (n=40) was treated with scheduled mannitol dosing, which could be escalated in the face of neurologic deterioration. Treatment was weaned at 96 hours or earlier if the patient awakened. There was no significant difference in 1-year mortality or morbidity between the groups, and these were comparable with contemporaneous outcome norms **(Ib/A)**. The mean ICP was 5.5mmHg higher in the monitor-based treatment group for both survivors and non-survivors. The authors suggested (but provided no evidence in support) that this difference in mean ICP may have confounded the study and that the results might have favored monitoring if the treatment threshold had been lower. This study is quite limited in its ability to prove a negative result because of its small sample size.

In 2005, Cremer *et al* published a retrospective study of 333 sTBI patients surviving for longer than 24 hours from two level I trauma centers in the Netherlands, both of which treated ICP, but only one of which employed ICP monitors [28]. At the center not using monitoring (n=122), ICP was treated based on CT findings and clinical observation, and mean arterial pressure was maintained at 90mmHg. At the center that monitored ICP (n=211), treatments targeted an ICP of less than 20mmHg and cerebral perfusion pressure (CPP) higher than 70mmHg. One-year morbidity and mortality figures were not significantly different between the two centers (34% vs. 33%, respectively) **(III/B)**. However, the monitored group received significantly more frequent use of sedatives, vasopressors, mannitol, and barbiturates, and survivors in this group underwent a significantly greater median number of ventilator days. The authors argued that ICP/CPP-targeted treatment increased treatment intensity without improving outcomes. Notably, only 67% of eligible patients at the 'monitoring' center were actually monitored, although all eligible patients were used in the analysis. The patients actually monitored appeared to have worse admission GCS motor scores and more frequent CT findings of diffuse injury (DI) with shift (DI IV pattern [29]), and more often required prehospital intubation. In addition, control of ICP in monitored patients may not have been optimal: 27% of those monitored for more than 24 hours had ICP higher than 20mmHg for more than 50% of the monitored period.

More recently, Shafi *et al* presented a retrospective study of 1,646 sTBI patients in the US National Trauma Data Bank (1994-2001) with sTBI (GCS ≤8) who survived for longer than 24 hours and stayed at least 3 days in the ICU [30]. They studied morbidity and mortality rates for 708 patients treated without ICP monitoring and 938 patients treated according to monitored ICP. Higher discharge mortality rates and worse discharge scores on the Functional Independence Measure were reported for the monitored group **(IIb/B)**. The authors concluded that ICP monitoring in accordance with (then) current Brain Trauma Foundation criteria [3] was associated with worse survival. Caveats regarding this study revolve around the retrospective use of a database designed for general trauma that lacks a number of important data points that are routinely controlled for in brain injury outcome studies (e.g., CT scan data

and pupillary status), and that this study had no means of controlling for confounding injury-related, physician-related, or prognosis-related rationales that might have been important in the decision to monitor individual patients.

Lane *et al* examined data from the Ontario Trauma Registry from 1989 to 1998 for patients with an Abbreviated Injury Scale score of more than 3 for the head region to determine the association between ICP monitoring and outcome [31]. This registry contains data on all patients with an Injury Severity Score of more than 12 admitted to level I trauma centers within the province of Ontario, Canada. The study identified 5,507 patients, of whom 541 (10%) had an ICP monitor placed. On univariate analysis, the use of an ICP monitor was significantly related to an increased risk of discharge mortality **(IIb/B)**. Multivariate analysis, controlling for injury mechanism, Abbreviated Injury Scale head, Injury Severity Score, and ICP monitoring, revealed that the use of an ICP monitor was significantly associated with a decrease in the death rate. This suggests that ICP monitoring had been used in more severely injured patients, but such monitoring was associated with decreased mortality. The authors felt these results might reflect a benefit from quantitative information available to direct therapy, selection of patients who appeared to have a better prognosis for monitoring, or more frequent use of monitoring at centers with increased aggressiveness in treating TBI, and were unable to differentiate between these possibilities.

Some of the strongest support for the efficacy of lowering intracranial hypertension in improving outcomes comes from a prospective randomized trial of high-dose barbiturate therapy for refractory intracranial hypertension reported by Eisenberg *et al* in 1988 [32]. They randomized 73 patients with refractory ICP elevation from multiple institutions to either high-dose pentobarbital ('barbiturate coma') or continuation of aggressive treatment without barbiturates. Control of refractory intracranial hypertension by any means was associated with improved outcomes **(Ib/A)**. Patients whose ICP responded had a 1-month mortality rate of 8%, whereas 83% of those who did not respond were dead at that point. Notably, however, although the authors looked at outcomes, their primary endpoint was ICP control in light of the ethical concern that patients in whom non-barbiturate therapy failed should be considered candidates to cross over and receive barbiturates (which occurred in 19/23 such non-responders). This weakened the study design with respect to clinical outcomes.

Decompressive craniectomy

Decompressive craniectomy for medically refractory intracranial hypertension also addresses the efficacy of lowering ICP in a similar specific group with intractable elevation and a very high likelihood of poor outcomes. Aarabi et al reported retrospectively on 50 consecutive adults undergoing decompressive craniectomy for severe brain swelling, 40 of whom manifested refractory ICP elevation before surgery [33]. Decompression lowered ICP from a mean of 23.9mmHg to 14.4mmHg in those 40 patients, and 85% of all patients had no postoperative ICP elevations **(III/B)**. Twenty patients (40%) had good outcomes (GOS score 4-5). The mortality rate was 28%.

Skoglund et al presented a retrospective study of 19 patients aged 7-46 years who underwent decompressive craniectomy for refractory intracranial hypertension [34]. Mean ICP was significantly reduced from a mean of 29.2mmHg before surgery to 11.1mmHg directly following decompression, and remained at 13.9mmHg 24 hours after the operation. Regression analysis demonstrated a significant correlation between the size of the craniectomy and the decrease in ICP **(III/B)**. Most patients (68%) recovered well (GOS score 4-5). The mortality rate was 10%.

Decompressive craniectomy has often been studied in children. Dam Hieu et al reported very high, uncontrollable ICP (120 and 90mmHg) in two children treated with early decompressive craniectomy, with favorable outcomes in both [35] **(III/B)**. ICP was recorded before, during, and after surgery, and decreased by 40 and 30mmHg during craniotomy alone; both children had easily controlled postoperative ICP courses.

Ruf et al also reported a correlation between the ability of decompressive craniectomy to normalize ICP and favorable outcomes in six children with refractory intracranial hypertension [36]. In all patients, ICP normalized immediately after surgery **(III/B)**. Although no standardized outcome scale was used, all of the children did well and there were no deaths.

Rutigliano et al reported that surgery was effective in normalizing refractory ICP elevation and producing favorable outcome in six patients younger than 20 years of age [37] **(III/B)**. One patient in whom simple decompression did not control the ICP was returned for debridement, which proved effective. Again, although a standardized outcome scale was not used, all patients appeared to have satisfactory outcomes.

Although it is performed for the treatment of intracranial hypertension and appears to effectively lower ICP in parallel with its effect on outcomes, there is evidence that decompressive craniectomy also favorably influences numerous other potentially important (and therefore confounding) physiological parameters. Kunze et al published a retrospective report on 28 patients aged 8-44 years who underwent decompressive craniectomy for uncontrollable ICP elevation [38]. They demonstrated decreased ICP (<25mmHg) and improved CPP (>75mmHg), cerebral blood flow, and microcirculation following surgery **(III/B)**. Good outcomes (GOS score 4-5) were reported in 56% of this group at 1 year. The mortality rate was 11%.

Although the above high-dose barbiturate and decompressive craniectomy studies deal with the specific subset of patients with refractory intracranial hypertension, and all reveal considerable variability in the success of the treatment, they do support the concept that lowering markedly elevated ICP that is refractory to more mundane treatment modalities can produce outcomes well outside of those expected for such groups. None of these studies was able to specifically determine if ICP lowering per se is the direct mechanism mediating improvement rather than serving as an indirect or secondary factor (such as might be the case if improvement of cerebral blood flow is the critical variable). It is also unclear if the beneficial action might generalize across brain injury

Table 1. Does ICP management improve outcomes following sTBI? *Continued overleaf.*

Reference	Design	Results	Evidence level/ recommendation
Becker *et al*, 1977 [9]	Retrospective study of 160 sTBI patients treated with a standard protocol that included ICP monitoring	3-month mortality: 30%	III/B
Jennett *et al*, 1977 [18]	Retrospective report of 700 sTBI patients treated without ICP monitoring in Scotland, the Netherlands, and the USA	6-month mortality: 52% (Scotland), 52% (the Netherlands), and 49% (USA)	III/B
Bowers and Marshall, 1980 [19]	Retrospective study of 200 consecutive sTBI patients admitted to five hospitals in the San Diego area	**Mortality in patients with admission GCS score 3-5** Monitored: 39% Not monitored: 62%	III/B
Miller *et al*, 1981 [20]	Prospective series of 225 sTBI patients treated with a uniform protocol including ICP monitoring	1-year mortality: 34% **ICP <20mmHg** Mortality: 18% Favorable outcome: 74% **ICP >20mmHg but reducible** Mortality: 26% Favorable outcome: 55% **Refractory ICP >20mmHg** Mortality: 92% Favorable outcome: 3%	III/B
Stuart *et al*, 1983 [21]	Retrospective study of 100 sTBI patients managed without ICP monitoring	Mortality: 34% Favorable outcome: 49%	III/B
Saul and Ducker, 1982 [22]	Prospective study of 127 sTBI patients treated at a threshold of 20-25mmHg and 106 patients subsequently treated at a threshold of 15mmHg	**Threshold of 20-25mmHg** Mortality: 46% **Threshold of 15mmHg** Mortality: 28%	IIb/B
Colohan *et al*, 1989 [23]	Prospective sTBI study comparing 822 patients treated in Virginia with 551 patients treated in India	Similar overall mortality when groups compared by GCS motor score Relative mortalities for patients who localized to painful stimuli (GCS_m=5) were better in Virginia (4.8% vs. 12.5%) Difference possibly related to ICP monitor-based treatment	IIb/B
Harris *et al*, 2008 [24]	Prospective TBI study comparing 632 patients from Georgia with 610 patients from two centers in Jamaica	sTBI mortality better in Georgia (32% vs. 57% and 54%) Attributed to treatment differences, including ICP monitoring	IIb/B

Chapter 33

Table 1. Does ICP management improve outcomes following sTBI? *Continued overleaf.*

Reference	Design	Results	Evidence level/ recommendation
Bulger *et al*, 2002 [25]	Analysis of prospective data from a UHC database on 182 sTBI patients from 34 level I and II trauma centers, with the centers divided into two groups according to monitoring of ICP in ≥50% of sTBI patients	All centers treated ICP with or without a monitor Centers monitoring in ≥50% of sTBI patients had lower discharge mortality (27% vs. 45%)	IIb/B
Ghajar *et al*, 1993 [26]	Prospective non-randomized study of consecutive sTBI patients monitored at the physician's discretion	**ICP monitoring (n=34)** Mortality: 12% Independent living: 59% **No ICP monitoring (n=15)** Mortality: 53% Independent living: 20%	IIb/B
Smith *et al*, 1986 [27]	Small prospective randomized trial of patients with ICP monitoring comparing 37 patients treated with mannitol for elevated ICP vs. 40 patients who received scheduled mannitol not based on measured ICP	No significant mortality difference between groups (35% vs. 42.5%) Study too small to support a negative result	Ib/A
Cremer *et al*, 2005 [28]	Retrospective study of 333 sTBI patients from a prospective database comparing sTBI patients from two centers, one of which did not monitor ICP	No significant difference in 1-year mortality (34% vs. 33%) ICP monitoring associated with significantly greater treatment intensity and number of ventilator days in survivors	III/B
Shafi *et al*, 2008 [30]	Retrospective study of 1,646 sTBI patients in the prospective National Trauma Data Bank comparing outcomes against use of ICP monitoring	Odds ratio for survival significantly worse (0.549) and FIM score lower (7.9 vs. 5.9) for monitored patients	IIb/B
Lane *et al*, 2000 [31]	Retrospective study of 5,507 sTBI patients in the prospective Ontario Trauma Registry, 541 of whom were monitored	Univariate analysis associated monitoring with increased discharge mortality Multivariate monitoring controlling for injury severity suggested monitoring was associated with decreased mortality	IIb/B
Eisenberg *et al*, 1988 [32]	Multicenter prospective randomized trial of high-dose barbiturates vs. continued standard therapy for refractory ICP elevation; cross-over to barbiturate group allowed for non-responders	Control of refractory intracranial hypertension by any means was associated with lower 1-month mortality (8% vs. 83%)	Ib/A

Table 1. Does ICP management improve outcomes following sTBI? *Continued.*

Reference	Design	Results	Evidence level/ recommendation
Aarabi *et al*, 2006 [33]	Retrospective study of 50 consecutive sTBI patients treated with decompressive craniectomy, 40 of whom were monitored before surgery	Decompression lowered the mean ICP from 23.9mmHg to 14.4mmHg Mortality of 28% and favorable outcome in 40% felt to be very good in light of severity of injuries	III/B
Skoglund *et al*, 2006 [34]	Retrospective study of 19 sTBI patients treated with decompressive craniectomy for refractory ICP elevation	Decompression lowered mean ICP from 29 to 11mmHg Mortality of 10% and favorable outcome in 68% felt to be very good in light of severity of injuries	III/B
Dam Hieu *et al*, 1996 [35]	Retrospective study of two pediatric sTBI patients treated with decompressive craniectomy for refractory ICP elevation	Decompression lowered mean ICP by 40 and 30mmHg Both had favorable outcomes	III/B
Ruf *et al*, 2003 [36]	Retrospective study of six pediatric sTBI patients treated with decompressive craniectomy for refractory ICP elevation	Decompression normalized ICP in all patients (one required a contralateral decompression) Three patients 'normal' and two with mild to moderate deficits at 6 months	III/B
Rutigliano *et al*, 2006 [37]	Retrospective case series of six sTBI patients <20 years of age treated with decompressive craniectomy for refractory ICP elevation	Decompression normalized ICP in five patients; one required debridement to normalize ICP Five of the six had FIM scores of independent or minimal assistance at discharge; the other remained dependent	III/B
Kunze *et al*, 1998 [38]	Retrospective study of 28 sTBI patients treated with decompressive craniectomy for refractory ICP elevation	Following surgery, ICP decreased to <25mmHg, cerebral perfusion pressure maintained at >75mmHg, and cerebral blood flow improved Mortality: 11% Favorable 1-year outcome: 56%	III/B
Taylor *et al*, 2001 [39]	Small prospective randomized trial of 27 pediatric sTBI patients with sustained ICP >20mmHg during the first 24 hours	Surgery appeared to modestly lower time-locked ICP by approximately 5mmHg more than controls Surgical patients had fewer episodes of ICP >20mmHg Non-significant trend toward improved 6-month outcome with surgery	Ib/A

GCS = Glasgow Coma Scale; FIM = Functional Independence Measure; ICP = intracranial pressure; sTBI = severe traumatic brain injury; UHC = University Hospitals Consortium

Chapter 33

types or if it is specific to certain pathophysiologic subsets of TBI.

One decompressive craniectomy trial addressed patients with 'sustained' rather than medically refractory intracranial hypertension. This was a pilot study by Taylor et al, and is also the only randomized controlled trial (RCT) attempted for decompressive craniectomy [39]. The investigators randomized 27 children older than 12 months with sTBI and intracranial hypertension within 24 hours of admission. Children who had sustained intracranial hypertension during the first day after admission (ICP 20-24mmHg for 30 minutes, 25-29mmHg for 10 minutes, or ≥30mmHg for 1 minute) or evidence of herniation (dilatation of one pupil or the presence of bradycardia) were eligible for randomization. Children received either standard management or standard management plus bitemporal decompressive craniectomy without duraplasty. ICP was modestly lower in the decompression group (8.98mmHg) than among controls (3.7mmHg) at 48 hours after randomization (p=0.057) and there were fewer episodes of ICP elevation. There was a trend toward improved 6-month outcome in the surgical group (p=0.046; p<0.0221 was required for statistical significance because of multiple sampling) **(Ib/A)**. Although this study had the most powerful statistical design among publications on decompressive craniectomy, it was greatly underpowered, did not accompany the craniectomies with duraplasties (possibly limiting their ameliorating effect on ICP), and studied a slightly different group from the other publications in that the ICP elevations were 'sustained' rather than medically intractable. The positive trends seen in this paper, however, give at least some support to the concept that the apparently linked effects of decompressive craniectomy on ICP and outcome may also apply to lesser degrees of intracranial hypertension.

Summary

Although the data are not very rigorous, they are rather consistent in suggesting that aggressive treatment including monitor-driven ICP management appears to be strongly associated with improved outcomes following sTBI. The independent contribution of monitoring to drive such management (rather than simply serving as a marker for aggressive treatment) remains undetermined. Although restricted by serious design limitations, studies such as those by Cremer et al, Shafi et al, and Stuart et al suggest that comparably favorable outcomes may be produced with concerted sTBI management (including ICP treatment) performed without the use of monitoring devices [21, 28, 30]. Given the very strong tendency for academic centers to include ICP monitoring as a part of their routine approach to sTBI and the absence of rigorous data suggesting that monitoring is harmful, there is little likelihood that studies will be forthcoming from such centers to address this particular shortcoming in the literature. The ongoing National Institutes of Health (NIH)-funded RCT of monitor-guided versus 'empiric' ICP management being conducted in Latin America will hopefully shed some light on the global benefit of ICP monitoring per se; this trial will address not only patient outcomes, but also issues such as resource utilization, ICU bed triage, and the utility of prognostic information. It may also be able to suggest whether there are specific subgroups of sTBI patients that clearly benefit (or not) from monitor-driven therapy.

The available studies that have asked 'Does ICP management improve outcomes following sTBI?' are summarized in Table 1.

Who is at risk for intracranial hypertension?

The question of who is at risk for intracranial hypertension interacts, of course, with the issue of what is/are the critical value(s) of ICP (see the next section). For the purposes of the present discussion, however, the widely employed range of 20-25mmHg is used to define intracranial hypertension.

Risks of monitor placement

The question of who should be monitored also involves the risk of placement of intracranial monitors. The review of ICP monitoring technology in the Brain Trauma Foundation's 2007 guidelines for the management of severe brain injury concluded that, for adults, ventriculostomy-based and parenchymal devices are most accurate, and that the literature suggests the complication rates of infection or insertion-related hemorrhage are similar and very low [2]. A similar conclusion was published for the pediatric population in 2003 [4]. Evidence published subsequent to the pediatric guidelines has suggested that the incidence of intracranial infection for parenchymal devices may approach zero [40] **(IIb/B)** and that ventriculostomy-related monitors have a higher (albeit still very low) incidence of clinically significant, insertion-related hemorrhage [41] **(III/B)**. The overall conclusions of the guidelines still appear to hold, however, in that the risk of monitoring is generally well below the risk of treating without quantitative ICP data (if one accepts that monitoring and treating are indicated; see above).

Who should be monitored: adults

Given the very low risk of monitoring, it is often argued that all sTBI patients should be considered candidates and that it is the decision not to monitor that should be studied. Since the early days of monitoring it has been apparent that clinical examination does not consistently correlate with the presence or absence of intracranial hypertension [6, 7, 20]. With the advent of readily available, acute CT imaging, this modality has become a critical consideration for screening for ICP monitoring. In a prospective report on 225 consecutive sTBI patients, Miller *et al* stated (but did not support with presented data) that the only group with an incidence below 25% of any degree of intracranial hypertension was ventilated patients with normal early CT imaging [20] **(III/B)**.

Lobato *et al* reinforced the negative predictive value of normal early CT imaging in a study of 46 sTBI patients, none of whom manifested sustained intracranial hypertension if their scans remained normal over 1-7 days post-injury [42] **(III/B)**. They noted, however, that lesions appeared on follow-up imaging in approximately one-third of patients with initially normal images, and stressed the utility of repeated imaging in sTBI patients.

Similar findings were reported in a prospective study of 94 sTBI patients by Poca *et al* [43], in which the authors correlated the occurrence of intracranial hypertension with the CT classification scheme of Marshall *et al* [29] **(III/B)**. There was no incidence of ICP elevation in the three patients with a DI I pattern (normal CT), although one of these patients subsequently developed a focal CT abnormality. Patients with DI II patterns (abnormal, no mass >25cc, basal cisterns normal, no midline shift >5mm) were the most variable, with 29% of patients (10/35) having some ICP elevations. Patients with DI III patterns (no mass >25cc, compressed or absent cisterns without midline shift >5mm) had an elevated ICP incidence of 63% (12/19 patients), and those with DI IV patterns (compressed cisterns with midline shift ≥5mm) all had refractory intracranial hypertension (three patients). Given the numbers in each group, this paper probably is most meaningful for DI II and DI III patients.

Narayan *et al* specifically investigated the question of predicting ICP elevations in 226 consecutive, predominantly adult (range 2-89 years, mean 31 years, median 25 years) patients with sTBI [44]. They reported a correlation between abnormalities on 'early' CT imaging (70% within approximately 6 hours) and the likelihood of intracranial hypertension. Patients with any abnormalities on CT had an incidence of raised ICP of 53-63%, and the degree of intracranial hypertension in such patients was relatively high (>40mmHg in 18-27%) and correlated with outcome. sTBI patients with normal 'early' CT imaging had an 87% incidence of a normal ICP course; 13% showed some degree of intracranial hypertension, although only 2% had ICP elevations above 40mmHg. In the 13% of patients with normal admission CT imaging and raised ICP, the presence of two or more predictive variables raised the likelihood of intracranial hypertension to a level similar to those patients with abnormal CT imaging. The variables were as follows **(III/B)**:

- Age older than 40 years.
- Systolic blood pressure of 90mmHg or less.
- Uni- or bilateral motor posturing.

Lee *et al* studied the ICP courses of 36 sTBI patients with CT evidence of diffuse axonal injury and

Table 2. Who is at risk for intracranial hypertension? *Continued overleaf.*

Reference	Design	Results	Evidence level/ recommendation
Jensen *et al*, 1997 [40]	Prospective study of 98 pediatric sTBI patients monitored with a parenchymal device Catheter tips cultured on removal; contrast CT follow-up; no prophylactic antibiotics	7% positive surveillance culture with no clinical or contrast CT evidence of infection Tip cultures were felt to represent contaminants	IIb/B
Anderson *et al*, 2004 [41]	Retrospective report of 80 pediatric patients monitored with ventriculostomy, parenchymal monitor, or both Monitors placed only with normal coagulation studies and maximum three passes for ventriculostomies	**Hemorrhages** Ventriculostomies: 17.6% Parenchymal devices: 6.4% (significant) **Incidence of hemorrhages that influenced clinical course or required surgical treatment** Ventriculostomies: 13.2% Parenchymal devices: 1.6% The overall risk of monitoring was felt to be acceptable	III/B
Lobato *et al*, 1986 [42]	Retrospective study of 46 sTBI patients with normal admission CT scans	No patient had sustained ICP elevations One-third of patients showed later development of CT pathology Suggested follow-up imaging but not routine monitoring in such patients	III/B
Poca *et al*, 1998 [43]	Prospective study of 94 sTBI patients Occurrence of intracranial hypertension correlated with Marshall CT classification	**Diffuse injury I (n=3)** ICP <20mmHg: 100% Controllable ICP: 0% Refractory ICP: 0% **Diffuse injury II (n=35)** ICP <20mmHg: 71% Controllable ICP: 26% Refractory ICP: 3% **Diffuse injury III (n=19)** ICP <20mmHg: 37% Controllable ICP: 32% Refractory ICP: 32% **Diffuse injury IV (n=3)** ICP <20mmHg: 0% Controllable ICP: 0% Refractory ICP: 100%	III/B

Table 2. Who is at risk for intracranial hypertension? *Continued.*

Reference	Design	Results	Evidence level/ recommendation
Narayan *et al*, 1982 [44]	Retrospective study of 226 consecutive monitored sTBI cases managed without ICP monitoring Studied predictors of ICP elevation	**Any admission CT abnormalities/normal admission CT** Incidence of ICP elevation: 53-63%/13% The presence of two or more of the following factors with a normal scan raised the incidence to approximately that of those with abnormal CT: ♦ age >40 years ♦ systolic blood pressure ≤90mmHg ♦ uni- or bilateral motor posturing	III/B
Lee *et al*, 1998 [45]	Retrospective study of 36 monitored sTBI patients with CT evidence of diffuse axonal injury	Only two patients required treatment for ICP elevation (for ventriculitis or hydrocephalus) However, 72% had at least one ICP value >20mmHg and 25% had maximal ICP >30mmHg (the authors felt this was generally due to extracranial causes, such as fever)	III/B
Català-Temprano *et al*, 2007 [48]	Retrospective review of 156 consecutive monitored pediatric TBI patients (113 sTBIs) All sTBI patients monitored by protocol	Mean initial ICP in sTBI children: 27mmHg 70% required treatment for intracranial hypertension Authors did not evaluate predictors	III/B

ICP = intracranial pressure; sTBI = severe traumatic brain injury

suggested that ICP monitoring may be considered optional in these cases [45]. Only two patients required treatment for intracranial hypertension, which in both cases was related to the development of hydrocephalus or ventriculitis. Nevertheless, only 10 of their patients (28%) had no ICP values above 20mmHg and nine (25%) had maximal values higher than 30mmHg (which the authors generally related to extracranial causes such as febrile episodes) **(III/B)**. Whether such an incidence and magnitude profile for ICP elevations supports routinely not monitoring such patients remains unclear.

Who should be monitored: pediatric patients

There is little information to guide decision-making regarding ICP monitoring in the pediatric population. The neurologic examination can vary with age or developmental stage and is therefore more difficult and less reliable. Examination of unfused sutures or open fontanels is not a reliable means by which to preclude ICP elevation [46]. Children may also experience late deterioration accompanied by ICP elevation in the absence of surgical lesions on CT imaging [47]. Català-Temprano *et al* retrospectively reviewed all 156 pediatric TBI patients who

Chapter 33

underwent ICP monitoring admitted to their institution over a 9-year period [48]. Of these, 113 were admitted with an initial GCS of 8 or less (one of the criteria for routine ICP monitoring), comprising the sTBI group. The mean initial ICP in these sTBI children was 27mmHg, and 70% required treatment for intracranial hypertension **(III/B)**. The authors did not provide information suggesting specific predictors of intracranial hypertension.

Summary

On the supposition that ICP monitoring should be used to guide ICP treatment and that a threshold of 20-25mmHg is acceptable, monitoring should be considered for patient groups with a 'high' incidence of intracranial hypertension wherein the risk of monitoring is acceptably lower than the adverse consequences of monitor insertion or of treating without monitoring. A precise definition of 'high' incidence has not been reached, and the risk-to-benefit ratio of treating with or without monitoring remains unclear.

Recognizing such caveats, consideration of the use of ICP monitoring to guide treatment would seem to be supported by limited class III evidence for adult sTBI patients (GCS score ≤8 after resuscitation) with abnormal CT scans. Class III evidence fairly consistently supports the consideration of ICP monitoring to guide the management of children and adolescents in general, and of adults with sTBI who have normal CT images and two or more of the following signs:

* Age older than 40 years;
* Systolic blood pressure of 90mmHg or less; and
* Uni- or bilateral motor posturing.

An incidence-based decision to monitor adult sTBI patients with a normal CT scan and without two of these risk factors, or not to monitor some patients with diffuse axonal injury patterns (especially open basal cisterns and no midline shift), remains without a contributory evidence base and is left to the discretion of the individual practitioner.

The available studies that have asked 'Who is at risk for intracranial hypertension?' are summarized in Table 2.

What is the proper intracranial pressure treatment threshold?

If intracranial hypertension is to be considered a treatable entity, the treatment threshold (i.e., the definition of intracranial hypertension) must be empirically established. This threshold will most likely differ between various categories of brain injuries. In addition, the value might change over time within a given injury subtype. The almost universally used threshold of 20-25mmHg originated from the earliest investigations of post-traumatic ICP, and became identified as the upper limit of normal. Most subsequent studies addressing the association between ICP and outcome and the influence of treatment on recovery have been conducted using data from patients in whom ICP-lowering treatments have been initiated at the 20-25mmHg threshold. This presents the following confounding questions:

* Do patients do better if their ICP is kept below the treatment threshold?
* Do they do worse because vigorous treatment of 'refractory' intracranial hypertension is hazardous?
* Or does such treatment directly or indirectly select a subset of responders?

Threshold for managing intracranial pressure

Patients can herniate at less than 20mmHg, in some part related to the location of the parenchymal injury [49] **(III/B)**. Conversely, satisfactory outcomes have been reported for patients with sustained ICP values above 40mmHg who continued to be treated aggressively and whose CPP was maintained above 60mmHg [50] **(III/B)**. While small and uncontrolled, such case series strongly suggest that the commonly used treatment threshold of 20-25mmHg requires formal analysis.

Marmarou *et al* analyzed data from 428 sTBI patients from the prospective Traumatic Coma Data Bank in whom ICP monitoring was initiated within 18 hours of trauma and continued for at least 60 hours [10]. The ICP course was analyzed by evaluating the proportion of ICP measurements greater than x, where x was 0-80mmHg, by increments of 5mmHg. Logistic regression analysis suggested that, after age, admission GCS motor score, and pupillary status on admission, the proportion of ICP measurements above 20mmHg was highly significant as the next most powerful outcome predictor **(IIb/B)**. The explanatory power of the ICP proportion variables with respect to outcome peaked at 20mmHg and was less for all other cut-off points.

As discussed previously, Saul and Ducker reported improved outcomes after altering their ICP treatment threshold from 25 to 15mmHg [22] **(IIb/B)**. The non-concomitant nature of their study, and other changes in their treatment protocol associated with the threshold change, greatly limit the implications of the reported relationship between ICP treatment threshold and outcomes.

Ratanalert *et al* performed a small prospective RCT of ICP/CPP management with 27 sTBI patients using ICP thresholds of 20 or 25mmHg [51]. CPP was kept above 70mmHg, and ischemia was avoided by keeping jugular venous oxygen saturation above 50mmHg and monitoring. Outcomes were similar between the two groups at 6 months **(Ib/A)**.

Pediatric patients

Pfenninger *et al* reported a retrospective analysis of outcome predictors in 24 pediatric sTBI patients treated at a threshold of 20mmHg [14]. Sustained ICP courses consistently below 20mmHg were predictive of good outcomes, while sustained (>3 minutes) intracranial hypertension above 40mmHg was predictive of death. Intermediate sustained ICP values were distributed across all survival groups **(III/B)**.

Esparza *et al* reported a retrospective outcome study with 56 pediatric sTBI patients treated using an ICP threshold of 20mmHg [52]. The rate of unfavorable

outcomes (GOS 1-3) was 7% for patients with ICP values of 20mmHg or less, 29% for those with values of 20-40mmHg, and 100% for those with values above 40mmHg **(III/B)**.

Influence of cerebral perfusion pressure

The issue of whether an ICP threshold is necessary *per se* or whether it may simply fold into the calculation of CPP has been addressed in two small RCTs. Robertson *et al* performed a prospective RCT with 89 patients whose treatment was focused on ICP control and 100 patients managed with a focus on CPP [53]. Both groups were treated to keep ICP below 20mmHg, primarily using mannitol. ICP management targeted CPP above 50mmHg and commonly employed hyperventilation to 25-30mmHg for ICP control. CPP management targeted CPP above 70mmHg and maintenance of euvolemia; hyperventilation was not used. The primary outcome measure was frequency of jugular venous desaturation, which was significantly less in the CPP group. There was no difference in the mean ICP between groups. Neurologic recovery was a secondary outcome variable, and there was no difference between groups. This was felt to be related to the following:

- Episodes of jugular venous desaturation were treated aggressively in both groups.
- The beneficial effects of fewer episodes of desaturation might have been offset by the significantly greater incidence of systemic complications related to CPP management (e.g., adult respiratory distress syndrome).

In addition, the study was only powered to detect a large (19%) difference in outcome at the 80% level. Considering the value of reducing the ischemic complications of sTBI, this study suggests that a great deal of the importance of ICP may actually arise from its contribution to CPP (mean arterial pressure minus ICP) **(Ib/A)**.

This same question was addressed in the pediatric population by a small prospective RCT reported by Prabhakaran *et al* in 2004 [54]. The study included 17

Table 3. What is the proper ICP treatment threshold? (Or, is there an actual set treatment threshold?)
Continued overleaf.

Reference	Design	Results	Evidence level/ recommendation
Marshall *et al*, 1983 [49]	Retrospective study of 15 monitored patients demonstrating oval pupils	ICP associated with oval pupil was 18-38mmHg in 14/15 patients Restoring ICP to <20mmHg was associated with return of pupil to round in 9/14 patients	III/B
Young *et al*, 2003 [50]	Case series of four patients with sTBI and sustained ICP >40mmHg who received continued treatment with CPP maintained at >60mmHg	All four patients had favorable recovery despite 'apparently lethal ICP levels'	III/B
Marmarou *et al*, 1991 [10]	Analysis of prospective data from the Traumatic Coma Data Bank on 428 monitored sTBI patients Analyzed ICP influence on outcome	Proportion of ICP measurements >20mmHg was a highly significant outcome predictor The explanatory power peaked at 20mmHg and was less for all other cut-off points	IIb/B
Saul and Ducker, 1982 [22]	Prospective study of 127 sTBI patients treated at a threshold of 20-25mmHg and 106 patients subsequently treated at a threshold of 15mmHg	**Threshold of 20-25mmHg** Mortality: 46% **Threshold of 15mmHg** Mortality: 28%	IIb/B
Ratanalert *et al*, 2004 [51]	Small RCT of ICP/CPP management using ICP thresholds of 20 or 25mmHg in 27 sTBI patients CPP maintained at >70mmHg	No difference in outcome at 6 months Study too small to support a negative result	Ib/A
Pfenninger *et al*, 1983 [14]	Retrospective study of 24 pediatric monitored sTBI patients Analyzed ICP vs. outcome	ICP consistently <20mmHg predicted good outcome ICP >40mmHg for ≥3 minutes was predictive of death	III/B
Esparza *et al*, 1985 [52]	Retrospective report on 56 pediatric sTBI patients treated using an ICP threshold of 20mmHg	**Unfavorable outcome (GOS 1-3)** <20mmHg: 7% 20-40mmHg: 29% >40mmHg: 100%	III/B
Robertson *et al*, 1999 [53]	RCT of 189 sTBI patients randomized to management groups focused on ICP or CPP (both groups targeted ICP <20mmHg) Jugular saturation was the primary outcome variable	CPP protocol associated with significantly fewer incidences of jugular venous desaturation CPP group had significantly more systemic complications No difference in outcome between groups Study powered only for a very large (19%) difference in outcomes, as measured by the Glasgow Outcome Scale	Ib/A

Table 3. What is the proper ICP treatment threshold? (Or, is there an actual set treatment threshold?)
Continued.

Reference	Design	Results	Evidence level/ recommendation
Prabhakaran *et al*, 2004 [54]	Small RCT of 17 sTBI children randomized to an ICP arm (ICP <20mmHg) or CPP arm (>70mmHg for those aged ≥2 years or >60mmHg for those <2 years)	No difference in outcome at 1 year Mean ICPs were not significantly different between the groups (ICP group 16.4mmHg, CPP group 22.3mmHg)	Ib/A
Chambers *et al*, 2005 [55]	Retrospective ICP and CPP data from first 6 hours of monitoring in 235 pediatric sTBI patients (treated at an ICP threshold of 20mmHg)	ICP threshold for 100% specificity for poor outcome was >20mmHg and differed by age (2-6 years: 37mmHg; 7-10 and 11-16 years: 29mmHg)	III/B
Chambers *et al*, 2001 [56]	Analysis of ICP and CPP data from 207 adult and 84 pediatric sTBI patients using ROC curves to determine outcome thresholds	CPP was more predictive of outcome The most predictive ICP threshold was 35mmHg for both groups, although the threshold was not sharply defined	IIb/B

CPP = cerebral perfusion pressure; GOS = Glasgow Outcome Scale; ICP = intracranial pressure; RCT = randomized controlled trial; ROC = random operating characteristic; sTBI = severe traumatic brain injury

Chapter 33

sTBI children, who were randomized to an ICP arm (goal ICP <20mmHg) or a CPP arm (goal CPP >70mmHg for those ≥2years and >60mmHg for those younger). Steroids and hyperventilation to 20-30mmHg were used routinely in the ICP group. There was no significant difference in 1-year outcomes between the groups **(Ib/A)**. The mean ICP was 16.4mmHg (median 17.5mmHg) for patients in the ICP group and 22.3mmHg (median 18mmHg) for those in the CPP group (not significant).

In a retrospective study of the ICP and CPP courses during the first 6 hours of monitoring in 235 pediatric sTBI patients, Chambers *et al* reported that the ICP threshold for 100% specificity for poor outcome was above 20mmHg and differed by age group [55]. The threshold was 37mmHg for patients 2-6 years, and 29mmHg for those 7-10 and 11-16 years. Both mean ICP and mean CPP were predictive of outcome **(III/B)**.

In another study, Chambers *et al* used receiver operating characteristic (ROC) curves to investigate the threshold levels for ICP and CPP in 207 adults

and 84 children with sTBI [56]. They studied the correlation of 2-minute rolling average values of maximum ICP (ICP$_{max}$) and minimum CPP (CPP$_{min}$) readings with outcome. CPP was more predictive of outcome. In both adults and children, an ICP$_{max}$ threshold value of 35mmHg was most predictive overall (although the predictive value only reached 61% by that value) **(IIb/B)**. There appeared to be some differences between injury subtypes (based on the Marshall CT classification [29]), with the ICP$_{max}$ threshold varying between 22 and 36mmHg. Of note, the ROC curves were very flat across the range of 20-50mmHg in adults and fairly flat across the same range in children, suggesting no sharply defined threshold. All patients in this study were admitted and monitored for treatment purposes, although neither the treatment threshold used nor the management protocols were described.

Summary

The inextricable confounding that complicates retrospective analysis of ICP treatment thresholds using data from clinical series that treated at a chosen ICP value has seriously limited our understanding of the interaction between ICP, treatment of intracranial hypertension, prognosis, and outcomes. There is a fair amount of evidence that the usual threshold range of 20-25mmHg is not secure across all treatment situations. (Indeed, there is little physiological evidence that it should be.) The uncertainty reflected in the body of evidentiary literature presented here supports the value of direct investigations of this question, as well as of physiological processes (e.g., cerebral compliance) that might contribute to or assist in defining such a threshold.

The available studies that have asked 'What is the proper ICP treatment threshold?' are summarized in Table 3.

Is it beneficial to monitor intracranial pressure while treating?

Despite the evidentiary weaknesses in the relationship between lowering elevated ICP and improving outcome (see above), the strong correlation between intracranial hypertension and morbidity and mortality makes ICP control an almost universal goal of sTBI management. In many centers in developed nations and in the vast majority of hospitals in the developing world, however, this is done without the use of ICP monitoring devices. The 'diagnosis' and estimated likelihood of intracranial hypertension is based on neurologic examination and CT imaging of the brain. Patients felt to be at risk of ICP elevation are placed on an empiric prophylactic/therapeutic regimen that includes some or all of the same treatments used for monitor-based care. Individual treatments are administered on a schedule, the duration of which is usually set at 5-10 days. Treatment is escalated based on neurologic or CT worsening. Less commonly, the treatment course is shortened based on improvement in these two parameters. In some instances, ICP monitors are desired but unavailable; in others, they are not felt necessary to improve outcomes or treatment; and in yet other centers, physicians are at equipoise with respect to the benefits of monitor-based treatment. It is at four of the latter centers in Latin America that I

and others are currently conducting an NIH-funded, prospective RCT of ICP monitor versus empirically based treatment of sTBI.

As discussed above, there is a literature base for treating without monitoring. The report by Cremer *et al* from the Netherlands suggests that the outcomes of empiric treatment may be equal to those with care based on monitored ICP values [28] **(III/B)**. The paper by Shafi *et al* suggests that the current management schemes used for treatment based on ICP monitoring may actually be deleterious [30] **(IIb/B)**. Both of these studies indicate that ICP monitoring increases parameters such as therapeutic intensity, duration of mechanical ventilation, and length of ICU stay without apparent benefit. It is notable that most of the modalities used in lowering ICP have toxic side effects. Prolonged sedation, immobilization, and mechanical ventilation increase ICU length of stay and the risk of iatrogenic complications [57, 58]. Hyperventilation may produce cerebral ischemia, and its use in a prophylactic fashion has been associated with worse outcomes [59]. Neuromuscular blockade increases the risk of ICU-related infections [60]. Mannitol can produce hypotension related to volume contraction and renal toxicity [61]. Barbiturates and hypothermia both increase the risk of hypotension and infection [32, 62, 63]. The increased scrutiny and treatment driven by displaying continuous quantitative ICP values necessarily represents a balance between better management feedback and the toxicities of overtreatment. Unfortunately, with the exception of the ongoing prospective RCT mentioned above, there have been no controlled studies of the benefit of using monitoring to guide ICP treatment.

Finally, with respect to the necessity of anchoring sTBI management on ICP monitoring, it is important to further understand the relative contributions of ICP toward determining outcome. At question is the place of ICP in terms of a direct role as a pathophysiologic entity versus an indirect influence on issues such as cerebral perfusion [64-66], the coupling between metabolism and delivery [67], and cerebral compliance [68, 69]. For instance, Rosner *et al* have argued that the actual value of ICP is its role in determining CPP [66]. To this end, it is interesting to note that the 'establishment' of 20mmHg as the management trigger occurred during a period when systemic hypertension was felt to be a risk factor for intracranial hypertension, patients were routinely kept 'dry', and CPP was not a monitored variable. Outside of the situation of frank herniation (for which there is no set ICP threshold), the question remains of exactly how sensitive the injured brain is to ICP *per se*.

Unfortunately, at present, this important aspect of the role of ICP monitoring in directing the management of sTBI patients remains without a substantial literature base.

Conclusions

Although ICP monitors now appear to be used to guide sTBI treatment in most trauma centers in resource-rich countries such as the USA, this remains an issue of clinical choice rather than scientific mandate [17]. At present, the adult 'Guidelines for the Management of Severe Brain Injury' [2] and the 'Guidelines for the Acute Medical Management of Severe Traumatic Brain Injury in Infants, Children, and Adolescents' [4] together can present only a single recommendation with respect to ICP monitoring based on class II evidence, with the remainder being limited to class III evidence.

At the current time, therefore, ICP treatment appears to be standard practice despite the evidentiary limitations. The use of ICP monitoring to guide such treatment seems to be supported by limited class III evidence for sTBI patients (GCS score ≤8 after resuscitation) with abnormal CT scans. Class III evidence fairly consistently supports the consideration of ICP monitoring to guide the management of children and adolescents with sTBI in general and of adults with sTBI, normal CT images,

and two or more of the following signs: age older than 40 years; systolic blood pressure of 90mmHg or less; and uni- or bilateral motor posturing.

It is disturbing that a modality so fundamental to our sTBI practice is so poorly fleshed out in the literature (despite the numerous pages published). The recognition of this shortcoming should be a clarion call for focused responsive research. However, the number of articles that appeared following the original publication of the 'Guidelines for the Management of Severe Head Injury' [1] to allow stronger or at least more definitive statements to be made in the two following revisions [2, 3] was startlingly low. Clearly, a number of aspects surrounding ICP monitoring and management require further investigation lest fundamental embedded errors in our basic management inhibit future developments. Such issues include the following:

- The necessity of monitoring ICP in specific injury types.
- Targeting ICP treatment protocols to specific injury types in terms of:
  - ICP treatment threshold;
  - the balance of focus on ICP itself versus its role in other parameters (e.g., CPP, cerebral blood flow, compliance);
  - evolution of the injury over time.
- The proper combination of therapies in treatment protocols.
- The utility of ICP for optimizing system variables and resource utilization, outside of direct patient care:
  - ICP as a prognostic indicator;
  - ICP as a tool for triage and resource allocation;
  - the value of proving the lack of intracranial hypertension in avoiding unnecessary treatment and shortening ICU LOS.

Chapter 33

Chapter 33

Recommendations

Recommendations	Evidence level
◆ Research consistently (but not exclusively) supports the efficacy of aggressive global management of sTBI patients, generally including monitor-assisted management of ICP, in improving outcomes.	II/B, III/B
◆ Research supports the use of ICP monitoring for the detection of intracranial hypertension and obtaining prognostic information.	II/B, III/B
◆ Research supports consideration of 20mmHg as the most generally applicable treatment threshold. However, the evidence also supports reconsidering the concepts of: 1) a fixed threshold for all types of sTBI; and 2) that the ICP threshold is independent of other indices (e.g., CPP).	II/B, III/B
◆ There is very limited evidence that ICP can be treated without an ICP monitor and produce acceptable outcomes. There is insufficient literature on the methods for doing this to support its recommendation.	-
◆ Consideration should be given to monitoring all sTBI patients if ICP is to be treated based on monitored data as part of a comprehensive approach to sTBI. The one group that may be considered to have a sufficiently low likelihood of developing intracranial hypertension to allow contemplation of not needing monitoring is patients with a GCS score ≤8 and normal CT images with ≤1 of the following indicators: 1) age >40 years; 2) systolic blood pressure ≤90mmHg; and 3) uni- or bilateral motor posturing.	III/B
◆ Inconsistencies among level II and III studies strongly support the need for more research to determine the efficacy and efficiency of current ICP management approaches in terms of outcomes and resource utilization.	-

References

1. Bullock R, Chesnut R, Clifton G, Ghajar J, Marion D, Narayan R, *et al*. Guidelines for the management of severe head injury. *J Neurotrauma* 1996; 13: 639-734.

2. Bratton S, Bullock R, Carney N, *et al*. Guidelines for the management of severe brain injury: 2007 Revision. *J Neurotrauma* 2007; 24(Suppl. 1): S1-106.

3. Bullock R, Chesnut RM, Clifton G, *et al*. Guidelines for the management of severe head injury: 2000 Revision. *J Neurotrauma* 2000; 17: 457-627.

4. Adelson PD, Bratton SL, Carney NA, *et al*. Guidelines for the acute medical management of severe traumatic brain injury in infants, children, and adolescents. *Pediatr Crit Care Med* 2003; 4(Suppl. 3): S1-71.

5. Aarabi B, Alden TD, Chesnut RM, *et al*. Guidelines for the management of penetrating brain injury. *J Trauma* 2001; 51(Suppl. 2): S1-86.

6. Lundberg N. Continuous recording and control of ventricular fluid pressure in neurosurgical practice. *Acta Psychiatr Neurol Scand* (Suppl) 1960; 149: 1-193.

7. Guillaume J, Janny P. Monometrie intracranienne continué; Intérêt physio-pathologique et clinique de la methode. *La Presse Medicale* 1951; 59: 953-5.

8. Narayan RK, Greenberg RP, Miller JD, *et al*. Improved confidence of outcome prediction in severe head injury. A comparative analysis of the clinical examination, multimodality evoked potentials, CT scanning, and intracranial pressure. *J Neurosurg* 1981; 54: 751-62.

9. Becker DP, Miller JD, Ward JD, Greenberg RP, Young HF, Sakalas R. The outcome from severe head injury with early diagnosis and intensive management. *J Neurosurg* 1977; 47: 491-502.

10. Marmarou A, Anderson RL, Ward JD, *et al*. Impact of ICP instability and hypotension on outcome in patients with severe head trauma. *J Neurosurg* 1991; 75(Suppl.): S159-66.

11. Marshall LF, Smith RW, Shapiro HM. The outcome with aggressive treatment in severe head injuries. Part I: the significance of intracranial pressure monitoring. *J Neurosurg* 1979; 50: 20-5.

12. Miller JD, Becker DP, Ward JD, Sullivan HG, Adams WE, Rosner MJ. Significance of intracranial hypertension in severe head injury. *J Neurosurg* 1977; 47: 503-16.

13. Schreiber MA, Aoki N, Scott BG, Beck JR. Determinants of mortality in patients with severe blunt head injury. *Arch Surg* 2002; 137: 285-90.

14. Pfenninger J, Kaiser G, Lutschg J, Sutter M. Treatment and outcome of the severely head injured child. *Intensive Care Med* 1983; 9: 13-6.

15. Jagannathan J, Okonkwo DO, Yeoh HK, *et al*. Long-term outcomes and prognostic factors in pediatric patients with severe traumatic brain injury and elevated intracranial pressure. *J Neurosurg Pediatr* 2008; 2: 240-9.

16. Ghajar J, Hariri RJ, Narayan RK, Iacono LA, Firlik K, Patterson RH. Survey of critical care management of comatose, head-injured patients in the United States. *Crit Care Med* 1995; 23: 560-7.

17. Hesdorffer DC, Ghajar J, Iacono L. Predictors of compliance with the evidence-based guidelines for traumatic brain injury care: a survey of United States trauma centers. *J Trauma* 2002; 52: 1202-9.

18. Jennett B, Teasdale G, Galbraith S, *et al*. Severe head injuries in three countries. *J Neurol Neurosurg Psychiatry* 1977; 40: 291-8.

19. Bowers SA, Marshall LF. Outcome in 200 consecutive cases of severe head injury treated in San Diego County: a prospective analysis. *Neurosurgery* 1980; 6: 237-42.

20. Miller JD, Butterworth JF, Gudeman SK, *et al*. Further experience in the management of severe head injury. *J Neurosurg* 1981; 54: 289-99.

21. Stuart GG, Merry GS, Smith JA, Yelland JD. Severe head injury managed without intracranial pressure monitoring. *J Neurosurg* 1983; 59: 601-5.

22. Saul TG, Ducker TB. Effect of intracranial pressure monitoring and aggressive treatment on mortality in severe head injury. *J Neurosurg* 1982; 56: 498-503.

23. Colohan AR, Alves WM, Gross CR, *et al*. Head injury mortality in two centers with different emergency medical services and intensive care. *J Neurosurg* 1989; 71: 202-7.

24. Harris OA, Bruce CA, Reid M, *et al*. Examination of the management of traumatic brain injury in the developing and developed world: focus on resource utilization, protocols, and practices that alter outcome. *J Neurosurg* 2008; 109: 433-8.

25. Bulger EM, Nathens AB, Rivara FP, Moore M, MacKenzie EJ, Jurkovich GJ. Management of severe head injury: institutional variations in care and effect on outcome. *Crit Care Med* 2002; 30: 1870-6.

26. Ghajar J, Hariri R, Patterson RH. Improved outcome from traumatic coma using only ventricular CSF drainage for ICP control. *Adv Neurosurg* 1993; 21: 173-7.

27. Smith HP, Kelly D Jr, McWhorter JM, *et al*. Comparison of mannitol regimens in patients with severe head injury undergoing intracranial monitoring. *J Neurosurg* 1986; 65: 820-4.

28. Cremer OL, van Dijk GW, van Wensen E, *et al*. Effect of intracranial pressure monitoring and targeted intensive care on functional outcome after severe head injury. *Crit Care Med* 2005; 33: 2207-13.

29. Marshall LF, Bowers-Marshall S, Klauber MR, *et al*. A new classification of head injury based on computerized tomography. *J Neurosurg* 1991; 75(Suppl.): S14-20.

30. Shafi S, Diaz-Arrastia R, Madden C, Gentilello L. Intracranial pressure monitoring in brain-injured patients is associated with worsening of survival. *J Trauma* 2008; 64: 335-40.

31. Lane PL, Skoretz TG, Doig G, Girotti MJ. Intracranial pressure monitoring and outcomes after traumatic brain injury. *Can J Surg* 2000; 43: 442-8.

32. Eisenberg H, Frankowski R, Contant C, Marshall L, Walker M, Centers CCNST. High-dose barbiturate control of elevated intracranial pressure in patients with severe head injury. *J Neurosurg* 1988; 69: 15-23.

33. Aarabi B, Hesdorffer DC, Ahn ES, Aresco C, Scalea TM, Eisenberg HM. Outcome following decompressive craniectomy for malignant swelling due to severe head injury. *J Neurosurg* 2006; 104: 469-79.

34. Skoglund TS, Eriksson-Ritzen C, Jensen C, Rydenhag B. Aspects on decompressive craniectomy in patients with traumatic head injuries. *J Neurotrauma* 2006; 23: 1502-9.

35. Dam Hieu P, Sizun J, Person H, Besson G. The place of decompressive surgery in the treatment of uncontrollable post-traumatic intracranial hypertension in children. *Childs Nerv Syst* 1996; 12: 270-5.

36. Ruf B, Heckmann M, Schroth I, *et al*. Early decompressive craniectomy and duraplasty for refractory intracranial hypertension in children: results of a pilot study. *Crit Care* 2003; 7: R133-8.

37. Rutigliano D, Egnor MR, Priebe CJ, *et al*. Decompressive craniectomy in pediatric patients with traumatic brain injury with intractable elevated intracranial pressure. *J Pediatr Surg* 2006; 41: 83-7.

38. Kunze E, Meixensberger J, Janka M, Sorensen N, Roosen K. Decompressive craniectomy in patients with uncontrollable intracranial hypertension. *Acta Neurochir* Suppl 1998; 71: 16-8.

39. Taylor A, Butt W, Rosenfeld J, *et al*. A randomized trial of very early decompressive craniectomy in children with traumatic brain injury and sustained intracranial hypertension. *Childs Nerv Syst* 2001; 17: 154-62.

40. Jensen RL, Hahn YS, Ciro E. Risk factors of intracranial pressure monitoring in children with fiberoptic devices: a critical review. *Surg Neurol* 1997; 47: 16-22.

41. Anderson RC, Kan P, Klimo P, Brockmeyer DL, Walker ML, Kestle JR. Complications of intracranial pressure monitoring in children with head trauma. *J Neurosurg* 2004; 101(Suppl. 1): 53-8.

42. Lobato RD, Sarabia R, Rivas JJ, *et al*. Normal computerized tomography scans in severe head injury. Prognostic and clinical management implications. *J Neurosurg* 1986; 65: 784-9.

43. Poca MA, Sahuquillo J, Baguena M, Pedraza S, Gracia RM, Rubio E. Incidence of intracranial hypertension after severe head injury: a prospective study using the Traumatic Coma Data Bank classification. *Acta Neurochir* Suppl 1998; 71: 27-30.

44. Narayan RK, Kishore PR, Becker DP, *et al*. Intracranial pressure: to monitor or not to monitor? A review of our experience with severe head injury. *J Neurosurg* 1982; 56: 650-9.

45. Lee TT, Galarza M, Villanueva PA. Diffuse axonal injury (DAI) is not associated with elevated intracranial pressure (ICP). *Acta Neurochir* (Wien) 1998; 140: 41-6.

46. Cho DY, Wang YC, Chi CS. Decompressive craniotomy for acute shaken/impact baby syndrome. *Pediatr Neurosurg* 1995; 23: 192-8.

47. Lobato RD, Rivas JJ, Gomez PA, et al. Head-injured patients who talk and deteriorate into coma. Analysis of 211 cases studied with computerized tomography [see comments]. *J Neurosurg* 1991; 75: 256-61.

48. Català-Temprano A, Claret Teruel G, Cambra Lasaosa FJ, Pons Odena M, Noguera Julian A, Palomeque Rico A. Intracranial pressure and cerebral perfusion pressure as risk factors in children with traumatic brain injuries. *J Neurosurg* 2007; 106(Suppl. 6): 463-6.

49. Marshall LF, Barba D, Toole BM, Bowers SA. The oval pupil: clinical significance and relationship to intracranial hypertension. *J Neurosurg* 1983; 58: 566-8.

50. Young JS, Blow O, Turrentine F, Claridge JA, Schulman A. Is there an upper limit of intracranial pressure in patients with severe head injury if cerebral perfusion pressure is maintained? *Neurosurg Focus* 2003; 15: E2.

51. Ratanalert S, Phuenpathom N, Saeheng S, Oearsakul T, Sripairojkul B, Hirunpat S. ICP threshold in CPP management of severe head injury patients. *Surg Neurol* 2004; 61: 429-34.

52. Esparza J, M-Portillo J, Sarabia M, Yuste JA, Roger R, Lamas E. Outcome in children with severe head injuries. *Childs Nerv Syst* 1985; 1: 109-14.

53. Robertson CS, Valadka AB, Hannay HJ, et al. Prevention of secondary ischemic insults after severe head injury. *Crit Care Med* 1999; 27: 2086-95.

54. Prabhakaran P, Reddy AT, Oakes WJ, King WD, Winkler MK, Givens TG. A pilot trial comparing cerebral perfusion pressure-targeted therapy to intracranial pressure-targeted therapy in children with severe traumatic brain injury. *J Neurosurg* 2004; 100 (5 Suppl. Pediatrics): 454-9.

55. Chambers IR, Stobbart L, Jones PA, et al. Age-related differences in intracranial pressure and cerebral perfusion pressure in the first 6 hours of monitoring after children's head injury: association with outcome. *Childs Nerv Syst* 2005; 21: 195-9.

56. Chambers IR, Treadwell L, Mendelow AD. Determination of threshold levels of cerebral perfusion pressure and intracranial pressure in severe head injury by using receiver-operating characteristic curves: an observational study in 291 patients. *J Neurosurg* 2001; 94: 412-6.

57. Girard TD, Kress JP, Fuchs BD, et al. Efficacy and safety of a paired sedation and ventilator weaning protocol for mechanically ventilated patients in intensive care (Awakening

and Breathing Controlled Trial): a randomised controlled trial. *Lancet* 2008; 371: 126-34.

58. Kress JP, Pohlman AS, O'Connor MF, Hall JB. Daily interruption of sedative infusions in critically ill patients undergoing mechanical ventilation. *N Engl J Med* 2000; 342: 1471-7.

59. Muizelaar JP, Marmarou A, Ward JD, et al. Adverse effects of prolonged hyperventilation in patients with severe head injury: a randomized clinical trial. *J Neurosurg* 1991; 75: 731-9.

60. Hsiang J, Chesnut RM, Crisp CB, Klauber MR, Blunt BA, Marshall LF, Editors. Early, routine paralyis for ICP control in severe head injury: is it necessary? Second International Neurotrauma Symposium, 1993. Glasgow, Scotland.

61. Chesnut RM, Gautille T, Blunt BA, Klauber MR, Marshall LF. Neurogenic hypotension in patients with severe head injuries. *J Trauma* 1998; 44: 958-63.

62. Clifton GL, Miller ER, Choi SC, et al. Lack of effect of induction of hypothermia after acute brain injury. *N Engl J Med* 2001; 344: 556-63.

63. Hutchison JS, Ward RE, Lacroix J, et al. Hypothermia therapy after traumatic brain injury in children. *N Engl J Med* 2008; 358: 2447-56.

64. Sharples PM, Matthews DS, Eyre JA. Cerebral blood flow and metabolism in children with severe head injuries. Part 2: Cerebrovascular resistance and its determinants. *J Neurol Neurosurg Psychiatry* 1995; 58: 153-9.

65. Sharples PM, Stuart AG, Matthews DS, Aynsley-Green A, Eyre JA. Cerebral blood flow and metabolism in children with severe head injury. Part 1: Relation to age, Glasgow coma score, outcome, intracranial pressure, and time after injury. *J Neurol Neurosurg Psychiatry* 1995; 58: 145-52.

66. Rosner MJ, Rosner SD, Johnson AH. Cerebral perfusion pressure: management protocol and clinical results. *J Neurosurg* 1995; 83: 949-62.

67. Cruz J. The first decade of continuous monitoring of jugular bulb oxyhemoglobinsaturation: management strategies and clinical outcome [see comments]. *Crit Care Med* 1998; 26: 344-51.

68. Shapiro K, Marmarou A. Clinical applications of the pressure-volume index in treatment of pediatric head injuries. *J Neurosurg* 1982; 56: 819-25.

69. Czosnyka M, Harris NG, Pickard JD, Piechnik S. CO_2 cerebrovascular reactivity as a function of perfusion pressure - a modelling study. *Acta Neurochir* (Wien) 1993; 121: 159-65.

Chapter 34

The role of decompressive hemicraniectomy in traumatic brain injury

Rajiv Saigal MD PhD, Neurotrauma Research Fellow 1
Atsuhiro Nakagawa MD PhD, Assistant Professor of Neurosurgery 1, 2
Geoffrey T Manley MD PhD, Professor of Neurosurgery and Vice-Chairman 1

1 DEPARTMENT OF NEUROSURGERY AND THE BRAIN AND SPINAL INJURY CENTER (BASIC), UNIVERSITY OF CALIFORNIA, SAN FRANCISCO, CALIFORNIA, USA
2 DEPARTMENT OF NEUROSURGERY, TOHOKU UNIVERSITY HOSPITAL, SENDAI, JAPAN

Introduction

More than 1.7 million Americans sustain a traumatic brain injury (TBI) every year; 50,000 of these people die and more than 80,000 experience long-term neurologic deficits, resulting in more than 5 million Americans currently living with chronic disability [1, 2]. Of those with severe brain injury, 60% will die or experience severe disability [3]. This dismal percentage increases to 80-85% when refractory intracranial hypertension is present [4, 5].

As described by the Monro-Kellie doctrine, the cranial cavity is a fixed space composed of brain, blood, and cerebrospinal fluid [6-8]. In some cases of TBI, edema and/or hemorrhage into this fixed space causes elevated intracranial pressure (ICP). Surgical decompression can relieve pressure by increasing intracranial compliance [6-8], and thus potentially spare normal brain parenchyma from secondary injury. However, as with any invasive procedure, decompression cannot be thought of as purely benign. Known risks include edema, hematoma formation, infarction, lack of protection against further trauma, and strangulation of cerebral tissue at the edge of the bone flap [9]. Promoted by Kocher as early as in 1901 [10], decompressive craniectomy (DC) fell

out of favor because of these risks before seeing a recent resurgence in the last few decades.

The creation of high-quality evidence to guide clinicians in weighing these risks and benefits has so far proved challenging. There are many causes of head trauma, giving each injury unique characteristics that are not easily captured by the traditional definitions of mild, moderate, and severe TBI (sTBI) [11, 12]. Evaluating the role of decompressive surgery in neurosurgical trauma is made difficult by the heterogeneity of disease processes. Currently, randomized controlled trials (RCTs) are considered the highest standard achievable. However, a fundamental requirement is that the patients being randomized are sufficiently similar to prevent subject-specific characteristics from overshadowing the treatment effect. Ongoing efforts to improve the classification of TBI may improve future clinical trials by helping to identify groups of patients who are most likely to benefit from specific treatments.

Methodology

We conducted a systematic review of the literature using Pubmed and the Cochrane database. Search terms included 'decompressive craniectomy,' 'decompressive hemicraniectomy,' and 'severe traumatic brain injury.' Key articles were used as sources for additional references. The most pertinent studies were included and the quality of their evidence was scored based on standard definitions by the US Preventive Services Task Force and the UK National Health Service.

High-quality evidence

In an extensive 2006 review of 154 published and unpublished trials on TBI for the Cochrane database [13], Sahuquillo and Arikan found only one study, published by Taylor *et al*, that satisfied the criteria for a high-quality trial based on randomization, independent and blind assessment of outcomes, number lost to follow-up, quality of control groups, and analysis based on intent-to-treat [5] **(Ib/A)**. This RCT was performed with 27 pediatric TBI patients (ages 1-14 years) who were randomized to bitemporal craniectomy plus medical management (n=13) or medical management alone (n=14) [5]. Bitemporal craniectomy was associated with a mean ICP reduction of 9.0mmHg, which was 5.3mmHg more than medical management alone. Overall, 54% of the decompression group versus only 14% of the control group reached a favorable Glasgow Outcome Scale (GOS) score, signifying mild disability or good recovery after 6 months. However, none of these reported differences reached statistical significance, and the study was further confounded by changes in management over its 7-year course. In addition, dura was left intact in the majority of patients or 'scarified' in a few, theoretically leading to suboptimal decompression. An attempt to mitigate these changes was made using a four-factor randomized block design. However, a larger, more consistent, and sufficiently powered randomized sample is needed to obtain definitive results.

DECRA

After the publication of the Cochrane review [13], the Decompressive Craniectomy (DECRA) trial was the first prospective multicenter RCT comparing bifrontal craniectomy (n=73) with standard non-surgical care (n=82) for patients with refractory intracranial hypertension [3, 14]. Conducted from 2002 to 2010, the trial involved patients aged 15-60 years with severe non-penetrating TBI treated in hospitals in Australia, New Zealand, and Saudi Arabia. Severe TBI was defined as a GCS of 8 of less or a Marshall CT score of III or higher (moderate diffuse injury) [12]. The primary outcome was initially the percentage of patients with a good outcome (score 5-8 on extended GOS [GOS-E]) at 6 months post-injury, and later changed to become the score on the GOS-E. Refractory intracranial hypertension was defined as 15 minutes of intermittent or continuous ICP elevation above 20mmHg in 1 hour despite first-tier medical management, such as mannitol, sedation, normalized pCO_2, hypertonic saline, external ventricular drainage, or paralysis. After randomization, allowable second-tier therapies included hypothermia to 35°C and barbiturates. Secondary outcomes included ICP, mortality, length of intensive care unit and hospital stay, and the proportion of survivors with poor outcomes (GOS-E 2-4). Exclusion criteria included penetrating intracerebral injury, concomitant spinal cord injury, prior craniectomy, hematoma requiring evacuation, intracerebral hematoma more than 3cm in diameter, GCS score of 3 with unreactive pupils, coagulopathy, and cardiac arrest at the scene. Despite fewer days in the intensive care unit (p<0.001) and improvements in ICP (p<0.001), the DC group had more unfavorable outcomes (odds ratio 2.21; p=0.02) and worse GOS-E scores (odds ratio 1.84; p=0.03). There was no significant difference in mortality (19% in the DC group vs. 18% with medical management) or length of hospital stay (28 vs. 37 days, respectively; p=0.82).

This study, which was carried out by a highly respected group of investigators, suffered from several significant issues inherent in small RCTs. Unfortunately, randomization did not yield equal distributions of patients between the groups (probably because of the small sample size) for important and validated prognostic variables such as Marshall CT scores and pupillary reactivity. Overall, 73% of DC patients had Marshall CT scores of III (compressed cisterns with midline shift <5mm) or IV (midline shift >5mm), compared with 65% of standard-care patients (p=0.39). In addition, 19 of 71 patients in the

DC group (27%) had bilateral non-reactive pupils compared with 10 of 80 patients in the standard-care group (12%; p=0.04). Pupillary reactivity is one of three major prognosticators (with age and motor score) in traumatic brain injury, as shown by the IMPACT study group [15].

Furthermore, the specific surgical techniques used differed from the original description by Polin *et al* (division of the sagittal sinus and falx to provide a large decompression) [4]. In addition, over the timespan taken to complete DECRA, many practicing neurosurgeons gradually transitioned to a large unilateral fronto-temoral-parietal DC, partly because of the higher complication rate associated with the bifrontal approach [16]. As the DECRA authors note, their results are only applicable to the specific surgical approach they employed [14]. The study screened 3,478 subjects with severe TBI during the study period and enrolled only 4%, reinforcing the fact that this study applies to only a small fraction of TBI patients.

The study used a liberal definition of refractory intracranial hypertension, defined as 15 minutes of ICP above 20mmHg within 1 hour. Median ICP in the 12 hours prior to randomization was only 20mmHg for both groups. Although there is no universally accepted trigger, surgical decompression is typically reserved as a final-tier therapy when sedation, cerebrospinal fluid drainage, and hyperosmolar treatment and paralysis have failed. The early use of DC in this trial is not consistent with the more modern clinical treatment algorithms used in current TBI trials such as ProTECT [17]. Thus, the remaining evidence-based finding of DECRA is that early bifrontal craniectomy for diffuse brain swelling after TBI should not be considered before maximal medical management and external ventrical drainage therapies have failed.

Key retrospective studies

Although not prospective RCTs, some well-conducted studies have offered additional insights into decompression. In a retrospective case-control study, Polin *et al* reported a significant improvement in ICP (p=0.0001 vs. preoperative; p=0.026 vs. control), increased survival (77% vs. 70%), and favorable outcomes (37% vs. 15%; p=0.014) in 35 patients undergoing bifrontal DC within 48 hours of injury for refractory cerebral edema in the absence of a mass lesion, compared with matched control patients from the Trauma Coma Data Bank [4] **(III/B)**. The results were more impressive for the subset of patients with ICP less than 40mmHg: in this population, 60% of patients (12/20) in the DC group experienced favorable outcomes compared with 18% of controls (p=0.001). Pediatric patients (n=18) showed a trend toward more favorable outcomes with decompression than adult patients (p=0.079). Of the 14 patients with a Glasgow Coma Scale (GCS) score of 4 or less at study entry, only one recovered. Unfortunately, subarachnoid bolts were routinely employed in lieu of ventriculostomy. The study also lacks data on intracerebral hematoma patients, who were excluded from the trial, and longer follow-up periods for non-operated control patients.

In a retrospective study of 57 head trauma patients treated from 1977 to 1997, Guerra *et al* reported that 60% of surgically decompressed patients (33/55 patients not lost to follow-up) achieved a favorable outcome (GOS 4-5) [18]. The mortality rate was only 19%, considerably lower than the rate of 58-82% reported for patients treated with barbiturates [18, 19] **(III/B)**. Decompression was the initial surgery for 38 patients and a second surgery for 17 patients who initially underwent evacuation of a space-occupying lesion (i.e., intraparenchymal hematoma, subdural hematoma, or epidural hematoma) and later developed malignant brain swelling; 58% and 65% of patients, respectively, reached a favorable outcome. Surgery was performed when patients suffered clinical deterioration that correlated with swelling on CT, decrease in GCS score, pupillary dilation, ICP higher than 30mmHg, or cerebral perfusion pressure (CPP) less than 45mmHg. Patients received either unilateral (n=31 total; 30 with follow-up data) or bilateral (n=26 total; 25 with follow-up) decompression, depending on the laterality of the swelling. Patients with a GCS score below 4 (initially and on post-traumatic day 2) or lack of brainstem reflexes were excluded from surgery. Conservative management before and after decompression included elevation of the head of the bed, sedation, analgesia, hyperventilation to a PCO_2 of 28-32mmHg, mannitol, tromethamine for acute rises in ICP, and burst suppression with barbiturates. Apart from its retrospective and non-controlled nature, the quality of the study suffered from different age exclusion criteria over time, ranging from those older than 30 years at study onset to those older than 50 years by study end. All six patients with an initial GCS score of 3 who recovered to no greater than a GCS score of 4 preoperatively had poor outcomes, emphasizing that patients in this group may not make good surgical candidates, assuming that the GCS score is related to the neurologic injury and not to sedation. The patients recovering to a GOS score of 5 (i.e., good recovery) had a mean age of 18.7 years, compared with 24.7 years or older for a GOS score of 1-4, giving credence to the idea that younger patients are more likely to do well with surgical decompression **(III/B)**.

Albanèse et al reported on a retrospective cohort study in which 40 of 816 patients with sTBI underwent DC if certain criteria were met: clinical signs of herniation correlating with a CT scan showing hematoma, swelling, and/or herniation [20]. Those with a mass lesion and a GCS score of less than 6 were operated on within 24 hours ('early DC group,' n=27) before ICP monitoring. In the absence of hematoma, surgery was indicated by an ICP above 35mm Hg, either unilateral or bilateral absence of pupillary reflexes, or CT showing swelling or herniation, with surgery performed after 24 hours ('late DC group,' n=13). Overall, 25% of patients experienced a good recovery (GOS 4-5): 18% in the early group and 38% in the late group **(III/B)**. In the early group, four out of five patients achieving a good recovery had an initial GCS score above 5, emphasizing its importance as a prognostic factor. Conversely, all eight patients in the early group with brainstem dysfunction on admission had poor outcomes, with seven dying and one living in a vegetative state. In the late group without mass lesion, 38% (five patients) survived with severe

disability or in a vegetative state. Unfortunately, these results cannot be used as evidence for the optimal timing of surgery because patients in the early and late groups had entirely different lesions. The study is further limited by a lack of statistical analysis.

Ucar et al compared outcomes in craniectomized patients according to the initial GCS score in a retrospective study of 100 sTBI patients [21]. Only 3.3% of patients with an initial GCS score of 4-5 (2/60 patients) attained a favorable outcome, compared with 35% of patients with an initial score of 6-8 (14/40 patients; p<0.05) **(III/B)**. A GCS score above 5 again served as an important prognostic line. Age was significantly associated with outcome, with a mean age of 27 years for those experiencing favorable outcomes, compared with 31 years for those experiencing unfavorable outcomes (p<0.05). Overall, decompression reduced mean ICP from 30 to 24mmHg (p<0.001). Only 11% of patients (4/37) with mass lesions improved to a GOS score of at least 4 compared with 20% (12/60) without mass lesions, although this finding did not reach statistical significance (p=0.058). These observations are consistent with those of Albanèse et al and much of the rest of the literature [20].

Coplin et al retrospectively compared craniotomy (n=17) with craniectomy and duraplasty (n=12) in 29 consecutive patients undergoing decompression for a midline shift greater than explainable by the mass effect of the hematoma alone [22]. Although the craniectomy group had lower preoperative GCS scores (mean±standard deviation 5±3 vs. 7±2; p=0.04) and more diffuse injury III and IV patients on the Marshall Scale [12], there was no difference between the groups in discharge GOS score, length of stay, or Functional Independence Measure score **(III/B)**. There was, however, an insignificant trend toward decreased mortality with craniectomy (25% vs. 41%; p=0.4). Reoperation was required in 18% of craniotomy patients compared with none of the craniectomy patients (p=0.2). Overall, 29% of patients underwent partial brain resection as part of their craniotomy. The authors concluded that craniectomy is safe as an initial procedure and does not need to be relegated to salvage therapy alone.

Kunze *et al* examined GOS scores after 1 year in another retrospective study of 28 patients with secondary craniectomy for sTBI and elevated ICP unresponsive to maximum medical treatment [23]. Excluding patients with central herniation, brainstem injury, ischemic infarction, and large primary lesions, 56% of patients achieved a positive outcome (GOS ≥4) **(III/B)**. ICP decreased in all patients from a mean of 42 to 21mmHg. Although this study provides interesting observational data, it lacked an internal control group and can only be compared with the literature at large.

Predictive factors for poor outcome

In patients who do undergo DC, a number of factors portend a poor outcome. In a retrospective study published in 2010, Lemcke *et al* followed 124 of 131 patients who underwent surgical decompression for head trauma at a single institution for a mean 49 months postoperatively [24]. The differences between patients with poor (GOS 1-3) and good (GOS 4-5) long-term outcomes were investigated. The following significant predictors of poor outcome following DC were identified **(III/B)**:

- Asymmetric pupil reactivity (p=0.002).
- Older age (38±20 vs. 27±17 years; p<0.001).
- Greater degree of midline shift (9.8±6.7 vs. 6.7±5.0mm; p=0.009).

The authors also noted a high percentage of poor outcomes in patients with an initial GCS score of 8 or less, clotting disorders, or obliteration of basal cisterns, but data were not reported. Interestingly, there was not a significant difference in time to surgery between the two groups (p=0.616).

Subtemporal decompression and temporal lobectomy

Gower *et al* compared pentobarbital coma (n=24) and subtemporal decompression (n=10) in 115 severe TBI patients treated for medically refractory intracranial hypertension at a single institution

between 1983 and 1987 [19]. Although decompressed patients had slightly lower initial GCS scores (mean±SD, 4.9±1.8 vs. 5.3±2.0), the authors found an 82% mortality rate with barbiturate coma versus 40% with decompression **(III/B)**. The mean±SD ICP reduced by 21%, from 24.1±12.9 to 19.1±7.4mmHg. Seven patients with refractory ICP on pentobarbital crossed over to the surgical decompression group. Four of these cross-over patients died, compared with a mortality rate of 82% among patients in a pentobarbital coma without subtemporal decompression, implying the benefit of surgical decompression as a salvage technique in treating otherwise refractory conditions. The large difference in mortality was probably biased by the 10 pentobarbital coma patients in whom therapy failed but who were not deemed candidates for surgery. Another major deficiency in the study is the lack of statistical analysis.

In a retrospective series by Lee *et al* of 29 patients with uncal herniation from contusion and acute subdural hematoma, temporal lobectomy (n=13; 10 patients with complete lobectomy and three with anterior lobectomy) was associated with significantly improved survival when provided in addition to subtemporal decompression and resection of contused brain alone (n=16) [25] **(III/B)**. With lobectomy, mortality decreased from 56% to 7.7% and mean±SD GOS scores improved from 2.2±0.4 to 4.0±0.4. Interestingly, all 10 complete lobectomy patients achieved good outcomes (GOS ≥4) while all three patients with anterior lobectomy had poor outcomes (GOS ≤2), corroborating the need for ample decompression. The study design was limited by its sequential nature; all lobectomy patients were treated subsequent to the subtemporal decompression group.

Nussbaum *et al* reported results following complete temporal lobectomy in a retrospective case series of 10 TBI patients aged 22-61 years with unilateral swelling and transtentorial herniation, but without subdural hematoma or epidural hematoma [26]. They found 30% mortality, 30% survival with minimal assistance, and 30% survival with functional independence, judged by the Barthel Index, a considerable improvement over the natural history of the disease **(III/B)**. As a case series the study is without a control group, but upholds other literature (such as the study of Lee *et al* [25]) showing good outcomes with complete lobectomy.

Evidence for improved ICP

Multiple studies have demonstrated ICP reductions following DC [21, 27-33]. In a retrospective series of 40 patients with sTBI, Howard *et al* reported significant reductions in mean±SD ICP (from 35.0±13.5 to 14.6±8.7mmHg; p<0.005) for 16 patients who underwent DC for intractable intracranial hypertension [28] **(III/B)**. This ICP-lowering effect has been used as an argument to perform DC early to prevent unnecessary increases in ICP and minimize the effects of secondary injuries associated with high ICP. Lowering ICP improves CPP. After DC is performed, CPP has been shown to increase and be maintained at ideal levels for maximal effect [23]. However, to date, there is no definitive evidence to support the early institution of DC before irreversible ischemia can occur.

Timofeev *et al* also reported significant and sustained reductions in ICP (from 36.4 to 12.6mmHg) in a retrospective series of 27 sTBI patients treated with an ICP-targeted-therapy protocol [30] **(III/B)**. They found a significantly lower mean arterial pressure was needed after DC to maintain optimum CPP levels, compared with the preoperative period (preoperative 99.5mmHg vs. postoperative 94.2mmHg; p=0.017), allowing a reduction of treatment intensity and weaning in most patients. The beneficial effect of DC on the control of ICP was also reflected in the amount of time ICP was above 25mmHg: this occurred only 2% of the time after DC, compared with approximately 30% of the time preoperatively.

Skoglund *et al* reported significant and sustained reductions in ICP in a retrospective series of 19 patients who underwent DC following a refractory ICP increase (mean±SD, 29.2±3.5mmHg preoperatively vs. 11.1±6.0mmHg postoperatively and 13.9±9.7mmHg at 24 hours after surgery) [31] **(III/B)**. In addition, there was a significant correlation between the size of the craniectomy and the decrease in ICP.

In a clinical study of 26 patients, Whitfield *et al* showed the amplitude of ICP waves was significantly reduced (p<0.02) and compensatory reserve increased (p<0.05) following DC for brain swelling after sTBI [32] **(III/B)**. In another retrospective analysis of 20 TBI patients undergoing bilateral DC and duraplasty, Yoo *et al* provided a quantitative analysis of the additional decompression provided by dural expansion [33]. Post-craniectomy, the mean±SD ICP decreased to 50.2±16.6% of the initial ICP. Subsequent dural opening further reduced the ICP to 15.7±10.7% of the initial pressure **(III/B)**. Illustrating the importance of ICP reduction, the authors reported 100% mortality when ICP persisted above 35mmHg postoperatively. ICP at postoperative day 1 was predictive of 6-month outcome.

In summary, the current literature provides consistent level III/B evidence that DC can reduce ICP. It also appears that this effect may be further enhanced by dural opening. However, there is still a need for more evidence that this reduction in ICP leads directly to improved clinical outcomes.

Evidence for improved perfusion

In a small observational study, Yamakami and Yamaura used single photon emission CT (SPECT) to show improved perfusion in five patients undergoing unilateral DC [34]. They did not, however, present data on non-craniectomized patients, who reportedly do not experience perfusion improvements **(III/B)**.

Extent of decompression

In a prospective RCT, Jiang *et al* studied the effect of standard (12x15cm unilateral frontotemporoparietal bone flap) versus limited decompression (6x8cm temporoparietal bone flap) in 486 patients with sTBI and refractory intracranial hypertension treated at five Chinese medical centers [35]. Favorable outcomes were achieved by 40% of patients who received the larger craniectomy compared with 29% in the limited-craniectomy group. Mortality was 35% (86/245) in the limited-craniectomy group and 26% (63/241) with larger decompression (p<0.05), thus supporting the use of larger craniectomy for more effective decompression **(Ib/A)**.

Does timing of decompression matter?

There is growing evidence supporting early decompression **(III/B)**. In the study by Polin *et al*, only patients operated on in the first 48 hours were found to receive any benefit from bifrontal DC [4]. Münch *et al* showed improved outcomes with early decompression in a retrospective study of 49 TBI patients [36]. Patients undergoing surgery at a mean of 4.5 hours post-trauma showed a mean±SD decrease in midline shift of 4.8±6.0mm (p=0.0001) compared with 0.4±6.3mm (p=0.4) in those having surgery at a mean of 56 hours post-trauma. Patients who underwent rapid decompression had significantly better outcomes, with a mean±SD GOS score of 3.1±1.9 versus 1.9±1.6 for delayed decompression (p=0.046). While these results support the use of early decompression, they do not support the use of DC as a prophylactic treatment for TBI.

Ongoing trials

An ongoing trial is seeking to address the lack of level I data regarding the use of DC in patients with TBI. The Randomised Evaluation of Surgery with Craniectomy for Uncontrollable Elevation of Intra-Cranial Pressure (RESCUEicp) trial is an ongoing European multicenter prospective RCT that to date has enrolled 235 of a target 600 patients [37]. Ventilated head trauma patients age 10-65 years who require ICP monitoring are eligible for the study. Patients in whom a first stage of medical management (ventilation, sedation, paralysis, elevation of head of bed, analgesia) fails are advanced to the second stage (mannitol, inotropes to keep CPP >60mmHg, hypertonic saline, cooling to 35-36°C, diuretics,

extraventricular drainage) if elevated ICP persists. Those in whom this second stage fails are randomized to continued medical management plus barbiturates (target n=300) or DC (target n=300), to be performed within 4-6 hours of randomization. Surgery is either unilateral or bilateral, depending on intracranial swelling pattern. Patients initially randomized to non-operative management can later be surgically decompressed if the patient's prognosis is felt to be compromised, such as in the setting of further deterioration. The main outcomes are GOS score at discharge and at 6 months; secondary measures include scores on the Short Form-36 questionnaire, ICP, time in intensive care, time to discharge, and health economic analyses.

Conclusions

As the field of neurotrauma awaits completion of ongoing prospective RCTs and high-quality cohort studies, the practicing neurosurgeon is left with lesser-quality data to make decisions about the use of DC. Although the field lacks grade A evidence, a great deal of grade B and C evidence can be brought to bear on clinical decision-making. Based on these data, decompressive surgery is effective in reducing ICP in many patients **(III/B)**. It also appears to be more beneficial when used earlier in the course of treatment in patients refractory to medical management **(III/B)**. Current surgical guidelines recommend DC for patients with parenchymal lesions causing progressive neurologic deterioration, contusions of greater than 20cm^3 with midline shift of 5mm or more, and effacement of basal cisterns [36] **(IV/C)**. As with most treatments for TBI, patients with a poor neurologic examination and advanced age do worse. However, the patient-specific factors that account for the improved outcome of TBI patients in many of these studies remain poorly defined. Clearly, there is a subset of TBI patients who benefit from DC. It is anticipated that ongoing efforts to improve the classification of TBI for targeted treatments will identify the patient groups most likely to benefit from DC.

Recommendations	Evidence level
◆ Pediatric patients with severe head injury are likely to benefit from DC.	Ib/A
◆ Early bifrontal craniectomy for diffuse brain swelling after TBI should not be considered before maximal medical management and external ventrical drainage therapies have failed.	Ib/A
◆ DC lowers ICP. Dural opening further enhances the ICP reduction.	III/B
◆ Younger age is correlated with improved outcomes following DC.	III/B
◆ Poor predictors of outcome following DC include low initial GCS score, older age, asymmetric pupil reactivity, increased midline shift, obliteration of basal cisterns, and the presence of clotting disorders.	III/B
◆ Early decompression gives a greater likelihood of good outcomes.	III/B
◆ Patients with a post-resuscitation GCS score of 3 are not good surgical candidates.	III/B
◆ When DC is performed, a larger extent of decompression is associated with improved outcomes.	Ib/A

References

1. Faul M, Xu L, Wald M, Coronado V. Traumatic Brain Injury in the United States: Emergency Department Visits, Hospitalizations, and Deaths. Atlanta: Centers for Disease Control and Prevention, National Center for Injury Prevention and Control, 2010.

2. Thurman DJ, Alverson C, Dunn KA, Guerrero J, Sniezek JE. Traumatic brain injury in the United States: a public health perspective. *J Head Trauma Rehabil* 1999; 14: 602-15.

3. Cooper DJ, Rosenfeld JV, Murray L, *et al*. Early decompressive craniectomy for patients with severe traumatic brain injury and refractory intracranial hypertension - a pilot randomized trial. *J Crit Care* 2008; 23: 387-93.

4. Polin RS, Shaffrey ME, Bogaev CA, *et al*. Decompressive bifrontal craniectomy in the treatment of severe refractory posttraumatic cerebral edema. *Neurosurgery* 1997; 41: 84-92.

5. Taylor A, Butt W, Rosenfeld J, *et al*. A randomized trial of very early decompressive craniectomy in children with traumatic brain injury and sustained intracranial hypertension. *Childs Nerv Syst* 2001; 17: 154-62.

6. Monro A. *Observations on the Structure and Function of the Nervous System*. Edinburgh: Creech and Johnson, 1823; 5.

7. Kellie G. An account of the appearances observed in the dissection of two of the three individuals presumed to have perished in the storm of the 3rd, and whose bodies were discovered in the vicinity of Leith on the morning of the 4th November 1821 with some reflecti. *Transactions of the Medico-chirurgical Society of Edinburgh* 1824: 1: 84-169.

8. Mokri B. The Monro-Kellie hypothesis: applications in CSF volume depletion. *Neurology* 2001; 56: 1746-8.

9. Valadka AB, Robertson CS. Surgery of cerebral trauma and associated critical care. *Neurosurgery* 2007; 61(1 Suppl.): 203-20; discussion 220-1.

10. Kocher T. Die Therapie des Hirndruckes. In: *Hirnerschütterung, Hirndruck und chirurgische Eingriffe bei Hirnkrankheiten*. Hölder A, Ed. Vienna: A. Hölder, 1901; 262-6.

11. Gennarelli TA, Spielman GM, Langfitt TW, *et al*. Influence of the type of intracranial lesion on outcome from severe head injury. *J Neurosurg* 1982; 56: 26-32.

12 Marshall L, Marshall S, Klauber M, *et al*. A new classification of head injury based on computerized tomography. *J Neurosurg* Suppl 1991; 75: S14-20.

13. Sahuquillo J, Arikan F. Decompressive craniectomy for the treatment of refractory high intracranial pressure in traumatic brain injury. *Cochrane Database Syst Rev* 2006; 1: CD003983.

14. Cooper DJ, Rosenfeld JV, Murray L, *et al*. Decompressive craniectomy in diffuse traumatic brain injury. *N Engl J Med* 2011; 364(16): 1493-502.

15. Steyerberg EW, Mushkudiani N, Perel P, *et al*. Predicting outcome after traumatic brain injury: development and international validation of prognostic scores based on admission characteristics. *PLoS Med* 2008; 5(8): e165.

16. Gooch MR, Gin GE, Kenning TJ, German JW. Complications of cranioplasty following decompressive craniectomy: analysis of 62 cases. *Neurosurg Focus* 2009; 26(6): E9.

17. Emergency Medicine Research Center. ProTECT III: Progesterone for Traumatic Brain Injury: Experimental Clinical Treatment: Phase III Clinical Trial. Available at: http://em.emory.edu/protect. Accessed 29 January, 2012.

18. Guerra WK, Gaab MR, Dietz H, *et al*. Surgical decompression for traumatic brain swelling: indications and results. *J Neurosurg* 1999; 90: 187-96.

19. Gower DJ, Lee KS, McWhorter JM. Role of subtemporal decompression in severe closed head injury. *Neurosurgery* 1988; 23: 417-22.

20. Albanèse J, Leone M, Alliez J, *et al*. Decompressive craniectomy for severe traumatic brain injury: evaluation of the effects at one year. *Crit Care Med* 2003; 31: 2535-8.

21. Ucar T, Akyuz M, Kazan S, Tuncer R. Role of decompressive surgery in the management of severe head injuries: prognostic factors and patient selection. *J Neurotrauma* 2005; 22: 1311-8.

22. Coplin WM, Cullen NK, Policherla PN, *et al*. Safety and feasibility of craniectomy with duraplasty as the initial surgical intervention for severe traumatic brain injury. *J Trauma* 2001; 50: 1050-9.

23. Kunze E, Meixensberger J, Janka M, Sörensen N, Roosen K. Decompressive craniectomy in patients with uncontrollable intracranial hypertension. *Acta Neurochir* Suppl 1998; 71: 16-8.

24. Lemcke J, Ahmadi S, Meier U. Outcome of patients with severe head injury after decompressive craniectomy. *Acta Neurochir* Suppl 2010; 106: 231-3.

25. Lee EJ, Chio CC, Chen HH. Aggressive temporal lobectomy for uncal herniation in traumatic subdural hematoma. *J Formos Med Assoc* 1995; 94: 341-5.

26. Nussbaum ES, Wolf AL, Sebring L, Mirvis S. Complete temporal lobectomy for surgical resuscitation of patients with transtentorial herniation secondary to unilateral hemispheric swelling. *Neurosurgery* 1991; 29: 62-6.

27. Aarabi B, Hesdorffer DC, Ahn ES, *et al*. Outcome following decompressive craniectomy for malignant swelling due to severe head injury. *J Neurosurg* 2006; 104: 469-79.

28. Howard JL, Cipolle MD, Anderson M, *et al*. Outcome after decompressive craniectomy for the treatment of severe traumatic brain injury. *J Trauma* 2008; 65: 380-5.

29. Olivecrona M, Rodling-Wahlström M, Naredi S, Koskinen LD. Effective ICP reduction by decompressive craniectomy in patients with severe traumatic brain injury treated by an ICP-targeted therapy. *J Neurotrauma* 2007; 24: 927-35.

30. Timofeev I, Czosnyka M, Nortje J, *et al*. Effect of decompressive craniectomy on intracranial pressure and cerebrospinal compensation following traumatic brain injury. *J Neurosurg* 2008; 108: 66-73.

31. Skoglund TS, Eriksson-Ritzén C, Jensen C, Rydenhag B. Aspects on decompressive craniectomy in patients with traumatic head injuries. *J Neurotrauma* 2006; 23: 1502-9.

32. Whitfield PC, Patel H, Hutchinson PJ, *et al*. Bifrontal decompressive craniectomy in the management of posttraumatic intracranial hypertension. *Br J Neurosurg* 2001; 15: 500-7.

33. Yoo DS, Kim DS, Cho KS, *et al*. Ventricular pressure monitoring during bilateral decompression with dural expansion. *J Neurosurg* 1999; 91: 953-9.

34. Yamakami I, Yamaura A. Effects of decompressive craniectomy on regional cerebral blood flow in severe head trauma patients. *Neurol Med Chir* 1993; 33: 616-20.

35. Jiang J, Xu W, Li W, *et al*. Efficacy of standard trauma craniectomy for refractory intracranial hypertension with severe traumatic brain injury: a multicenter, prospective, randomized controlled study. *J Neurotrauma* 2005; 22: 623-8.

36. Münch E, Horn P, Schürer L, *et al*. Management of severe traumatic brain injury by decompressive craniectomy. *Neurosurgery* 2000; 47: 315-22.

37. Hutchinson P, Kirkpatrick P. The RESCUEicp Study. Available at: www.rescueicp.com. Accessed January 29, 2012.

Chapter 34

Chapter 34

Chapter 35

Timing of surgery for spinal cord injury

David W Cadotte MSc MD, Neurosurgery Resident
Julio C Furlan MD MBA MSc PhD, Neurology Resident
Michael G Fehlings MD PhD FRCSC FACS, Professor of Neurosurgery

DIVISION OF NEUROSURGERY, UNIVERSITY OF TORONTO, TORONTO, ONTARIO, CANADA

Introduction

Over the course of the last several decades a number of important discoveries have been made with regard to the pathophysiology of traumatic spinal cord injury (SCI). Perhaps the largest paradigm shift in how clinicians think about SCI has related to primary versus secondary injury. Primary injury can be defined as damage to neural tissue as a result of the mechanical forces of the traumatic event, whether a motor-vehicle accident, diving accident, or otherwise. These forces can result in compression, distraction, laceration, or shear stress that directly damages the extremely fragile neural tissue. Unfortunately, little can be done outside the realm of prevention to minimize the sequelae of these events.

Secondary injury can be defined as the body's response to primary injury. More specifically, secondary injury is a combination of molecular and cellular events that occur in the hours, days, and weeks following the primary injury. The exact mechanisms and cellular cascades that occur during the secondary stage of SCI have been the focus of intense research during the past several decades – and researchers are continuing to learn a great deal.

Edema, inflammation, ischemia, and free-radical-mediated damage constitute the end results of a complex array of cellular cascades. The focus of treatment strategies for SCI has been on minimizing the deleterious effects of secondary injury and providing the spinal cord with the optimal environment for recovery. A number of such translational strategies have either made their way into clinical practice or are the subject of ongoing clinical trials to determine their safety, efficacy, and ability to provide tangible benefits to patients who find themselves suffering from neurologic deficit.

Surgical decompression is a non-pharmacologic therapy that aims to reduce the neurologic deficit occurring as a result of secondary damage. The underlying theory for this therapeutic modality rests in the notion that ongoing compressive forces contribute to secondary damage. It is important to consider the fact that there may be several indications for surgery following traumatic SCI. First and foremost is spinal instability caused by torn ligaments and bony fracture. There is little controversy over the need for surgical stabilization in this setting. The other, and the focus of this evidence-based review, is surgical decompression that aims to improve neurologic outcomes without a strong indication for the treatment of spinal column instability. As mentioned above, physical compression of the spinal cord triggers an ongoing series of deleterious cascades, and surgical decompression aims to relieve this compression. An extension of the question of whether surgical decompression offers benefits is the timing of such decompression. Clearly, decompression of the spinal cord years after the initial injury would be expected to offer little or no benefit. Intuition tells us that early surgical decompression may offer a better chance at neurologic improvement, but the exact timing threshold is unknown. Evidence is mounting for improved outcomes with decompressive surgery and for the timing threshold associated with these outcomes. This chapter presents the current evidence in these areas.

Methodology

Outline of research questions

Given the aforementioned background information, a knowledge gap is identified that has been addressed by a number of preclinical and clinical research studies. These studies have focused on many different aspects of surgical treatment for SCI, and their results have varied. The aim was to systematically integrate this information. Two questions were framed:

- Do preclinical studies confirm the biological basis for surgical decompression after SCI?
- What are the neurologic and functional outcomes following early surgical decompression in the clinical setting?

Literature search strategy

The primary literature search was carried out using the Medline, Cinahl, Embase, and Cochrane databases. A secondary search strategy incorporated articles referred to in meta-analyses and systematic and non-systematic reviews that were identified in the primary search strategy. We selected all original articles that examined the potential effects of duration of compression or the timing of surgical

decompression of the spinal cord on outcomes in the setting of traumatic SCI. Case reports, editorials, and meeting abstracts were excluded.

The literature searches addressed publications from 1966 to April 2009. The search strategy included the following specific words or phrases: 'surgical decompression,' 'decompression,' 'spinal cord compression,' 'time,' and 'timing.' Those specific key words were paired with the following medical subject headings: 'spinal cord injury,' 'SCI,' 'tetraplegia,' 'quadriplegia,' and 'paraplegia.' The literature search was limited to English-language papers only. The search results were divided into preclinical studies (animal SCI models) and clinical studies.

Data abstraction and synthesis

Articles were selected that fulfilled the inclusion and exclusion criteria. Disagreements were resolved by debate and consensus. A research assistant extracted the relevant data from each selected article. Subsequently, all clinical studies were examined with regard to the extracted data to determine the level of evidence according to Sackett et al [1]. In addition, the methodologic quality of each article was assessed using the criteria of Downs and Black [2]. Divergences during these steps were resolved by consensus.

Results

Overview of preclinical studies

A total of 198 abstracts were captured in the original search. Of these, 19 experimental studies using different animal SCI models fulfilled the inclusion and exclusion criteria [3-21]. In brief, the preclinical studies developed spinal cord compression or contusion models in dogs (eight studies), rats (six studies), cats (three studies), or monkeys (two studies). Outcome measures included electrophysiologic testing (12 studies), behavioral tests (11 studies), histopathological examination of spinal cord tissue (seven studies), spinal cord blood flow assessment (four studies), and spinal cord concentration of energy-related metabolites (one study).

Overview of clinical studies

The primary search of clinical studies yielded 153 abstracts, from which three review papers were used for the secondary search. A total of 22 clinical studies fulfilled the inclusion and exclusion criteria [22-43]. Most of the clinical studies compared at least two patient groups who underwent early or later decompressive surgery of the spinal cord (20 studies), whereas two studies examined only the feasibility and safety of early surgical decompression of the spinal cord without group comparisons [22, 23]. While the vast majority of the clinical studies provided level III evidence, two provided level IIb evidence. The scores for methodologic quality varied from 7 to 25, with a mean value of 12.41 and a median of 11.5.

Preclinical animal models

Most of the preclinical animal model studies stated that either the degree of compression (i.e., the amount of weight applied during a compression study) or the length of time the spinal cord was compressed directly correlated to the degree of recovery. Keeping in mind that these are animal experiments conducted under ideal circumstances, we review the preclinical literature with regard to the timing of decompression following traumatic SCI in three domains:

- Histopathological correlation between the injury model and the damage caused to the spinal tissue.
- Animal models that did not show a functional benefit of early decompression.

Table 1. Preclinical animal studies examining the electrophysiologic or histologic consequences of spinal cord compression with a fixed duration of time.

Reference	Species (n)	Injury model	Timing of decompression	Study conclusions
Brodkey et al, 1972 [3]	Cats (5)	Weight was applied over the dorsal surface of the spinal cord and intact dura	Time since SCC and/or aortic clamping to CEP effects	Direct pressure to the spinal cord and hypotension result in additive deficits, as recorded by CEP
Kobrine et al, 1978 [5]	Macaque monkeys (10)	SCC (right, lateral) using a Fogarty catheter in the epidural space	1 hour	Mechanical forces of compression, rather than ischemia, are mainly responsible for the loss of neural conduction in such a model
Bohlman et al, 1979 [4]	Dogs (14)	Compression model: transducer Contusion model: Allen weight-drop device	4-8 weeks until neurologic recovery ceased to improve	Of the eight pressure-induced SCIs that recovered, microscopic examination was normal in two, central gray necrosis occurred in two, peripheral demyelinization in two, and lacerations in three Pathological findings associated with significant paralysis: mild anterior horn gray matter necrosis in two, laceration of the ventral white and gray matter in three, and no microscopic evidence of cord damage in one The CEP response closely paralleled the degree of initial SCI either from contusion or compression, as well as the neurologic recovery of the animals

CEP = cortical evoked potential; SCC = spinal cord compression; SCI = spinal cord injury

Table 2. Animal studies that demonstrated no benefit from early decompression following spinal cord injury. *Continued overleaf.*

Reference	Species (n)	Injury model	Timing of decompression	Study conclusions
Croft *et al*, 1972 [6]	Cats (15)	Weight was applied over the dorsal surface of the spinal cord and intact dura	Graded weight (18-58g) and graded time (5-20 minutes)	Graded pressure (38g for 5-20 minutes and 58g for 20 minutes) on the spinal cord produced reversible blocking of SSEPs
Thienprasit *et al*, 1975 [7]	Cats (28)	A no. 3 French Fogarty catheter was passed through an L2 laminectomy extradurally in the cephalic direction for 6cm, inflated with 0.6-0.9cc of air, and immediately deflated	No treatment vs. laminectomy at 6 hours after SCI vs. laminectomy at 6 hours after SCI + cooling of spinal cord for 2 hours	In more severely injured animals (based on return of CEP response), surgical decompression and cooling offered improved outcomes
Aki and Toya, 1984 [8]	Dogs (33)	SCC: weight placement	30 or 60 minutes	With increasing compressive weights (6-60g), SEP amplitudes were progressively more reduced and latencies more prolonged. Following release of compression, amplitudes and latencies recovered at the lower weights, but were more likely to reflect greater conduction deficits with progressively greater weights. Pathologic findings: hemorrhage and necrosis were not found in the gray and white matter in the groups weighted with 6 and 16g, whereas small petechial hemorrhages and tissue necrosis were observed in the center of the gray matter in the groups weighted with 36 and 60g. There were no distinct findings in the white matter with higher weights
Delamarter *et al*, 1991 [9]	Dogs (30)	Circumferential constriction of the cauda equina with a nylon electrical cable	2-3 seconds, 1, 6, and 24 hours, and 1 week	All 30 dogs developed caudal equina syndrome after constriction and all recovered significant motor function 6 weeks after decompression (recovered to walking [Tarlov grade 5] with bladder and tail control at 6 weeks after SCI). Immediately after compression, all five groups demonstrated >50% deterioration of the posterior tibial nerve SSEP amplitudes. At 6 weeks after decompression, all five groups had a mean amplitude recovery of 20-30%. There was no difference in recovery of SSEPs among the groups. All groups demonstrated scattered Wallerian degeneration and axonal regeneration. There were no significant differences in the histologic findings among the groups

Table 2. Animal studies that demonstrated no benefit from early decompression following spinal cord injury. *Continued.*

Reference	Species (n)	Injury model	Timing of decompression	Study conclusions
Hejcl *et al*, 2008 [10]	Rats (23)	Spinal cord transection	HEMA-MOETACl hydrogel was inserted immediately (acute group) or 1 week (delayed group) after SCI	There was no significant difference in the spinal cord between the acute and delayed implantation groups on histopathological examination There were no significant differences between the two treatment groups with regard to BBB scores

BBB = Basso, Beattie, and Bresnahan; CEP = cortical evoked potential; SCC = spinal cord compression; SCI = spinal cord injury; SEP = spinal evoked potential; SSEP = somatosensory evoked potential

♦ Animal models that did show a functional benefit of early decompression.

Histopathological correlation

Three studies examined either the electrophysiologic or histologic consequences of spinal cord compression with a fixed duration of time (Table 1) [3-5]. The collective results of these early investigations into SCI suggest that direct pressure to the spinal cord, probably resulting in direct damage to the neural cell membranes, combined with hypotension and resultant ischemia, results in loss of neurologic function. Animals that showed recovery following injury demonstrated either a normal spinal cord under microscopic examination or evidence of central gray necrosis, peripheral demyelinization, or laceration. Animals that failed to recover had more pronounced evidence of damage to the neuroanatomic circuits of the spinal cord at the level of the anterior horn cells or laceration of either the gray or white matter.

No benefit from early decompression

Five studies failed to demonstrate a benefit of early decompression following SCI. This generalized conclusion is closely linked to the experimental design of each of these studies (Table 2). Of those that compared time of compression with outcome [6-8], the maximum time of compression was 2 hours. Croft *et al* found that with a graded pressure and time up to a maximum of 58g for 20 minutes, the electrophysiologic changes observed (somatosensory evoked potentials) were completely reversible [6]. The weakness of this investigation was that no statistical analysis was carried out. Thienprasit *et al* subjected a group of cats to a compression model of SCI and then stratified the animals into those that demonstrated electrophysiologic recovery within 6 hours and those that did not [7]. Each group was then randomized to receive no treatment, decompression, or decompression plus hypothermia. Of the animals that showed electrophysiologic recovery, there was no difference in behavioral recovery between the control group and the groups that received decompression or decompression plus cooling. Of the animals that showed no electrophysiologic recovery, there was no difference between the control group and the group that received early decompression; however, animals in the early decompression plus cooling group did show better behavioral outcomes, suggesting a possible neuroprotective role for hypothermia after SCI. Aki and Toya, using a dog model, showed that compression for either 30 or 60 minutes resulted in similar electrophysiologic and histologic outcomes [8].

Of the remaining two studies that failed to demonstrate a correlation between time of compression and outcome, the first attempted to model cauda equina injury [9] and the second studied a novel hydrogel [10], with the hypothesis that this agent would act as a scaffold

Table 3. Animal studies that demonstrated a benefit from early decompression following spinal cord injury. *Continued overleaf.*

Chapter 35

Reference	Species (n)	Injury model	Timing of decompression	Study conclusions
Kobrine *et al*, 1979 [11]	Macaque monkeys (18)	SCC (right, lateral) using a Fogarty catheter in the epidural space	1, 3, 5, 7, or 15 minutes	Data suggested that the cause of neural dysfunction after balloon compression is physical injury of the neural membrane, irrespective of blood flow changes. Recovery is related to length of time of compression
Dolan *et al*, 1980 [12]	Rats (91)	Spinal cord clip compression	3, 30, 60, 300, or 900 seconds (15 minutes)	Functional recovery decreased as the duration and force of compression increased
Guha *et al*, 1987 [13]	Rats (75)	Spinal cord clip compression	15, 60, 120, or 240 minutes	The major determinant of recovery was the intensity of compression applied to the spinal cord. The time until decompression also affected recovery, but only for the lighter compression forces (2.3 and 16.9g)
Nystrom and Berglund, 1988 [14]	Rats (81)	SCC: weight placement	1, 5, and 10 minutes	Both the amount of weight and the duration of placement affected the animals' ability to recover – a heavier weight and longer duration of placement were associated with less recovery
Zhang *et al*, 1993 [15]	Rats (not disclosed)	SCC: graded weight compression	5 minutes of compression with varied weight Group 1: no compression, control Group 2: 9g weight Group 3: 35g weight Group 4: 50g weight	In groups 2 and 3, lactate levels increased to six to seven times the basal levels in the first fraction. Group 2 levels normalized within about 30 minutes, while group 3 levels were slower in recovering Group 4 lactate levels increased 10-fold in the second fraction. Only partial recovery was seen in the 2-hour period No significant change in pyruvate levels was seen in any of the groups Inosine levels rose by 0.7-0.9μM in groups 2 and 3, and by 1.4μM in group 4 Inosine recovery was faster than lactate recovery, with group 4 recovering completely in about 40 minutes Recovery of hypoxanthine was slower compared with other metabolites. Complete recovery took almost 80 minutes
Delamarter *et al*, 1995 [16]	Dogs (30)	Circumferential constriction of the caudal spinal cord with a nylon electrical cable to 50% of the diameter of the spinal canal	2-3 seconds, 1, 6, and 24 hours, and 1 week	The dogs with immediate decompression generally recovered neurologic function within 2-5 days. Animals that were compressed for ≥6 hours showed no significant motor recovery after decompression of the spinal cord Discrete areas of Wallerian degeneration and demyelination were seen in the spinal cords of animals decompressed either immediately or at 1 hour. In contrast, there was severe central necrosis in the spinal cords of animals decompressed at ≥6 hours
Carlson *et al*, 1997 [17]	Dogs (12)	SCC: hydraulic loading piston	5 minutes, 3 hours	Regional spinal cord blood flow was reduced at the site of piston compression. In the sustained-compression group, no recovery of SSEP occurred and blood flow remained significantly lower than baseline at 30 and 180 minutes after maximum compression Spinal cord decompression was associated with early recovery of blood flow and SSEP recovery. By 3 hours, blood flow was similar in both the compressed and decompressed groups, even though SSEP recovery occurred only in the decompressed group

Table 3. Animal studies that demonstrated a benefit from early decompression following spinal cord injury. *Continued.*

Reference	Species (n)	Injury model	Timing of decompression	Study conclusions
Carlson *et al*, 1997 [18]	Dogs (21)	Cord compression	Spinal cord displacement was maintained for 30 (n=7), 60 (n=8), or 180 minutes (n=6) after lower-extremity SSEP amplitudes were reduced by 50% of baseline	SEP recovery was seen in 6/7 dogs in the 30-minute group, 5/8 dogs in the 60-minute group, and 0/6 of dogs in the 180-minute compression group Regional spinal cord blood flow at baseline decreased after stopping dynamic compression. Reperfusion flows after decompression were inversely related to the duration of compression Reperfusion flows, measured as the interval change in blood flow between the time dynamic compression was stopped to 5, 15, or 180 minutes after decompression, were significantly greater in dogs that recovered SEP (p<0.05) Spinal cord decompression within 1 hour of SEP loss resulted in significant electrophysiological recovery after 3 hours of monitoring
Dimar *et al*, 1999 [19]	Rats (42)	Contusion injury: impactor	0, 2, 6, 24, and 72 hours	Progressively more severe central and dorsal cavitation were seen as the time of SCC increased Midsagittal sections demonstrated progressive cephalad and caudal cord necrosis and cavitation, which worsened with the duration of compression. These changes were most severe in the 24- and 72-hour specimens
Carlson *et al*, 2003 [20]	Dogs (16)	SCC: hydraulic piston	Spinal cord displacement was maintained for 30 (n=8) or 180 minutes (n=8) after SSEP amplitudes were reduced by 50% of baseline	A shorter time of compression was associated with better neurologic function at both early and late time points Lesion volumes, as assessed with MRI, were smaller in the 30-minute vs. the 180-minute compression group (p=0.04) The 30-minute compression group showed smaller lesion volume (p<0.001) and a greater percentage of residual white matter (p=0.005) compared with the 180-minute compression group
Rabinowitz *et al*, 2008 [21]	Dogs (18)	Circumferential constriction of the thoracolumbar junction with a nylon electrical cable	Group 1: decompression at 6 hours + methylprednisolone Group 2: decompression at 6 hours + sham Group 3: methylprednisolone only	Decompression within 6 hours (groups 1 and 2) was associated with significant neurologic improvement when compared with no decompression (group 3) Methylprednisolone did not significantly affect outcomes There was no statistical difference in the percentage of cord involvement histologically between the three groups; group 3 showed greater involvement below the level of the lesion

SCC = spinal cord compression; SEP = spinal evoked potential; SSEP = somatosensory evoked potential

for neural repair following transection. Neither demonstrated an effect of early treatment.

Benefit from early decompression

The number of animal studies that have shown benefit from early decompression far outweighs those that have not (Table 3). Using a primate model of SCI, Kobrine *et al* showed that the duration of compression correlated to the neurologic outcome of these animals, and that physical injury to the neuronal membrane could account for a lack of recovery [11]. In a rat model that used five times as many animal subjects, Dolan *et al* showed that the degree of functional recovery was directly proportional to the duration and force of compression, with greater recovery observed with lower forces and less time of compression [12]. Guha et al further delineated this observation using a rat model and concluded that the major determinant of recovery was the intensity of compression and that the time of compression was important only with lighter compressive forces [13]. These results were echoed by a similar study conducted 1 year later [14]. Zhang et al expanded on this notion by measuring concentrations of energy-related metabolites in the spinal cord after injury [15]. They concluded that animals subjected to a larger compressive force showed higher concentrations of lactate and inosine in the extracellular compartment of the spinal cord and that these higher concentrations were associated with less neurologic recovery. Delamarter et al used a canine model to show that compression of the cauda equina for 6 hours or longer resulted in a lack of significant motor recovery despite decompression [16]. This lack of recovery was associated with central necrosis of the spinal cord.

In a set of two experiments using a canine model of SCI, Carlson et al demonstrated that the duration of compression could be correlated to electrophysiology recordings and spinal cord blood flow, with a shorter duration of compression associated with return of blood flow and recovery of somatosensory evoked potential [17, 18]. Dimar et al added that a longer duration of compression was associated with an extension of the injury in a cephalad and caudal direction, resulting in more pronounced cavitation and necrosis of the spinal cord [19]. As technology improved, Carlson et al made use of MRI to further our knowledge with regard to lesion volumes relative to the time of spinal compression [20]. They demonstrated a significant difference in MRI-based lesion volumes between 30- and 180-minute compression groups. Perhaps the most hypothesis-driven study of recent times was carried out by Rabinowitz et al, who compared not only the timing of decompression but also the use of methylprednisolone [21]. Using a randomized design in a canine model, the authors demonstrated that surgical decompression with or without methylprednisolone administration offered greater neurologic improvement than methylprednisolone alone. This is an important study that made a head-to-

head comparison of two therapies at the forefront of human treatment. The authors rightfully commented on the value of such a trial.

In summary, this collection of animal studies demonstrates a significant body of evidence, across many species, that both the initial force and the duration of compression are related to the degree of neurologic improvement.

Clinical trials: strength of evidence

Level I

No level I evidence exists to guide clinicians with regard to the timing of surgical decompression following SCI.

Level II

We identified two level II studies (Table 4) [24, 26]. Vaccaro et al studied 62 patients who presented with an SCI between C3 and T1 [24]. They defined early surgery as treatment within 72 hours and late surgery as treatment after 5 days. The authors found no difference between the groups with regard to length of stay (LOS) in the intensive care unit (ICU) or inpatient rehabilitation, or in American Spinal Injury Association (ASIA) motor scores **(IIb/B)**.

In contrast, Cengiz et al studied 27 patients who sustained a traumatic SCI from T8 to L2 [26]. They defined early and late surgery as occurring within 8 hours of injury and late surgery as occurring 3-15 days after injury. There were several differences between the groups at follow-up. The early surgery group demonstrated greater improvements on the ASIA impairment scale, no complications in hospital, and a shorter hospital and ICU LOSs **(IIb/B)**. Four patients in the later surgery group experienced complications: three cases of lung failure and one case of sepsis. The authors concluded that there are statistically significant differences between patients treated early and those treated late, both with regard to neurologic improvement and overall morbidity. There were no mortalities in either group.

Table 4. Level IIb studies of the timing of surgical decompression following spinal cord injury.

Reference	Study population	Timing of intervention	Study conclusions	Quality assessment[a]
Vaccaro *et al*, 1997 [24]	n=62 Level of injury: C3-T1 **Early surgery group, n=34** Mean age: 39.79 years 24 males, 10 females **Late surgery group, n=28** Mean age: 39 years 22 males, 6 females	Early: ≤72 hours Late: >5 days	No significant differences were seen in LOS in the acute postoperative ICU, length of inpatient rehabilitation, or improvement in AIS or ASIA motor score between the early vs. late surgery groups (no p values reported)	12
Cengiz *et al*, 2008 [26]	n=27 Level of injury: T8-L2 Mean age: 41.4 years (range 23-68 years) 18 males, 9 females **Early surgery group, n=12** Mean age: 39.7 years 8 males, 4 females **Late surgery group, n=15** Mean age: 41.4 years 10 males, 5 females	Early: ≤8 hours Late: 3-15 days	The groups were comparable regarding AIS and type of fracture AIS significantly increased from before to after surgery in the early (p=0.004) and late (p=0.046) surgery groups, but the postoperative AIS of the early group was better than that of the late group (p<0.011) 83.3% of individuals in the early surgery group vs. 26.6% in the late surgery group showed improvement in the AIS No patients in the early surgery group experienced complications, vs. three cases of lung failure and one of sepsis in the late surgery group. There were no deaths in either group The early surgery group had significantly shorter hospital (p<0.001) and ICU (p=0.005) LOS than the late surgery group	25

[a] = assessed using the criteria of Downs and Black [2]. AIS = ASIS impairment scale; ASIA = American Spinal Injury Association; ICU = intensive care unit; LOS = length of stay

Level III

Most clinical studies that have attempted to address the question of timing of decompression following traumatic SCI represent level III evidence. The following sections provide an overview of investigations that outline the following:

* Hospital LOS.
* Medical complications following SCI.
* Neurologic outcomes.

Length of hospital stay

When attempting to study the effect of early surgery on SCI, a relatively easy metric to follow is the length of time a patient spends in the ICU or inpatient unit. This measurement considers not only the severity of the injury, but also the accessibility of the medical system in terms of stabilizing the patient and allowing him or her to proceed with rehabilitation. Of the 22 clinical studies identified in this review, nine level III studies measured LOS (Table 5) [27-35]. Early surgical

Chapter 35

Table 5. Level III studies of the timing of surgical decompression following spinal cord injury: length of hospital stay.

Reference	Study population	Timing of intervention	Mean length of stay (days)		p-value	Quality assessment[a]
			Early surgery	Late surgery		
Levi et al, 1991 [35]	n=103 Cervical SCI	Early surgery: ≤24 hours Delayed surgery: >24 hours	38.7	45.2	<0.05	10
Campagnolo et al, 1997 [27]	n=64 All levels SCI	Early spinal stabilization: ≤24 hours Late spinal stabilization: >24 hours	37.5	54.7	0.01	12
Mirza et al, 1999 [28]	n=30 C2-C7 injury	Early surgery: ≤72 hours Late surgery: >72 hours	21.9	36.8	0.04	10
Croce et al, 2001 [29]	n=291 All levels SCI	Early surgical fixation: ≤3 days Late surgical fixation: >3 days	19.3 9.9[b]	28.0 15.9[b]	0.001[a]	14
Chipman et al, 2004 [31]	n=146 Thoracolumbar spinal column injury	Early surgery: <72 hours Late surgery: >72 hours	ISS <15: 8.1 ISS <15: 2.9[b] ISS ≥15: 11.5 ISS ≥15: 4.1[b]	ISS <15: 15.5 ISS <15: 4.7[b] ISS ≥15: 20.7 ISS ≥15: 10.5[b]	<0.001 NS[b] <0.001 0.003[b]	15
McKinley et al, 2004 [32]	n=779 All levels SCI	Early surgery: ≤72 hours Late surgery: >72 hours	-	-	<0.01	18
Kerwin et al, 2005 [33]	n=299 All levels SCI	Early surgery: ≤3 days Late surgery: >3 days	14.3 7.2[b]	21.1 7.9[b]	0.0005 NS[b]	12
Schinkel et al, 2006 [34]	n=298 Thoracic spine injuries	Early surgery: ≤72 hours Late surgery: >72 hours	22 (median) 8 (median)[b]	31 (median) 16 (median)[b]	0.048 0.001[b]	12

[a] = ICU and hospital LOS; [b] = ICU LOS; ICU = intensive care unit; ISS = Injury Severity Score; LOS = length of stay; NR = not reported; NS = not significant

decompression offered a statistically significant shorter hospital LOS in all nine studies (although Guest et al reported no p values [30]), and shorter ICU LOS in one study [34] **(III/B)**. A subset of studies further subdivided overall LOS into duration of stay in the ICU, and found that this time point was also shorter in patients receiving early decompressive surgery [29-31, 33] **(III/B)**. Only one study that measured these values found no correlation between the timing of surgical decompression and ICU LOS [33] **(III/B)**. An obvious extension of this metric is the rate at which patients are readmitted to hospital. This was measured in only one study, in which there was no difference between the early and late surgical intervention groups [32] **(III/B)**.

Medical complications

The following complications were recorded in eight of the 22 studies: respiratory complications, wound infections, decubitus ulcers, cardiac complications, urinary tract infections, gastrointestinal hemorrhage, deep vein thrombosis (DVT), and death. Four studies showed no difference in the rate of medical complications between early and late surgical groups [27, 35-37] **(III/B)**, whereas four studies showed fewer complications overall in those receiving early surgical decompression [28, 29, 31, 32] **(III/B)**. Specifically, the following results were reported:

- Mirza *et al* reported significantly fewer complications in persons receiving surgery within 72 hours of injury [28] **(III/B)**.
- Croce *et al* reported lower rates of pneumonia and DVT in persons receiving surgery within 24 hours [29] **(III/B)**.
- Chipman *et al* reported a lower frequency of all complications in patients with an Injury Severity Score above 15 receiving surgery within 72 hours of injury (although this same group reported an equal number of medical complications in persons with an Injury Severity Score <15, regardless of the time of decompression) [31] **(III/B)**.
- McKinley *et al* report higher rates of pneumonia in the late surgery group (>72 hours after injury), but equal rates of other complications (i.e., DVT, pulmonary embolism, ulcers) in the early and late groups [32] **(III/B)**.

Neurologic outcomes

Thirteen of 20 studies were powered for and directly reported on the recovery of neurologic function after surgical intervention. The remainder of the studies (seven of the 20 level III studies) were powered to investigate other aspects of acute spine trauma such as time to reach the hospital, feasibility of early surgery, and inpatient complications. Early surgical decompression was associated with better neurologic outcomes in four studies:

- Clohisy *et al* reported that surgical decompression within 48 hours was associated with significant improvements on the modified Frankel Scale [38] **(III/B)**.
- McLain and Benson reported better neurologic improvement (no p value reported) with surgical decompression within 24 hours [36] **(III/B)**.
- Mirza *et al* found that surgery within 72 hours, but not after this time, was associated with significant improvements in the ASIA motor score [28] **(III/B)**.

- Papadopoulos *et al* found that patients who received surgical decompression within 12 hours (±1.3 hours) of injury experienced significantly greater neurologic improvements than those with surgery outside this time window [39] **(III/B)**.

Despite these findings, seven studies with the same level of evidence reported no neurologic benefit to early surgical decompression [29, 30, 32, 35, 40-42] **(III/B)**. Two studies showed equivocal results [37, 43] **(III/B)**.

Conclusions

Do preclinical studies confirm the biological basis for surgical decompression after SCI?

While somewhat limited in their ability to directly answer clinically relevant questions regarding human SCI, animal models provide overwhelming evidence for two aspects of injury pathophysiology: both the degree of spinal cord compression and the timing of that compression have a negative impact on the ability to recover neurologic function.

What are the neurologic and functional outcome effects of early surgical decompression in the clinical setting?

Early surgical decompression following SCI has been demonstrated to be feasible. Early decompression is associated with shorter hospital stays and fewer medical complications than delayed surgery. The evidence for neurologic improvement after early surgical decompression is mixed. While it is unlikely that this treatment strategy alone will result in marked clinical improvements, there is certainly a trend toward better outcomes following early decompression.

Chapter 35

Recommendations	Evidence level
◆ While somewhat limited in their ability to directly answer clinically relevant questions regarding human SCI, animal models provide overwhelming evidence for two aspects of injury pathophysiology: both the degree of spinal cord compression and the duration of compression have a negative impact on the ability to recover neurologic function.	-
◆ Early surgical decompression following SCI is feasible. Early decompression is associated with shorter hospital LOS and fewer medical complications than delayed surgery.	III/B
◆ The evidence for neurologic improvement after early surgical decompression is mixed. While it is unlikely that this treatment strategy alone will result in marked clinical improvement, there is certainly a trend toward better outcomes following early decompression.	IIb/B, III/B

References

1. Sackett DL, Straus SE, Richardson WS, Rosenberg WM, Haynes RB. *Evidence-based Medicine: How to Practice and Teach EBM*. Toronto, ON: Churchill Livingstone, 2000.

2. Downs SH, Black N. The feasibility of creating a checklist for the assessment of the methodological quality both of randomised and non-randomised studies of health care interventions. *J Epidemiol Community Health* 1998; 52: 377-84.

3. Brodkey JS, Richards DE, Blasingame JP, Nulsen FE. Reversible spinal cord trauma in cats. Additive effects of direct pressure and ischemia. *J Neurosurg* 1972; 37: 591-3.

4. Bohlman HH, Bahniuk E, Raskulinecz G, Field G. Mechanical factors affecting recovery from incomplete cervical spinal cord injury: a preliminary report. *Johns Hopkins Med J* 1979; 145: 115-25.

5. Kobrine AI, Evans DE, Rizzoli H. Correlation of spinal cord blood flow and function in experimental compression. *Surg Neurol* 1978; 10: 54-9.

6. Croft TJ, Brodkey JS, Nulsen FE. Reversible spinal cord trauma: a model for electrical monitoring of spinal cord function. *J Neurosurg* 1972; 36: 402-6.

7. Thienprasit P, Bantli H, Bloedel JR, Chou SN. Effect of delayed local cooling on experimental spinal cord injury. *J Neurosurg* 1975; 42: 150-4.

8. Aki T, Toya S. Experimental study on changes of the spinal-evoked potential and circulatory dynamics following spinal cord compression and decompression. *Spine* 1984; 9: 800-9.

9. Delamarter RB, Sherman JE, Carr JB. 1991 Volvo Award in experimental studies. Cauda equina syndrome: neurologic recovery following immediate, early, or late decompression. *Spine* 1991; 16: 1022-9.

10. Hejcl A, Urzikova L, Sedy J, *et al*. Acute and delayed implantation of positively charged 2-hydroxyethyl methacrylate scaffolds in spinal cord injury in the rat. *J Neurosurg Spine* 2008; 8: 67-73.

11. Kobrine AI, Evans DE, Rizzoli HV. Experimental acute balloon compression of the spinal cord. Factors affecting disappearance and return of the spinal evoked response. *J Neurosurg* 1979; 51: 841-5.

12. Dolan EJ, Tator CH, Endrenyi L. The value of decompression for acute experimental spinal cord compression injury. *J Neurosurg* 1980; 53: 749-55.

13. Guha A, Tator CH, Endrenyi L, Piper I. Decompression of the spinal cord improves recovery after acute experimental spinal cord compression injury. *Paraplegia* 1987; 25: 324-39.

14. Nystrom B, Berglund JE. Spinal cord restitution following compression injuries in rats. *Acta Neurol Scand* 1988; 78: 467-72.

15. Zhang Y, Hillered L, Olsson Y, Holtz A. Time course of energy perturbation after compression trauma to the spinal cord: an experimental study in the rat using microdialysis. *Surg Neurol* 1993; 39: 297-304.

16. Delamarter RB, Sherman J, Carr JB. Pathophysiology of spinal cord injury. Recovery after immediate and delayed decompression. *J Bone Joint Surg Am* 1995; 77: 1042-9.

17. Carlson GD, Minato Y, Okada A, *et al*. Early time-dependent decompression for spinal cord injury: vascular mechanisms of recovery. *J Neurotrauma* 1997; 14: 951-62.

18. Carlson GD, Warden KE, Barbeau JM, *et al*. Viscoelastic relaxation and regional blood flow response to spinal cord compression and decompression. *Spine* 1997; 22: 1285-91.

19. Dimar JR 2nd, Glassman SD, Raque GH, Zhang YP, Shields CB. The influence of spinal canal narrowing and timing of decompression on neurologic recovery after spinal cord contusion in a rat model. *Spine* 1999; 24: 1623-33.

20. Carlson GD, Gorden CD, Oliff HS, Pillai JJ, LaManna JC. Sustained spinal cord compression: part I: time-dependent effect on long-term pathophysiology. *J Bone Joint Surg Am* 2003; 85-A: 86-94.

21. Rabinowitz RS, Eck JC, Harper CM Jr, *et al*. Urgent surgical decompression compared to methylprednisolone for the treatment of acute spinal cord injury: a randomized prospective study in beagle dogs. *Spine* (Phila Pa 1976) 2008; 33: 2260-8.

22. Botel U, Glaser E, Niedeggen A. The surgical treatment of acute spinal paralysed patients. *Spinal Cord* 1997; 35: 420-8.

23. Tator CH, Fehlings MG, Thorpe K, Taylor W. Current use and timing of spinal surgery for management of acute spinal surgery for management of acute spinal cord injury in North America: results of a retrospective multicenter study. *J Neurosurg* 1999; 91: 12-8.

24. Vaccaro AR, Daugherty RJ, Sheehan TP, *et al*. Neurologic outcome of early versus late surgery for cervical spinal cord injury. *Spine* 1997; 22: 2609-13.

25. Ng WP, Fehlings MG, Cuddy B, *et al*. Surgical treatment for acute spinal cord injury study pilot study #2: evaluation of protocol for decompressive surgery within 8 hours of injury. *Neurosurg Focus* 1999; 6: e3.

26. Cengiz SL, Kalkan E, Bayir A, Ilik K, Basefer A. Timing of thoracolomber spine stabilization in trauma patients; impact on neurological outcome and clinical course. A real prospective (RCT) randomized controlled study. *Arch Orthop Trauma Surg* 2008; 128: 959-66.

27. Campagnolo DI, Esquieres RE, Kopacz KJ. Effect of timing of stabilization on length of stay and medical complications following spinal cord injury. *J Spinal Cord Med* 1997; 20: 331-4.

28. Mirza SK, Krengel WF 3rd, Chapman JR, *et al*. Early versus delayed surgery for acute cervical spinal cord injury. *Clin Orthop Relat Res* 1999; 359: 104-14.

29. Croce MA, Bee TK, Pritchard E, Miller PR, Fabian TC. Does optimal timing for spine fracture fixation exist? *Ann Surg* 2001; 233: 851-8.

30. Guest J, Eleraky MA, Apostolides PJ, Dickman CA, Sonntag VK. Traumatic central cord syndrome: results of surgical management. *J Neurosurg* 2002; 97: 25-32.

31. Chipman JG, Deuser WE, Beilman GJ. Early surgery for thoracolumbar spine injuries decreases complications. *J Trauma* 2004; 56: 52-7.

32. McKinley W, Meade MA, Kirshblum S, Barnard B. Outcomes of early surgical management versus late or no surgical intervention after acute spinal cord injury. *Arch Phys Med Rehabil* 2004; 85: 1818-25.

33. Kerwin AJ, Frykberg ER, Schinco MA, Griffen MM, Murphy T, Tepas JJ. The effect of early spine fixation on non-neurologic outcome. *J Trauma* 2005; 58: 15-21.

34. Schinkel C, Frangen TM, Kmetic A, Andress HJ, Muhr G. Timing of thoracic spine stabilization in trauma patients: impact on clinical course and outcome. *J Trauma* 2006; 61: 156-60.

35. Levi L, Wolf A, Rigamonti D, Ragheb J, Mirvis S, Robinson WL. Anterior decompression in cervical spine trauma: does the timing of surgery affect the outcome? *Neurosurgery* 1991; 29: 216-22.

36. McLain RF, Benson DR. Urgent surgical stabilization of spinal fractures in polytrauma patients. *Spine* 1999; 24: 1646-54.

37. Krengel WF 3rd, Anderson PA, Henley MB. Early stabilization and decompression for incomplete paraplegia due to a thoracic-level spinal cord injury. *Spine* 1993; 18: 2080-7.

38. Clohisy JC, Akbarnia BA, Bucholz RD, Burkus JK, Backer RJ. Neurologic recovery associated with anterior decompression of spine fractures at the thoracolumbar junction (T12-L1). *Spine* 1992; 17(Suppl. 8): S325-30.

39. Papadopoulos SM, Selden NR, Quint DJ, Patel N, Gillespie B, Grube S. Immediate spinal cord decompression for cervical spinal cord injury: feasibility and outcome. *J Trauma* 2002; 52: 323-32.

40. Sapkas GS, Papadakis SA. Neurological outcome following early versus delayed lower cervical spine surgery. *J Orthop Surg* (Hong Kong) 2007; 15: 183-6.

41. Chen L, Yang H, Yang T, Xu Y, Bao Z, Tang T. Effectiveness of surgical treatment for traumatic central cord syndrome. *J Neurosurg Spine* 2009; 10: 3-8.

42. Pollard ME, Apple DF. Factors associated with improved neurologic outcomes in patients with incomplete tetraplegia. *Spine* 2003; 28: 33-9.

43. Duh MS, Shepard MJ, Wilberger JE, Bracken MB. The effectiveness of surgery on the treatment of acute spinal cord injury and its relation to pharmacological treatment. *Neurosurgery* 1994; 35: 240-8.

Timing of surgery for spinal cord injury